Prostate Cancer

THIS VOLUME
IS ONE OF A SERIES

International Perspectives In Urology

EDITED BY
John A. Libertino, M.D.

NEW AND FORTHCOMING TITLES

McDougal and Persky
TRAUMATIC INJURIES OF THE GENITOURINARY SYSTEM

Javadpour
RECENT ADVANCES IN UROLOGIC CANCER

deVere White
ASPECTS OF MALE INFERTILITY

Bennett
MANAGEMENT OF MALE IMPOTENCE

Roth and Finlayson
STONES: CLINICAL MANAGEMENT OF UROLITHIASIS

International Perspectives In Urology

Volume 3

John A. Libertino, M.D.
series editor

Prostate Cancer

Edited by

Günther H. Jacobi, M.D.

Professor of Urology, Department of Urology, University of
Mainz, Federal Republic of Germany

Rudolf Hohenfellner, M.D.

Professor and Chairman, Department of Urology, University
of Mainz, Federal Republic of Germany

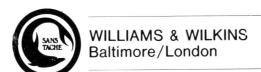

WILLIAMS & WILKINS
Baltimore/London

Copyright, © 1982
Williams & Wilkins
428 E. Preston Street
Baltimore, MD 21202, U.S.A.

Made in the United States of America

Library of Congress Cataloging in Publication Data

Main entry under title:

Prostate cancer.

   (International perspectives in urology; v. 3)
   Includes index.
   1. Prostate gland—Cancer. I. Jacobi, Günther H. II. Hohnfellner, Rudolf. III. Series.
[DNLM: 1. Prostatic neoplasms. W1 IN827K v. 2 / WJ 752 P9653]
RC280.P7P74   616.99'463   81-14784
ISBN 0-683-04354-4   AACR2

Composed and printed at the
Waverly Press, Inc.
Mt. Royal and Guilford Aves.
Baltimore, MD 21202, U.S.A.

Series Editor's Foreword

The management of cancer of the prostate is enigmatic. During the past decade, the advocates of radical prostatectomy have jousted with the opponents of external beam radiotherapy and interstitial radiation treatment. These academic debates have created confusion in the minds of the practicing urologist. Obviously if there are this many solutions to the problem, the issues remain unresolved.

In an attempt to help with the resolution of the dilemma confronting the clinical urologist, we have invited Professors Jacobi and Hohenfellner to edit this volume entitled, *Prostate Cancer.* Professor Jacobi is eminently qualified to carry out this task as he is one of the major forces in the EORTC (European Organization for Research on Treatment of Cancer). His area of special interest is prostatic adenocarcinoma. Professor Hohenfellner is the Chairman of the Department of Urology at the University of Mainz in West Germany. An authority on both pediatric and adult urology, his department, under his guidance, has given forth many Urology Department chairmen and is a potent force in European urology.

Doctors Jacobi and Hohenfellner have obtained the participation of many of the outstanding urologists in the world to contribute to their monograph on carcinoma of the prostate. This in no small measure is a reflection of the esteem with which Drs. Jacobi and Hohenfellner are held. The book is divided into two sections, one clinical and the other experimental. This is done in an effort to address both the clinical challenges that confront the practicing urologist as well as to stimulate the younger urologists to explore new horizons in the field of prostatic cancer. Doctors Jacobi and Hohenfellner have brought their intellect, energy, and enthusiasm to the task. They have created a contemporary, comprehensive textbook on adenocarcinoma of the prostate with a truly international perspective.

JOHN A. LIBERTINO, M.D.

Preface

When the editor of this series asked us to compile an edition on prostate cancer we were rather concerned whether we (or anyone else) would be able to put together all the different and rapidly changing parameters into a meaningful and valuable volume. Together with the tremendous (and prompt) help of 22 authors and their associates from seven European countries and Japan, all authorities in their individual field of prostate cancer, we have undertaken to fulfill this goal.

The issue of prostate cancer is multifaceted, involving speculations, illusions, differing experiences, philosophies, commonplaces, rigid dogmas, as well as new horizons. With this work, we hope to present the reader with a deeper understanding of this complex field of medical science.

We would like to address the reader's attention to *Chapter 3*, which defines the point of view of the editors and replaces the extensive introduction usually encountered in a detailed foreword. Most chapters are supplemented by an *Editorial Comment*, which reflects the personal view of the editors, and which in some instances tries to update the most recent literature that appeared during the editing process of this work.

We are indebted to all contributors and hope this work achieves the widespread exposure merited by the issue of prostatic carcinoma.

GÜNTHER H. JACOBI, M.D.
RUDOLF HOHENFELLNER, M.D.

Contributors

J. E. Altwein, M.D.
Chapter 11
Professor and Chairman,
Department of Urology, Armed
Forces Hospital, D-7900 Ulm,
Federal Republic of Germany

L. Andersson, M.D.
Chapter 13
Professor and Chairman,
Department of Urology,
Karolinska Hospital
S-10401 Stockholm, Sweden

S. Baba, M.D.
Chapter 2
Assistant Professor, Department
of Urology, National Defense
Medical College, Saitama-Ken
359, Japan

K. Bandhauer, M.D.
Chapter 12
Professor and Chairman,
Department of Urology, Klinik
für Urologie am Kantonsspital,
CH-9007 St. Gallen, Switzerland

G. Bartsch, M.D.
Chapter 23
Associate Professor of Urology,
Department of Urology,
University of Innsbruck Medical
School, A-6020 Innsbruck,
Austria

A. Binder, Ph.D.
Chapter 24
Hytec-System, D-6104 Seeheim-
Jugenheim, Federal Republic of
Germany

**G. D. Chisholm, Ch.M.,
F.R.C.S., F.R.C.S.E.**
Chapter 7
Professor of Surgery, University
of Edinburgh. Honorary
Consultant Urological Surgeon,
Western General Hospital,
Edinburgh. Honorary Senior
Lecturer, Institute of Urology,
London. Head of the
Department of Surgery/Urology
University of Edinburgh Medical
School, Edinburgh EH 8 9AG,
Great Britain

G. Dhom, M.D.
Chapter 6
Professor and Chairman,
Department of Pathology,
University of the Saarland
Medical School, Director of the
German Prostate Cancer
Registry, D-6650
Homburg(Saar), Federal
Republic of Germany

F. Edsmyr, M.D.
Chapter 13
Professor of Radiology,
Radiumhemmet, Karolinska

Hospital, Director of the WHO
Collaborating Centre for
Research and Treatment of
Urinary Bladder and Prostatic
Cancer,
S-10401 Stockholm, Sweden

W. Ehrenthal, M.D.
Chapter 8
Department of Clinical
Chemistry, University of Mainz
Medical School, D-6500 Mainz,
Federal Republic of Germany

P.-L. Esposti, M.D.
Chapter 5
Associate Professor for Oncology
and Radiotherapy,
Karolinska Hospital,
Radiumhemmet, S-10401
Stockholm, Sweden

P. Faul, M.D.
Chapter 4
Professor of Urology, Chief of
the Division of Urology, City
Hospital, D-8940 Memmingen,
Federal Republic of Germany

H. G. W. Frohmüller, M.D.
Chapter 9
Professor and Chairman,
Department of Urology,
University of Würzburg Medical
School, D-8700 Würzburg,
Federal Republic of Germany

K. Griffiths, B.Sc., Ph.D.
Chapter 21
Professor and Director of the
Tenovus Institute for Cancer
Research, The Welsh National
School of Medicine,
Cardiff CF4 4XX, Great Britain

D. Gupta, F.R.C. Path.
Chapter 19

Professor and Director of the
Department of Diagnostic
Endocrinology, University of
Tübingen Medical School,
D-7400 Tübingen, Federal
Republic of Germany

M. E. Harper, B.Sc., Ph.D.
Chapter 21
Tenovus Institute for Cancer
Research, The Welsh National
School of Medicine,
Cardiff CF4 4XX, Great Britain

Ch. Hohbach, M.D.
Chapter 6
Associate Professor, Department
of Pathology, University of the
Saarland Medical School,
German Prostate Cancer
Registry,
D-6650 Homburg(Saar), Federal
Republic of Germany

R. Hohenfellner, M.D.
Chapter 3
Professor and Chairman,
Department of Urology,
University of Mainz Medical
School, D-6500 Mainz, Federal
Republic of Germany

M. Hümpel, Ph.D.
Chapter 14
Head of the Department of
Pharmacokinetics, Research
Laboratories of Schering AG,
D-1000 Berlin (West) Federal
Republic of Germany

G. H. Jacobi, M.D.
Chapters 3, 15, 22
Professor of Urology,
Department of Urology,
University of Mainz Medical
School, D-6500 Mainz, Federal
Republic of Germany

K. F. Klippel, M.D.
Chapter 18
Professor of Urology,
Department of Urology,
University of Mainz Medical
School, D-6500 Mainz, Federal
Republic of Germany

I. Könyves, M.D., Ph.D.
Chapter 13
Director of the Department of
Cancer Chemotherapeutics and
Hormones, AB Leo, S-25109
Helsingborg, Sweden

K. H. Kurth, M.D.
Chapter 24
Chef de Clinic, Department of
Urology, Erasmus University of
Rotterdam Medical School, 3015
GD Rotterdam, The Netherlands

W. Leistenschneider, M.D.
Chapter 25
Associate Professor of Urology,
Department of Urology, Free
University of Berlin Medical
School, Klinikum Charlottenburg,
D-1000 Berlin (West), Federal
Republic of Germany

F. Neumann, Vet.D.
Chapter 14
Professor of Veterinarian
Medicine, Head of the Main
Department of Endocrine
Pharmacology, Research
Laboratories of Schering AG,
Staff Member of the Faculty of
Veterinarian Medicine at the
Free University of Berlin,
D-1000 Berlin (West), Federal
Republic of Germany

M. Pavone-Macaluso, M.D.
Chapter 16
Professor and Chairman,

Department of Urology
University of Palermo Medical
School, Chairman of the
EORTC Urological Group,
I-90141 Palermo, Italy

W. Prellwitz, M.D.
Chapter 8
Professor of Internal Medicine,
Head of the Department of
Clinical Chemistry, University of
Mainz Medical School, D-6500
Mainz, Federal Republic of
Germany

H. P. Rohr, M.D.
Chapter 23
Professor of Pathology, Institute
of Pathology of the University of
Basel Medical School, CH-4056
Basel, Switzerland

Th. Senge, M.D.
Chapters 14, 15
Professor and Chairman,
Department of Urology
University of Bochum Medical
School, Marienhospital,
D-4690 Herne, Federal Republic
of Germany

B. Schenck, M.D.
Chapter 14
Hospital Bergmannsheil, D-4600
Bochum, Federal Republic of
Germany

F. H. Schröder, M.D.
Chapter 17
Professor and Chairman,
Department of Urology, Erasmus
University of Rotterdam Medical
School, 3015 GD Rotterdam,
The Netherlands

F. Schultze-Seemann, M.D.
Chapter 1
Archivar of the German Society

of Urology, D-1000 Berlin
(West), Federal Republic of
Germany

F. J. W. ten Kate, M.D.
Chapter 24
Institute of Anatomic Pathology,
Erasmus University of
Rotterdam Medical School, 3015
GD Rotterdam, The Netherlands

U. Tunn, M.D.
Chapters 14, 15
Associate Professor of Urology,
Department of Urology
University of Bochum Medical
School, Marienhospital,

D-4690 Herne, Federal Republic
of Germany

H. J. de Voogt, M.D.
Chapter 20
Professor and Chairman,
Department of Urology, Free
University of Amsterdam
Medical School, 1007 MB
Amsterdam, The Netherlands

B. van der Werf-Messing, M.D.
Chapter 10
Professor and Chairman, The
Rotterdam Radio-Therapeutic
Institute, 3075 EA Rotterdam,
The Netherlands

Contents

SECTION 1 (*Clinical*)

1
Section

Clinical

1

The Historical Contribution of European Urology to Scientific Progress in the Field of Prostatic Neoplasia

F. Schultze-Seemann, M.D.

A review of early European medical literature reveals no significant reports on the prostate and its diseases. This is possibly attributable to the fact that life expectancy was relatively short and only few reached the so-called "prostatic" age. The name "prostata", *i.e. glandula pro stata*, is ascribed to Herophilos of the Alexandrian school (*ca.* 300 B.C.), while Oribasius first described constriction at the bladder neck in 360 A.D. and proposed a perineal approach to transsection to achieve free urine flow. Of the large collection of dissertations written in the Latin language in Germany and France between 1580 and 1820, not one was on prostate diseases—the same being true for dissertations in French appearing up to 1850. It was with increasing knowledge of microscopic techniques, during the 19th century, that the distinction between prostatic carcinoma and prostatic hypertrophy began.

One of the first treatises on prostatic cancer, entitled *"Carcinomatöse Degeneration der Vorsteherdrüse"* ("Carcinomatous Degeneration of the Prostate Gland"), was published in 1822 in Berlin by Beling,[1] while the Englishman Home,[2] who had been the first to describe in detail the enlargement of the middle lobe of the prostate 11 years earlier, had made no mention of prostatic cancer. As a result of the scarcity and inaccuracy of microscopic examinations, prostatic carcinoma was a virtual rarity up to *ca.* 1850.

Statistics compiled by the Frenchman Tanchou[3] in 1844 were long considered authoritative for the incidence of prostate cancer. He had listed all cancer deaths recorded in the death registries of Paris and its suburbs between 1830 and 1840, including what was believed to be the primary seat of the disease, naming only one organ for each case. Of 1,904 deceased men, there were only five cases of prostatic disease—most likely an underestimate considering that the data were taken from ordinary death registries. Nevertheless, many authors of the time quoted these statistics, with the result that prostate cancer was further considered a rare disease. As a result, only single case reports appeared in the literature in subsequent years.

An example of this was Heyfelder's case,[4] which appeared in Finland in 1855. He described a 34-year-old sailor with a history of lues, who had suffered from urinary retention at age 33, and developed again urinary obstruction as well as a perineal tumor 1 year later, which was then punctured. A few days afterward he died of urosepsis. At autopsy the kidney was twice its original size and contained abscess cavities full of pus. "The dorsal portion of the prostate was considerably thickened and indurated as in scirrhus; towards the ventral part it was encompassed by a sac which held a turbid, pulpy, acrid mass. Microscopic examination revealed a fibrosarcoma"—possibly luetic gumma??

From this description of a prostatic section, the difficulty in deciding, on the basis of reports of the time, whether this is actually a case of prostatic malignancy, can clearly be seen. As *every* prostatic induration was referred to as "*scirrhus*" in those days, from our point of view this could indicate either cancer or prostatitis or tuberculosis as well. This was pointed out by the renowned London urologist, Henry Thompson, in his Monograph written in 1858 entitled, *The Enlarged Prostate, Its Pathology and Treatment* (Fig. 1.1.),[5] as well as by the Swiss anatomist, E. Kaufmann, in 1902.[6]

Thompson's Monograph was a milestone in the research on prostate diseases being done in England at that time—begun by Home in 1811 and carried on by Coulson, Stafford, and Adams. Thompson mentions the statistics compiled by Tanchou, but based on experience of his own, comes to the conclusion that the incidence of prostatic carcinoma arrived at by Tanchou "is very much smaller than the true number." In Thompson's opinion, "a certain small proportion of instances is lost sight of among the very large number of cases assigned to senile hypertrophy." Referring to the 72 cases of bladder cancer listed by Tanchou, he writes: "It is not unreasonable to suppose that some of these may have been prostatic in their origin."

In particular, Thompson notes the "notoriously loose and indefinite manner in which the term scirrhus has been commonly employed," often to describe an "extreme hardness of the prostatic substance." He therefore adheres to an earlier statement made by Walshe[7] that "the evidence of the occurrence of true scirrhus of the prostate is defective," and stresses the significance of expert microscopical examination. This lacking, he

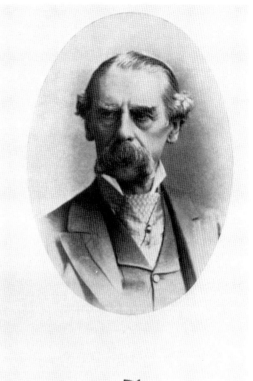

Figure 1.1 *Sir Henry Thompson* and the title page of his pioneer monograph published in 1858 in London. Portrait taken from the "Galerie hervorragender Ärzte und Naturforscher," a Supplement to the *Münchener Medizinische Wochenschrift*, Blatt 151. J. F. Lehmann Verlag, München, around 1905.

concludes, "We must not hesitate to deny the admission to a category so designated, of any case, not accurately and intelligently observed."

An additional difficulty was the diagnosis of prostate cancer in the living. At the time of his writing, in 1858, malignant disease had "been observed only in childhood and at advancing age. No authenticated cases are on record between the ages of eight and forty-one." It had been shown that "encaphaloid deposit may sometimes take place into a prostate previously hypertrophied, and already the cause of obvious symptoms of urinary obstruction." But it was difficult to verify these conditions during life: "nevertheless, if, the existence of enlarged prostate having been ascertained some years ago, exacerbation of symptoms rather rapidly occurs, with manifest increase in the size of the tumor, attended by cachexia, above all by enlargement of the lymphatic glands in the neighborhood, we may pretty safely conclude that malignant action has supervened."

According to Thompson, cancerous changes of the prostate first present the symptoms common to other prostatic obstructions, but develop more rapidly than senile hypertrophy. It displays a "more severe pain, often very intense; occasional, often frequent, haemorrhages; and more or less constitutional cachexia. The pain is felt in the rectum, or in the region of the sacrum, and shooting down the thighs, either the anterior or posterior aspect."

In cases of a doubtful nature, the urine should, in Thompson's opinion, be examined for the presence of malignant cells: "Some observers state that they have verified cancer-cells in the urine. Others have failed to do so after close and repeated examinations. A good deal of debris may usually be seen in advanced cases, its presence appears to indicate that the growth has fungated, and throws off more or less of its elements in the condition of sloughly detritus."

At the end of his chapter, Thompson presents 18 cases of cancer of the prostate in tabular form selected from English and French authors up to 1858, which he considered to be substantiated by sufficient evidence. All cases—with the exception of one "*scirrhus*"—were characterized as "*encephaloid*," the type of cancer most common to the prostate.

These commonly recognized characteristics were the subject of detailed discussion by the Swiss pathologist E. Kaufmann in his chapter entitled "Die Verletzungen und Krankheiten der Prostata." ("Injuries and Diseases of the Prostate") contained in Socin and Burckhardt's *German Surgery*, which appeared in 1902.[6] The term "*scirrhus*," as Kaufmann points out, had been used by Thompson's contemporaries for any hardness of the prostate, and particularly for senile hypertrophy. In Kaufmann's opinion, the expression "*encephaloid of the prostate*," also in frequent use, could refer to both a medullar carcinoma or a round cell sarcoma. In addition, every description of a prostate cancer which had appeared since the beginning of the 19th century had undergone arbitrary renaming by later authors attempting tabular comparisons of its frequency. For example, Langstaff[8] had described a "*fungus haematodes*" of the prostate in 1817 which was later changed by Wyss[9] to "encephaloid," which meant to him, cancer.

These arbitrary changes make it difficult for us today to draw clear conclusions concerning the pathological anatomy of the individual cases and the frequency of prostatic carcinoma at that time. For the earlier writers of the 19th century, it was not particularly important for therapy if they were dealing with a carcinoma or sarcoma of the prostate. Furthermore, such differentiation was almost always uncertain with the microscopic knowledge available at the time.

For many decades this uncertainty remained the reason for the scarcity of reports on prostate cancer, despite numerous publications in all other fields of medicine, as well as for the continued belief that prostate cancer was a rare disease. According to Kaufmann,[6] in 1902, the allegations of older authors were very uncertain and doubtful, and Thompson had been the first, in 1858, to present 18 "most probably" substantiated observations of prostate cancer.

That prostate cancer was found only rarely is confirmed by the following figures: Wyss[9] (1866) described 28 cases including two of his own; Jolly[10] reported more than 45 definite cases in 1869; Jullien[11] more than 55 in 1880; and finally, Engelbach,[12] in 1888, compiled a very thorough report containing 114 cases, although several of them were not definite.

As late as 1893, the old master of French urology, Guyon, still spoke of prostatic carcinoma as being a rare affection, like renal cancer, in contrast to the frequent bladder cancer. He claimed that a prostatic tumor is only rarely located in one prostatic lobe or results in early and extensive "degeneration of the pelvic lymph nodes." Furthermore, the appearance of cancer cells in the urine was of no absolute importance, as errors could result from changes in the bladder epithelium.

The end of the 19th century, however, marks a turning point in the estimate of prostatic carcinoma frequency, due to the increasing accuracy of microscopic techniques. Kaufmann had already claimed that prostatic carcinoma was "not so rare": Observations of it had increased considerably—owing at least in part to the fact that it was no longer unusual to find a prostatic cancer at autopsy of such minimal size that it had escaped macroscopic detection. Very important was the increasing awareness, mentioned by Thompson almost half a century earlier, that prostatic cancer could be mistaken for a case of simple hypertrophy. Moreover, it was now recognized that the malignant disease showed a preference for bone metastases, which had not been commonly known before.

Decisive for the latter was the work of von Recklinghausen,[14] a pathologist from Strassburg who wrote on *osteoplastic carcinosis* for the Festschrift in honor of Rudolf Virchow's 71st birthday in 1891 (Fig. 1.2). He had observed that the primary prostatic focus was usually small and insignificant in comparison to the numerous and often far advanced bone metastases, and that precisely this diffuse, cancerous infiltration in the skeleton was highly characteristic of prostatic carcinoma. To counter any possible doubts on his material, he referred—as early as 1891—to an analogy with mammary carcinoma, *i.e.* in "vertebral bone cancer" of the female, the usually very small original focus of the disease can be found in the breast. Von Recklinghausen thereby provided the decisive impetus toward directing attention at autopsy to the prostate in cases of vertebral metastases.

After the appearance of this significant work, cases of prostatic carcinoma were confirmed with greater frequency, so that in 1899 the Viennese urologist, von Frisch[15] expressed his full support of von Recklinghausen's results. According to von Frisch, the primary cancer in both prostatic and breast carcinoma can only rarely be seen macroscopically; it appears to be merely an indurated nodule and seldom leads to necrolysis. Only the typical regional lymph node involvement is conspicuous and facilitates diagnosis.

At the end of the 19th century, therapy was purely palliative and consisted primarily in relieving urinary retention. For radical treatment, total extirpation of the prostate was recommended as the most appropriate procedure. It was first practiced in Germany by Küchler on the cadaver, and on the living by Billroth around 1860. These pioneers used the perineal approach, and patients even remained continent sometimes.

Because of the more accurate microscopic examinations in use by the

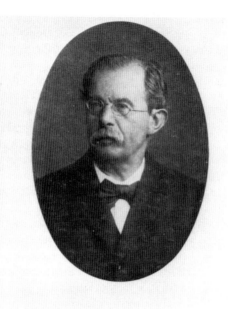

FESTSCHRIFT

Die fibröse oder deformirende Ostitis, die Osteomalacie und die osteoplastische Carcinose in ihren gegenseitigen Beziehungen.

RUDOLF VIRCHOW

ZU SEINEM 71. GEBURTSTAGE

Von

GEWIDMET

Prof. F. v. Recklinghausen
in Strassburg

VON

DEN FRÜHEREN UND JETZIGEN ASSISTENTEN
DES BERLINER PATHOLOGISCHEN INSTITUTS

(Mit 5 Tafeln.)

F. v. Recklinghausen   1

BERLIN
DRUCK UND VERLAG VON GEORG REIMER
1891

Figure 1.2 *Von Recklinghausen*, Professor of Pathology at Straßburg, and the title paper of his chapter on osseous metastasis and prostate cancer, which appeared in the "Festschrift in Honor of Rudolf Virchow's 71st Birthday", published in 1891 in Berlin. Portrait taken from the "Galerie hervorragender Ärzte und Naturforscher", a Supplement to the *Münchener Medizinische Wochenschrift*, Blatt 147. J. F. Lehmann Verlag, München, around 1903.

end of the 19th century, prostatic carcinoma was no longer considered a rarity. Von Frisch[15] published a review of the literature in 1899, stressing that the etiology was unknown in all cases and that there was complete agreement among all authors that inflammation was not a predisposing factor.

In 1900, Albarran and Hallé[16] of France also confirmed Sir Thompson's earlier claim: in more than 10% of their cases, classified clinically as common prostatic hypertrophy, the histological picture showed unmistakable signs of malignancy—a fact subsequently substantiated by numerous other authors. From this point on, prostatic carcinoma was no longer a rare disease.

Concerning therapy at the end of the 19th century, a connection between prostate enlargement and sex hormones was gradually being suspected, after it had been known for centuries that the prostate of steers could reduce in size following castration. As a result, the first attempts at castration treatment of prostatic carcinoma were already being done before the turn of the century.[17]

Acknowledgement. I should like to express my sincere thanks to Mrs. Susan Hensel (Mainz) for her translation work and help with the preparation of this chapter.

REFERENCES

1. Beling, A. Carcinomatöse Degeneration der Vorsteherdrüse. *Arch. Med. Erfahrung (Berl) 1:* 443, 1822.
2. Home, E. *Practical Observations on the Treatment of the Diseases of the Prostate Gland.* G.W. Nicol, London, 1811.
3. Tanchou, S. Recherches sur le Traitement Médical des Tumeurs Cancéreuses du Sein. Univ. Dissertation, Paris, 1844, pp. 256–261.
4. Heyfelder, J. F. Scirrhus prostatae. *Dtsch. Klin. 7:* 505, 1855.
5. Thompson, H. *The Enlarged Prostate, Its Pathology and Treatment.* John Churchill, London, 1858.
6. Kaufmann, E. Pathologisch-anatomischer Beitrag. *Die Verletzungen und Krankheiten der Prostata,* In *Deutsche Chirurgie,* edited by A. Socin and E. Burckhardt. Verlag Enke, Stuttgart, 1902.
7. Walshe, W. H. *The Nature and Treatment of Cancer.* Taylor & Walton, London, 1846, p. 414.
8. Langstaff, G. Case of fungus haematodes with observations. *Med. Chir. Transact. (Lond) 8:* 279, 1817.
9. Wyss, O. Die heterologen Neubildungen der Vorsteherdrüse. *Virchows Arch. 35:* 378, 1866.
10. Jolly, J. Essai sur le cancer de la prostate. *Arch. Gen. Med. (Paris) 1:* 577, *2:* 61, 1869.
11. Jullien, L. Etude sur le cancer de la prostate. *N. Dict. Med. Chir. Prat. (Paris) 29:* 697, 1880.
12. Engelbach, P. Les Tumeurs Malignes de la Prostate. Thesis, Paris, 1888.
13. Guyon, F. *Leçons Cliniques sur les Maladies des Voies Urinaires,* 3 Vol. Paris, 1894, 1896, and 1897. German Translation: *Klinik der Krankheiten der Harnblase und Prostata.* 1st Edition, Verlag August Hirschwald, Berlin, 1893, Ch. 3, pp. 304–316.
14. von Recklinghausen, F. Die fibröse oder deformirende Ostitis, die Osteomalacie und die osteoplastische Carcinose in ihren gegenseitigen Beziehungen. In *Festschrift Rudolf Virchow zu seinem 71. Geburtstage.* Georg Reimer Publ., Berlin, 1891, pp. 22–35, 81–85.
15. von Frisch, A. Die Krankheiten der Prostata. In *Spezielle Pathologie und Therapie,* edited by H. Nothnagel. Alfred Hölder, Wien, 1899.
16. Albarran, B., and Hallé, A. Hypertrophie et néoplasies épithéliales de la prostate. *Ann. Mal. Org. Gen.-Urin.* Red. Adm. St. George, Paris, 1900.
17. Cabot, A. T. The question of castration for enlarged prostate. *Ann. Surg. 24:* 265, 1896.

2

Epidemiology of Cancer of the Prostate: Analysis of Countries of High and Low Incidence

S. Baba, M.D.

Despite the fact that the prostate is the second commonest site of cancer affecting males in the United States[1] and the third commonest site in the Federal Republic of Germany[2] as well as in England and Wales,[3] the etiology of the tumor remains unknown. Relatively few of the related etiological factors are established. However, it is clear that cancer of the prostate increases steadily with age from 40 to 50 and rarely occurs under the age of 40.[3,4] For some unknown reason it has been reported to be comparatively rare in the East, particularly among the Japanese.[3] The relatively lower mortality rate reported from Eastern as opposed to Western European countries is also of interest.[5]

There are two principal sources of data which may be drawn upon to establish epidemiological patterns in neoplastic disease. For lethal neoplasms, the annual mortality statistics are an important and accurate source of information. However, they have some disadvantages for less lethal diseases, because the incidence of these diseases is not directly reflected in the mortality rates. The other important sources can be provided by regional and national cancer registries which unfortunately as yet cover only a limited part of the world population.[6]

Besides these two main sources of data contributing to vital statistics, pathological data obtained from autopsy records have been assessed statistically, since the most reliable information about real incidence of cancer of the prostate is obtained from careful microscopic examination of the materials.[7]

AUTOPSY DATA

During the 19th century, cancer of the prostate was considered only a medical rarity. Since Albarran and Hallé[8] reported a higher incidence of this cancer in 14 of 100 surgical specimens of benign prostatic enlargement, cancer of the prostate has been generally accepted as an important independent etiological entity (see Chapter 1).

Many authors have since reported on the incidence of this cancer in routine autopsy specimens.[7,9-11] Alexejew and Dunajewski[9] examined the pathological data in autopsy records of 37,899 males chosen at random and reported the incidence of this cancer as 0.85%. Horstmann[10] investigated autopsy material of 10,030 males who died of various diseases and found the incidence of this cancer to be 2.5%.

Besides the cancer which is diagnosed clinically, there is a type not detectable before death because it produces no clinical evidence of the disease. This type of cancer is not easily found macroscopically on cut surface of the autopsy specimens and can be found only incidentally or by the step-section technique. In 1935, Rich[11] and Moore[12] independently reported the pathological incidence of this cancer, based on careful histological examination at autopsy. This type of nonclinical cancer was first described by Rich[11] as "occult carcinoma," which was later called more appropriately "latent carcinoma" by Andrews[13] (see Chapter 6). The prevalence of latent cancer of the prostate has been reported from several countries.[14-18] Comparisons of these reports are complicated by differences in technique, diagnostic criteria, intensity of diagnostic work-up, and age distribution of the autopsy populations (Table 2.1). It is easily accepted that small carcinomatous foci can be detected much more frequently when the entire prostate is examined at intervals of 3 to 4 mm. This method was termed "*step section*" by Moore[12] but must not be confused with serial sectioning, from which the most reliable information

Table 2.1
Incidence of Latent Prostatic Cancer (%)[a]

Age	Routine Autopsy		Step Section			
	U.S.A.[11]	Germany[10]	Austria[12]	Austria[21]	Canada[19]	Japan[20]
40–49		0%	17.4%	4.9%	4.3%	4.5%[b]
		(0/12)	(4/23)	(6/112)	(1/23)	(1/20)
50–59	5.4%	4.5%	13.8%	10.4%	9.7%	6.6%
	(7/130)	(1/22)	(9/65)	(25/241)	(3/31)	(5/76)
60–69	8.1%	4.3%	24.3%	17.3%	18.5%	13.6%
	(8/98)	(1/35)	(18/77)	(54/312)	(10/54)	(12/88)
70–79	20.3%	16.7%	20.6%	28.3%	25.0%	35.8%
	(12/59)	(6/36)	(13/63)	(67/237)	(12/48)	(19/53)
80–89	0%	0%	29.2%	38.8%	17.6%	45.5%
	(0/5)	(0/9)	(7/24)	(38/98)	(3/17)	(10/22)
Total	9.2%	10.5%	20.2%	19.0%	16.8%	18.1%
	(27/292)	(12/114)	(51/252)	(190/1000)	(29/173)	(25/229)

[a] Figures in parentheses refer to the number of cases with latent cancer divided by the number of examined cases.
[b] Data obtained from males over 45 years old.

about the prevalence of latent cancer can be obtained. Gaynor,[21] studying the autopsy material by step section method, found a steady increase of latent prostatic cancer from 4.9% in the 40 to 49-year-old group, to a maximum of 38.8% in the 80 to 89-year-old group (see Chapter 3). Walthard[22] examined by serial section 100 prostates taken from individuals over 40 years of age and found cancer in 30%. Rullis et al.[23] reported that the prevalence of prostatic cancer, obtained from 57 autopsies in males 80 years of age and older, was 66.7% by the serial section method.

With step section method, no clear difference in the prevalence of latent cancer has been demonstrated between Japanese and other groups, which makes a great contrast to that yielded by morbidity and mortality rates based on vital statistics. It has been a matter of discussion whether or not the latent cancer remains biologically inactive and some "trigger mechanism" is necessary to provide stimulus to further growth and extension.[17, 19] Grading of the latent cancer is particularly difficult; however, available evidence suggests that well-differentiated tumors do not have to become poorly differentiated to grow or become biologically active and clinically manifest.[17]

Akazaki and Stemmermann[24] carefully studied latent cancer of the prostate in 239 Japanese and 158 Japanese immigrants in Hawaii who were more than 50 years old with special focus on its prevalence and histologic features. These data failed to demonstrate any important or statistically significant difference in the prevalence of latent cancer between the two groups. Nevertheless, in Japanese immigrants latent cancer tended to proliferate and invade, suggesting that the prevalence of the proliferative type of latent cancer was higher in the immigrants. It was reported recently that the rate of proliferative latent cancer among Japanese immigrants in Hawaii was intermediate between the rates of Japanese in Japan and white males in the United States.[25] These observations obtained from autopsy data suggest that the cause of prostatic cancer is present in almost equal force in every population; however, the factors promoting its growth might be attributed to some environmental factors.

It must be recalled that latent cancer of the prostate is not synonymous with clinical cancer, and it covers a wide biological range from inactive small foci to anaplastic invasive types. The lesion has attained greater clinical importance recently with a rising life expectancy and better diagnostic means, although the extent to which latent cancer is included may vary with great availability of medical care.

INCIDENCE AND MORBIDITY DATA

Two main sources of data are available to assess the incidence and morbidity rates. The one source is obtained from *hospital-based* cancer records and the other from *population-based* cancer registries.

Hospital-Based Clinical Incidence

The major contribution to cancer morbidity statistics comes from hospital records, although these data give a rather incomplete picture of the incidence of cancer for the whole population.

There appeared a great body of literature on the clinical incidence of prostatic cancer in patients undergoing prostatectomies,[26-29] the rates ranging from 11.9 to 31.3%. As for the small nodules or foci of the cancer confined to the prostate ($T_{0-1}N_xM_0$ categories of the tumor, node, metastasis (TNM) system, see Chapter 8), the possibility for discovery is entirely dependent on the technique and frequency of biopsy or on the method of prostatectomy. The incidence of preoperatively unsuspected cancer (T_0 or A_{1-2} of the American system) in prostatectomy specimens has been reported to be about 6.5% in the United States,[30-32] and varies with the care of preoperative rectal examination.

In Japan, where latent cancer is found almost as frequently as in other countries by autopsy materials, the incidence of clinically manifest cancer among patients has been reported to be much lower than expected. As pointed out by Ravich[33] recently, some reports on the clinical incidence of prostatic cancer from Japan are computed as the ratio of this cancer to the total number of male patients of a given urological hospital population, which differs from the method based on the ratio to the total number of patients with any prostatic disease. In fact, reported clinical incidence rates in Japan have been much lower than the rate in the United States, ranging from 0.26 to 0.93% in Japan *versus* a mean value of 20% in the United States. The former figures are calculated with reference to the number of male outpatients.[34,35] However, available hospital data in Japan show the ratio to be 14.8% in 280 hospitalized patients with prostatic lesions (Unpublished data, Keio University Hospital, Tokyo). Furthermore the incidence of clinically unsuspected cancer ($T_0N_0M_0$) at prostatectomy in Japan has been reported to be 5.3%, which does not differ substantially from the incidence reported in the United States.[36] These observations obtained from clinical experiences suggest that the incidence for this type of prostate cancer among Japanese patients lies in the range of that of other populations.

The lower incidence of clinically manifest cancer of the prostate has been reported also among Jews. In Ravich's survey of prostatic operations, cancer associated with benign prostatic lesions occurred in only 1.7% of Jews, compared to nearly 20% of non-Jews[28]. However, Gibson[37] later investigated this matter extensively and found that the rate among Jews for this cancer was not significantly lower (13.24%) than the rate in Gentiles (18.2%).

The incidence of clinical prostate cancer, thus calculated as the number of patients with prostatic lesions, seems to vary in accordance with the rate of latent cancer included. If latent cancer of the prostate is a reservoir of potential clinical cases, it is plausible to assume that the rate of clinically encountered cancer should parallel autopsy data. Lilien et al.[26] studied the clinical incidence of prostatic cancer in 115 patients undergoing perineal prostatectomy for benign hyperplasia. Statistical analysis of the distribution of cancer cases according to age groups failed to show any increasing incidence with age, but indicated a frequency related to the number of prostatectomies performed per age group. This report suggests that, if twice as many prostatectomies for benign obstruction were carried out in a given age group as are performed in another age group, approximately twice as many carcinomas will be found in the former group. This concept seems especially important when the incidence that occurs in different countries is compared as the number of prostatectomies performed differs greatly from one country to another.

Population-Based Cancer Registry

Although the ratio of clinically encountered prostatic cancer appears to be similar in different racial groups, the population-based incidence varies greatly, because it is calculated on the basis of a given population from the total number of newly diagnosed cases in a designated area. The incidence for clinically manifest prostatic carcinoma is 78 among nonwhite and 46 for white males per 100,000 population per year in the United States.[38,39] These figures are approximately three times higher than the corresponding mortality rates reported in the U.S. In both of these racially different populations, age-specific rates begin to rise sharply after the age of 50 (Table 2.2). However, between 50 and 84 years of age incidence rates of nonwhites are roughly twice as high as those of white males. Based on the *Cancer Registry of Birmingham*, Waterhouse[40] reported similar age-specific incidence rates as compared to white males in the United States, increasing steadily from about 20 per 100,000 population per year at age 55 to about 500 at age 85. On the other hand, African Negroes seem to have a much lower rate for this cancer than those in the United States.[41] These data suggest the presence of unknown etiological factors, which are more common to the nonwhite males in the United States than to the white males.

The rate of occurrence of prostate cancer is also high among the Northern and Western European countries. In Norway for the period between 1964 and 1966, prostate cancer accounted for 19% of new male cancer registrations[42] and in Sweden it accounted for 20.3% of all male cancer cases in 1970.[43] The incidence in Hamburg (Germany) is reported to be as high as that of Birmingham[41] (see Chapter 4).

Compared with the high incidence among Northern and Western European countries, the incidence in Hungary appeared relatively low, comprising only 8% of all types of cancer affecting the male.[7] Wynder *et al.*[4] stated that the low incidence among Jews in the United States

Table 2.2
Age-adjusted Prostate Cancer Incidence (1969–1971): Rates per 100,000 per year[a]

Age	White	Nonwhite
45–49	5	7
50–54	17	36
55–59	52	118
60–64	127	270
65–69	255	465
70–74	431	785
75–79	658	926
80–84	829	1,275
>85	889	866

[a] From G. B. Hutchinson.[39]

appeared to be related to the lower rate among immigrants from Eastern Europe, since Jewish immigrants to this country have come mainly from Russia and Poland, countries with a generally low incidence.

Unfortunately it is not possible to compare the population-based cancer registries among all the geographic areas in the world. However, according to Doll *et al.*,[41] the incidence of prostate cancer adjusted to a world standard population, per 100,000 per year, is 33.9 for the United States (Connecticut), 26.5 for Sweden, 17.4 for England (Birmingham), 16.5 for Germany (Hamburg), 12.6 for Japanese immigrants (Hawaii), 3.8 for Japan (Miyagi), and 0.9 for Chinese (Singapore). From these figures it could be assumed that the risk of manifest prostatic cancer affecting males living in Japan is extremely low, although the histological incidence of "incidental" or "latent" cases among Japanese with benign prostatic diseases does not substantially differ from that of other populations. A clue to understanding this discrepancy might be the evidence that *invasive* or *proliferative* (*i.e.*, biologically highly active) latent cancer of the prostate seems relatively rare among Japanese living in Japan.[24, 25] However, the reason why such biologically active cancer is not common among Japanese males remains unexplained.

MORTALITY STATISTICS

There appear to be large geographical and ethnic differences not only in morbidity but also in mortality statistics. The mortality rate for prostate cancer is highest for nonwhite males in the United States, while it is extremely low among Japanese[3, 4] (Figure 2.1). It is of great interest that other hormone-related sites, such as breast, ovary, and endometrium, are also uncommon sites for cancer among Japanese (Table 2.3). Wynder *et al.*[44] demonstrated that the mortality rate of prostatic cancer correlated well with that of breast cancer except in the Jewish population. Among the Jews, however, the rate of mortality for uterine cancer is relatively low, as is that for prostatic cancer. In Eastern Europe the mortality rates for cancer of the prostate were reported as being relatively low in 1964 to 1965 (*e.g.* Poland, 7.34; Czechoslovakia, 9.18; Yugoslavia, 5.78).[5]

Time Trends

During the past few decades an increased mortality from cancer of the prostate has been observed in most countries.[3] In the United States mortality for both white and nonwhite males increased during the decade of 1930 to 1940, after which time the rate for whites decreased slightly, while the rate for nonwhites continued to increase.[45] In Germany, the rate has increased during the last two decades from 15.3 in 1955 to 22.9 in 1975[2, 46] (Fig. 2.2). Although the rate for the age group older than 64 was 22.1 times as high as that for age 35 to 64 in 1955, the rate for the older age group increased to 26.9 times as high as the rate for the younger population in 1975 (Fig. 2.2).

Although the mortality has been constantly low for Japanese males,

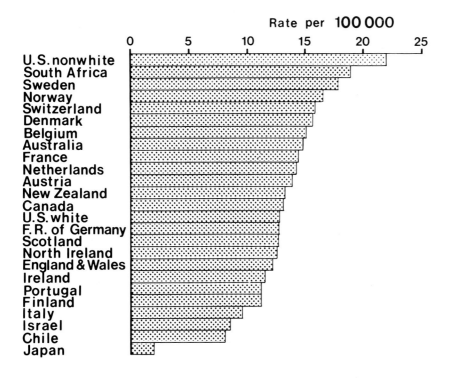

Rate per 100 000

0	5	10	15	20	25

U.S. nonwhite
South Africa
Sweden
Norway
Switzerland
Denmark
Belgium
Australia
France
Netherlands
Austria
New Zealand
Canada
U.S. white
F.R. of Germany
Scotland
North Ireland
England & Wales
Ireland
Portugal
Finland
Italy
Israel
Chile
Japan

Table 2.3
Age-adjusted Mortality Rates for Different Sites of Cancer per 100,000 Population (1964–1965)[a]

		U.S. Nonwhite	U.S. White	Germany	Israel[b]	Japan
Male	Prostate	21.97	12.72	12.70	8.45	1.85
	Stomach	17.99	9.42	37.05	18.20	68.57
Female	Breast	20.03	21.76	17.53	20.98	3.80
	Uterus	23.44	10.25	12.69	6.18	13.47
	Ovary and Endometrium	5.95	7.33		6.87	1.74

[a] The data adjusted to a standard population in 46 countries around 1950.
[b] Israel includes the Jewish population only. From M. Segi et al.[3]

the age-adjusted mortality rates have increased sharply from 1950 to 1965, especially in the older age group[47] (Fig. 2.3). It is not clear whether this change is due to a real increase in the number of cases, or merely due to the increased number of newly diagnosed cases.

Migration

If the differences between countries are due to environmental factors, they should be affected by immigration. Haenszel[48] analyzed more than 34,000 cancer deaths recorded for foreign-born immigrants in the United States during 1950 and observed that the standardized mortality rate for

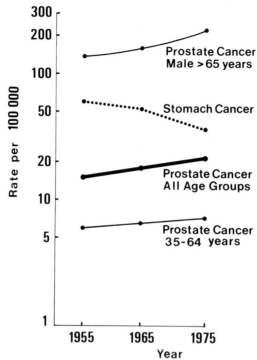

Figure 2.2 Age-adjusted mortality rates for cancer of prostate and stomach in the Federal Republic of Germany. (Reproduced with permission from R. Frentzel-Beyme et al.[46])

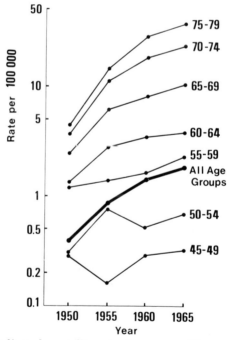

Figure 2.3 Age-adjusted mortality rates for cancer of the prostate in Japan. (Reproduced with permission from Segi et al.[3,47])

prostatic cancer was significantly higher in Irish and German immigrants, but lower in the groups from Austria, Poland, Italy, and USSR, as compared to the native-born whites in the United States. In addition, the importance of environmental factors in the ethnic and international patterns of this cancer is suggested by rising rates among groups immigrating to the United States from low-risk countries.

The studies on Polish[49] and Japanese immigrants[50,51] in the United States have offered attractive advantages for cancer research, because they demonstrate great contrasts in cancer risks between the native countries and United States for several sites, including breast, prostate, stomach, colon, and rectum. According to Haenszel and Kurihara,[50] the first generation of Japanese immigrants (*Issei*) in the United States had a higher mortality rate for prostatic cancer, but nowhere near the incidence of whites in the United States (Table 2.4). These findings are in agreement with those made on Polish immigrants,[49] except that the degree of assimilation to the host population has been less complete among Japanese.[50]

Quality of Death Certificates

While the availability and quality of medical facilities and death certificates vary around the world, data on cancer deaths in developed countries represent a virtually complete coverage of the population.[6] However, even in these countries the quality of data may vary, depending on the statistical systems in operation. One possible factor which may cause the variation of mortality statistics may be derived from religious or cultural differences among countries. In Japan, there is a legal requirement for submission of the death certificate in order to get a cremation permit. The prompt preparation of the death certificate makes it sometimes difficult to obtain autopsy permission.[52]

The numbers of deaths ascribed to senility without mention of accurate causes may also dilute the mortality rates for cancer of the prostate. Table 2.5 shows the numbers of the deaths ascribed to such unknown causes in selected countries.[53] As shown in this table, there is no correlation of these figures and corresponding mortality rates.

It is also not plausible to assume that all of the differences in mortality for this cancer have been brought about by the numbers of deaths due to unknown causes.

Even taking the above-mentioned possible sources of error into account, there seem to remain large differences in the mortality rates

Table 2.4
Age-adjusted Mortality Rates among Japanese Immigrants in U.S.A.[a]

	65–75 yr	75 yr and Older
Japanese in Japan	11.6	28.0
Immigrants (Issei)	40.2	130.9
U.S. whites	92.6	307.5

[a] From W. Haenszel and M. Kurihara.[50]

Table 2.5
The Rate of Unknown Death Cause (1963–1965) (per 100,000 Population)[a]

Finland	8.5	Italy	37.7
England and Wales	10.2	Austria	45.3
Sweden	10.2	Japan	66.3
South Africa (white)	11.0	Germany	72.8
United States	12.1	Poland	82.2
Israel (Jews)	19.1	Phillipines	95.7
Czechoslovakia	20.1	France	151.9

[a] From Demographic Year Book 1966.[53]

between countries with high and low incidences, that these differences can be confidently accepted.

Geographic Patterns

The relative incidence of particular causes based on mortality rates has been successfully visualized by geographic area, permitting an insight into the "cancer scenery" of several countries.[46,54,55]

The Atlas of Cancer Mortality among U.S. Counties: 1950–1969 demonstrated clusters of counties with elevated mortality of cancer of the prostate in the northcentral and northeastern states.[54] Blair and Fraumeni[56] studied age-adjusted mortality from prostatic cancer during 1950 to 1969 in the United States, correlating the demographic, industrial, and agricultural data from 3,056 U.S. counties. They found an elevated mortality in counties with a high percentage of residents of Scandinavian and German descent, in counties with metal-using and textile industries, and in regions with high consumption of high-fat diet.

Recently Frentzel-Beyme et al.[46] illustrated maps of cancer mortality in the Federal Republic of Germany using data from 1955 to 1975. In the course of the 2 decades the mortality rates for prostatic cancer in the 35 to 64-year-old age group increased sharply and steadily in Northrhine-Westphalia and two southern German states (Bavaria, Baden-Württemberg). In Hamburg, where the occupational composition of the working population comprises 38.7% from industry,[57] the mortality rates have not changed remarkably in this age group; however, the rates for the older age group have been constantly high in these decades. Thus Hamburg had the highest mortality rate for all age groups (24.2 per 100,000) next to Baden-Württemberg (25.0) in 1975 (Figure 2.4).

This information obtained from geographic patterns of cancer mortality suggests some unknown environmental or occupational pollutants in the etiology and/or pathogenesis of prostatic cancer. Cadmium exposure[58,59] and certain jobs in the rubber industry[60] have been reported as possible risk factors.

SOME ETIOLOGICAL FACTORS

Endocrinological Considerations

Since hormones were shown to have stimulatory effects on the development and growth of the prostate, they have been considered to play an important role in the pathogenesis of its cancer disease.

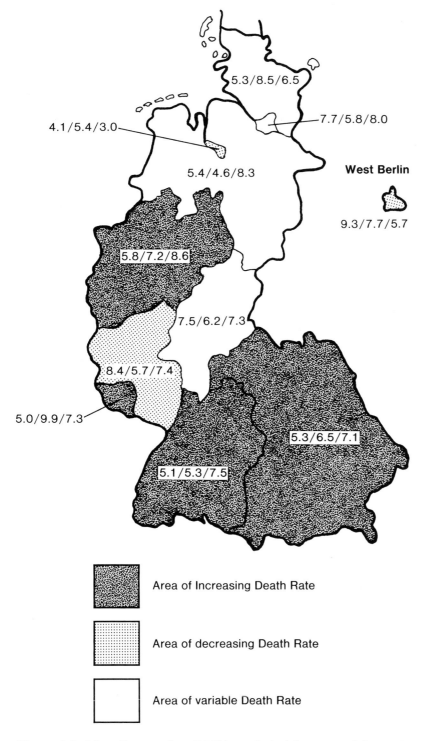

5.3/8.5/6.5

4.1/5.4/3.0

7.7/5.8/8.0

5.4/4.6/8.3

West Berlin

9.3/7.7/5.7

5.8/7.2/8.6

7.5/6.2/7.3

8.4/5.7/7.4

5.0/9.9/7.3

5.3/6.5/7.1

5.1/5.3/7.5

Area of Increasing Death Rate

Area of decreasing Death Rate

Area of variable Death Rate

Figure 2.4 Mortality rates (per 100,000 population) for cancer of the prostate in 35 to 64-year-old age group in the Federal Republic of Germany for the periods of 1955, 1965, and 1975. (Reproduced with permission from R. Frentzel-Beyme *et al.*[46])

The main role played by androgens may be to stimulate the development and maintenance of the prostate epithelium so that a sufficient number of cells is present in which malignant change may occur.[61] However, cancer of the prostate has been reported to occur in five adolescents[62-65] and in a patient with Klinefelter's syndrome.[66] Furthermore, Sharkey and Fischer[67] reported a case of prostatic cancer in a 59-year-old white male, occurring 22 years after orchiectomy and x-ray therapy for seminoma of the testis, in whom no testicular tissue could be demonstrated at autopsy. These observations indicate that such hormonal secretion, at least of the testicular origin, is not in all cases essential for the development of this cancer.

Groups of patients with liver cirrhosis have been studied to determine whether estrogen has any effect on the incidence of cancer of the prostate. An autopsy study by Glantz[68] demonstrated that there was a lower incidence of prostate cancer in cirrhotics (3.3%) than in noncirrhotics (9.0%). Similar findings were reported by Robson,[69] who stated that the incidence of this malignancy was 8.3% in cirrhotics and 11.7% in noncirrhotics. These studies suggest that prolonged exposure to high estrogen levels could prevent or delay the development of cancer in the prostate.

The Japanese have been thought to be an ideal group to study for endocrinological factors since the mortality rate for this carcinoma is apparently lower in the Japanese than in other populations. However, no significant difference has been demonstrated in levels of plasma testosterone or urinary gonadotropins between Japanese and American males.[70-72]

A possible drawback to the studies in this field is that most have been performed after the disease has been established, while critical changes might have taken place many years before the diagnosis was made. In this regard, Greenwald et al.[73] studied physical features of men before developing cancer of the prostate. In this prospective study 268 men, who later died of cancer of the prostate, were compared with 536 ethnically and socioeconomically homogenous controls. No significant differences, however, were demonstrated for any physical indices of somatotype, gynandromorphy, androgyny, baldness, and pilosity. A similar study was performed by Wynder et al.[4] in patients with prostatic cancer, suggesting no significant differences from the control group in hair distribution, weight, and height.

The relationship between cancer and benign hypertrophy of the prostate has also been studied extensively. Edwards et al.[19] examined 173 prostates from subjects 40 or more years of age by multiple sections and found malignant change in 27 of 97 hypertrophic prostates (27.8%), but in only eight of 75 nonhypertrophic prostates (10.8%). It has been a subject of debate whether, or not, there exists any etiological interrelationship between cancer and benign hypertrophy. Since both pathological changes occur progressively with age, a random coincidence is also conceivable.

Recently two well-controlled investigations have been performed in this area. Armenian et al.[74] have conducted prospective and retrospective studies to investigate the relationship between these two diseases. In their prospective study, 296 patients with hypertrophy and 299 age-adjusted controls were followed up for at least 7 years.

The death rate from prostatic cancer among the patients who had hypertrophy was 3.7 times higher than the control groups. In the retrospective study, hospital records of 290 prostate cancer patients and 290 age-matched controls were compared. A matched pair analysis of the previous hospital histories revealed 87 possible admissions due to hypertrophy among the cancer subjects, while only 21 such admissions were found among the controls. These findings from both studies revealed clearly a high risk of prostatic cancer in patients with hypertrophy.

Greenwald et al.[75] followed 838 patients with a previous history of prostatectomy because of benign hypertrophy for a period of about 11 years and compared the rate of development of cancer of the prostate in these patients with 802 age-matched controls. They found no significant difference in cancer risk between the two groups, suggesting that the previous prostatectomy had reduced the risk of cancer.

Although benign hyperplasia is not generally regarded as a precancerous lesion, it seems possible that cancer and benign hyperplasia may coexist in the same individual and share some unknown etiological factors.

Socioeconomic Status

Because there are marked racial differences in the occurrence of prostatic cancer, a study of the socioeconomic status of these patients seems attractive. Most of the previous studies, however, have been confined to white and nonwhite populations in the United States.[4, 76, 77]

Ross et al.[77] studied the socioeconomic status of patients with testicular and prostatic cancers in Los Angeles. They found that both sites had higher rates of occurrence among upper occupational and social class groups. On the other hand, the study by Hakky et al.[78] has shown a higher incidence of prostatic cancer in lower social classes in England. As yet, there seems to be no clear relationship between prostatic cancer and socioeconomic status.

Sexual Factors

The association between a previous history of gonorrhea and prostatic cancer has been investigated, since gonococcus was suspected to facilitate entry of virus into the prostatic cell with subsequent development of cancer. This concept of a venereally transmitted agent in the etiology of prostatic carcinoma was supported by an animal study in which prostate carcinoma was induced in vitro by SV 40 oncogenic virus.[79] Findings of virus-like particles in human prostatic cancer cells lend more support to this hypothesis.[80]

In a retrospective study of 75 cancer patients and 75 age-matched controls, Heshmat et al.[81] demonstrated a statistically significant association between gonorrheal infection and subsequent development of prostate cancer.

Negroes with a higher percentage of gonorrhea than a white population were observed in both cancer and control groups.[4] Because patients with prostatic cancer are reported to be more sexually active than controls,[82,83] it seems possible that a sexually transmitted disease might be an etiologic factor for this cancer.

Genetic Factors

Woolf[84] reported a higher incidence of this cancer among relatives of prostate cancer patients than in control white males. Bourke and Griffin[85] reported a higher frequency of blood type A among patients with this cancer, however Wynder et al.[4] failed to confirm it. Terasaki et al.[86] studied the frequencies of 25 HLA antigens in cancer patients and healthy controls among whites in the United States and found higher association of HLA-A28 and HLA-BW22 with patients of prostatic cancer.

The Effect of Radiation

It has been reported that radiant energy has a long-term carcinogenic potential on the rodent prostate.[87,88] Bean et al.[52] examined the occurrence of adenocarcinoma among men, most of whom were in Hiroshima or Nagasaki at the time of the atomic bomb explosion. Cancer of the prostate was present in 118 of 1,357 routine autopsies (8.7%). This lesion was found in 58 of 213 prostates, which were systematically studied by the multiple step section method. This intensive study, however, failed to show a significant relationship between the prevalence of prostatic cancer and radiation exposure.

SUMMARY AND CONCLUSION

Autopsy studies by the step section method suggest that latent cancer of the prostate develops at an incidence of between 15 and 20% equally among every population from age 40 to 90. Although it has been assumed that the frequency of clinically encountered cancer of the prostate based on hospital cancer records varies widely among ethnic populations, this concept has been probably distorted by different medical facilities and computation systems. When the rates of the clinical incidence for this cancer are based on a satisfactory series of patients with prostatic lesions, the rates seem to appear within the 11 to 30% range.

The population-based incidence obtained from several cancer registries seems to have a similar range of variation to the corresponding mortality rate. The population-based incidence in the United States is approximately three times as high as the mortality rate. The incidence and mortality can be accepted as accurate reflections of the underlying biologic phenomena of this malignancy.

The striking lack of correlation between the pathological incidence of latent cancer and the mortality for prostatic cancer in Japan remains unexplained. The discrepancy in the prevalence of proliferative, or biologically active latent cancer between native Japanese and their immigrants in the United States seems attractive. Some environmental factors which provide stimulus to further growth may be a clue to this problem.

Conventional investigations of critical hormonal factors among patients with prostate cancer have failed to demonstrate any significant differences.

Continuous efforts to demonstrate a possible relationship between viruses and cancer of the prostate are warranted.

Socioeconomic studies have been controversial; however, further study should be concentrated on more specific etiological factors related to sexual activities and dietary patterns.

Occupational exposure may account for one of the etiological factors of this disease. A possible lead can be obtained from geographic patterns of mortality, permitting evaluation of various demographic and environmental factors in each country.

Acknowledgements. The author is grateful to Dr. M. Murai and Prof. H. Tazaki for kindly supplying some statistical data from Japan. The author also thanks Prof. H. Nakamura for permission to quote the unpublished data. This work was supported by the *Alexander von Humboldt Foundation*, Bonn, Federal Republic of Germany.

REFERENCES

1. Cutler, S. J., and Young, J. L. Third national cancer survey: incidence data. *Natl. Cancer Inst. Monogr.* 41, 1975.
2. Oeser, H.: *Krebs: Schicksal oder Verschulden?* Georg Thieme Verlag, Stuttgart, 1979, pp. 14–15.
3. Segi, M., Kurihara, M., and Matsuyama, T. Cancer Mortality for Selected Sites in 24 Countries, No. 5 (1964–1965), p. 120. Department of Public Health, Tohoku University School of Medicine, Sendai, Japan, 1969.
4. Wynder, E. L., Mabuchi, K., and Whitmore, W. F. Epidemiology of cancer of the prostate. *Cancer 28:* 344, 1971.
5. Silverberg, E., and Holleb, A. I. Cancer statistics, 1971. *Cancer 21:* 13, 1971.
6. Cancer Statistics. *WHO Tech. Rep. Ser.* 632, Geneva, 1979.
7. Balogh, F., and Szendröl, Z. *Cancer of the Prostate.* Akadémiai Kiado; Budapest, 1968, p. 18.
8. Albarran, J., and Hallé, N. Hypertrophie et neoplasies épithéliales de la prostate. *Ann. Mal. Org. Genito-urin. 18:* 113 and 225, 1900.
9. Alexejew, M., and Dunajewski, L. Prostatakarzinom im Kindesalter. *Z. Urol. Chir. 1:* 64, 1930.
10. Horstmann, W. Pathologisch-anatomische Untersuchungen über geschwulstartige Erkrankungen der Prostata, insbesondere über das Karzinom. *Z. Urol 45:* 50, 1952.
11. Rich, A. R. On the frequency of occurrence of occult carcinoma of the prostate. *J. Urol. 33:* 215, 1935.
12. Moore, R. A. The morphology of small prostatic carcinoma. *J. Urol. 33:* 224, 1935.
13. Andrews, G. S. Latent carcinoma of the prostate. *J. Clin. Pathol. 2:* 197, 1949.
14. Franks, L. M. Latent carcinoma of the prostate. *J. Pathol. 68:* 603, 1954.
15. Karube, K. Study of latent carcinoma of the prostate in the Japanese on necropsy materials. *Tohoku J. Exp. Med 74:* 265, 1961.
16. Hirst, A. E., and Bergman, R. T. Carcinoma of the prostate in men 80 or more years old. *Cancer 7:* 136, 1954.
17. Scott, R., Mutchnik, D. L., Laskowski, T. Z., and Schmalhorst, W. R. Carcinoma of the prostate in elderly men: incidence, growth characteristics and clinical significance. *J. Urol. 101:* 602, 1969.
18. Tazaki, H. Pathological studies on the prostate glands of Japanese with special reference to latent malignancy. *Keio J. Med. 11:* 253, 1962.

19. Edwards, C. N., Steinthorsson, E., and Nicholson, D. An autopsy study of latent prostatic cancer. *Cancer, 6:* 531, 1953.
20. Oota, K. Latent carcinoma of the prostate among the Japanese. *Acta Un. Int. Cancer 17:* 952, 1961.
21. Gaynor, E. D. Zur Frage des Prostatakrebses. *Virchows Arch. Pathol. Anat. 301:* 602, 1938.
22. Walthard, B. Die Häufigkeit und Histogenese des Prostatakarzinoms. *Z. Urol. Chir. Gynäk. 43:* 483, 1937.
23. Rullis, I., Shaeffer, I. A., and Lilien, O. M. Incidence of prostatic carcinoma in the elderly. *Urology 4:* 295, 1975.
24. Akazaki, K., and Stemmermann, G. N. Comparative study of latent carcinoma of the prostate among Japanese in Japan and Hawaii. *J. Natl. Cancer Inst. 50:* 1137, 1973.
25. Akazaki, K., 1972 (cited by Akazaki and Stemmermann, 1973).
26. Lilien, O. M., Schaefer, J. A., Kilejan, V., and Andaloro, V. The case for perineal prostatectomy. *J. Urol. 99:* 79, 1968.
27. Ray, E. H. Endocrine therapy of prostatic carcinoma. *J.A.M.A. 163:* 1008, 1957.
28. Ravich, A. The relationship of circumcision to cancer of the prostate. *J. Urol. 48:* 298, 1942.
29. Van Buskirk, K. E., and Kimbrough, J. C. Carcinoma of the prostate. *J. Urol. 71:* 742, 1954.
30. Bauer, W. C., McGavran, M. H., and Carlin, M. R. Unsuspected carcinoma of the prostate in suprapubic prostatectomy specimens. A clinopathological study of 55 consecutive cases. *Cancer 13:* 370, 1960.
31. Smith, G. G., and Woodruff, I. M. Development of cancer of prostate after subtotal prostatectomy. *J. Urol. 63:* 1077, 1950.
32. Turner, R. D., and Belt, E. Study of 229 consecutive cases of total perineal prostatectomy for cancer of prostate. *J. Urol. 77:* 62, 1957.
33. Ravich, A. Point of view, misleading reports on Japanese incidence of prostatic cancer. *Urology 11:* 542, 1978.
34. Kato, T., and Okada, K. Clinical statistics of prostate carcinoma. Urol. Dept. of Kyoto Univ., Japan. *Nihonrinsho 32:* 2309, 1974.
35. Kobayashi, T., Mishina, T., Miyakoda, K., Araki, H., Fujiwara, T., Maekawa, M., and Watanabe, H. Clinical and statistical observations on 64 cases of prostatic cancer. *J. Nishinippon Urol. 41:* 487, 1979.
36. Takayusu, H., Ogawa, A., Koiso, K., Komine, Y., and Ishii, Y. Results of the treatment of prostatic cancer. *Jpn. J. Urol. 69:* 426, 1978.
37. Gibson, E. C. Carcinoma of the prostate in Jews and circumcised Gentiles. *Br. J. Urol. 26:* 227, 1954.
38. National Cancer Institute. Third National Cancer Survey, 1961–1971 Incidence, Advanced Three Year Report. Bethesda, Md., Natl. Inst. Health., 1974.
39. Hutchinson, G. B. Epidemiology of prostatic cancer. *Semin. Oncol. 3:* 151, 1976.
40. Waterhouse, J. A. H. *Cancer Handbook of Epidemiology and Prognosis.* Churchill, Livingstone, London, 1974.
41. Doll, R., Payne, P., and Waterhouse, J. *Cancer Incidence in Five Continents, A Technical Report. International Union Against Cancer (U.I.C.C.),* Springer-Verlag, Berlin, 1966.
42. Pedersen, E. The incidence of cancer in Norway 1964–1966. Norwegian Cancer Society, Oslo, 1966.
43. Skeet, R. G. Epidemiology of urogenital tumors. In *Scientific Foundations of Urology,* Vol. 2, edited by I. W. David and D. C. Geoffrey, William Heinemann Medical Books, London, 1976, pp. 199–211.
44. Wynder, E. L., Hyams, L., and Shigematsu, T. Correlation of international cancer death rates. *Cancer 20:* 113, 1967.
45. Ernster, V. L., Selvin, S., and Winkelstein, W. Cohort mortality for prostatic cancer among United States non-whites. *Science 200:* 1165, 1978.
46. Frentzel-Beyme, R., Leutner, R., Wagner, G., and Wiebelt, H. Cancer mortality in the states of the Federal Republic of Germany 1955–1975. In *Cancer Atlas of the Federal Republic of Germany.* Springer-Verlag, Berlin, 1979.
47. Segi, M., Kurihara, M., and Matsuyama, T. Cancer Mortality in Japan. Department of Public Health, Tohoku Univ. School of Medicine, Sendai, Japan, 1965.

48. Haenszel, W. Cancer mortality among the foreign-born in the United States. *J. Natl. Cancer Inst. 26:* 37, 1961.

49. Staszewski, T., and Haenszel, W. Cancer mortality among the Polish-born in the United States. *J. Natl. Cancer Inst. 35:* 291, 1965.

50. Haenszel, W., and Kurihara, M. Studies of Japanese migrants. *J. Natl. Cancer Inst. 40:* 43, 1968.

51. Buell, P., and Dunn, J. E. Cancer mortality among the Japanese Issei and Nissei of California. *Cancer 18:* 656, 1965.

52. Bean, M. A., Yatani, R., Lui, P. I., Fukazawa, K., Ashley, F. W., and Fujita, S. Prostatic carcinoma at autopsy in Hiroshima and Nagasaki Japanese. *Cancer 32:* 498, 1973.

53. Mortality statistics. In *Demographic Year Book 1966*, 18th issue. United Nations, New York, 1967.

54. Mason, T. J., McKay, F. W., Hoover, R., *et al.* Atlas of Cancer Mortality among U.S. Counties: 1950–1969. Natl. Inst. Health, DHEW Publ., No.(NIH)75-780, Washington D.C., U.S. Govt. Print. Off., 1975.

55. Segi, M. *Atlas of Cancer Mortality for Japan by Cities and Countries, 1969-1971.* Daiwa Health Foundation, Tokyo, 1977.

56. Blair, A., and Fraumeni, J. F. Geographic patterns of prostatic cancer in the United States. *J. Natl. Cancer Inst. 61:* 1379, 1978.

57. *Statistisches Jahrbuch 1975 für die Bundesrepublik Deutschland.* W. Kohlhammer GmbH, Stuttgart, 1975.

58. Kipling, M. D., and Waterhouse, J. A. M. Cadmium and prostatic cancer. *Lancet 1:* 730, 1967.

59. Potts, C. L. Cadmium proteinuria— the health of battery workers exposed to cadmium oxide dust. *Ann. Occup. Hyg. 8:* 55, 1965.

60. McMichael, A. J., Spirtis, R., and Kupper, L. L. An epidemiologic study of mortality within a cohort of rubber workers, 1964–1972. *J. Occup. Med. 16:* 458, 1974.

61. Franks, L. M. Some comments on the long-term results of endocrine treatment of prostatic cancer. *Br. J. Urol. 30:* 383, 1958.

62. Chiu, C. L., and Weber, D. L. Prostatic carcinoma in young adults. *J.A.M.A. 230:* 724, 1974.

63. Gardner, S. J., and Cummins, M. T. Prostatic carcinoma in a youth. *J.A.M.A. 58:* 1282, 1912.

64. Kimbrough, J. C., and Lewis, E. L. Carcinoma of prostate in young adults. *J. Urol. 68:* 626, 1952.

65. Nicholson, N. J. Carcinoma of the prostate in a youth. *Br. J. Surg. 32:* 533, 1945.

66. Arduino, L. J. Carcinoma of the prostate in sex chromatin positive Klinefelter's syndrome. *J. Urol. 98:* 234, 1967.

67. Sharkey, D., and Fischer, E. R. Carcinoma of the prostate in the absence of testicular tissue. *J. Urol. 83:* 468, 1960.

68. Glantz, G. M. Cirrhosis and carcinoma of the prostate gland. *J. Urol. 91:* 291, 1964.

69. Robson, M. C. Cirrhosis and prostatic neoplasms. *Geriatrics 21:* 150, 1966.

70. Kobayashi, T., Lobotsky, J., and Lloyd, C. W. Plasma testosterone and urinary 17-ketosteroids in Japanese and Occidentals. *J. Clin. Endocrinol. Metab. 26:* 610, 1966.

71. Motohashi, K., and Nishikawa, M. *Endocrinology*, Vol. 2, edited by G. Miyake and K. Yamamoto. Tokyo, Asakura-shoten, 1964, p. 1600.

72. Heller, A., and Shipley, R. A. Endocrine studies in aging. *J. Clin. Endocrinol. Metab. 11:* 945, 1951.

73. Greenwald, P., Damon A., Kirmss, V., and Polan, A. K. Physical and demographic features of men before developing cancer of the prostate. *J. Natl. Cancer Inst. 53:* 341, 1974.

74. Armenian, H. K., Lilienfeld, A. M., Diamond, E. L., and Bross, D. J. Relation between benign prostatic hyperplasia and cancer of the prostate. *Lancet 2:* 115, 1974.

75. Greenwald, P., Kirmss, V., Polan, A. K., and Dick, V. S. Cancer of the prostate among men with benign hyperplasia. *J. Natl. Cancer Inst. 53:* 335, 1974.

76. Graham, S., Levin, M., and Lilienfeld, A. M. The socioeconomic distribution of cancer of various sites in Buffalo, N.Y., 1948–1952. *Cancer 13:* 180, 1960.

77. Ross, R. K., McCurtis, J. W., Henderson, B. E., Menck, H. R., Mack, T. M., and Martin, S. P. Descriptive epidemiology of testicular and prostatic cancer in Los Angeles. *Br. J.*

Cancer 39: 284, 1979.

78. Hakky, S. I., Chisholm, G. D., and Skeet, R. G. Social class and carcinoma of the prostate. *Br. J. Urol. 51:* 393, 1979.

79. Paulson, D. E., Robson, A. J., and Fraley, E. E. Viral transformation of hamster prostate tissue in vitro. *Science 159:* 200, 1968.

80. Tannenbaum, M., and Lattimer, J. K. Similar virus-like particles found in cancers of the prostate and breast. *J. Urol. 103:* 471, 1970.

81. Heshmat, M. Y., Kovi, J., Herson, J., Jones, G. W., and Jackson, M. A. Epidemiologic association between gonorrhea and prostatic carcinoma. *Urology 6:* 457, 1975.

82. Steele, R., Lees, R. E. M., Kraus, A. S., and Rao, C. Sexual factors in the epidemiology of cancer of the prostate. *J. Chronic Dis. 24:* 29, 1971.

83. King, H., Diamond, E., and Lilienfeld, A. M. Some epidemiological aspects of cancer of the prostate. *J. Chronic Dis. 16:* 117, 1963.

84. Woolf, C. M. An investigation of the familial aspects of carcinoma of the prostate. *Cancer 13:* 739, 1960.

85. Bourke, J. B., and Griffin, J. P. Blood groups in benign and malignant prostatic hypertrophy. *Lancet 2:* 1279, 1962.

86. Terasaki, P. I., Perdue, S. T., and Mickey, M. R. HLA frequencies in cancer: a second study. In *Progress in Cancer Research and Therapy. Vol. 3: Genetics of Human Cancer.* Raven Press, New York, 1977, p. 321.

87. Brown C. E., and Warren, S. Carcinoma of the prostate in irradiated parabiotic rats. *Cancer Res. 38:* 159, 1978.

88. Hirose, F., Takizawa, S., Watanabe, H., and Takeichi, N. Development of adenocarcinoma of the prostate in ICR mice locally irradiated with X rays. *Gann 67:* 407, 1976.

89. Baba, S., and Jacobi, G. H. Epidemiology of prostate cancer. *Akt. Urol. 11:* 277, 1980.

Editorial Comment to Chapter 2

The Western versus Eastern discrepancy as well as ethnic variations are evident (Ahluwalia *et al.*, 1981). Although its nature is still unclear, it is nevertheless statistically documented. However, Niijima and Koiso (1980) have reported a recent increase of appearance in Japan,

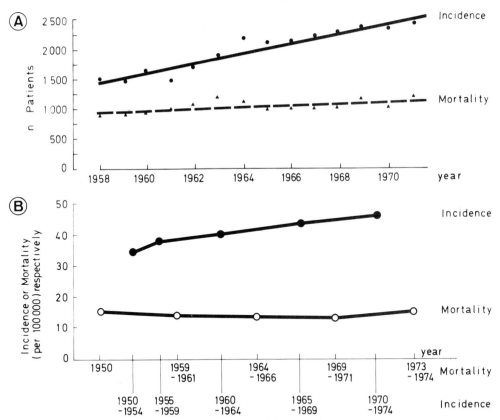

Figure 2.5 Comparative data on increasing incidence and unchanged mortality of prostatic carcinoma from Scandinavia and America. *A*, Absolute figures for Sweden. *B*, Relative values from the U.S.A. Data compiled and drawn according to figures given by Trasti *et al.*, 1979 (*A*) and Schottenfeld, 1981 (*B*).

a country of known low incidence. Data from Trasti *et al.* (1979) and Schottenfeld (1981) show that in Europe as well as in America the incidence of prostate cancer has increased, while the mortality has remained essentially unchanged (Fig. 2.5). Is it not reasonable that substances we eat, breathe, or touch are, as co-factors, responsible for this increasing appearance of prostate cancer? A recent analysis of Nasca *et al.* (1981) of foreign-born in New York State indicates that immigrants from certain European countries have a higher incidence of prostate cancer when compared with a cancer-of-origin standard. This finding, together with endocrine data compatible with factors other than the genetic makeup of the population (Ahluwalia *et al.*, 1981), suggests a major environmental component for this malignancy.

G. H. J.
R. H.

References

Ahluwalia, B., Jackson, M. A., Jones, G. W., Williams, A. O., Rao, M. S., and Rajguru, S. Blood hormone profiles in prostate cancer patients in high-risk and low-risk populations. *Cancer 48:* 2267, 1981.

Nasca, P. C., Greenwald, P., Burnett, W. S., Chorost, S., and Schmidt, W. Cancer among the foreign-born in New York state. *Cancer 48:* 2323, 1981.

Niijima, T., Koiso, K. Incidence of prostatic cancer in Japan and Asia. *Scand. J. Urol. Nephrol. Suppl. 55:* 17, 1980.

Schottenfeld, D. The epidemiology of cancer: an overview. *Cancer 47:* 1095, 1981.

Trasti, H., Nilsson, S., and Peterson, L.-E. Applied diagnostic techniques: a decisive factor in the long-term T-year survival rate in prostatic carcinoma. *Br. J. Urol. 51:* 135, 1979.

3

Staging, Management, and Post-treatment Re-evaluation of Prostate Cancer: Dogma Questioned

G. H. Jacobi, M.D.
R. Hohenfellner, M.D.

STAGING AND EVALUATION OF TUMOR AND DISEASE

How Far Must Staging Go?

The most obvious question that cancer patients ask themselves and their doctor is "How far advanced is my tumor?", a question which, nowadays, most of them immediately connect with the question of how great their chances of cure may be.

For prostatic carcinoma, the answer to these questions are imprecise and range widely: at one extreme of the spectrum there may be precise information on a small cancer nodule with histologically confirmed negative lymph nodes and with a lack of distant spread ruled out by highly sophisticated isotope scan techniques, computerized imaging procedures, and specific laboratory methods. At the other extreme, there could be a rather vague impression of a so-called locally far advanced lesion with a single scintigraphic hot spot at the lumbar spine along with a pre-existing spondylarthrosis. The case illustrated in Figure 3.1 shows the x-ray study of a patient suffering from anemia, severe bone pain, and urinary obstruction. In light of an histologically confirmed prostatic carcinoma, the answer given to this patient would be rather clear.

Since the responsibility for the extent of the evaluation of tumor stage is ours, the question that we have to ask ourselves in each new case is a

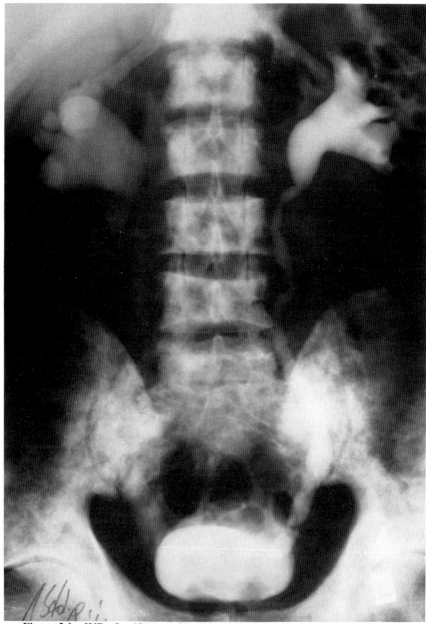

Figure 3.1 IVP of a 68-year-old patient with hormone-resistant prostatic carcinoma (stage $T_3N_xM_1$) 1 hour after injection of contrast medium. Note diffuse osseous metastases with severe bone pain and bilateral upper tract dilatation due to extensive local tumor mass (several factors of poor risk in the same patient, see page 47). In this case there is no need for any further staging procedure!

simple one, namely, what sort of essential information on tumor extent is obligatory to be able to introduce the most individual and rational treatment strategy to the particular patient.

The main factor which warrants extensive staging is the possible curative intent of treatment, a situation which justifies the engagement of all diagnostic measures to rule out lymphatic and distant spread, regardless of invasiveness or cost. There is no doubt that the young patient without distant metastases, who would be a candidate for radical prostatectomy, needs prior surgical lymphostaging. There is, however, only weak evidence given by Barzell and co-workers[1] and Zincke et al.[2] that excision of small nodal metastases limited to the periprostatic area might be of more than staging value and render the patient into the node-negative category. On the other hand, the aggressive node dissectors among us have to reflect upon whether in stage C or even D_1 lesions, with an expected rate of lymphatic spread of up to 80%, this invasive procedure really does influence further treatment strategy.

For the unsuspected stage A lesion, it is obviously not sufficient to satisfy the patient and ourselves with the feeling of a clinically unsuspected "early" carcinoma. In contrast, we must accept the fact that a number of stage A tumors (T_0- International Union against Cancer (UICC)), are multifocally or diffusely occupying what we thought to be a benign prostatic hypertrophy (BPH) specimen. The tumor volume as well as grade of differentiation of these lesions may reflect a bad cancer.[3]

How to Improve Staging Procedures

The goal of innovations or refinements of already established staging procedures is to improve specificity and sensitivity. Ultrasonography may discriminate T_3 from T_4 (C versus D_1) tumors (Fig. 3.2), while multiple biopsies may reveal cancer tissue from two or three areas where the palpating finger only detects one nodule. Lymphography combined with CT-scanning may improve sensitivity of each one when applied alone, and selective fine needle biopsy under ultrasonographic guidance may prevent an otherwise performed staging operation.

With the introduction (and premature?) wide acceptance of radioimmunologic techniques for acid phosphatase determination, many of us thought we finally had a tool for early tumor detection. In terms of a screening test, Kiesling and Watson[4] are correct in their reservedness, but there is another side of the issue. A paramount clinical question in every patient who undergoes invasive therapy with curative intent is, how much can we rely on a negative bone scan? Does open skeletal diagnosis with biochemical and morphological bone marrow work-up add anything to this dilemma?

With the help of a newly developed nonisotope enzyme immunoassay (ELISA) for specific prostate acid phosphatase, we were recently able to investigate the serum of 136 patients with M_0 disease determined by bone scan plus x-ray survey.[5] Thirty-five patients had elevated ELISA-phosphatase despite negative bone scans, and the question arose as to whether these patients had preclinical perhaps exclusively biochemical evidence of early osseous spread. Of 50 patients reevaluated 2 to 15 months after the initial study, 29 now had bone scans positive for metastases (Table 3.1). Thus, technical innovations applied with a rational goal and a clinically relevant question may prove to their benefit.

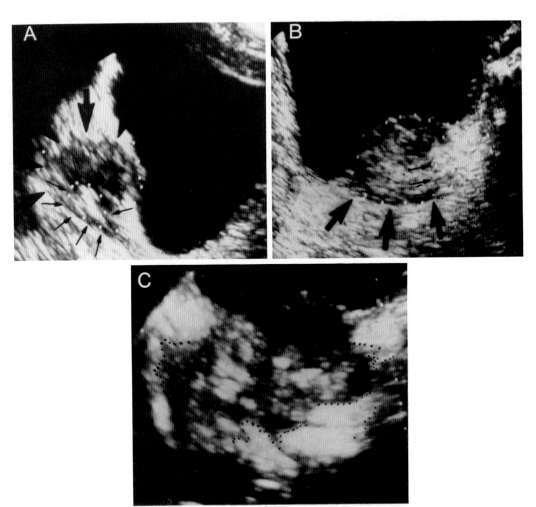

Figure 3.2 Suprapubic transvesical sonographic scanning of the prostate for staging of carcinoma. Transversal (*A*) and longitudinal (*B*) sections through prostate staged by rectal examination as T_2-carcinoma nodule. *A*, Well defined organ boundary on left side and dorsal aspect (*large arrows*); clearly documented pericapsular tumor penetration from right lobe (*small arrows*). *B*, Tumor growth is not clearly defined to prostate at cranial organ boundary. *C*, Ultrasonography of a prostatic carcinoma keyed as "small T_3" at rectal examination; tumor extends far beyond prostatic capsule into periprostatic tissue. In our hands the suprapubic transvesical approach is at least as accurate as transrectal sonography with the significant advantage of a noninvasive procedure.

ANOTHER CLINICAL PROBLEM

A simple hot spot on the scintiscan, reconfirmed by x-ray as an osteoplastic lesion, automatically puts this patient into the category M_1 (stage D), independent of the remaining distant status. It must, however, be expected that different quantities of metastatic deposits, *i.e.* total tumor mass, do affect response to treatment as well as prognosis.

The Veterans Administration Cooperative Urological Research Group suggested, in order to assess the extent of osseous metastatic spread, a

Table 3.1
Sensitivity Study of Newly Developed Enzyme Immunoassay (ELISA-PSAP) for Specific Prostate Acid Phosphatase in Serum[a]

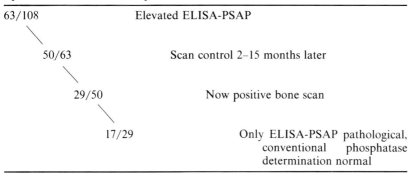

63/108	Elevated ELISA-PSAP
50/63	Scan control 2–15 months later
29/50	Now positive bone scan
17/29	Only ELISA-PSAP pathological, conventional phosphatase determination normal

[a] This study was performed in 136 patients with prostate cancer without scintigraphic and roentgenographic evidence of osseous metastases. Early biochemical evidence of preclinical osseous spread considered exclusively by a pathological ELISA-PSAP study was given in 17 of 29 cases (58.6%). From G. H. Jacobi et al.[5]

Table 3.2
Substaging of Osseous Metastases According to Quantitative Bone Involvement (<50% versus >50%) in Five Skeletal Regions Determined at Isotope Scan.[a]

Region Quantity	Metastatic Involvement per Region	
	Up to 50%	More than 50%
Skull	73	12
Shoulder girdle and thorax	66	11
Vertebra	66	23
Pelvic girdle	58	18
Thighs	48	22
Any area	72 (n = 88)	21 (n = 18)

[a] As a prognostic factor, the *3-year-survival rates* in percent are given for 106 patients with metastases. In a control group of 74 patients without distant metastases prospectively followed during the same period, 3-year survival was 80%; in all skeletal areas investigated, the quantitative substaging of bony metastases revealed a significantly different prognosis. From G. H. Jacobi et al.[20]

system of quantification based on roentgenographic analysis of the skeleton in four grades of metastatic involvement at eight sites.[6] We have recently applied a modified system to the isotope scan and have found that patients initially presenting with high degrees of focality and/or regional quantity of metastases have a poor prognosis (Table 3.2). Thus, differentiated applications of already established staging procedures can significantly improve our information on the extent of tumor disease.

Development from Tumor Classification to Clinical Staging

A variety of tumor classifications still (and increasingly!) obscures the urological literature, thus impeding the daily communication among colleagues and making the interinstitutional comparison of therapy results difficult. The original American *ABCD-staging system* has been repeatedly subdivided whenever a prognostic significance for such substaging became evident. The American staging system for prostate cancer allocates the loco-regional and distant extent of the tumor disease to known anatomical structures or areas. The tumor, node, metastasis (TNM) classification introduced by the UICC[7] (see Chapter 7) clearly does not do more, although the TNM categories much more precisely describe tumor extent. The TNM classification and the American staging system are not readily interconvertible, although this is common practice. A slightly modified version of the comparison of both systems published by Murphy and co-workers[8] is given in the "Editorial Comment to Chapter 7."

It should clearly be stated that the TNM system is *not a staging system* and the UICC does not, at present, recommend a clinical staging for prostate cancer. What we are presently dealing with is the anatomy-related characterization of the extent of cancer disease by the categories *T, N, M* and *G*. From T_{0-4}, N_{0-4}, and M_{0-1}, up to 50 TNM combinations are theoretically possible, and for each of the TNM categories more or less strictly defined minimal requirements are recommended. Therefore, we must come to some sort of grouping system in which we combine certain T, N, and M categories and allocate these to clinically relevant prognostic features. Such a combined anatomical-clinical staging could eventually lead to differentiated therapy strategies. An anatomy-oriented characterization of the evaluable tumor is bound to be incomplete, since our limited staging procedures will always be describing the tip of an iceberg (Fig. 3.3).

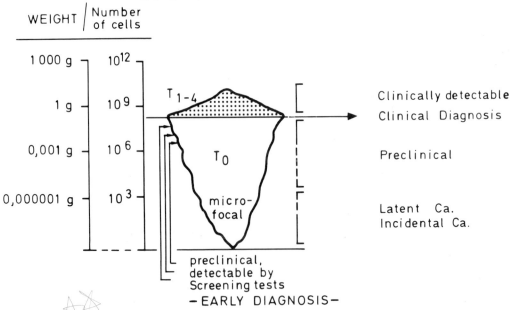

Figure 3.3 "Iceberg-Situation" in prostatic carcinoma: the clinically detectable part of the tumor is categorized as T1–4; preclinical tumors (not palpable = T_0) are the *incidental carcinoma* (stage A) at prostatectomy for BPH or *the latent carcinoma* at autopsy. Effective screening tests including repeated rectal examination in risk populations should be able to detect early prostatic carcinoma at the transition point from T_0 to T_1 (stage A–stage B).

INDIVIDUALIZED TREATMENT STRATEGIES

With the introduction of contrasexual measures for treatment of prostate cancer, an era began lasting decades, during which orchiectomy and/or estrogens were almost dogmatically applied to almost all patients in whom prostatic cancer was even considered by rectal palpation. The sometimes dramatic clinical responses have seduced urologists (and do still some of us) to prescribe such treatment irrespective of tumor extent. However, androgen depletion was considered originally by Huggins and his associates as *palliative* treatment, and many physicians have abused the purpose for which this treatment was originally designed. In this era of modern medical alternatives summarized by Smith,[9] and in anticipation of the information given in Chapters 9 to 16 of this volume, some remarks on the subject seem appropriate.

Predetermination of the Intention of Treatment

Some of the current therapy concepts for prostate cancer are based on empirically deduced data from animal studies, some derived from the experiences with other cancer lesions (eradication by surgery or radiation), and only a few are deducted from controlled clinical trials. The ultimate goal of any cancer treatment is cure. The definition of cure in prostatic carcinoma is, however, difficult to assess. Periods of 5 or 10 years of follow-up without tumor recurrence are usually indicative of cure; 5 or 10 years of survival without information on the evidence of residual or recurrent disease are *not*. If, after ablative therapy (surgery, radiation), new tumor growth occurs, are we then dealing with a recurrence or with residual disease?

We believe that any treatment strategy on prostate cancer should be oriented to the following questions:

1. Are we dealing with a tumor limited to the prostate that could be classified as *curable by local means*, or has the cancer overcome the organ boundaries and become a loco-regional growth requiring pelvic treatment?
2. Is the tumor already in its widespread status with the attributes of a *cancer disease* which then requires *systemic* treatment?
3. Does the patient suffer from local or distant tumor burden requiring *palliative* measures?
4. If biological markers (biochemical, immunological, cytomorphological) known to be associated with an unfavourable treatment response are present, is this, then, the case for *adjunct* treatment modalities to improve the chance of local tumor control?
5. Has our intent of treatment and the therapy modalities chosen been oriented to the patient's age, his general performance status, and his individual personal requirements?

The keystone of any oncological strategy—that the *local tumor* requires a *local attack*, whereas disseminated *tumor disease* requires *systemic measures*—is also true for prostate cancer. Most of these questions are left to the doctor's discretion, and in general the patient's belief in either cure or palliation largely depends on how we convince him of the *pros* and *cons* (and sometimes the absolute necessity) of the different treatment modalities. If we then ask ourselves the patient's question, the answer of *"what is the best treatment"* remains all too often obscure.

To Treat or Not to Treat

Some of us have believed that the frequent finding of clinically unsuspected prostatic cancer foci at autopsy of men who died of other causes would be proof for the thesis that most prostate cancers are of low biological potential. This latent type of prostatic carcinoma has been characterized as *silent* or *dormant* and has been compared with a domestic animal—present, but tame.

Without doubt latent prostate cancer is of no individual clinical relevance, since the patient is already dead, so why the controversy? Extensive pathological studies, summarized by Bouffioux,[10] have revealed that a large number of so-called clinically *unsuspected* lesions were, in fact, clinically *undiagnosed*, not exclusively focal in nature, in some studies of an extent to be diagnosed even macroscopically during routine autopsy, and histologically not necessarily different from manifest prostatic carcinoma. There is ample evidence that in the dynamic natural history of prostatic cancer the true latent lesion is not a special entity, but simply an early lesion as can be the incidental stage A type of prostatic carcinoma (Fig. 3.4). Thus, Hudson and co-workers[11] have stated that "many of the

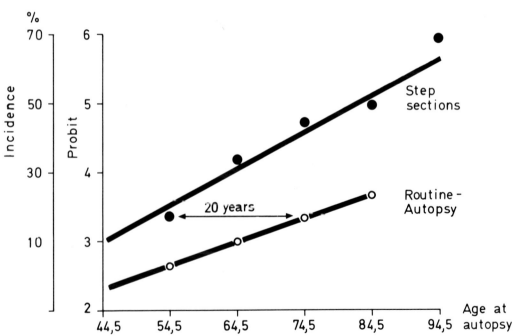

Figure 3.4 Time correlation between the locally advanced prostatic carcinoma detected macroscopically at routine autopsy and the true latent carcinoma detected by step-sections at autopsy. The time gap of 20 years possibly reflects the period a beginning carcinoma needs for clinical manifestation. (Reproduced with permission from Chr. Bouffioux.[10])

38   PROSTATE CANCER

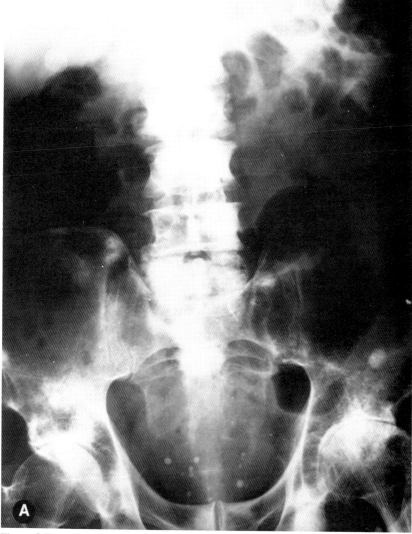

Figure 3.5 *A*, X-rays demonstrate an unusual example of spontaneous remission of bone metastases in an 81-year-old patient who only underwent *local* radiotherapy for palliation.

metastatic prostatic cancers of 1953 would have been 'occult cancer at autopsy' in 1933." The question arising from this fact is whether all prostatic carcinoma being clinically manifest or incidentally detected need definitive treatment.

In the past we have relied heavily on one of the most significant prognosticators, the grade of tumor differentiation, and have thought of watchful waiting and deferred treatment usually in the case of a small and highly differentiated tumor nodule. From very recent studies, however, we learn that the tumor grade derived from biopsy represents, in only 33%, the true grade of the entire tumor,[12] and that in more than half of the cases operated for a biopsy-proven well to moderately differentiated adenocarcinoma, the tumor is biologically undergraded as compared to

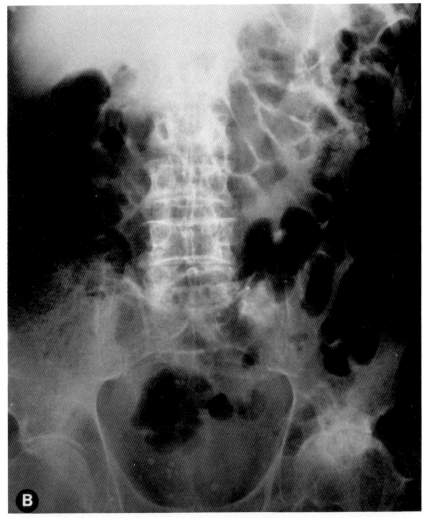

Figure 3.5 *B*, X-ray taken 23 months after that shown in Figure 3.5*A*.

the entire surgical specimen.[13] Thus, the decision of whether to treat or not to treat made on the basis of the grading result of a biopsy seems at the least questionable. The biopsy result simply reflects the momentary picture of the tumor in its entirety. The circumstances under which deferred treatment for even widespread but asymptomatic carcinoma is justified are outlined in Chapter 11. Maintenance of the tumor extent or stable disease can be achieved. Spontaneous tumor remission, as demonstrated in Figure 3.5, however, remains a very rare event.

Is Radiotherapy as a Treatment Modality Being Correctly Evaluated?

Local high-voltage radiotherapy is being increasingly applied to localized tumors with the intention of cure, and this treatment is widely offered to the patient as a comparably effective alternative to radical surgery. Who would doubt that the patient whose x-ray study is shown in Figure

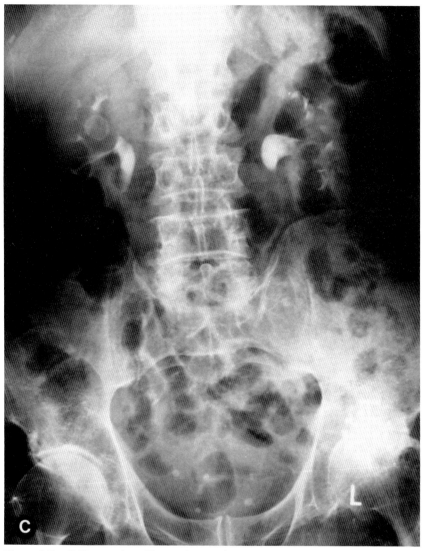

Figure 3.5 *C*, X-ray taken 50 months after that shown in Figure 3.5*A*.

3.6, and who is without evidence of disease 9 years after radiotherapy, had been given cure by this treatment? We have, however, information that almost half of the patients undergoing external beam radiotherapy given with "curative intention" will not experience local tumor control as determined by repeated postirradiation biopsies.[14, 15] Thus, we have to be careful in offering some sort of alternative therapy without yet having objective data from long-term clinical studies available for comparison. Parameters indicating radiation failure are discussed later in this chapter and in the "Editorial Comment to Chapter 10."

The So-called Controlled Randomized Clinical Trial

This approach is a prerequisite for the proof of a new (or old but not yet objectively reconfirmed) treatment modality as being superior to a

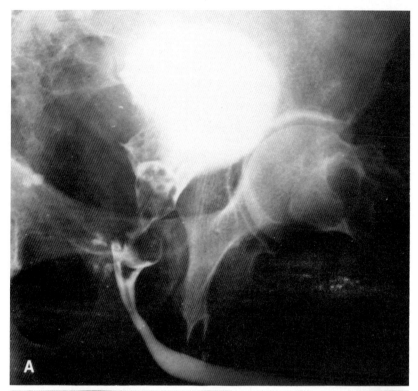

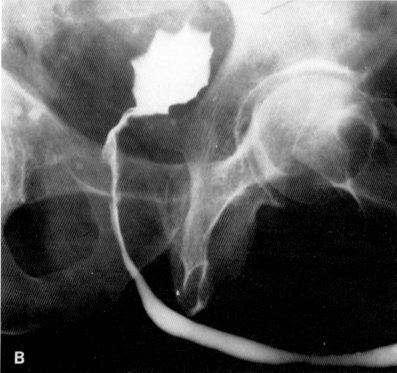

Figure 3.6 Patient, 74 years old, with locally advanced, moderately differentiated adenocarcinoma of the prostate (stage T_3, N_X, M_0). *A*, Retrograde urethrogram at diagnosis with tumor infiltrating into prostatic urethra. *B*, Same study 9 months after local high-voltage radiotherapy (7600 r) to the area of the small pelvis. Two years after radiotherapy, transrectal aspiration biopsy was negative for residual tumor; the patient is without evidence of disease 9 years after radiotherapy as the sole treatment.

standard therapy. In such so-called *phase-III* studies, the response to treatment is prospectively investigated under randomized conditions.

Several practical, ethical, and legal problems are involved, however, in such studies which bear the status of a "scientific experiment."

1. How do we define the standard treatment for prostate cancer, against which the new therapy regimen is to be compared? Is it the one currently still considered to be the best or is it the one most widely accepted?

2. Which assessment of response to treatment is reliable? How reproducible are the response criteria in use? How can we define a complete objective response, and under which circumstances is subjective improvement, *i.e.* improvement of quality of life (the main goal of any palliative treatment), of more value than the measurable shrinkage of a soft-tissue metastasis?

3. How reliable is randomization when in multicentric trials surgical procedures and apparative modalities are compared from institution to institution? How far can standardization of such therapies be achieved?

4. How are results from patients who are failures in one therapy arm and require treatment modification to be well evaluated?

5. Is it ethical to withhold a patient from the standard treatment that he would be given elsewhere and, instead of this, treat him with something that might turn out to be less effective?

6. To what extent do we need informed consent from the patient for the randomization? There is considerable debate as to whether the patient needs to know that his treatment is chosen by computer (or even by tossing a coin).

7. How straightforward must our arguments be to justify a nontreated control arm in any stage of prostatic carcinoma?

In studies which are designed to evaluate the long-term efficacy of *one* given modality judged by survival, the retrospective investigation may, under certain circumstances, be of comparable value with the prospective trial (Fig. 3.7).

Hormone Autonomy

Numerous synonyms are in use for the situation of primary or secondary unresponsiveness of prostatic cancer to androgen depletion treatment. Terms such as *estrogen resistance, hormone relapse,* or *estrogen escape phenomenon* either incompletely or incorrectly characterize the situation, and the attributes "initial" *versus* "acquired" are wrong as well when seen from a tumor-biological point of view. We believe that the term *"hormone autonomy"* best describes the mechanism by which prostatic cancer is to some degree initially or secondarily unresponsive to withdrawal of androgens. The tumor itself harbors, from the beginning of treatment on, two cell components: a certain volume of cells living only by dependence on androgens, another quantity of cell clones growing autonomously of androgens. These cells will be keyed herein as *androgen-deaf.* The pro-

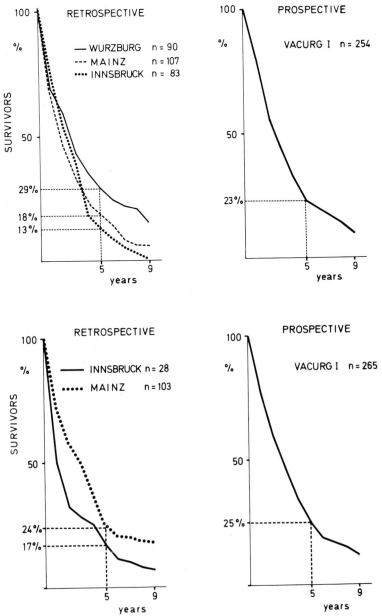

Figure 3.7 The comparison of survival data either *prospectively* followed by the VACURG (*right side*) or *retrospectively* analyzed by three European centers (*left side*). Survival data of the upper part refers to orchiectomy plus long-term estrogens, the lower part to estrogen treatment only. (Reproduced with permission from H.G.W. Frohmüller et al.[24])

portion of these two components is, even by sophisticated androgen-receptor assays, not yet assessible prior to treatment (see Chapter 20). From clinical experience we know, however, that it is the well differen-tiated adenocarcinoma which obviously needs to be fed with androgens for maintenance or further growth. Since almost two-thirds of all prostatic neoplasms are pluriform in architecture (see Chapter 6) and are apparently composed of differing tumor quantities of variable androgen dependence or autonomy, it becomes clear that by contrasexual means, only part of the tumor entity is hit, while the other continues to grow. Not fitting into this concept is the observation that in some patients the criteria of tumor relapse are predominantly *objective* (local tumor, distant metastases progressive in size and number), while in others a *subjective* relapse (bone pain) becomes evident.[16]

To further influence prostatic carcinoma of patients who no longer respond to androgen depletion is one of our greatest challenges. It would seem logical to apply to every prostatic carcinoma which requires systemic treatment, two types of treatment in combination—the *contrasexual* one to hit androgen-sensitive cells, and the *nonhormonal* one (perhaps chemotherapy) to hit the hormone-autonomous cells.[17]

CONTINUOUS RE-EVALUATION— RESPONSE TO TREATMENT AND PHYSICIAN'S QUALITY CONTROL

It is never only a question of whether the patient is doing well under the treatment given, but always a matter of whether the doctor has done it or is still doing it well. There are three possibilities for the patient never seen again by his urologist after initiation of therapy: he is either doing very well, he has changed doctors, or he is dead. The possible change of response to medical treatment, the uncertainty of the so-called local tumor control after definitive therapy, residual or recurrent tumor, late complications, drug toxicity, and the biological change of the individual carcinoma are altogether a *sine qua non* for continuous evaluation.

Monitoring of Local Tumor Response

In Chapter 5, Dr. Esposti has nicely developed the concept of the paramount value of aspiration biopsy in following patients after treatment. If the material obtained by fine-needle aspiration biopsy is investigated and cytological criteria of regression are applied, a reproducible regression grading can be established.

The great value of the studies performed by Leistenschneider and Nagel[18] is that they were able to correlate such regression grading to the clinical course of the disease. From Table 3.3 it is easily seen that patients with a carcinoma that shows an excellent or good cytological regression almost never experience progressive tumor disease. On the other hand, 85% of patients whose tumor shows a poor cytological regression will subsequently develop clinical tumor progression. The same authors have shown that rectal palpation alone is not reliable in this regard. Of 208 patients under hormonal treatment with a clinically favorable course and excellent to moderate signs of tumor regression on cytology, 66% had palpable findings not attributable to a good local response.[18]

Table 3.3
Correlation between Local Tumor Regression Cytologically Verified by Aspiration Fine Needle Biopsy and the Clinical Course of the Disease in 131 Patients[a]

Grade of Regression		No.	Clinical Progression	
			No.	%
0	Very good	23	1	4.3
II	Good	16		
IV	Sufficient	26	2	7.7
VI	Moderate	46	6	13.1
VIII	Poor	20	17	85.0

[a] The grades of regression are based on cytomorphological criteria during a 1- to 3-year follow-up (also see Chapter 6). From W. Leistenschneider and R. Nagel.[18]

Table 3.4
The 2-Year Biopsy after Local Radiotherapy as a Prognostic Index with Clinical Relevance (Response to Irradiation *versus* Failure)[a]

Biopsy	Metastases after Radiotherapy					
	At 2 Years		Total	At 4 Years		Total
	M$_0$	M$_1$		M$_0$	M$_1$	
Tumor negative	59	1(1.6%)	60/98(61.2%)	32	7(18%)	39/64(60.9%)
Tumor positive	31	7(18.4%)	38/98(38.8%)	9	16(64%)	25/64(39.1%)
Total	90(92%)	8(8%)	98(100%)	41(64%)	23(36%)	64(100%)

[a] Two years after radiation as sole treatment, 98 patients had transrectal aspiration biopsy (tumor positive/negative) and isotope bone scan (M$_0$/M$_1$); the results of isotope scan at 4-years (64 of 98 patients from the 2-year follow-up = 65.3%) are correlated to the biopsy result at 2 years after irradiation.

Repeated aspiration biopsy is also of enormous value in following patients after radiotherapy. It is only the biopsy control by which the local response to radiation can be determined and by which tumor residuals, *i.e.* failures, can be detected. According to our own most recent statistics on the clinical value of biopsy data after radiation, 18.4% of patients with a biopsy-proven residual tumor 2 years after radiation will, at the same time, have or quickly develop distant metastases, this rate being 64% after 4 years (Table 3.4).

Re-evaluation of Distant Spread

Monitoring the skeletal status by bone scan has, besides its limited specificity due to the high sensitivity, another pitfall. We do not know how to interpret the situation when in one site metastatic deposits disappear while at other sites new spots of increased isotope activity appear. As long as under this so-called *mixed response* the patient remains asymptomatic, the case is easy (unless this response is to be rated in a clinical trial). If minimal positive or even negative changes in bone scan are associated with the onset of bone pain, the question of whether subjective or objective response would be of more clinical relevance comes up.

On x-ray, most bone metastases from prostate cancer appear as osteo-sclerotic or osteoplastic lesions. The detection of discrete sclerotic areas during therapy in what appeared to be normal bone, may in fact represent the healing of previously unsuspected metastases rather than a manifestation of new metastatic disease (Fig. 3.8).

A question frequently raised during the recent debate on cost reduction in medical care is whether we really need the annual intravenous pyelogram (IVP) in following up prostatic carcinoma patients. Our answer is *no*! Wahner and co-workers[19] were able to show that with the evaluation of the imaging of the upper urinary tract during bone scan, almost all significant changes of interest in prostatic carcinoma patients can be detected. We have reconfirmed this observation by comparing urinary tract findings of bone scan and IVP in a prospective fashion and found good correlation in 88%.[20] An example of how nicely the upper tract can be imaged at bone scan is given in Figure 3.9.

Factors Determining Prognosis

The term prognosis includes three principal parameters: the possibility of cure (*prognosis quoad sanationem*), the influences of tumor or treatment on survival (*prognosis quoad vitam*), or the effects of both on the quality of the remaining life span in the presence of the incurable tumor (*prognosis quoad palliationem*). For the last two parameters of prognosis, Berry and co-workers[21] have characterized the following clinical factors as being negatively associated: diagnosis after the age of 65, rapid development of metastases, metastatic bone pain, poor performance status, pleural effusion, marked anemia, elevated serum acid phosphatase, and pathological liver function tests. Some of these factors of poor risk are also present in an ancillary score system designed by Kvols et al.,[22] which is helpful in predetermining prognosis and in assessing response to treatment.

In our own material of 670 patients followed for 3 to 30 years (mean observation at risk, 11 years), the following clinical features have been evaluated in a partially retrospective, mainly prospective fashion in order to assess possible risk factors[23]

1. Upper urinary tract dilatation
2. Elevated serum acid phosphatase
3. Age at first diagnosis
4. Multiplicity of osseous metastases
5. Duration of symptoms at the time of first diagnosis.

Since, in the majority of cases, a uniform treatment strategy has been employed, this analysis was performed irrespective of the individual therapy. For evaluating prognosis among the five mentioned primary risk patterns, the number of deaths and survivors and the mean time of survival or follow-up have been determined. As a prognostic index, the statistics were computed on the number of deaths divided by total number of months of follow-up expressed in deaths/1000 patient months. Based on these criteria, 612 patients were evaluated. The death rate of this total group was 29.5. Primary clinial patterns associated with death rates

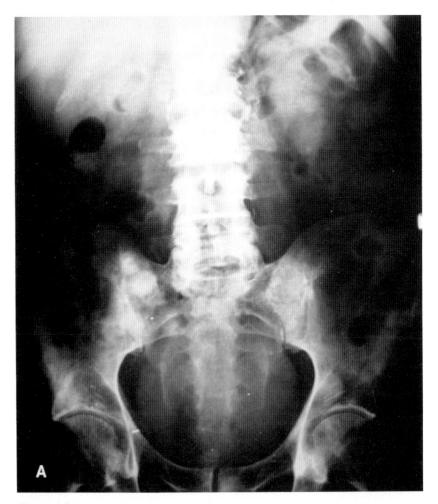

Figure 3.8 *A*, Example of sclerotic restitution of osseous bone lesions under treatment; 72-year-old patient with stage $T_3N_3M_1$ poorly differentiated carcinoma with bone pain. At X-ray multiple osseous metastases are seen at pelvic girdle.

significantly poorer than the total group are illustrated on the lefthand side, those patterns with death rates insignificantly differing from the total group are on the righthand side of Figure 3.10. Of the eight patterns with death rates significantly higher than the total group, the following five were investigated against each other, since some of these factors could also be present coincidentally:

1. Upper tract dilatation
2. Elevated serum acid phosphatase
3. Age greater than 70 years at diagnosis
4. Multiple bone metastases
5. Duration of symptoms less than 3 months at diagnosis.

In Table 3.5, these five primary patterns have been correlated to each other, and the number of patients per group with only one of these

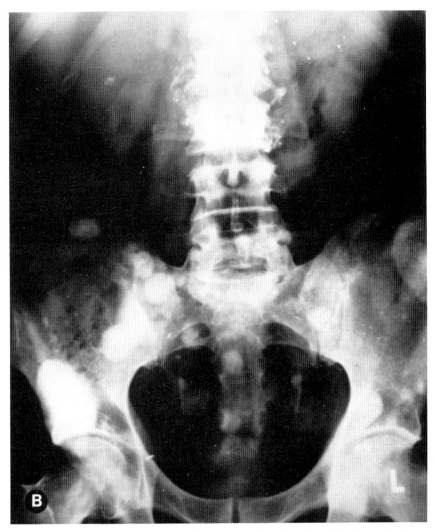

Figure 3.8 *B*, After orchiectomy plus estramustine phosphate (450 mg IV/day for 7 days, oral continuation thereafter) there is improvement of bone pain within 4–6 days. Osseous metastases with sclerotic changes representing the healing process are seen. Due to the calcification of the lesions under treatment they now appear much more prominent at x-ray (here keyed as "*snow ball-like appearance.*" The regression of bone metastases was reconfirmed histologically in punch biopsy material taken from the right iliac crest by Jamshidi needle. The patient is alive and asymptomatic 6 years after first diagnosis.

primary patterns has been determined. Furthermore, already established risk factors, such as loco-regional advanced stages C and D_1 (T_{3-4}, N_{1-2} M_0; UICC) and poor grade of differentiation (G_{3+4}) were also related to the primary patterns.

In summarizing the cumulative data given in Table 3.5, the following conclusions can be drawn:

    1. *Upper tract dilatation per se* cannot be considered as a risk factor.

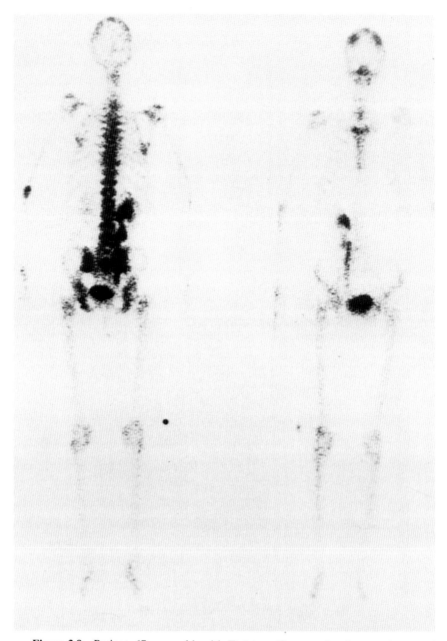

Figure 3.9 Patient, 67 years old, with T_3 (stage C) prostatic adenocarcinoma of right prostatic lobe. At isotope scan, there is no evidence of osseous metastases, but marked upper tract dilatation of the right side is seen with ectasia of the ureter and renal pelvis. In our experience a follow-up IVP often is unnecessary.

Almost one-third of patients have coincident multiple osseous metastases and are more than 70 years old at diagnosis, both factors related with a significantly elevated death rate (Fig. 3.10). Only three patients in this group had this primary pattern as a single unfavorable sign. Furthermore,

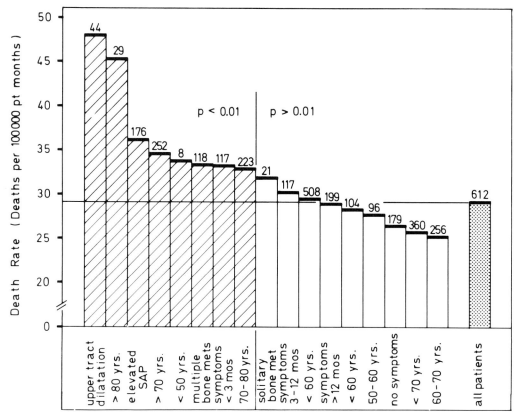

Figure 3.10 Death rate computed as number of deaths divided by total patients' months of follow-up expressed as death per 1,000 patient months for the clinical features of: upper tract dilatation, elevated serum acid phosphatase (SAP), patients' age at diagnosis, osseous metastases, and duration of symptoms in 612 evaluable patients. The far most right-hand column represents the death rate for the entire group. The clinical patterns are divided by whether they are significantly superior or insignificantly different in their death rate when compared to the death rate of the entire group.

a significantly higher number of patients with this clinical sign have a locally advanced tumor stage and grade, presumably as cause of upper tract dilatation.

2. An *elevated serum acid phosphatase per se* cannot be considered as a risk factor. Every second patient had coincident multiple bone metastases, as the presumable underlining condition and/or was more than 70 years of age. Only every seventh patient in this group had this primary pattern as single factor associated with increased death rate. Poor local tumor stage or grade seems unrelated to an elevated serum acid phosphatase; the rates for both are comparable with those of the total group.

3. Patient's *age of more than 70 years* at diagnosis, a primary pattern associated with the death rate of 34.9 as compared to 29.5 of the entire group (Fig. 3.10), seems for itself to be a factor of poor risk alone, since every second patient in this group presented with this primary pattern

Table 3.5
Evaluation of Primary Pattern (Fig. 3.10) versus Secondary Pattern in Relation to Tumor Stage and Grade as Additional Factors

Primary Pattern		Secondary Pattern					Pts. with Prim. Pattern Only		Additional Factors	
		Upper Tract Dilatation	Elevated SAP	Older than 70 yr of Age	Multiple Bone Metastases	Duration of Symptoms <3 mo	n	%	Local Stage $T_{3+4}(C+D_1)$ (69.2%)[a]	Grade of Diff. G_{3+4} (47.4%)[a]
Upper tract dilatation	n	44	8	15	13	11	3	6.8	36	37
	%	100	18.2	34.1	29.5	25			81.8	84.1
Elevated SAP	n	20	176	77	98	50	24	13.6	108	89
	%	11.4	100	43.7	55.7	28.4			61.4	50.6
Older than 70 yr of age	n	11	76	252	57	51	89	50.6	192	99
	%	4.4	30.2	100	22.6	20.2			76.2	39.3
Multiple bone metastases	n	6	84	19	118	35	39	33.1	103	60
	%	5.1	71.2	16.1	100	29.7			87.3	50.8
Duration of symptoms <3 mo	n	10	43	32	35	117	16	13.7	91	47
	%	8.5	36.8	27.3	29.9	100			77.8	40.2

[a] Percent of total group (n = 612).

only. However, 22.6% of these patients also had multiple bone metastases, and 32% had elevated serum acid phosphatase. Unexpectedly, this group of patients was not associated with an overproportional rate of advanced local tumor stages or poor grade of differentiation.

4. *Multiple bone metastases*, in contrast to solitary lesions, are, in itself, a sign of poor prognosis. One-third of all patients in this group had this primary pattern alone, two-thirds presented coincidentally with elevated serum acid phosphatase, and almost every third patient reported a short duration of symptoms of less than 3 months. A significantly increased number of patients also had a locally far advanced tumor lesion. These results are consistent with the data given in Table 3.2 (page 35).

5. A short *duration of symptoms of less than 3 months* can, in itself, not be considered as a factor of poor risk, although the death rate of this group significantly exceeds that of the entire tumor population (Fig. 3.10). Nearly every third patient had coincident multiple bone metastases, with elevated serum acid phosphatase in 36.8% of cases. Local tumor stage or grade were not discriminating factors with respect to the short duration of symptoms.

In conclusion, multiple osseous metastases is the predominant risk factor among the parameters studied. Age over 70 years at diagnosis, elevated serum acid phosphatase in the absence of detectable metastases, and a locally far advanced stage with upper tract dilatation as co-factors negatively affect prognosis in terms of the evaluable death rate.

After completion of this study, we were able to select 86 of 118 patients with multiple bone metastases of which prospectively followed data on *bone pain* were available. Twenty-seven patients (31.4%) suffered from metastatic bone pain; the death rate of 49.2 exceeded those of the primary pattern investigated (Fig. 3.10). From the remainder, 59 patients without initial bone pain, including 19 (32.2%) without any primary treatment, had a death rate of 30.8, which does not differ significantly from the entire original group of patients (Fig. 3.10). Thus, patients initially presenting with multiple osseous metastases *and* bone pain experience a poor course of their disease.

It seems logical to offer prompt contrasexual means possibly combined at the onset with chemotherapy to those patients who present with factors of poor risk when first diagnosed.

CLOSING REMARKS

In light of innovations in the primary work-up, management, and re-evaluation during and after treatment of prostatic carcinoma, the practicing urologist is highly dependent on the experience of institutions in which the different issues of this cancer can be evaluated in a large number of patients. Problems concerning the technical and statistical requirements, and the organization of personnel for this responsibility are a challenge for every large urological department. Retrospective analyses or therapeutic trials can be enjoyable for the co-ordinator but are usually boring for the physicians completing these forms. Significant innovations by a single scientist are usually supported by an institution. In our rather small urological community any urological institution should make every effort to supply all of us with new data capable of improving the patient's outcome. This challenge is an international one, and the communication can never be unilateral.

Despite geographic separations, our "urological language" should be the same, and the Editors of this Volume hope that it will contribute to this task.

REFERENCES

1. Barzell, W., Bean, M. A., Hilaris, B. S., and Whitmore, W. F., Jr. Prostatic adenocarcinoma: relationship of grade and local extent to the pattern of metastases. *J. Urol. 118:* 278, 1977.
2. Zincke, H., Fleming, T. R., Furlow, W. L., Myers, R. P., and Utz, D. C. Radical retropubic prostatectomy and pelvic lymphadenectomy for high-stage cancer of the prostate. *Cancer 47:* 1901, 1981.
3. Cantrell, B. B., de Klerk, D. P., Eggleston, J. C., Boitnott, J. K., and Walsh, P. C. Pathological factors that influence prognosis in stage A prostatic cancer: the influence of extent versus grade, *J. Urol. 125:* 516, 1981.
4. Kiesling, V., Jr., and Watson, R. A. A closer look at serum prostatic acid phosphatase as screening test. *Urology 16:* 242, 1980.
5. Jacobi, G. H., Ehrenthal, W., Engelmann, U., Grimm, D., Riedmiller, H., Prellwitz, W., and Hohenfellner, R. Immunological determination of serum acid phosphatase in patients with prostate cancer. II. Serum studies with the enzyme-immunoassay ENZYGNOST-PAP. *Akt. Urol. 12:* 283, 1981.
6. Hovsepian, J. A., Byar, D. P., and The Veterans Administration Cooperative Urological Research Group. Carcinoma of prostate, correlation between radiologic quantitation of metastases and patient survival. *Urology 6:* 11, 1975.
7. *UICC: TNM Classification of Malignant Tumors,* 3rd Ed. Springer, Berlin, 1978.
8. Murphy, G. P., Gaeta, J. F., Pickren, J., and Wajsman, Z. Current status of classification and staging of prostatic cancer. *Cancer 45:* 1889, 1980.
9. Smith, P. H. Medical management of prostatic cancer. *Eur. Urol. 6:* 65, 1980.
10. Bouffioux, Chr. Cancer de la prostate. *Acta Urol. Belg. 47:* 201, 1979.
11. Hudson, P. B., Finkle, A. L., Hopkins, J. A., Sproul, E. E., and Stout, A. P. Prostatic cancer. XI. Early prostatic cancer diagnosed by arbitrary open perineal biopsy among 300 unselected patients. *Cancer 7:* 690, 1954.
12. Müller, H.-A., Ackermann, R., and Frohmüller, H. G. W. The value of perineal punch biopsy in estimating the histological grade of carcinoma of the prostate. *Prostate 1:* 303, 1980.
13. Kastendieck, H. Morphologie des Prostatacarcinoms in Stanzbiopsien und totalen Prostatektomien. *Pathologe 2:* 31, 1980.
14. Kurth, K. H., Altwein, J. E., Skoluda, D., and Hohenfellner, R. Follow-up of irradiated prostatic carcinoma by aspiration biopsy. *J. Urol. 117:* 615, 1977.
15. Jacobi, G. H., Riedmiller, H., and Hohenfellner, R. Lokale Hochvoltbestrahlung des Prostatakarzinoms: Analyse von 214 Fällen. *Verh. Ber. Dtsch. Ges. Urol.* Springer, Berlin, 1981, pp. 185–187.
16. Stone, A. R., Hargreave, T. B., and Chisholm, G. D. The diagnosis of oestrogen escape and the role of secondary orchiectomy in prostatic cancer. *Br. J. Urol. 52:* 535, 1980.
17. Jacobi, G. H., and Hohenfellner, R. Palliativtherapie des Prostatakarzinoms durch kontrasexuelle Massnahmen und Zytostatika. *Therapiewoche 31:* 7713, 1981.
18. Leistenschneider, W., and Nagel, R. Zytologisches Regressions—Grading und seine prognostische Bedeutung beim konservativ behandelten Prostatakarzinom. *Akt. Urol. 11:* 263, 1980.

19. Wahner, H. W., Maher, H. T., Hattery, R. R.: Prostatakarzinom: Diagnose von Harnabflußstörungen mit Hilfe der Knochenszintigraphie. *Akt. Urol. 8:* 261, 1977.
20. Jacobi, G. H., Loebnau, M., and Hahn, K. Mainzer Prostatakarzinom-Kartei: IV. Quantitative Beurteilung des Ganzkörper-Skelettszintigramms. (Unpublished observation)
21. Berry, W. E., Laszlo, J., Cox E., Walker, A., and Paulson, D. Prognostic factors in metastatic and hormonally unresponsive carcinoma of the prostate. *Cancer 44:* 763, 1979.
22. Kvols, L. K., Eagan, R. T., and Myers, R. P. Evaluation of melphalan. *Cancer Treat. Rep. 61:* 311, 1977.
23. Jacobi, G. H., Seifert, U., Riedmiller, H., and Hohenfellner, R. Mainzer Prostatakarzinom-Kartei: III. Analyse Klinischer Risikofaktoren. (Unpublished observation)
24. Frohmüller, H. G. W., Ackermann, R., Altwein, J. E., Bartsch, G., and Jacobi, G. H. Kontroverse Aspekte der endokrinen Therapie des fortgeschrittenen Prostata-Carcinoms. *Verh. Ber. Dtsch. Ges. Urol.,* Springer, Berlin, 1981, pp. 162–164.

4

Experience with the German Annual Preventive Checkup Examination

P. Faul, M.D.

Inspired by the efforts of C. E. Alken, preventive cancer checkups were introduced in Germany in 1971 and are now supported and financed by the state insurance programs.[1]

All men 45 years and older have the right to a free checkup every year. The aim of the checkup primarily is the early diagnosis of prostatic carcinoma, but also of other diseases of the urogenital-anal region, as well as the initiation of an appropriate therapy, preferably at an early stage of the disease.

The preventive checkup for men currently includes a detailed history-taking, clinical examination of the outer genitals, rectum, regional lymph nodes and skin, rectal palpation of the prostate and ampulla recti for the detection of anorectal malignancies, a screening test for blood in the stool, and screening for arterial hypertension.

Herein I would like to discuss the benefits and liabilities of the preventive examination in relation to prostatic carcinoma.

AIMS OF THE PREVENTIVE EXAMINATION

The demand for a routine preventive cancer checkup is based on the oncological principle that all diseases have a better chance of cure if they are detected and thus treated at an early stage. In addition, the principle also applies that every carcinoma has a clinically silent stage in which it can be cured if discovered incidentally.

For prostatic carcinoma it can be said that, as a rule, by the time a patient visits a doctor because of suspicious complaints, the local cancer is often far advanced or metastases are already present. Schwartz *et al.*[2] therefore describe the early diagnosis not as a goal in itself, but as a means of implementing early therapy.

With the aid of appropriate follow-up, the aim is to prevent personal suffering, invalidity, and premature death. Prophylactic treatment may even be possible in the early stages of the disease, before the patient has reached the age at which the morbidity and mortality of prostatic carcinoma is known to increase: the age at diagnosis therefore plays a relatively significant role.

UNDERLYING EPIDEMIOLOGICAL FACTORS

Factors underlying the need for establishing programs for the early detection of prostate cancer are:

1. Prostatic carcinoma represents about 8% of all cancer diseases in the male and almost every third malignant tumor of the male urogenital tract.[3]
2. Both in Germany and in the United States, prostatic carcinoma is the third most common cancer after carcinoma of the respiratory and digestive organs.[4, 5]
3. According to the Federal Bureau of Statistics in the Federal Republic of Germany, about 6,000 deaths per year attributed to prostatic cancer were registered in 1972 and 1973 (9.5% of all cancer deaths); this figure has increased to 7,300 per year thereafter.[6] According to the most recent death statistics, malignancies of the lung, gastrointestinal tract, and prostate account for about two-thirds of all male cancer deaths, prostatic cancer ranging third with 10.3% (Fig. 4.1).
4. In the U.S.A., 19,000 deaths due to prostatic cancer are reported each year,[4] and the prostate is the second most common site of cancer.[5] Further information on the world-wide differences in prostate cancer epidemiology, *i.e.* morbidity, mortality, and the variations in statistical sources of epidemiological data are outlined in Chapter 2.
5. In the Federal Republic of Germany, the death rate for prostatic carcinoma in men under 45 years of age is reported to be 0.1%, while for men under 60 years, it is 3.3% per year.[6] The highest prostatic carcinoma mortality is seen in the 8th decade and shows a clearly rising tendency after the age of 60.

These figures document the dire need for early tumor recognition measures.

PROS AND CONS OF THE MALE PREVENTIVE CHECKUP

Despite these impressive figures—which underline the significance of prostatic carcinoma disease—the relevance of the male preventive checkup has recently been the subject of critical debate in Germany.[7] Wide press publicity has triggered off uncertainty among the general public and even among members of the medical profession.

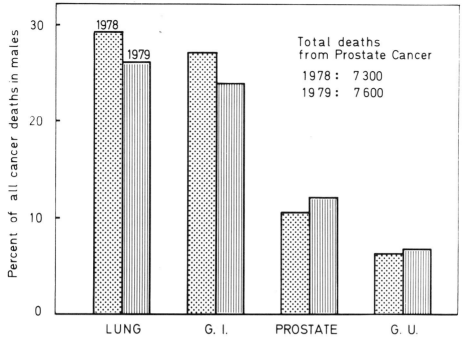

Figure 4.1 Death rate for prostate cancer in the Federal Republic of Germany (death certificates) in 1978 and 1979 in comparison to other, and in relation to all male cancer deaths. Overall cancer deaths (male and female) in 1978 were 155,062 or 21.4% of all deaths, in 1979 about 154,600 or 21.7%, respectively. While relative death rates for lung and G.I. malignancies showed a decrease of 2.4 or 3.0%, respectively, for prostate cancer, an increase of 1.9% was calculated for 1979. (Data taken from the official death statistics of the Federal Bureau of Statistics, Federal Republic of Germany, 1980)

The critics' central objections are to the rectal examination and in particular to the biopsy, *i.e.* their demand is for the abolition of the only dependable method of diagnosing prostatic carcinoma currently available.[3, 8] They also mention the cost *versus* benefit relationship and their general skepticism of the diagnostic measures in use, such as the biopsy, even in cases of suspicious palpatory findings.

One must indeed admit that the preventive checkup might have some weak points: (1) rectal palpation as a routine screening method; (2) the lack of sensitivity of all biochemical serum markers to detect early prostate cancer; (3) the lack of practicability of bringing the entire male population over 45 years of age, in a country with 66 million people, to a preventive checkup (cost *versus* benefit relation); (4) motivation of the male population to undergo such a checkup in an asymptomatic, healthy state.

PROSTATIC GROWTH ITSELF AS A DILEMMA

Rectal palpation has a sensitivity of 44 to 76% and a specificity of 69 to 81%.[9] These figures, however, largely depend upon the skill of the investigator.

In our own material consisting of 350 patients with a suspicious palpation finding, biopsy confirmed prostatic carcinoma in only 26%, while in 34.3%, chronic prostatitis was discovered by histological or cytological means.[10]

In the U.S.A., investigators promoting arbitrary *open* biopsy even provocatively "reject, then, in its entirety, the concept that prostate cancer detection by rectal palpation is adequate for discovery of the disease—or even the suspicion that it exists . . . ."[11] Suspicion of carcinoma on the basis of rectal palpation, particularly in the early clinical stages of the disease, is highly uncertain. Depending on the source quoted, from 14 to 45% of the male population over 50 have latent carcinoma—and these are not palpable (see Chapter 2). In the material of the *German Prostate Cancer Registry* (also see Chapter 6), Dhom[8] found latent prostatic carcinoma in 36.4% of all men older than 45 years of age. The impression that only 5 to 10% of all latent tumors will become manifest life-threatening carcinoma[12, 13] is a matter of speculation. Hudson and co-workers[11] correctly stated that, "many of the prostatic cancers of 1953 would have been 'occult cancer at autopsy' in 1933."

If the postoperative staging categories are used, life expectancy for those subjected to a radical operation in stages pT_{0-1} (stages A and B_1 according to the American system) is virtually identical with that of an age-adjusted cohort of the general male population. Possible advantages can be expected, particularly for men under 70 years of age with stage T_2 tumors in whom lesions not exclusively well-differentiated are treated. This limited target group for a definitively curative radical operation, *i.e.* all grades of differentiation except for the exclusively highly differentiated ones (nodule limited by the organ capsule), and the moderate diagnostic accuracy of this group permit only limited hopes for the value of an early recognition program.

SENSITIVE SERUM MARKERS AS A LIMITATION

It was enthusiastically expected in recent years that with the development of specific and sensitive radioimmunological methods of phosphatase determination a powerful tool for the early discrimination between malignant and benign prostatic enlargement and localized and early metastasizing prostatic cancer would become available (see Chapter 8). However, Foti and co-workers[14] found elevated RIA phosphatases in up to 14% of cases with BPH, in 35 to 50% of patients with stage A, and, in up to 18% an elevation of this marker even in patients after prostatectomy. Thus, serum phosphatases determined by radioimmunoassay (and all other biochemical tests available today) do not fulfill the requirements of a screening method in a preventive checkup program. For further information on the issue of phosphatase determination, see Chapter 8.

THE PROBLEM OF COST *VERSUS* BENEFIT RELATION

According to Schwartz,[15] as well as Barker and Rose,[16] determination of the value of preventive programs is difficult in chronic diseases, such as malignant growths, which usually become manifest at a quite advanced age. The diagnostic characteristics of the test are described by such terms as sensitivity, specificity, and prediction, whereby the value of early therapy is primarily oriented to mortality data.

The number of general practitioners, surgeons and internists currently in practice would probably be in the position to handle the rectal examination of all 9 million men over 45 years of age living in the Federal Republic of Germany. However, it seems hypothetical to suppose that the number of biopsies necessary for the verification of suspicious palpation findings could be managed by the 1,200 practicing urologists in Germany to date. According to Melchior,[17] this would only be possible after all the urologists in training have completed their training.

However, according to Oeser and Rauch,[18] only one prostatic carcinoma was found in 1000 preventive checkups; Biersack et al.[19] discovered 20 in 1000 (2%). Discussion of the value of the checkup, however, must also consider the detection of a series of other diseases, as pointed out by Sommerhoff (in reference 19) and depicted in Table 4.1.

DOES THE BIOPSY OF A CANCEROUS PROSTATE PROMOTE TUMOR SPREAD?

The claim by Krokowski[7] that prostate biopsy bears the danger of provoking tumor seeding or even metastases has not yet been scientifically substantiated.[20-22] In our own material of more then 1,000 transrectal fine needle aspiration biopsies, not one instance of local tumor seeding was confirmed. In addition, Swedish investigators who have had the most

Table 4.1
Pathologic Findings of 1000 Preventive Checkup Examinations in Males Over 45 Years of Age[a]

Pathological Finding	No. (%)
High blood pressure	252 (25.2%)
Breast cancer	1 (0.1%)
Inguinal hernia	8 (0.8%)
Pathological genital findings Phimosis (2), balanitis (1) Induratio penis plastica (1) Meatal stenosis (1) Epididymitis (2), varicocele (1) Urethral stricture (1) Spermatocele (6), hydrocele (3)	18 (1.8%)
Pathological urinalysis Infection (14), Tbc (2) Urinary calculi (5) G.U. tumors (3)	24 (2.4%)
Pathological rectal findings Anal fissure and hemorrhoids (20) Prostatitis (18) Benign prostatic hyperplasia (121) Prostatic carcinoma (20)	179 (17.9%)

[a]M. Sommerhoff, Bonn, 1979. From H. J. Biersack et al.[19]

extensive experience with this technique (see Chapter 5) impressively showed that tumor cell seeding did not occur after transrectal fine needle biopsy.[21, 22]

The claim made by several critics that even routine rectal palpation could be responsible for some seeding of tumor cells into the blood circulation with subsequent widespread cancer disease is nothing but an unproven speculation. Other forms of prostatic massage, such as a hard stool or bicycle riding, would then probably have the same effect.

CURRENT RESULTS OF THE CHECKUP PROGRAM IN THE FEDERAL REPUBLIC OF GERMANY

Of the preventive checkups performed in Germany from 1972 to 1976, 77.9% were performed by general practitioners and internists, 14.6% by urologists, 2.5% by general surgeons, and 1.4% by dermatologists (dermatology traditionally covers andrology in Germany).

As urology was not, for a long time, one of the specialties included in the German Medical Board Examination, and the rectal examination did not belong to the standard general medical checkup, a certain margin of error, *i.e.* a certain number of false negative diagnoses by the general practitioners and internists must be expected. Participation by the urologists is 100%, whereby one urologist does about 300 checkups each year.[6]

Participation in the preventive program by the male population over 45 years of age is currently still not more than 20% of a total of almost 9 million entitled to it. This figure, however, includes a certain number of male individuals whose intent to participate in the checkup program is not *prevention* but the clarification of urogenital *complaints.* These patients have usually not taken advantage of the program on an annual basis. The aim of the program is that each male undergo the checkup annually, even if he feels asymptomatic. In Austria this preventive measure is therefore more correctly called a "checkup of the healthy."

The highest rate of participation is found among men in the 48 to 52-year age group; of those, about every fourth entitled to the test took part in it. With increasing age, participation falls, resulting in an inverse proportion between participation and the age-dependent prostatic cancer risk.

Analysis of the urological findings in the period 1972 to 1976 revealed only a low percentage of significant findings in the entire preventive checkup program, which could tend to question its effectiveness.

The first analysis performed by the BMKV, a federal association of the Social Security Services in Germany, in 1976, *i.e.* 5 years after introduction of the checkup program, revealed only 1.7% suspicious prostatic findings and 2.05% indications of occult diseases of the kidney, urinary collecting system, rectum, and skin; this is a total of 3.75% significant findings (Fig. 4.2). Numerically there were 22,585 suspicious prostatic cases, 3,125 pathological findings of the outer genitalia, 4,720 pathological rectal processes, and 17,344 pathological urinalyses (Fig. 4.3). Unfortunately, data on the histological verification of these findings are not generally

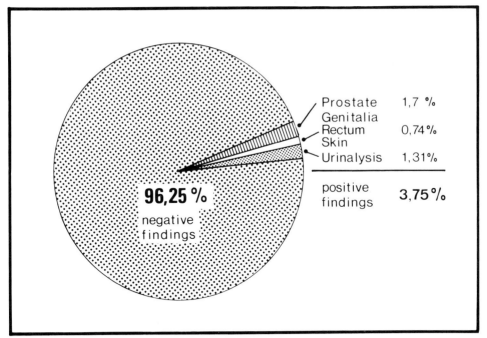

Figure 4.2 Rates of significant pathological findings of 1,328,863 annual preventive checkup examinations between 1972 and 1976. Significant findings were encountered in 49,626 patients (3.75%). (Data taken from the Federal Association of the Social Security Services (BMKV), Cologne, Federal Republic of Germany.[6])

available, since a centralized evaluation is not included within this checkup.

At the discretion of the urologist, however, a certain rate of cases are sent to the *German Prostatic Cancer Registry*. According to Dhom, 87% of 4,305 carcinomas detected by the preventive checkup were less than highly differentiated or pluriform, *i.e.* they had a high biological activity, while only 13% were highly differentiated, *i.e.* they displayed a relatively low malignancy (Chapter 6).

Furthermore, of a group of approximately 600,000 suspicious cases of prostate cancer investigated within 4 years, one-sixth were positively confirmed by biopsy. Further information on the data bank of the *German Prostate Cancer Registry* is outlined in Chapter 6.

According to the *Central Institute of the Social Security Service* in Germany, a preventive checkup was performed on 1.5 million men in 1978. Of these, an isolated induration of the prostate was palpated in 0.98% (14,976 cases) and a totally indurated prostate in 0.41% (6,332 cases). These figures demonstrate, in conjunction with Figure 4.3, that in 1978 alone an almost equal number of cases with a tentative prostatic carcinoma diagnosis was detected as in the entire time interval of 1972 to 1976, *i.e.* the initial period of the checkup program.

From the 1977 data, a total of 15,011 cases suspected of prostate cancer were centrally recorded.[2] In 13.4% the diagnosis of prostatic carcinoma

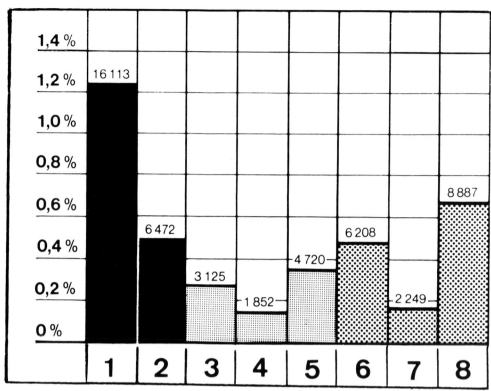

Figure 4.3 Differentiation of all pathological findings obtained from 49,626 male patients by the annual preventive checkup examination between 1972 and 1976 in the Federal Republic of Germany. (Data taken from BMKV, Cologne, Germany.[6]) *1*, isolated prostatic induration; *2*, total prostatic induration; *3*, outer genitalia; *4*, skin; *5*, rectum; *6*, proteinuria; *7*, glucosuria; *8*, hematuria (micro-).

was reconfirmed histologically (Fig. 4.4). This, however, does not imply that the rest of the palpatory findings were tumor-negative; these prostates were either not biopsied or the results were not forwarded to the Central Institute.

A decisive advantage of the preventive checkup examination and the intensive diagnosis of a disease is that an increased number of cases are detected. In our own material the result was that the annual rate of cases treated for prostatic carcinoma showed a sharp increase after the introduction of the transrectal fine needle biopsy for cytological confirmation of the tumor. During 1968 and 1969, only 3.4 patients were hospitalized each month for treatment, while in 1970 and 1971 this figure had increased to an average of nine patients per month.[23] This represents, on an annual basis, an increase in the number of patients with prostatic carcinoma of 60%, and can be explained by the fact that every even minimally suspicious palpatory finding was checked by biopsy.

In the *German Prostate Cancer Registry* (Homburg/Saar), the number of newly diagnosed prostatic cancer cases detected annually—and consequently the incidence rate—also more than doubled between 1970 and 1976.[24] This, however, does not imply a nationwide doubling of the

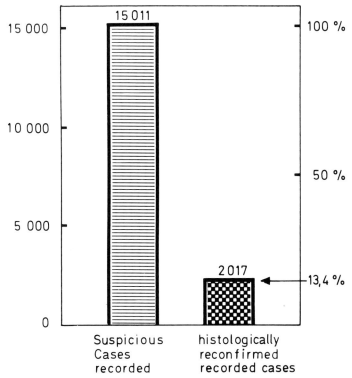

Figure 4.4 Results of the annual preventive checkup for prostate cancer in Germany for 1977; neither the 13.4% histological reconfirmations of the entire number of suspected cases of prostate cancer reflects the true rate of cancer cases detected by the checkup program, nor does the absolute number of 2,017 reflect the true number of prostate cases newly diagnosed in 1977 in Germany. (Drawn according to data from F. W. Schwartz *et al.*[2])

incidence. Nevertheless, an increase in the number of younger patients or earlier stages of the disease was not registered, a criticism of the checkup raised by its opponents.[7] One would expect that with the early detection of prostatic carcinoma the age of the individuals in whom the tumor is found by routine examination would decrease, but 8 years after initiation of the program, this seems not yet to be the case. In 1978, a total of 1,951 histologically confirmed prostatic carcinomas were recorded and the age distribution, presented in Figure 4.5, does not seem significantly different from data obtained in earlier years in Germany or elsewhere.

The preventive checkup is not able to detect the only true early form of prostatic cancer, namely latent carcinoma. A tentative diagnosis is first possible in stage T_1, *i.e.* early stages B according to the American Staging system.

Biersack *et al.*[19] however, report that osseous metastases are already present in 7.1% of the patients in this stage; in stage T_3, this rate increases to 19.3%. Of 121 patients 55 years old and younger reported by Dhom and Kopper,[24] 10% had skeletal metastases at the time of first diagnosis. Reduction of the number of prostatic carcinoma already metastasized at the time of diagnosis is one purpose of the preventive checkup.

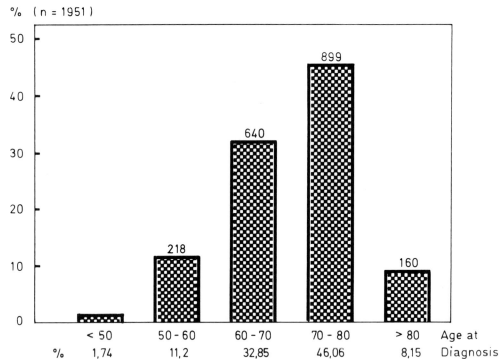

Figure 4.5 Age distribution of 1,951 cases of prostate cancer recorded in Germany in 1978 in conjunction with the annual preventive checkup. (Unpublished data taken from the BMKV, Cologne, Germany.)

We could show on the basis of 496 patients with prostatic carcinoma who underwent estrogen treatment, that the biological activity of the growth is largely dependent on the grade of differentiation, and this in turn influences the clinical stage.[25] While, however, the histological grade of differentiation of a clinically manifest carcinoma is not basically different from that of latent carcinoma, they vary considerably in the percentile distribution of the various grades.

The main task of the preventive checkup is the early recognition of rapidly proliferating less differentiated carcinoma. Without timely treatment, these tumor types lead to an agonizing, fatal disease.

We share Dhom and Kopper's opinion[24] that, on the basis of careful consideration of the clinical stage and morphological, *i.e.* histological or cytological grading, we are today able to make a usually reliable evaluation of the prognostic course of a given prostatic carcinoma. This in turn makes possible the decision not to treat certain types of prostatic carcinoma, but rather to subject such a patient to careful controls, or "watchful waiting."

In addition to clinical stage and morphological grading, the patient's age—and with that his life expectancy—must always be taken into consideration. As the latter is today, as a rule, so high, slowly proliferating tumors with a high degree of differentiation may still become life threatening after years. To label various prostatic malignancies as "good" or "bad" cancers, at least on the basis of one or two biopsies, is dangerous.

While Krokowski[7] advocates that the only target group which can be considered for the preventive checkup is the stage B (T_{1-2}) prostatic carcinoma, and that only for this group can a benefit from the checkup be expected, we disagree. Even for a locally advanced tumor, *i.e.* stage T_{3-4} (C) without metastases in a 70-year-old man, the checkup can have important consequences. If we are dealing with a primarily well or moderately well differentiated tumor without detectable metastases and symptoms of the local carcinoma, then contrasexual treatment with estrogens will not necessarily be initiated. This elderly patient could possibly be more endangered by such treatment than by the biologically relatively inactive prostatic carcinoma.

At the present time it is not possible to make a definitive statement whether the checkup has altered the fateful outcome of the disease by early detection of the tumor, or whether survival has improved. This is partly due to the fact that only 20% of the male population eligible for the checkup has actually taken part in it. A statistically reliable success of the cancer checkup is therefore not yet possible.[24] In judging the effectiveness of the examination, however, it is necessary to bear in mind the fate of each individual.

To achieve better participation in the preventive checkup program, the efforts at providing the public with intelligent information must not cease so that as many potential patients as possible will obtain knowledge of the favorable chances of tumor cure in the early stages. Only in this manner can the "fear of the feared diagnosis" be reduced and trust in the medically recommended measure inspired.

What today in the majority of developed countries is possible (and effective) in checkup programs during pregnancy, in early childhood, in pedodontics, or for early detection of genital cancer of the female should also be possible for prostate cancer. Everything takes time and patience.

REFERENCES

1. Alken, C. E. Krebsvorsorge beim Mann. *Dtsch. Ärztebl. 29:* 2233, 1970.
2. Schwartz, F. W., Holstein, H., and Brecht, J. G. *Öff. Gesundheitswes. 41:* 347, 1979.
3. Faul, P. Die Vorsorgeuntersuchung beim Mann. *Z. Allg. Med. 7:* 365, 1976.
4. Kirchheim, D. Das Prostatakarzinom. *Dtsch. Ärztebl. 13:* 807, 1980.
5. Klein, L. A. Prostatic carcinoma. *N. Engl. J. Med. 300:* 824, 1979.
6. Knipper, W. Praktische Erfahrungen mit der Vorsorgeuntersuchung in der Urologie. *Urologe B 19:* 49, 1979.
7. Krokowski, E. Was leistet die Prostatakrebsvorsorge? *Therapiewoche 28:* 9893, 1978.
8. Dhom, G. Das Prostatakarzinom und die Bedeutung seiner Früherkennung. *Med. Unserer Zeit 2:* 134, 1978.
9. Eschenbach, A. C., and Johanson, D. E. Adenocarcinoma of the prostate. *Compr. Ther. 4:* 18, 1978.
10. Faul, P., and Schmiedt, E. Cytologic aspects of diseases of the prostate. *Int. Urol. Nephrol. 5:* 297, 1973.
11. Hudson, P. B., Finkle, A. L., Hopkins, J. A., Sproul, E. E., and Stout, A. P. Prostatic cancer. XI. Early prostatic cancer diagnosed by arbitrary open perineal biopsy among 300 unselected patients. *Cancer 7:* 690, 1954.
12. Basset, M. L., and Goulston, K. J. Colorectal cancer: the challenge of early detection. *Med. J. Aust. 1(9):* 489, 1978.
13. Lent, V., and Meyer, M. Zur Treffsicherheit der rektalen Palpation bei der Früherkennung des Prostatakrebses. *Dtsch. Med. Wochenschr. 103:* 335, 1978.

14. Foti, A. G., Cooper, J. F., Herschmann, H., and Halvaez, R. R. Detection of prostatic cancer by solid-phase radioimmunoassay of serum prostatic acid phosphatase. *N. Engl. J. Med. 297:* 1357, 1977.
15. Schwartz, F. W. Krebsfrüherkennung in der gesetzlichen Krankenversicherung. German Cancer Congress, March 1980.
16. Barker, J. P., and Rose, G. *Epidemiology in Medical Practice.* Churchill & Livingstone, Edinburgh, 1976.
17. Melchior, H. J. Neue Aspeket der Krebsbekämpfung. Symposium, Kassel, Germany, 1978.
18. Oeser, H., and Rauch, K. Die Effektivität einer präventiven Krebsbekämpfung. *Dtsch. Med. Wochenschr. 94:* 2015, 1969.
19. Biersack, H. J., Wegener, G., Distelmaier, W., and Krause, U. Bedeutung der Vorsorgeuntersuchung beim Prostatakarzinom. *Dtsch. Ärztebl. 42:* 2758, 1979.
20. Hermanek, P., and Klosterhalfen, H. Fernmetastasierung durch Biopsie und Operation? *Urologe A 18:* 49, 1979.
21. Engzel, U., Esposti, P. L., Rubio, C., Sigurdson, A., and Zajicek, J. Investigation of tumor spread in connection with aspiration biopsy. *Acta Radiol. [Ther.]* (Stockh.) *10:* 385, 1971.
22. Zajicek, J. Die transrektale Aspirationsbiopsie der Prostata. Diagnostik und Therapie des Prostatakarzinoms. *Beitr. Urol.* 1: 30, 1979.
23. Faul, P. Die klinische Bedeutung der Prostatazytologie. *Münch. Med. Wochenschr. 116:* 15, 1974.
24. Dhom, G., and Kopper, B. Probleme der Früherkennung des Prostatakarzinoms. German Cancer Congress, March 1980.
25. Faul, P., Schmiedt, E., and Kern, P. Die prognostische Bedeutung des zytologischen Differenzierungsgrades beim östrogenbehandelten Prostatacarcinom. *Urologe A 17:* 377, 1978.

Editorial Comment to Chapter 4

From this Chapter three main questions arise: *First*, are the operatives for screening given by Miller (1981), *i.e.*–the cancer screened for being an important cause of cancer mortality or morbidity; the screening test being of sufficient sensitivity and specificity and acceptable to the patient; treatment results at tumor stages detected by the screening being superior to treatment at later stages–attributable to prostatic carcinoma?

We think that they are! Kiesling and Watson (1980) correctly state that:

> "With regard to the initial detection of prostate carcinoma, the most economical and most reliable probe for detection remains not a needle in the patient's arm, but the gloved finger of the physician engaged in a thorough rectal examination of the prostate."

Thus, if *every* male in the prevalence age group for prostate cancer undergoes a thorough annual rectal examination with biopsy control of any even trivial induration we should in the future be able to shrink part of the "tumor iceberg" illustrated in Figure 3.3 (page 36).

Second, how can we increase the number of participants in the annual prostate cancer checkup? This "advertising to increase the number of persons who request screening" has been listed by Eddy (1981) as one out of 13 factors which any screening program director should take into account.

This question is closely associated with all patients' delay in cancer conditions, a truly social phenomenon, and Moore (1973) even questions the value of an obligatory checkup. As long as 10 to 20% of all cancer patients would never consult a physician about their *symptoms*, a figure derived from 563 cancer patients including prostatic carcinoma (Hackett *et al.*, 1973), how can we ever expect the majority of elderly men to undergo some regular screening in an *asymptomatic* state.

Third, how can we control costs for such a screening program? This is not only a question of the extent and frequency of the checkup but also a question of who should perform it—the doctor or the specially trained cancer detection nurse (Miller, 1976).

We feel that accurate evaluation of all the possible findings deriving from a thorough rectal examination requires a great number of differential diagnostic considerations with the sometimes *ad hoc* decision for further diagnostic procedures. Thus, a checkup program for prostatic carcinoma should remain in the hands of urologists or trained general practitioners.

The individual value of the early detection of a prostate cancer amenable to possibly curative treatment cannot be analyzed "cold heartedly" on the basis of the relative costs of one such case per a certain number of cancer-negative checkups (Eddy, 1981). It is a divine fortune that we cannot buy health; thus, early detection and treatment are our most important goals.

G. H. J.

REFERENCES

Eddy, D. M. The economics of cancer prevention and detection: getting more for less. *Cancer 47:* 1200, 1981.

Hackett, T. P., Cassem, N. H., and Raker, J. W. Patient delay in cancer. *N. Engl. J. Med. 289:* 14, 1973.

Kiesling, V., Jr., and Watson, R. A. A closer look at serum prostatic acid phosphatase as screening test. *Urology 16:* 242, 1980.

Miller, D. G. What is early diagnosis doing. *Cancer 37:* 426, 1976.

Miller, D. G. Principles of early detection of cancer. *Cancer 47:* 1142, 1981.

Moore, F. D. Hesitation and delay as a social phenomenon. *N. Engl. J. Med. 289:* 40, 1973.

5

Aspiration Biopsy and Cytological Evaluation for Primary Diagnosis and Follow-up

P.-L. Esposti, M.D.

INTRODUCTION

Among the various methods of biopsy proposed for diagnosis of prostatic lesions, transrectal aspiration biopsy of the prostate, introduced by Franzén et al.[1] at Radiumhemmet, has won general recognition as a fast, safe, and accurate procedure. At Radiumhemmet, Karolinska Hospital, transrectal aspiration biopsy of the prostate with Franzén's instrument has become routine and more than 15,000 cytological diagnoses of prostatic aspirates have been performed in the last 20 years.[2]

The aim of the present report is to assess the value of aspiration biopsy and cytology in the diagnosis and management of prostatic carcinoma. The following aspects of the problem have been analyzed: the diagnostic accuracy of transrectal aspiration biopsy of the prostate; the incidence and types of complications after transrectal aspiration biopsy of the prostate; the prognostic significance of cytological grading of tumor differentiation in aspirates from patients with prostatic carcinoma receiving hormonal therapy; the importance of such cytological grading in monitoring choice of therapy; the possibility of improving the diagnostic accuracy in aspirates by means of quantitative cytophotometric techniques.

BIOPSY OF THE PROSTATE: GENERAL REMARKS

The anatomical site of the prostatic gland, situated behind the pubes, at the base of the bladder, anterior to the rectum and surrounding the proximal part of the urethra, has resulted in a large variety of biopsy procedures.

Some of the most frequently used methods of prostatic biopsy together with the routes of approach and the type of diagnosis intrinsic to each method are listed in Table 5.1.

Open Perineal Biopsy

A high accuracy for the method has been claimed.[3, 4] It is, however, a major surgical operation which is best left in the hands of skilled specialists, and the possibility of incontinence and impotence must be considered.

Transurethral Biopsy

This is generally considered an inadequate method. Since prostatic carcinoma is most often found in the posterior part of the gland, it would be necessary, at least in early cases, to remove by resectoscope a large portion of the gland before reaching the cancer.

Needle Biopsy (Punch Biopsy)

Various instruments in the form of needles having a cutting end have been devised in order to obtain cores of prostatic tissue for histological diagnosis. Various types of needles have been proposed: Vim-Silverman, Turkel, Veenema, and Travenol are the most common ones.

The *perineal route* and the Vim-Silverman needle have been used by Kaufman *et al.*[4] who reported an accuracy of 61% in early stages of prostatic carcinoma (stage I and II), of 72% in stage III, and of 90% in stage IV.

The *transrectal route* for thick needle biopsy of the prostate was first introduced by Astraldi.[5] The method was judged as essentially devoid of serious complications, and an accuracy of 50% in palpable nodules and of 85% in advanced cases with metastases was reported.[6]

Needle Biopsy: Aspiration Biopsy with Fine Needle

Aspiration biopsy by *perineal route* was first described by R. S. Ferguson.[7] He used an ordinary syringe with a 15-cm long, 18-gauge needle

Table 5.1
Techniques of Prostatic Biopsy

Method	Route	Type of Morphological Diagnosis
Open biopsy	Perineal	Histological
	Rectal	Histological
Endoscopic biopsy	Transurethral	Histological
Needle biopsy	Transperineal	Histological
Punch biopsy	Transrectal	Histological
Needle biopsy	Transperineal	Cytological
Aspiration biopsy	Transrectal	Cytological
Prostatic massage		Cytological

which was inserted into the prostate transperineally. In 70% of aspirations it was possible to secure tissue from the prostate for examination. The smear, consisting mainly of sheets of cells or showers of isolated cells, was examined by a pathologist who had become familiar with the particular morphology of aspirated material. However, notwithstanding the admirable work of these pioneers, the method did not win general acceptance.

Aspiration biopsy by *transrectal route* utilized in the present study will be given a more detailed description in the following section.

Cytology of Prostatic Secretions

The reports of Mulholland[8] and Papanicolaou[9] stimulated interest in the possibilities of cytodiagnosis, utilizing cells exfoliated in prostatic secretions after prostatic massage. The method enjoyed popularity during the 1950s but soon fell into discredit: apart from the fact that many physicians considered it inadvisable to submit patients to a thorough massage of a prostate suspected for malignancy, it was seen that the accuracy of the method was poor in early cases of prostatic carcinoma, while often in late cases no secretions at all could be obtained from stony hard, fixed glands.[10]

TRANSRECTAL ASPIRATION BIOPSY: THE RADIUMHEMMET'S EXPERIENCE

Method

THE INSTRUMENT

The *instrument* consists of a syringe, a needle, and a needle guide (Fig. 5.1). A special handle on the syringe permits a one-hand grip during aspiration. The needle is 20 cm long, fine (22 gauge), and flexible, except in its proximal end. The needle guide is a metal tube having the same length as the thin part of the needle. It is slightly curved to fit the line of the palpating finger. The proximal end of the guide is funnel-shaped to facilitate introduction of the needle. On the distal end of the guide a steering ring for the index finger is fitted. An adjustable metal plate midway along the guide supports the instrument by resting on the operator's thenar. The apparatus is sterilized before use. Gloves for both hands, a finger-cot for the palpating finger, and lubricating jelly are required, which also should be sterile.

THE PROCEDURE

The patient is placed in lithotomy position. Previous preparation of the bowel is as a rule not necessary. Anaesthesia is not required. The instrument is arranged on the operator's left hand (Fig. 5.2). After lubrication with sterile jelly the finger is carefully introduced into the rectum. A firm pressure of the tip of the finger establishes a good contact with the suspected tumor area in the prostate through the rectal wall. The needle is then advanced into the lesion (Fig. 5.3). The plunger of the

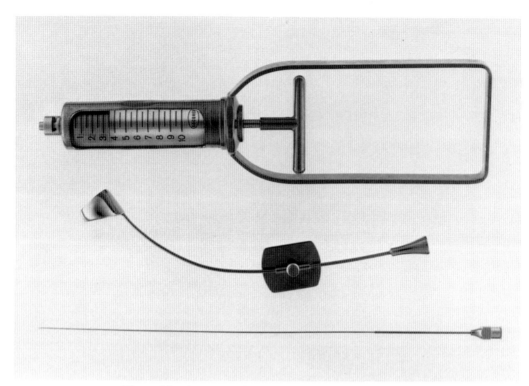

Figure 5.1 Apparatus for transrectal aspiration biopsy: syringe with a special handle, needle guide, and needle.

syringe is quickly retracted by the right hand, creating a vacuum in the system, while the needle is moved back and forth in the target area three or four times. The pressure on the syringe is equalized by allowing the plunger to return to its neutral position. Only then is the needle pulled out of the prostate and back into the guide.

THE SMEAR

The aspirated material in the needle is expressed onto a glass slide. If the aspirate is predominantly fluid it must be spread rapidly with a coverslip as for a blood smear. Large tissue fragments are gently squeezed by flat pressure with a coverslip. The smear is then dried in the air and stained with May-Grünwald-Giemsa stain, or fixed in methanol and stained according to Papanicolaou. The choice of methods for fixing and staining aspirated cell material has given rise to discussion. It is generally agreed that wet fixation and staining with hematoxylin-eosin or Papanicolaou stain give good nuclear detail and readily permit comparisons with corresponding cells in tissue sections. For good quality in such smears it is essential that they are rapidly fixed while still wet. Even a minimum of air drying causes distorting of cell details and inconsistency of pattern. Cell material in aspirates often dries very rapidly while the smears are being prepared, with resultant variability of quality. Consequently, we

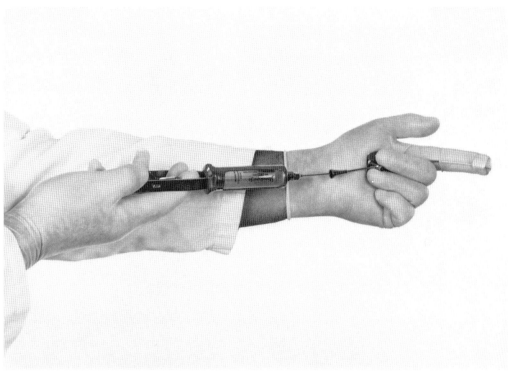

Figure 5.2 Apparatus arranged on the hand as during biopsy. The instrument rests on the thenar of the left hand. The plunger of the syringe is retracted by the right hand.

prefer to use methods developed for air-dried smears, mainly the May-Grünwald-Giemsa (MGG) stain, which has long been a standard in hematology.

THE RATIONALE OF FRANZÉN'S TECHNIQUE

Histological studies with step-section technique have shown that the majority of carcinomatous foci in the prostate are located under the capsule and in nearly 75% of cases in the posterolateral aspect of the gland.[11, 12] As these foci are usually of higher consistency than the rest of the gland, malignancy can be suspected by rectal palpation of an indurated nodule. The guiding of the biopsy needle transrectally by the palpating finger constitutes, therefore, the most direct method of those available to reach a prostatic nodule.

The thin needle (22 gauge) minimizes trauma; as a consequence several needlings are possible at one examination, and several repeat biopsies may be performed within a short period without causing discomfort to the patient. The special handle adapted to the syringe renders the suction movement performed by the right hand quick and effective and relieves the operator of the need of assistance. For these reasons transrectal aspiration biopsy with fine needle has met general favor, and there are now several publications on the subject, most, however, emerging from Europe.[13-38]

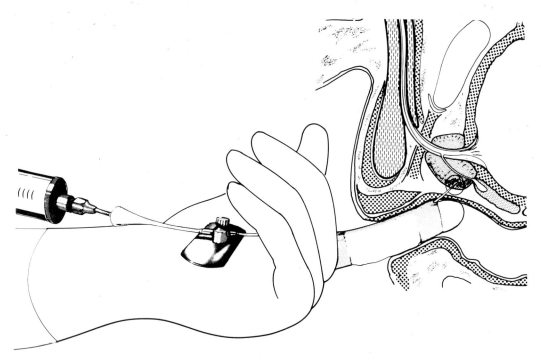

Figure 5.3 Sagittal section of the prostate showing the needle inserted into the target.

Complications

Traumatic complications following prostatic biopsies with thick needle (punch biopsies) are known from the review of the literature: severe bleeding, hematomas, and rectal fistulas have been reported; several cases of death following biopsies were registered due to anuria, pulmonary embolism, and coli-sepsis.[39–41]

None of these serious complications were seen when reviewing the first 3,000 transrectal aspiration biopsies with fine needle performed at Karolinska Hospital between 1956–1966. The incidence of complications was less than 0.5%, consisting of two cases of transient hematuria, two cases of epididymitis, three cases of hemospermia, and five cases of transient febrile reactions.[18] In the following years, however, when the number of needle biopsies sharply increased to more than 14,000 cases, four cases of severe sepsis were registered, one with a fatal outcome.[42] In general, febrile reactions were found to be more common in patients referred for cytological confirmation of prostatitis (1.5%). Patients with rheumatic disease (chronic polyarthritis) seemed to run a higher risk of complication after transrectal aspiration biopsy of the prostate, mainly in the form of severe, acute hyperthermia with chills; the frequency of complications was found to be 6.5% in a relatively small group of 63 patients.

In conclusion, while biopsy with fine needle can still be considered, in comparison with other types of prostatic biopsies, as a relatively safe procedure, the remote possibility of more severe complications such as sepsis should, in our opinion, limit its use to cases with a clinical suspicion of malignancy.

Accuracy of the Method

The cytological findings at first biopsy, after reviewing 4,630 patients examined from 1956 to 1968[2] are shown in Table 5.2. The percentage of unsatisfactory smears is less than 1%. Under the above-mentioned period transrectal aspiration biopsy of the prostate was performed at Karolinska Hospital by a permanent staff of three senior physicians, including the author. The results obtained express the possibilities of the method in the hands of skilled personnel.

The incidence of prostatic carcinoma is 30%. The relative significance of cancer incidence in transrectal aspiration biopsy of the prostate must be pointed out. The number of carcinoma cases reported depends on variable factors, such as the principles for selection of cases and the threshold of suspicion. A careful selection of cases will give a high incidence of positive biopsies but increase the risk that patients with carcinoma are not submitted to biopsy. On the contrary, a low incidence of positive cases can be explained by the fact that too many patients with palpatorily benign glands have been referred to biopsy.

In fact, one might consider that prostatic carcinoma was found at first biopsy only in one of 175 cases with a benign gland at rectal palpation (Table 5.3). In general, the higher the degree of clinical suspicion, the higher was the incidence of carcinoma detected at first biopsy. By repeating the biopsy more cases of carcinoma are detected in the clinically suspected groups but none in the palpatory benign glands (Table 5.4). One might conlcude that: (1) transrectal aspiration biopsy is not an effective method for detection of latent prostatic carcinoma; (2) in cases with equivocal palpatory findings, if the first cytological report was benign, a repeat aspiration biopsy is mandatory.

It is, however, only by comparison with histological reports that the accuracy of aspiration biopsy technique can be correctly evaluated.[2, 13] As Table 5.5 shows, 350 patients submitted to aspiration biopsy of the prostate had some kind of histological control. The cytological examination showed benign lesions in 140 of these patients and carcinoma in 210. Nine patients (6.0%) in the cytologically benign group were diagnosed at the subsequent histological examination as having carcinomas: in at least four of them the malignancy was growing predominantly in the anterior part of the gland and was easily detected by transurethral resection. In

Table 5.2
Cytological Findings at First Biopsy in 4,630 Patients

Cytology	No. of Patients	%
Unsatisfactory	33	0.7
Benign prostatic cells	2780	60.0
Suspicious for cancer	325	7.0
Prostatic cancer	1410	30.5
Other malignancy	82	1.8

five (2.0%) of the cytologically malignant group, the histological examination failed to demonstrate carcinoma; the histological specimen was obtained by transurethral resection in four and by perineal needle biopsy in one case. The "early" nodule in the posterior part of the gland was detected by transrectal aspiration biopsy but not by the other biopsy procedures. Clinical follow-up did not contradict the cytological diagnosis of carcinoma in any of the five cases. It might be worth mentioning that of a group of 18 patients with early carcinoma cytologically detected and submitted to radical prostatectomy, the diagnosis of malignancy was confirmed histologically in all of them.

A false positive cytologic diagnosis is not to be feared when the diagnostic work-up is performed by a trained staff. An overall accuracy of 94% is to be expected if aspiration biopsy is repeated in clinically suspected but cytologically negative cases.

CYTOLOGICAL PATTERN IN PROSTATIC ASPIRATES

Benign Lesions

Aspirated material from benign prostatic tissue consists of a drop of blood or prostatic fluid containing macroscopically visible fragments of

Table 5.3
Clinical Groups and Cytological Diagnosis of Cancer at First Biopsy.

Clinical Group[a]	Frequency of Cancer	%
1) Benign	1/175	0
2) Atypical	44/261	17
3) Suspicious	90/133	68
4) Malignant	143/146	98

[a] Findings at rectal palpation.

Table 5.4
Cancer Found at Second Biopsy in Cases with Benign or Inconclusive Findings at First Biopsy

Clinical Groups[a]	Frequency of Cancer	%
1) Benign	0/39	0
2) Atypical	4/57	7
3) Suspicious	5/33	15
4) Malignant	3/3	100

[a] Findings at rectal palpation.

Table 5.5
Cytological versus Histological Diagnosis in 350 Patients Submitted to Transrectal Aspiration Biopsy of the Prostate

Cytological Diagnosis	No. of Patients	Histological Diagnosis	
		Benign	Cancer
Benign	140	131 (94%)	9 (6%)
Cancer	210	5 (2%)	205 (98%)

epithelium. Microscopically the epithelial aggregates are arranged in large nonstratified sheets or as pluristratified clusters (Fig. 5.4*A*). The nuclei are regularly shaped and the cytoplasmic/nuclear ratio appears constant. The nucleoli are barely visible. In nonstratified sheets intercellular borders can be brought into focus and give the cells a polygonal appearance. In May-Grünwald-Giemsa stained smears, variably sized granuli can be seen in the cytoplasm (Fig. 5.4*B*). Pluristratified clusters often exhibit quasi-papillary, irregular structures and may arouse suspicion of malignancy. Higher magnification, however, shows that the nuclei are fairly regular and the amount of cytoplasm constant. Free cells are relatively few and have the same appearance as the aggregated cells; nuclear atypia is absent.

In the experience of the author, it is not possible to recognize, by aspiration biopsy of a benign gland, the presence of *benign prostatic hyperplasia.* The aspirated epithelial plugs exhibit the same morphological characteristics in biopsies from young patients as from older men with enlarged, hyperplastic glands.

In *acute prostatitis* the diagnosis, suggested by the clinical history, is usually confirmed by rectal examination: the gland is swollen and tender to palpation. Due to increased risk for complications one should refrain from biopsy when such a clinical picture is present. If a biopsy is performed, the aspirated material, often a viscous fluid with the macroscopic appearance of pus, will contain inflammatory cells, mainly leukocytes, cellular debris, and occasional clusters of prostatic epithelium, often exhibiting regressive changes. In *chronic prostatitis* the gland is usually deformed with areas of variable induration. Aspiration biopsy yields most often scant material, consisting of a droplet of fluid containing a few clusters of epithelial cells and a few inflammatory cells. In many cases of *granulomatous prostatitis* the presence at rectal examination of a painless, hard nodule in the prostate will suggest a carcinoma. However, microscopy of the aspirate will show inflammatory cells, mostly neutrophilic and eosinophilic granulocytes with some plasma cells and histiocytes, together with clusters of epitheloid cells and polynucleated giant cells. Occasionally, clusters of prostatic epithelium may exhibit various degrees of nuclear atypia suggesting malignancy. Clinical follow-up and repeat aspiration biopsies are in these cases advisable. The author has registered four cases of granulomatous prostatitis coexisting with prostatic carcinoma.

Prostatic Carcinoma: Cytological Diagnosis and Malignancy Grading

In prostatic carcinoma the aspirates generally are rich in cells, which only occasionally are mixed with blood. The high cellularity and absence of blood give a distinctive "granulated" appearance to dried, unstained smears. At microscopy the main characteristics of a carcinoma are evident: nuclear atypia with prominent nucleoli, decreased cytoplasmic/nuclear ratio, and reduced mutual adhesiveness of the cells. According to the degree of deviation from the normal epithelial structure, prostatic carcinoma can be grouped in highly, moderately, and poorly differentiated types.[43]

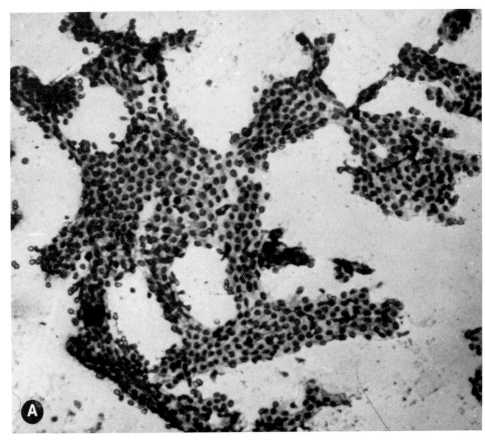

Figure 5.4 Needle aspirate from benign prostate. MGG stain. *A*, Nonstratified layers of epithelial cells with regular nuclei. ×120.

GRADE *1* OR HIGHLY DIFFERENTIATED CANCER

Nuclear polymorphism is of moderate degree; single cells are infrequent. The most typical feature of the highly differentiated carcinoma is the microadenomatous complex. The cytoplasm of the malignant cells is crowded into a central mass, while the enlarged nuclei are arranged in a peripheral circle. When this pattern is repeated throughout the smear without noteworthy nuclear polymorphism, the picture can be regarded as pathognomonic of well differentiated prostatic adenocarcinoma.

GRADE *2* OR MODERATELY DIFFERENTIATED CANCER

The general pattern is similar to that of grade *1*; however, the number of free cells is higher and nuclear polymorphism is more pronounced (Fig. 5.5).

GRADE *3* OR POORLY DIFFERENTIATED CANCER

The aspirate consists predominantly of dissociated cells, with polymorphic, often bizarre nuclear forms and greatly enlarged nucleoli (Fig. 5.6).

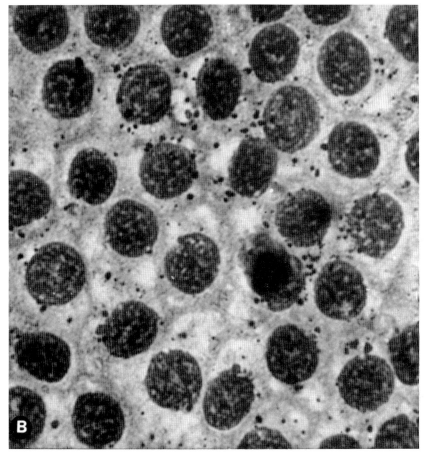

Figure 5.4 Needle aspirate from benign prostate. MGG stain. *B*, Sheet of benign epithelial cells at large magnification. Notice distinct cellular borders and cytoplasmic granuli. ×800.

A tendency to form patterns reminiscent of the glandular structures is as a rule present. More seldom an anaplastic variant is seen with dissociated cells resembling immature cells, *e.g.* of acute leukemia. In the present study this variant has been grouped together with grade *3* tumors. The cytological degree of differentiation was remarkably constant in all slides from the individual tumors. In the rare instances in which two degrees of atypia coexisted, the most undifferentiated degree determined the malignancy grading.

There is no fundamental difference in criteria of differentiation of prostatic carcinoma in aspirated cell material and histological sections. The histological diagnosis of carcinoma rests mainly on two criteria: cytological abnormalities of individual cells and abnormalities in the size, configuration, and arrangement of the acini. When such criteria are adopted, comparisons of malignancy grades of prostatic carcinoma in aspirated material and in histological sections become possible. The correlation between cytological and histological grades of differentiation in 36 cases of prostatic carcinoma[43] showed the following results: the five

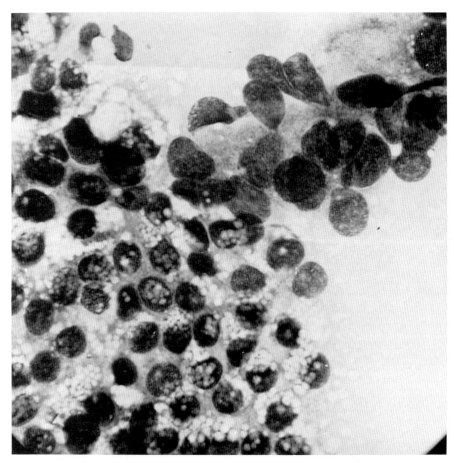

Figure 5.5 Needle aspirate from prostate carcinoma. Clusters of malignant cells with acinar structures at the top. The difference in the nuclear size with benign epithelium (*below*) is striking. Due to the nuclear atypia the carcinoma was graded as moderately differentiated. MGG stain. ×800.

tumors cytologically classified as highly differentiated received the same histological diagnosis. In 15 of the 18 cytologically moderately differentiated tumors the histological grading was likewise moderate and in three it was poor. In 12 of 13 cytologically poorly differentiated tumors the histological classification was the same, and one was reported as moderately differentiated. Similar results are reported by others.[15, 16]

PROGNOSTIC SIGNIFICANCE OF CYTOLOGICAL MALIGNANCY GRADING AND ITS THERAPEUTICAL INFERENCE

The data reported here are based on a study of 469 patients with prostatic carcinoma diagnosed by transrectal aspiration biopsy and cytologically graded according to cell differentiation.[43] All the patients received the same type of hormone therapy and had a clinical follow-up for

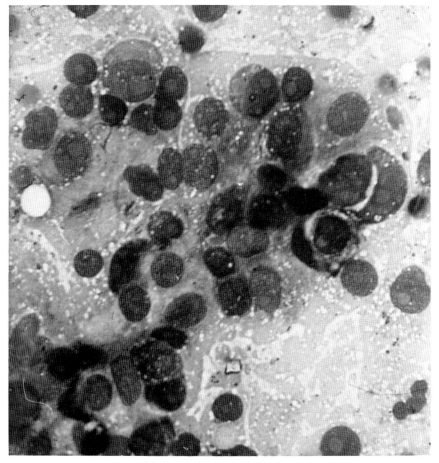

Figure 5.6 Needle aspirate from poorly differentiated prostatic carcinoma: mostly single cells with enlarged nucleoli. MGG stain. ×800.

at least 5 years. Of these, 131 patients (28%) had a tumor graded as highly differentiated, 265 (56%) were graded as moderately differentiated, and 73 (16%) were graded as poorly differentiated. The crude 5-year survival rates according to cytological grading are shown in Figure 5.7. The total survival rate was 52%: it was 68% in highly differentiated, 55% in moderately differentiated, and 11% in poorly differentiated tumors. The following considerations are possible:

1. The survival rate of patients with highly differentiated tumors is only slightly worse than the expected survival of a population of men around 67 years of age.

2. The rate of survival in the group of moderately differentiated tumors occupies an intermediate position between highly and poorly differentiated cases. However, a more detailed analysis of this group[44] revealed its biological if not morphological heterogeneity. Some of these cases responded as well to therapy as cases having a highly differentiated tumor, while others behaved in a similar fashion to poorly differentiated carcinomas;

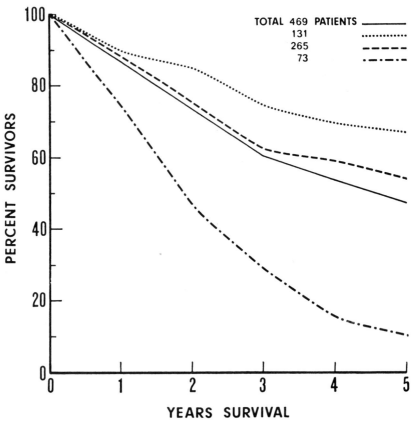

Figure 5.7 Cytologic differentiation grading of prostatic carcinoma and crude survival rates in 453 patients. (Reproduced with permission from P. L. Esposti.[43])

3. The low survival rate of poorly differentiated tumors indicates that the given therapy was not effective in these carcinomas, which behaved very aggressively.

As a consequence, the following therapeutical principles have been adopted at Karolinska Hospital: asymptomatic well differentiated carcinomas of the prostate are not actively treated but kept under clinical and cytological control. Cytologically moderately differentiated carcinomas are treated with hormones. Poorly differentiated carcinomas without distant metastases are primarily irradiated. Total prostatectomy is considered in patients not older than 65 years of age, in good general health, with a moderately or poorly differentiated carcinoma still confined to the gland.

OTHER MALIGNANCIES IN THE PROSTATE

By aspiration biopsy it is possible to detect malignancies in the prostate different from the primary prostatic adenocarcinoma. When 4,630 cases submitted to aspiration biopsy of the prostate were reviewed[2] malignancies other than prostatic adenocarcinoma were found in 82 cases. The majority consisted of urothelial carcinomas, easily recognized by the absence of acinar clusters and the presence of strongly atypical individual cells exhibiting abundant cytoplasm which is dense and homogeneous and with sharp borders. In most of the cases the urothelial carcinoma originated in the urinary bladder and invaded the prostatic gland. But in some cases no tumor was found in the bladder, the malignancy originating from the periurethral glands.[45] Other malignancies found in the prostate were squamous cell carcinomas, malignant lymphomas, and malignant mesenchymal tumors (also see Chapter 6).

PITFALLS IN THE CYTOLOGICAL DIAGNOSIS OF PROSTATIC ASPIRATES

A correctly performed transrectal aspiration biopsy of the prostate is often the basis for an accurate cytological diagnosis. It is assumed that,

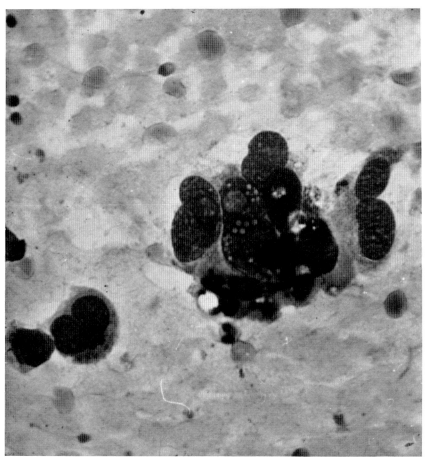

Figure 5.8 Needle aspirate from seminal vesicles. Epithelial cells showing hyperchromatic, polymorphic nuclei. Notice coarse pigment granuli in the cytoplasm and spermatozoa in the background. Clinical diagnosis: prostatovesiculitis. MGG stain. ×800.

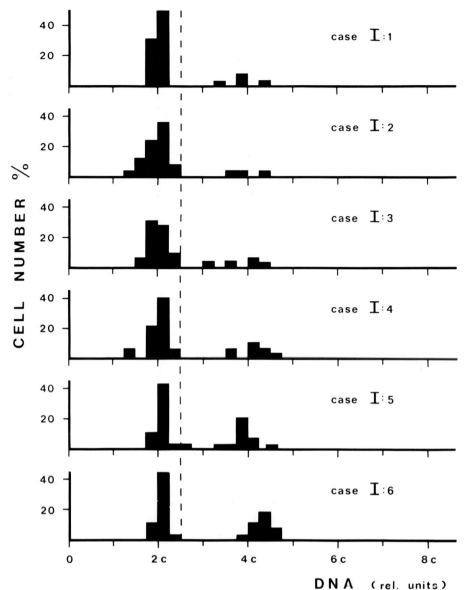

Figure 5.9 Frequency histogram of nuclear DNA content. Each histogram (*A* and *B*) is based on the analysis of 50 to 100 cancer cells. The DNA values are expressed in relation to the mean values of the internal staining control for each preparation (the granulocytes of the smear), which were given the arbitrary value 2 c (diploid DNA content). The *broken line* represents the upper limit value (2.5 c) of the diploid staining control. *A*, Six patients of group *I* (low degree of malignancy). The histogram shows that a substantial proportion of cell nuclei exhibited a diploid amount of DNA. (Reproduced with permission from A. Zetterberg and P. L. Esposti.[49])

regardless of the site of origin in the gland, prostatic carcinoma spreads distally beneath the capsule.[12, 46] In the experience of the author the majority of the nodules of early carcinoma will be found in the lower lateral part of the prostatic lobe, near the apex and the lateral sulcus; an

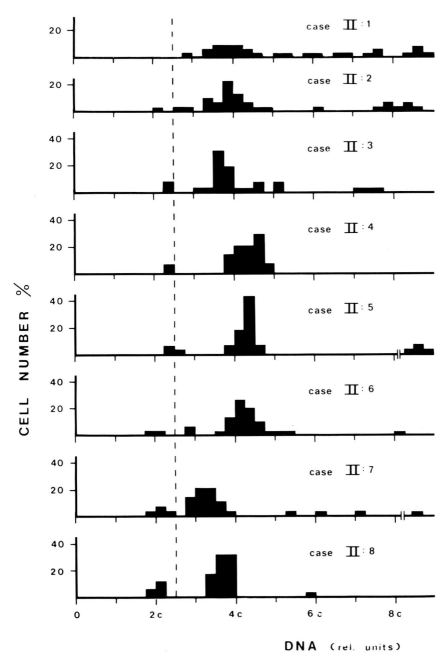

Figure 5.9 *B,* Frequency histogram of nuclear DNA content as in previous figure. Eight patients of group *II* (high degree of malignancy). The histogram shows a clear hyperploid distribution pattern. (Reproduced with permission from A. Zetterberg and P. L. Esposti.[49])

aspiration performed in this area and just under the capsule will yield abundant cellular material, consisting exclusively of carcinoma cells. If the needle is pushed too deeply into the gland, the benign, hyperplastic part of the gland will be penetrated, and the aspirate will consist mainly of sheets of benign epithelium, possibly intermingled with a few clusters exhibiting microacinar structures. These clusters might originate from a microscopic area of latent carcinoma, from atrophic prostatic tissue or from atypical epithelial proliferation of a benign gland. It is a rule at Karolinska Hospital not to report malignancy unless the whole smear contains predominantly carcinoma cells, thus minimizing the risk of false positive reports. If the biopsy is performed in the upper part of the gland, the aspirate might contain clusters of strongly atypical epithelial cells, suggesting malignancy. However, a few spermatozoa in the background, and the presence of coarse granuli of pigment in the cytoplasm will indicate that the cell material has been aspirated from a seminal vesicle (Fig. 5.8). It is a known fact that vesicular epithelium contains a strongly degenerated cellular element with bizarre nuclei which must not be erroneously identified as carcinoma cells.[47, 48]

If, at the end of the biopsy, the negative pressure present in the system is not completely equalized before withdrawal of the needle from the target, rectal content will enter the needle. As a result, fecal material and bacteria will be identified in the background of the smear, while prostatic cell material will be intermingled with clusters of rectal mucosal cells; the

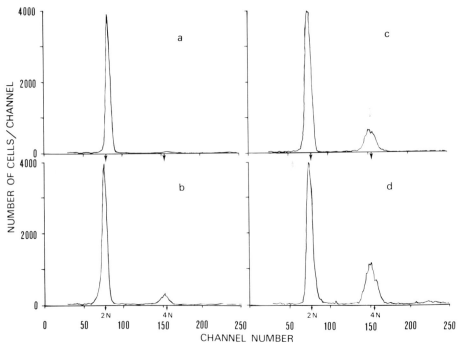

Figure 5.10   DNA histograms from flow-cytophotometry of aspirated cells. *a*, A case of benign prostate. *b–d*, Hormone-treated prostatic carcinomas. Abscissa: channel number corresponding to the amount of DNA in each cell. Ordinate: number of cells per channel. The largest peaks on the left represent diploid G1 cells (*2N*). In section *a* the peak on the right represents normal tetraploid G2 cells (*4N*). Sections *b*, *c*, and *d* show aneuploid cell lines with increasing percentages of cells in the tetraploid region. (Reproduced with permission from B. Tribukait *et al.*[51])

diagnosis is rendered difficult or impossible. This is one of the most common mistakes of the inexperienced operator.

PROSTATIC ASPIRATES IN RESEARCH WORK

The epithelial plugs obtained by aspiration biopsy constitute an ideal material for enzymatic analysis of the epithelial component of the prostate. Quantitative determination of acid phosphatase has been performed in prostatic carcinoma and compared to the content in other tumors[13]; cells from prostatic carcinoma exhibited lower enzymatic activity than the benign prostatic cells. Acid phosphatase activity in benign as well as malignant prostatic epithelial cells, however, was always higher than that observed in cells aspirated from nonprostatic tumors.

Increased DNA content in aspirated cells, expressing chromosomal

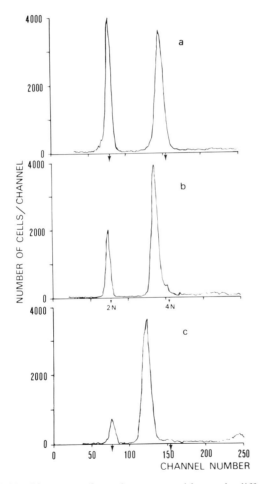

Figure 5.11 DNA histograms from three cases with poorly differentiated prostatic carcinoma, showing different degrees of aneuploidy in the tri- to tetraploid region. For further explanation see the legend to Figure 5.10. (Reproduced with permission from B. Tribukait *et al.*[51])

abnormality, can be assessed by cytophotometry. The cytochemical analysis of individual cells, based on quantitative cytophotometric measurements of Feulgen-stained nuclei, showed that nuclei from benign lesions exhibited the normal diploid amount of DNA. Contrary to this, cells from prostatic carcinomas were characterized by various degrees of heteroploidy. A general correlation between degree of heteroploidy and degree of clinical and cytological malignancy seems to exist.[44] In order to assess the prognostic significance of nuclear DNA levels in prostatic carcinoma, a method was developed by which old MGG-stained smears could be used for quantitative cytophotometric DNA determinations after destaining. A retrospective study was thus possible on 43 patients with a cytological diagnosis of prostatic carcinoma of different malignancy grading.[49] The patients were selected on the basis of the clinical response to hormonal therapy; patients of group *I* showed a good response with survival without evidence of cancer for at least 5 years. Patients of group *II* showed a poor response with death from cancer within 3 years. Most of the carcinomas belonging to patients of group *I* were characterized by a diploid or combined diploid-tetraploid DNA distribution pattern, while in carcinomas from patients of group *II* most of the cancer cells contained abnormally increased DNA amounts (Fig. 5.9).

At present research work is in progress using flow-cytofluorometric DNA analysis of cell material as already done with other urological tumors.[50, 51] DNA determinations of a large number of cells is possible (Figs. 5.10 and Fig. 5.11). In the opinion of the author, the use of these two complementary methods, *i.e.* the quantitative DNA determination of a limited number of Feulgen-stained, morphologically well identified cells and the rapid-flow cytophotometry of a large amount of cells, will increase knowledge of the biological properties of the tumor and offer additional information to morphological analysis in the malignancy grading and management of prostatic carcinoma (also see Chapter 25).

REFERENCES

1. Franzén, S., Giertz, G., and Zajicek, J. Cytological diagnosis of prostatic tumours by transrectal aspiration biopsy: a preliminary report. *J. Urol. 32:* 193, 1960.
2. Esposti, P. L. Aspiration Biopsy Cytology in the Diagnosis and Management of Prostatic Carcinoma. Thesis, Karolinska Institute, Stockholm, 1974
3. Hudson, P. B., Finkle, A. L., Jost, H. M., Trifilio, A., and Stout, A. P. Prostatic cancer X. Comparison of open and "punch" biopsy techniques. *A.M.A. Arch. Surg. 70:* 508, 1955.
4. Kaufman, J. J., Rosenthal, M., and Goodwin, W. E. Methods of diagnosis of carcinoma of the prostate: a comparison of clinical impression, prostatic smear, needle biopsy, open perineal biopsy and transurethral biopsy. *J. Urol. 72:* 450, 1954.
5. Astraldi, A. Biopsie des tumeurs de la prostate. *Arch. Urol. Necker 5:* 151, 1925.
6. Emmett, J. L., Barber, K. W., Jr., and Jackman, R. J. Transrectal biopsy to detect prostatic carcinoma: a review and report of 203 cases. *J. Urol. 87:* 460, 1962.
7. Ferguson, R. S. Prostatic neoplasms, their diagnosis by needle puncture and aspiration. *Am. J. Surg. 9:* 507, 1930.
8. Mulholland, S. W. A study of prostatic secretion and its relation to malignancy. *Proc. Staff Meetings Mayo Clin. 6:* 169, 1931.
9. Papanicolaou, G. N. Cytology of the urine sediment in neoplasms of the urinary tract. *J. Urol. 57:* 375, 1947.
10. Frank, I. N. The cytodiagnosis of prostatic cancer. *J.A.M.A. 209:* 1698, 1969.

11. Gaynor, E. P. Zur Frage des Prostatakrebses. *Virchows Arch. [Pathol. Anat.] 301:* 602, 1938.

12. Moore, R. A. The morphology of small prostatic carcinoma. *J. Urol. 33:* 224, 1935.

13. Esposti, P. L. Cytologic diagnosis of prostatic tumours with the aid of transrectal aspiration biopsy. A critical review of 1,110 cases and a report of morphologic and cytochemical studies. *Acta Cytol. (Baltimore) 10:* 182, 1966.

14. Bachmann, K. F. Cytodiagnostische Untersuchung der Prostata mit transrectaler Aspirationspunktion. *Schweiz. Med. Wochenschr. 96:* 1225, 1966.

15. Andersson, L., Jönsson, G., and Brunk, U. Puncture biopsy of the prostate in the diagnosis of prostatic cancer. *Scand. J. Urol. Nephrol. 1:* 227, 1967.

16. Ekman, H., Hedberg, K., and Persson, P. S. Cytological versus histological examination of needle biopsy specimens in the diagnosis of prostatic cancer. *Br. J. Urol. 39:* 544, 1967.

17. Williams, J. P., Still, B. M., and Pugh, R. C. B. The diagnosis of prostatic cancer: cytological and biochemical studies using the Franzén biopsy needle. *Br. J. Urol. 39:* 549, 1967.

18. Esposti, P. L., Franzén, S., and Zajicek, J. The aspiration biopsy smear. In *Diagnostic Cytology and Its Histopathologic Bases*, 2nd Ed., edited by L. G. Koss. J. B. Lippincott, Philadelphia, 1968, p. 565.

19. Alfthan, O., Klintrup, H.-E., Koivuniemi, A., and Taskinen, E. Comparison of thin-needle and Vim-Silverman-needle biopsy in the diagnosis of prostatic cancer. *Duodecim 84:* 506, 1968.

20. Kelami, A., and Kirstaedter, H. J. Erste Erfahrungen mit der Franzén-Nadel in der Diagnose des Prostatakarzinoms. *Urol. Int. 24:* 560, 1969.

21. Rheinfrank, R. E., and Nulf, T. H. Fine needle aspiration biopsy of the prostate. *Endoscopy 1:* 27, 1969.

22. Schnürer, L.-B., Fritjofsson, Å., Lindgren, A., Magnusson, P.-H., and Pettersson, S. Fine needle versus coarse needle in punction diagnosis of prostatic carcinoma. *Acta Pathol. Microbiol. Scand. 76:* 150, 1969.

23. Sparwasser, H., and Lüchtrath, H. Die transrectale Saugbiopsie der Prostata. *Urologe 9:* 281, 1970.

24. Faul, P., Klosterhalfen, H., and Schmiedt, E. Erfahrungen mit der Feinnadelbiopsie (Saug- bzw. Aspirationbiopsie nach Franzén) der Prostata. *Urologe 10:* 120, 1971.

25. Hendry, W. F., and Williams, J. P. Transrectal prostatic biopsy. *Br. Med. J. 4:* 595, 1971.

26. Schulte-Wissermann, H., and Lüchtrath, H. Aspirationsbiopsie und Cytologie beim Prostatacarcinom. *Virchows Arch. [Pathol. Anat.] 352:* 122, 1971.

27. Sunderland, H., and Lederer, H. Prostatic aspiration biopsy. *Br. J. Urol. 43:* 603, 1971.

28. Linsk, J. A., Axilrod, H. D., Solyn, R., and Delaverdac, C. Transrectal cytologic aspiration in the diagnosis of prostatic carcinoma. *J. Urol. 108:* 455, 1972.

29. Faul, P., and Praetorius, M. Die cytologische Diagnose des Prostatacarcinoms und seine verschiedenen Malignitätsgrade. *Urologe A 12:* 259, 1973.

30. Faul, P. *Prostata-Zytologie.* Dietrich Steinkopf-Verlag, Darmstadt, 1975.

31. Epstein, N. A. Prostatic biopsy. A morphologic correlation of aspiration cytology with needle biopsy histology. *Cancer 38:* 2078, 1976.

32. Spieler, P., Gloor, F., Egle, N., and Bandhauer, K. Cytological findings in transrectal aspiration biopsy on hormone- and radio-treated carcinoma of the prostate. *Virchows Arch. A Pathol. Anat. Histol. 372:* 149, 1976.

33. Bishop, D., and Oliver J. A. A study of transrectal aspiration biopsies of the prostate, with particular regard to prognostic evaluation. *J. Urol. 117:* 313, 1977.

34. Kline, T. S., Kelsey, D. M., and Kohler F. P. Prostatic carcinoma and needle aspiration biopsy. *Am. J. Clin. Pathol. 67:* 131, 1977.

35. Nienhaus, H. Aspiration biopsy cytology of prostate carcinoma. *Recent Results Cancer Res. 60:* 53, 1977.

36. Leistenschneider, W., and Nagel, R. Komplikationen bei transrektaler Stanz- und Feinnadelbiopsie. *Therapiewoche 28:* 1963, 1978.

37. Lin, B. P. C., Davies, W. E. L., and Harmata, P. A. Prostatic aspiration cytology. *Pathology 11:* 607, 1979.

38. Zajicek, J. Prostatic gland and seminal vesicles. Aspiration biopsy cytology Part 2.

Monogr. Clin. Cytol. 7: 129, 1979.

39. Bertelsen, S. Transrectal needle biopsy of the prostate. *Acta Chir. Scand. 226* (Suppl.): 357, 1966.

40. Davison, P., and Malament, M. Urinary contamination as a result of transrectal biopsy of the prostate. *J. Urol. 105:* 545, 1971.

41. Wendel, R. G., and Evans, A. T. Complications of punch biopsy of the prostate gland. *J. Urol. 97:* 122, 1967.

42. Esposti, P. L., Elman, A., and Norlén, H. Complications of transrectal aspiration biopsy of the prostate. *Scand. J. Urol. Nephrol. 9:* 208, 1975.

43. Esposti, P. L. Cytologic malignancy grading of prostatic carcinoma by transrectal aspiration biopsy. *Scand. J. Urol. Nephrol. 5:* 199, 1971.

44. Zetterberg, A., and Esposti, P. L. Cytophotometric DNA-analysis of aspirated cells from prostatic carcinoma. *Acta Cytol. (Baltimore) 20:* 46, 1976.

45. Mostofi, F. K., and Price, E. B., Jr. Tumors of the male genital system. *Atlas of Tumor Pathology*, 2nd series, fasc. 8. Armed Forces Institute of Pathology, Washington, D.C., 1973.

46. Hinman, F., Jr. The early diagnosis and radical treatment of prostatic carcinoma. *Calif. Med. 68:* 338, 1948.

47. Koivuniemi, A., and Tyrkkö, J. Seminal vesicle epithelium in fine-needle aspiration biopsies of the prostate as a pitfall in the cytologic diagnosis of carcinoma. *Acta Cytol. (Baltimore) 20:* 116, 1976.

48. Droese, M., and Voeth, C. Cytologic features of seminal vesicle epithelium in aspiration biopsy smears of the prostate. *Acta Cytol. (Baltimore) 20:* 120, 1976.

49. Zetterberg, A., and Esposti, P. L. Prognostic significance of nuclear DNA levels in prostatic carcinoma. *Scand. J. Urol. Nephrol.*, Suppl. *55:* 53, 1980.

50. Tribukait, B., Gustafson, H., and Esposti, P. L. Ploidy and proliferation in human bladder tumors as measured by flow-cytofluorometric DNA-analysis and its relations to histopathology and cytology. *Cancer 43:* 1742, 1979.

51. Tribukait, B., Esposti, P. L., and Rönström, L. Tumour ploidy for characterization of prostatic carcinoma: flow-cytofluorometric DNA studies using aspiration biopsy material. *Scand. J. Urol. Nephrol.*, Suppl. *55:* 59, 1980.

Editorial Comment to Chapter 5

Everybody should keep in mind that in more than 20 years the Karolinska Sjukhuset, Radiumhemmet in Stockholm became somewhat of a *Mecca* for a great number of people fascinated by Franzén and Zajicek and their disciples, authorities in the field of cytological prostate cancer detection and follow-up.

It is not a matter of sticking some aspiration fine needle into any organ or structure percutaneously. The fact (and not the question) is that with the refined technology described in this chapter we acquire better information by less troublesome means.

R. H.

6

Pathology and Classification of Prostate Malignancies: Experience of the German Prostate Cancer Registry

G. Dhom, M.D.
Ch. Hohbach, M.D.

The histological or cytological evaluation of a suspicious rectal finding today is one of the indispensable diagnostic steps for the detection or exclusion of prostatic carcinoma. Yet, introduction of the punch biopsy into the diagnostic checkup has confronted pathologists with previously unknown problems of diagnosis and differential diagnosis. They are compelled to pronounce a definite diagnosis of tremendous consequence for the patient from a few glandular groups or cells. By introducing a nationwide annual checkup program in the Federal Republic of Germany in 1971 (see Chapter 4), it was anticipated that the number of biopsies and thus the diagnostic problems would rapidly increase at many institutions. These expectations were indeed fulfilled. Therefore, in 1972 at the suggestion of C. E. Alken, a histopathological *Prostate Cancer Registry* was established, compiling biopsies and being accessible for consultation by pathologists in uncertain cases.[1, 2] The *Registry* was completed and fully operating in 1975. Until then 13,387 biopsies were recorded including 6,758 clinical prostatic carcinomas corresponding to 50.4% of the total biopsies submitted. Since then the *Registry* has continued to operate as a consultative service and is concerned with the diagnosis and classification of prostatic carcinoma. The *Registry* is not a central institution performing all biopsy work-up for the Annual Preventive Checkup

Program (Chapter 4). All data discussed in this chapter were recorded between 1972 and 1975.

CLASSIFICATION OF PROSTATIC CARCINOMA AND DISTRIBUTION OF ITS VARIOUS SUBTYPES

The variety of histological and cytological patterns of prostatic carcinoma is known, as well as its completely different growth behavior: on the one hand the aggressive tumor extending beyond the prostate margins and often associated with distant metastases, on the other hand the tumor remaining latent throughout life and not influencing life expectancy. Thus, it was necessary to establish a histological classification which could be correlated with growth behavior and prognosis. Yet, such an effort was faced with the problem that in one particular carcinoma several histological patterns would be found, side by side, and that one biopsy would not reflect in every case the total spectrum of the tumor architecture. This should be taken into consideration when classifying a single tumor biopsy.

In order to account for the variety of histological features and to keep the individual error limited, we divide the ordinary types of the prostate carcinoma into *uniform* and *pluriform* subtypes (Table 6.1). Within the uniform types we differentiate those with pure glandular patterns. Thus, the highly differentiated adenocarcinoma is a tumor still forming rather regular glands, showing only slight nuclear anaplasia and frequently a light cytoplasm. The poorly differentiated adenocarcinoma forms totally irregular, often extremely small glands with tiny lumina. They show pronounced nuclear anaplasia with multiple enlarged nucleoli. The cy-

Table 6.1
Classification and Distribution of Prostatic Carcinoma[a]

Ordinary Prostatic Carcinoma	n	%
A. Carcinoma with uniform pattern		
1. Highly differentiated adenocarcinoma	924	13.67
2. Poorly differentiated adenocarcinoma	1057	15.64
3. Cribriform carcinoma	470	6.95
4. Undifferentiated, solid carcinoma	526	7.78
B. Carcinoma with pluriform pattern		
1. Highly and poorly differentiated adenocarcinoma	463	6.85
2. Cribriform and solid carcinoma	408	6.04
3. Cribriform pattern in other types	1707	25.26
4. Other combinations	1046	15.48
Special Carcinoma		
1. Endometrioid carcinoma	8	0.12
2. Urothelial (transitional cell) carcinoma	126	1.86
3. Squamous cell carcinoma	14	0.21
4. Mucous carcinoma	9	0.13
Total	6758	100

[a] *German Prostate Cancer Registry*, Homburg/Saar (1972–1975). From Ch. Hohbach and G. Dhom.[39]

toplasm is frequently basophilic. The cribriform pattern is an intraglandular cell proliferation. However, it should not be confused with an *in situ carcinoma*. Despite the distinct demarcation of single nests to the surrounding connective tissue it can form extensive infiltrating tumor masses. The nuclear anaplasia and cytoplasmic structure are quite variable. The solid "anaplastic" carcinoma very often derives directly from the cribriform carcinoma (Figs. 6.1 to 6.5). The four basic patterns described are often mixed to different degrees to form "Carcinoma with pluriform pattern." Three of these combinations are included in the classification scheme (Table 6.1). If one intends to follow the rule "*a potiori fit denominatio*," the main tumor structure can be used for classification, "predominantly glandular pattern," "predominantly solid cribriform pattern" and so on.[3, 4] Although the tumor architecture is the primary consideration for classification, the cytologic, especially the caryologic features become important for the prognostic assessment of prostatic carcinoma. This must be kept in mind when transferring classification into a tumor grading, as will be discussed later in this chapter. Rare or extraordinary tumors must also have their place in such a classification. Regarding prostate carcinoma, these lesions are the urothelial carcinoma, squamous cell carcinoma, endometrioid carcinoma, and mucous carcinoma.

The distribution of the two main groups of prostatic carcinomas in our classification is as follows:

1. Carcinomas with uniform differentiation constitutes 46% of the material in our *Registry*.

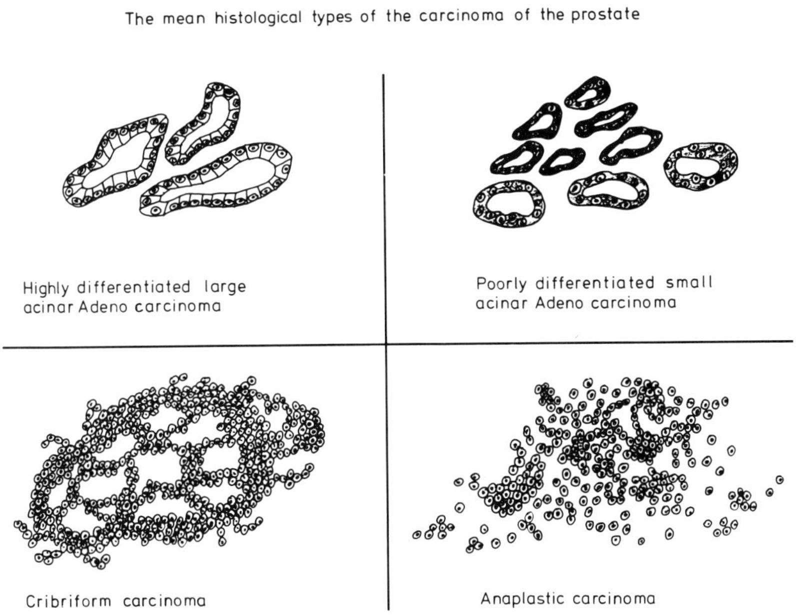

The mean histological types of the carcinoma of the prostate

Highly differentiated large acinar Adeno carcinoma

Poorly differentiated small acinar Adeno carcinoma

Cribriform carcinoma

Anaplastic carcinoma

Figure 6.1 Basic histologic pattern of uniform and pluriform prostatic carcinoma. (Modified from G. Dhom.[20])

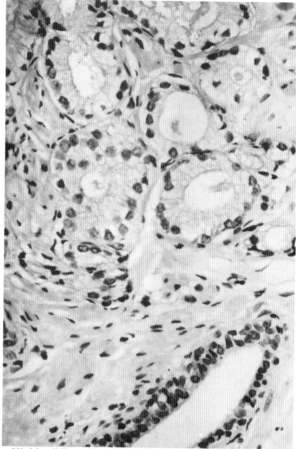

Figure 6.2 Highly differentiated carcinoma: well differentiated glands with loss of basal cells as compared to normal glands, enlarged nuclei, few enlarged nucleoli (hematoxylin and eosin. (HE), ×360)

2. Pluriform carcinomas that are made up of several basic types account for 54% (Table 6.1).

Pure adenocarcinomas predominate in the first group with 29%. There are no significant differences in the number of well and poorly differentiated adenocarcinomas. The same is true for uniform cribriform and solid carcinomas. Pure cribriform tumors are found only occasionally.

Among the special carcinomas, *urothelial carcinoma* of the prostate has a particular position. It originates from the prostatic urethra, the periurethral or the peripheral glands. It is associated in every second case with an urothelial carcinoma of the urinary bladder or with typical prostatic carcinoma,[5] thus lacking sensitivity to conservative treatment. *Squamous cell* cancers are rare tumors, as well. They may develop after a long-term estrogen therapy of an ordinary adenocarcinoma. The *endometrioid* carcinomas grow intraductally in adenomatous and papillary patterns. They are believed to derive from the prostatic utricle. The

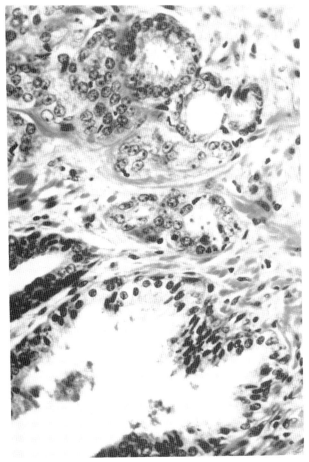

Figure 6.3 Poorly differentiated adenocarcinoma: irregularly arranged small glands with marked nuclear anaplasia and multiple enlarged nucleoli. (HE, ×360)

localization, however, can normally not be verified from the biopsy material. Distinct *mucin-secreting* prostate carcinomas are rare. In contrast, a slight mucin secretion is frequently observed in cribriform tumors. The infiltration of a carcinoma from the rectum into the prostate should be excluded in every instance.

In the group of pluriform carcinoma the rate of cribriform tumors, which amounts to 31%, is remarkable. The numerical distribution within our classification is based mainly on punch biopsies or on specimens from transurethral resections, that account for 57 and 28% of tumor-positive biopsies, respectively. At this point, one must keep in mind, that the whole differentiation pattern of prostatic carcinoma can be *undergraded* in some cases of pure adenocarcinomas, as was shown by the histologic evaluation of the total prostatectomy specimen compared with the foregoing biopsy. Thus, the real number of pluriform tumors is surely greater than expressed in our data.

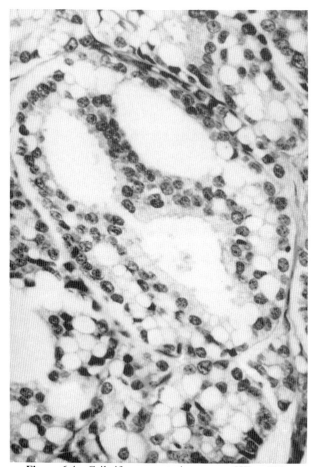

Figure 6.4 Cribriform prostatic cancer. (HE, ×400)

JUVENILE CARCINOMA OF THE PROSTATE

Prostatic cancer is generally considered a carcinoma of advanced age. From the cases in the *Registry* 52% of carcinomas are found in the group of men between 65 and 74 years of age (Fig. 6.6). There is no general agreement as to the age limit up to which one can still talk about juvenile prostatic carcinoma. This age limit has been set arbitrarily at 56 years[6] or at 50 years.[7, 8, 9]

The incidence of juvenile prostatic carcinoma, given as percentage of the total number of carcinomas examined, varies between 1.1%,[7] 4.3%,[9] and 6.5%.[6] In our own material carcinomas were found in 137 men younger than 55 years of a total of 4,137 men recorded in the *Registry*, corresponding to 3.3%. There are only sporadic cases in young men between 25 and 39 years of age. Among all juvenile carcinoma 5.8% are found between 40 and 44 years of age, 19% between 45 and 49 years, and 72% between 50 and 54 years of age at diagnosis.

At the time of diagnosis the distribution of the various clinical stages shows only minor differences between juvenile carcinomas and the tumors

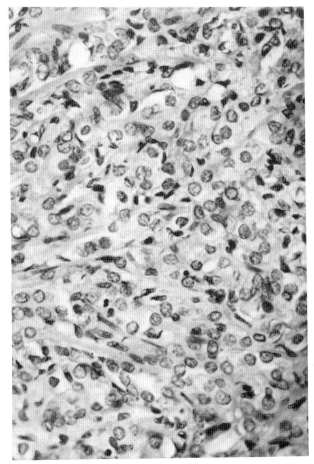

Figure 6.5   Undifferentiated solid carcinoma of the prostate. (HE, ×400)

of men older than 55 years of age, which constitute the bulk of our *Registry* cases (Table 6.2). The majority of cases, both in younger men (72%) as well as in the elderly (82%), show already the advanced tumor stages B$_2$ through D.[10] This is in agreement with the data reported by Johnson and associates.[9] However, there is no doubt that the true rate of stage D lesions is underestimated in our *Registry*, because the staging procedures are—with respect to widespread disease—usually incomplete at the time of the submission of the biopsy. Only stage B$_1$ is more frequently found in younger men (22%) as compared to 11% in the elderly. This, however, is not due to the more frequent participation of this age group in the federal program for early prostate cancer detection, as outlined in Chapter 4.

In stage A no significant differences are encountered between the different age groups in the *Registry*. Its rate though is distinctly below the value of 10.7% given by Silber and McGavren.[6] Taking into account the fact that prostatic carcinoma is often understaged on rectal examination,[10, 11] we have to assume a much higher percentage of advanced tumor stages

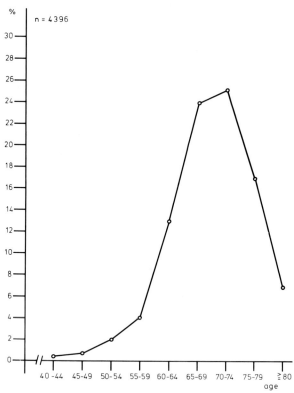

Figure 6.6 Age distribution of prostatic cancer at the *German Prostate Cancer Registry* (1972–1975); n = 4396, 52% of the patients are between the age of 65 and 74, whereas 3.3% are younger than 55 years. (Modified from Ch. Hohbach and G. Dhom.[39])

Table 6.2
Clinical Stage of Prostatic Carcinoma in Different Age Groups at Initial Diagnosis (Predominance of the Advanced Stages B$_2$ to D, 1972–1975)

Stage		n	%
American Classification	UICC		
Younger than 55 yr			
A	T_0	7	5.8
B$_1$	T_1	27	22.3
B$_2$	T_2	30	24.8
C	T_{3+4}	44	36.4
D	N+ M$_1$	13	10.7
Total		121	100
Older than 55 yr			
A	T_0	222	7
B$_1$	T_1	347	11
B$_2$	T_2	1004	31.9
C	T_{3+4}	1202	38.2
D	N+ M$_1$	376	11.9
Total		3151	100

in young men, too. There is no general agreement as to the prognosis of juvenile carcinoma of the prostate. Byar and Mostofi[8] stated that it corresponds to that of older patients, while Johnson et al.[9] found a worse prognosis in their group of younger individuals with this malignancy.

No doubt, the statistically longer life expectancy of younger tumor patients in comparison with the majority of the aged population with tumor disease is, in itself, a factor contributing to an unfavourable prognosis of the carcinoma, i.e. a longer time span during which the tumor can progress and/or become resistant to treatment (Details on this issue are provided in Chapter 3). Early recognition of prostatic carcinoma and the problematic question as to its ideal treatment strategy is therefore, of particular interest in younger patients.

COMPARISON OF STAGES AND HISTOLOGY OF PROSTATIC CARCINOMA

This comparison is made to answer the question whether the clinical stage and histopathologic grade of prostatic carcinomas represent merely descriptive informations or whether there is a definite relationship between the morphology of prostatic carcinoma and its clinical course. In the advanced stages B_2 to D which, as already mentioned, account for 82% of the total *Registry* material, cribriform and solid carcinomas, including combinations with other subtypes, predominate. In stage B_1 the number of these unfavorable tumors equals that of the pure adenocarcinomas which have a better prognosis. It is only in stage A that we find a majority of well differentiated adenocarcinoma. The proportion of prostatic tumors with a poor prognosis to pure adenocarcinoma with a better prognosis is *1.7:1* in our material (Fig. 6.7). In juvenile carcinoma, too, the more rapidly proliferating tumors prevail with a ratio of *1.3:1* and apparently are responsible for the predominance of advanced tumor stages at the time of diagnosis (Table 6.2, Fig. 6.7).

These findings do not support the assumption, that a given prostatic carcinoma necessarily changes from a well differentiated into a poorly differentiated tumor in its course of development.[12] If this were the case, we might expect to find in old patients only advanced stages and poorly differentiated tumors. We find in contrast in all age groups from the onset carcinomas of various grades of differentiation with a predominance of rapidly proliferating pluriform tumors with cribriform and solid pattern (Fig. 6.8). They show, depending on the type of tumor, an individual grade of malignancy that distinctly determines the further clinical course. Thus, the survival rate in cases of purely well differentiated adenocarcinomas closely approximates that of the normal age-adjusted life expectancy, whereas cribriform and solid carcinoma are associated with a high cancer mortality.[13] With increasing dedifferentiation the grade of malignancy and the expansion of prostatic carcinoma increases. As a rule, the clinical stage is more advanced at the time of diagnosis, independent of the patient's age. The stage of the tumor, therefore, is basically the

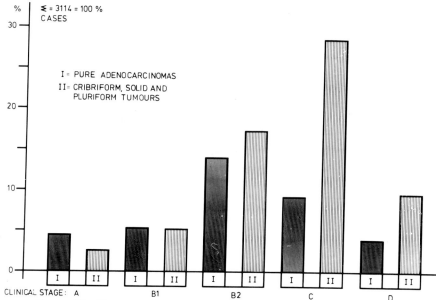

Figure 6.7 Tumor morphology and clinical stage: predominance of prognostic unfavorable tumors in stages B_2 to D. (Modified from Ch. Hohbach and G. Dhom.[39])

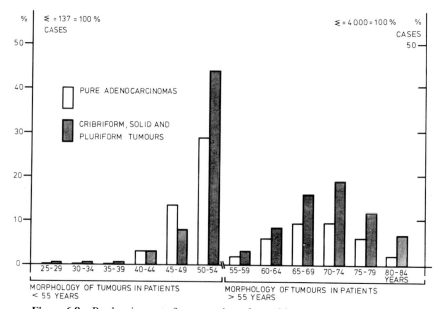

Figure 6.8 Predominance of prognostic unfavorable tumor-types in older as well as in younger men. (Modified from Ch. Hohbach and G. Dhom.[39])

function of its biologic growth behavior, which again is equivalent to its morphology. The histologic differentiation with determination of the grade of malignancy of prostatic carcinoma therefore becomes the most important prognostic criterion.

GRADING OF PROSTATIC CARCINOMA

Since Broders[14] there were numerous attempts to arrange the morphological patterns of prostate carcinoma into a grading system.[15] It is the aim of each grading system to define the degree of malignancy in order to obtain a prognostic assessment of every single case.[4, 15, 16] In this regard prostatic carcinoma raises special problems. The variety of its histological pattern *per se* and the usually small and nonrepresentative segment of the entire tumor in biopsy material limits the practicability of any grading system, and may render the information given to the clinician questionable.

The criteria available for morphological grading of prostate cancer are the *degree of differentiation* of the tumor and the *degree of anaplasia* of the single tumor cell. In case of differentiation tumors still capable of forming glands can be compared with those forming only solid tumor masses, the cribriform carcinoma ranging in between. For the degree of anaplasia the difference of each individual tumor cell from the normal cell is evaluated, especially the variety of nuclear pattern, the size, and the number of nucleoli.

Furthermore, some grading systems also include the local growth behavior. Whether or not a grading system is practicable depends upon its reproducibility and whether it can be correlated with the survival rates or other prognostic criteria. Within the systems proposed for the grading of prostatic carcinoma reproducibility can only partially be achieved.[4] Since the degree of subjective evaluation is quite large, every effort has to be made to introduce objective criteria into the grading by means of morphometric and cytophotometric techniques (see Chapters 23 and 25). Yet, these laboratory tests at present, are of limited use when applied to routine diagnosis. They are however, useful to examine and to more objectively reconfirm the basis for a grading system.[17] The Veterans Administration Cooperative Urological Research Group (VACURG) has proposed a system combining the histological degree of differentiation and clinical stage.[18] In this grading, however, the degree of cellular anaplasia is neglected and the subjective margins of its denomination seem extensive. Therefore, a simple and reproducible grading system, *combining differentiation and anaplasia* was proposed by Mostofi[15]:

Grade 1. The tumor forms glands lined by epithelial cells which show slight nuclear anaplasia.

Grade 2. The tumor forms glands lined by epithelial cells which show moderate nuclear anaplasia.

Grade 3. The tumor forms glands lined by cells which show marked nuclear anaplasia, or the tumor is undifferentiated (*i.e.* no glands are formed).

The cribriform pattern is not expressively included in this system. Yet, since these patterns are often closely correlated with the undifferentiated, solid carcinoma and with a poor prognosis, we propose to consider it as a *grade 3 carcinoma.* According to our classification, the highly or well differentiated adenocarcinoma corresponds to *grade 1 carcinoma.* The *grade 2 carcinoma* is a carcinoma with poor glandular differentiation and pronounced nuclear anaplasia: Poorly differentiated adenocarcinoma, or the combination of highly and poorly differentiated adenocarcinoma. *Grade 3 carcinomas* include cribriform and solid carcinomas and their combinations with marked nuclear anaplasia.

Böcking[17] also combined the histological growth pattern with the degree of nuclear anaplasia in his system. Four stages of the growth pattern are defined: (1) highly differentiated adenocarcinoma; (2) poorly differentiated adenocarcinoma; (3) cribriform carcinoma; and (4) solid-anaplastic carcinoma. This growth pattern is then combined with three degrees of nuclear anaplasia: 0, low nuclear anaplasia; 1, moderate nuclear anaplasia; 2, marked nuclear anaplasia. The final grade of malignancy of a prostatic carcinoma results from the numerical addition of its histological growth pattern and the grading figure of its nuclear anaplasia. The tumor is graded according to its component getting the highest score from the combined histological and cytological grading. The score *0–1* corresponds to the *grade I of malignancy, 2–3 to grade II*, and *more than 3* to *grade III of malignancy* (see tabulation given in the Editorial Comment). In total, this grading system corresponds to the one proposed by Mostofi[15] and includes our modifications. Mostofi[15] as well as Böcking[17] were able to show that the degree of malignancy correlates well with the patient's survival.

The degree of cell anaplasia and the ability or inability to form intact cell units can finally be estimated from the cytological slides of aspiration biopsies and thus can be introduced into a grading system (see Chapter 5). The success of such an approach depends upon the quality of the cytological preparation and the experience and skill of the cytologist; both factors are of utmost importance in obtaining good correlation between histologic and cytologic analysis.[19]

MORPHOLOGIC CRITERIA OF TUMOR REGRESSION

In regard to treatment the aid of the pathologist is limited to identify, characterize, and grade the therapeutic effects in cases treated by conservative means or radiotherapy. These tumors frequently show useful diagnostic and prognostic morphologic changes. The normal prostatic epithelium shows a different reaction: Focal squamous cell metaplasia after estrogen treatment, pronounced atrophy after orchiectomy or antiandrogenic treatment with cyproterone acetate, and atrophy and nuclear pleomorphism after radiotherapy. In contrast, both contrasexual hormone treatment with or without orchiectomy, as well as high voltage irradiation, result in rather similar cytologic alterations in therapy-sensitive carcinoma: Vacuolar swelling of the cytoplasm, nuclear vacuoles and pyknosis, and stromal edema with subsequent sclerosis (Figs. 6.9 and 6.10). Quite often individual therapy results in a significant quantitative reduction of the carcinoma. Altogether these quantitative and qualitative parameters can be used for histologic grading of treated carcinoma in order to specify success or failure of therapy by means of repeated biopsies, in intervals of 6 months to 1 year.[20–23] With respect to therapy-induced tumor regression,

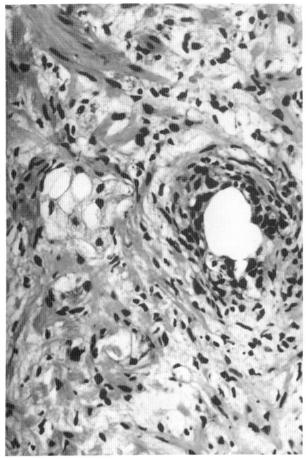

Figure 6.9 Undifferentiated prostatic carcinoma after local irradiation, with marked regression, vacuolar swelling of cytoplasm, pyknosis of nuclei, atrophy and pleomorphism of normal epithelium. (HE, ×400)

we use a scheme with a 10 point scale: The untreated tumor is given 10 points, the degree of regression is indicated by a substraction in 2-point decrements (Table 6.3).

In our experience prostatic carcinomas show a different reaction to conservative treatment. Up to now more than 300 patients with different types of prostatic carcinoma were followed clinically and by repeat punch biopsy. Fifteen percent of pure adenocarcinomas did not respond to hormonal therapy or showed only slight and focal regression, whereas 50% of pluriform and poorly differentiated tumors reacted in this way 1 year after diagnosis. In case of combined hormonal and irradiation treatment *all* adenocarcinomas demonstrated histological signs of regression with only 5% showing slight and focal regression. On the contrary, in 32% of the pluriform and poorly differentiated tumors there was no or insufficient response to treatment (see also Editorial Comment to Chapter 10).

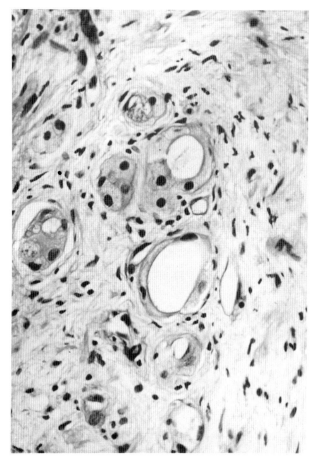

Figure 6.10 Estrogen-induced regression of poorly differentiated adenocarcinoma; few shrunken glands with pyknotic nuclei and vacuolated cytoplasm. (HE, ×400)

Table 6.3
Morphologic Criteria of Treated Prostatic Carcinoma for Grading of Tumor Regression (*Regression Grading*) in Biopsy Material

Grade 10	No regression
Grade 8	Tumor of great extension, only focal regression
Grade 6	Tumor of great extension, increased regression
Grade 4	Few tumor nests, increased regression
Grade 2	Minute shrunken cells, hardly recognizable as cancer
Grade 0	No tumor

INCIDENTAL AND LATENT CARCINOMA

Carcinoma of the prostate that is found at autopsy in patients dying from other diseases is called *latent* cancer.[12, 24] *Occult* carcinomas, on the other hand, are those with metastases detected before the primary tumor is discovered. In our unselected autopsy material latent carcinoma of the prostate is found in 36.4% of all men older than 45 years (Table 6.4). Beyond the age of 75 the incidence increases to 51.6% which is comparable to data reported by other investigators[25] as outlined in Chapter 2.

Extensive histologic studies of the entire prostate gland show that, with increasing age, there is not only an increase in the incidence of latent carcinoma, but also an increase in number and size of the individual tumor foci.[26] One third of all latent carcinomas at our institution were greater than 1 cm in diameter (Table 6.4). Small tumors are found with a constant incidence of about 11% in all age groups. Large latent carcinomas, however, are more frequent in areas where the morbidity and mortality of manifest prostatic cancer are high, as for example in Sweden, Germany, or Jamaica. They are rare in regions with a low morbidity and mortality, such as Singapore or Israel.[27] With advancing age and increasing tumor spread latent carcinomas tend to dedifferentiation and aggressive behavior. Latent carcinoma, like clinically manifest carcinoma, grows predominantly and usually as multifocal tumors in the outer gland. The inner parts of the gland become involved only when the tumor grows. Tumors with a primarily inner gland development occur in only 4% of latent carcinomas, this feature being comparable with manifest tumors.[27, 28] There is no predilection of the dorsal portion of the prostate, but the ventrolateral lobe shows the same tumor incidence.[29] In regard to morphology, highly differentiated pure adenocarcinoma predominates with 57.7% (Table 6.5). All other tumor types are observed as well, but their frequency is of no great importance.

Table 6.4
Latent Carcinoma of the Prostate (Institute of Pathology, Homburg/Saar, 1972-1975): Frequency, Age Prevalence and Tumor Size[a, b]

Age	n	Latent Carcinoma	Tumors $\phi > 1$ cm
45–54	43	8 (18.6%)	1
55–64	49	20 (40.8%)	6
65–74	50	19 (38.0%)	6
>75	31	16 (51.6%)	8
Total	173	63 (36.4%)	21 (33.3%)

[a] From G. Dhom.[29].

[b] Of the 173 autopsies performed, latent carcinoma was detected in 63 cases (36.4%); in 21 instances (33.3% of latent lesions) tumor extension was larger than 1 cm in diameter.

Table 6.5
Incidence of Highly Differentiated Pure Adenocarcinoma in the Various Tumor Classes[a]

Type of Tumor Detection	n (100%)	Highly Diff. Adenocarcinoma	
		n	%
Clinical prostatic carcinoma of the Registry (1972–75)	6,758	924	13.67
Incidental prostatic carcinoma	141	59	41.8
Latent prostatic carcinoma	116	67	57.7

[a] *German Prostate Cancer Registry*, Homburg/Saar, 1972–1975. From Ch. Hohbach and G. Dhom.[39]

An intermediate position between clinically manifest aggressive carcinoma and latent carcinoma is occupied by prostatic tumors that are discovered incidentally, usually in a specimen of transurethral resection performed for benign prostatic hyperplasia. These lesions are classified as *stage A* or *category* T_0 (UICC).[10, 30] They are designated as *incidental carcinomas.*[31, 32] Their incidence of 7% in the material of the *Registry* is somewhat lower than in other series.[33] Their age distribution is largely identical with that of manifest carcinoma[34] (Fig. 6.11).

In a previous analysis of 141 incidental carcinoma of the *Registry* we found quite variable morphologic patterns and considerable differences of the extension within the prostate.[32] Only 29.8% were true focal microcarcinoma occupying less than 10% of the tissue volume, whereas in 15.6% the entire BPH prostatectomy specimen was invaded by the exclusively pluriform and low differentiated tumor (Table 6.6). With regard to this, Jewett[10] suggested that we subdivide incidental carcinoma in *stage A_1* (microcancer) and *stage A_2* tumors (multifocal or diffuse incidental carcinomas). In the UICC staging system the multifocal A_2-tumor can only incorrectly be keyed a $T_{0(m)}$.[30] The proportionality between the degree of differentiation and local extension of the tumor evidently holds true not only for manifest prostatic carcinomas, but also for incidental carcino-

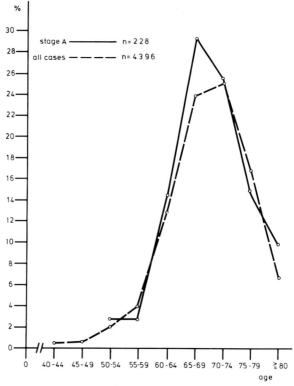

Figure 6.11 Age distribution of prostatic cancer (1972–1975) at the *German Prostate Cancer Registry,* Homburg (Saar). (Modified from Ch. Hohbach and G. Dhom.[39])

mas.[35] Accordingly, we found well differentiated pure adenocarcinomas predominantly among the true focal microcarcinomas. While in the total material of the *Registry* only 13% are pure (well differentiated) adenocarcinomas; the rate is 22% for stage B_1 and 41.8% for stage A (Table 6.5). The clinical course of incidental carcinoma is determined by the tumor type. Multifocal and/or poorly differentiated carcinoma have a poor prognosis,[33, 34, 36] whereas well differentiated tumors usually are locally defined lesions without a significant risk of cancer mortality.[35, 37, 38]

Grading of incidental carcinoma offers a morphological basis for clinical experience. This was demonstrated by us in a recent study of 78 cases of stage A tumors which were graded according to Mostofi.[15] Among the 35 A_1 tumors there were 29 (83%) G_1 carcinomas with low malignancy, only (17%) G_2 tumors, and no G_3 tumor. On the contrary, we found 23 (53.5%) G_2 and G_3 carcinomas in stage A_2 (Table 6.7). With regard to their clinical course, there is no doubt that the majority of stage A_1 tumors are slow growing carcinomas. We should consider them as potential latent carcinomas, which would have been diagnosed at autopsy if the patient would have died before his operation for benign hyperplasia of the prostate.

SUMMARY

Between 1972 and 1975 more than 13,000 prostate biopsies were recorded in the *German Prostate Cancer Registry*. Among these were 6,758 carcinomas. We distinguish in our classification between "ordinary" and

Table 6.6
Relative Volume (in %) of BPH Specimen Involved be Incidental Prostatic Carcinoma (Clinical Stage A, T_0, Respectively)[a]

	Cases	%
· Less than 10%	42	29.8
· More than 10%	68	48.2
· Total specimen involved	22	15.6
· Adequate assessment not possible	9	6.4
Total	141	100.0

[a] From G. Dhom and B. Hautumm.[32]

Table 6.7
Incidental Carcinoma of the Prostate (Stage A, T_0, Respectively), Histological Grading of 78 Cases (Institute of Pathology, Homburg/Saar, 1972–1975)

Grade	A_1 (T_0)		A_2 ($T_{0(m)}$)[a]		Total	
	n	%	n	%	n	%
G1	29	83	20	46.5	49	62.8
G2	6	17	14	32.6	20	25.6
G3			9	20.9	9	11.6
Total	35	44.9	43	55.1	78	100

[a] Pathologically determined multifocality.

"special" prostatic carcinomas. *Ordinary carcinomas* include four basic types: the highly and poorly differentiated adenocarcinoma, as well as the cribriform and undifferentiated solid carcinoma. Sixty-four percent are of uniform histologic pattern, while 54% are of pluriform differentiation with combinations of the various subtypes. *Special tumors* are endometrioid, urothelial, squamous cell, and mucous carcinomas. The prognosis of prostatic carcinoma is expressed by the *grade of malignancy*, which includes not only the histological differentiation of the tumor, but also the degree of anaplasia of the single tumor cell. It should be emphasized that criteria of grading must be *reproducible* and must correlate with the survival rate of the patients. Grading is not only confined to the prognostic assessment of the untreated carcinoma, but can also be applied to follow the course of the disease by biopsy control. Tumors which are sensitive to contrasexual therapy show a distinct morphologic pattern which allows a grading of the therapy-induced tumor regression. Of the patients recorded in the *Registry* 52% are between the age of 65 and 75, whereas 3.3% are younger than 55 years and thus, belong to the group of juvenile prostatic carcinoma. The latter show only minor differences in the distribution of their tumor stage, as compared to the majority of elderly men. In the older age group a predominance of the advanced stages B_2 to D, which are rapidly proliferating, usually pluriform in their architecture and portend a poor prognosis. All histologic features are found in the younger as well as in older men. Highly differentiated adenocarcinomas with low malignancy prevail in stage A (incidental carcinoma), which accounts for only 7% of our total material and in latent carcinomas, which are found in 36.4% of autopsies of men older than 45 years. The incidence, the number of tumor foci, and the extension of latent carcinomas in the prostate increases with age.

REFERENCES

1. Dhom, G. Differentialdiagnostische Probleme des Prostatacarcinoms (Erfahrungen mit dem Prostatacarcinom-Register). *Beitr. Pathol.* 153: 203, 1974.
2. Dhom, G., and Kopetzky, C. D. Ein Jahr Prostata-Carcinom-Register. *Urologe A 13*: 96, 1974.
3. Kastendieck, H. Cyto- and histomorphogenesis of the prostate carcinoma. A comparative light and electron-microscopic study. *Virchows Arch. Pathol. Anat. 370*: 207, 1976.
4. Kastendieck, H. Prostatic carcinoma, aspects of pathology, prognosis, and therapy. *J. Cancer Res. Clin. Oncol. 96*: 131, 1980.
5. Dhom, G., and Mohr, G. Urothel-Carcinome in der Prostata. *Urologe A 16*: 70, 1977.
6. Silber, J., and McGavren, M. H. Adenocarcinoma of the prostate in men less than 56 years old: a study of 65 cases. *J. Urol. 105*: 283, 1971.
7. Tjaden, H. B., Culp, D. A., and Flocks, R. H. Clinical adenocarcinoma of the prostate in patients under 50 years of age. *J. Urol. 93*: 618, 1965.
8. Byar, D. P., and Mostofi, F. K. Cancer of the prostate in men less than 50 years old: an analysis of 51 cases. *J. Urol. 102*: 726, 1969.
9. Johnson, D. E., Lanieri, J. P., Jr., and Ayala, A. G. Prostatic adenocarcinoma occurring in men under 50 years of age. *J. Surg. Oncol. 4*: 207, 1972.
10. Jewett, H. J. The present status of radical prostatectomy for stages A and B. *Urol. Clin. North Am. 2*: 105, 1975.
11. Byar, D. P., and Mostofi, F. K. Carcinoma of the prostate: prognostic evaluation of certain pathologic features in 208 radical prostatectomies. *Cancer 30*: 5, 1972.
12. Kastendieck, H. *Ultrastrukturpathologie der menschlichen Prostatadrüse.* Cyto- und Histomorphogenese von Atrophie, Hyperplasie, Metaplasie, Dysplasie und Carcinom.

Prog. Pathol., Vol. 106, edited by W. Büngeler, M. Eder, K. Lennert, G. Peters, W. Sandritter, and G. Seifert. Fischer Verlag, Stuttgart, 1977.

13. Schröder, F. H. Prostatic carcinoma—comments on radical surgical treatment. In *II. International Symposium on the Treatment of Carcinoma of the Prostate*, edited by A. Rost and U. Fiedler. Klinikum Steglitz, Berlin, 1980, p. 172.

14. Broders, A. C. Carcinoma, grading and practical application. *Arch. Pathol. 2*: 376, 1926.

15. Mostofi, F. K. Problems of grading carcinoma of prostate. *Semin. Oncol. 3*: 161, 1976.

16. Murphy, G. P., and Whitmore, W. F. A report of the workshops on the current status of the histologic grading of prostate cancer. *Cancer 44*: 1490, 1979.

17. Böcking, A. *Grading des Prostatakarzinoms.* Habilitationsschrift, Freiburg 1980.

18. Gleason, D. F., Mellinger, G. T., and the Veterans Administration Cooperative Urological Research Group. Prediction of prognosis for prostatic adenocarcinoma by combined histological grading and clinical staging. *J. Urol. 111*: 58, 1974.

19. Ackermann, R., and Müller, H. A. Retrospective analysis of 645 simultaneous perineal punch biopsies and transrectal aspiration biopsies for diagnosis of prostatic carcinoma. *Eur. Urol. 3*: 29, 1977.

20. Dhom, G. Classification and grading of prostatic carcinoma. *Tumors of the Male Genital System. Recent Results Cancer Res. 60*: 14, 1977.

21. Alken, C. E., Dhom, G., Straube, W., Braun, J. S., Kopper, B., and Rehker, H. Therapie des Prostata-Carcinoms und Verlaufskontrolle (II). *Urologe A 14*: 112, 1975.

22. Alken, C. E., Dhom, G., Kopper, B., Rehker, H., Dietz, R., Kopp, S., and Ziegler, M. Verlaufskontrolle nach Hochvolttherapie des Prostatacarcinoms. *Urologe A 16*: 272, 1977.

23. Jacobi, G. H., Kurth, K.-H. and Hohenfellner, R. Local high voltage radiotherapy with curative intent for prostatic carcinoma: report of a selected series. *Akt. Urol. 10*: 291, 1979.

24. Franks, L. M. Latent carcinoma of prostate. *J. Pathol. 68:* 603, 1954.

25. Schlenzka, R. Das latente Prostatakarzinom, Inauguraldissertation der Medizinischen Fakultät der Universität des Saarlandes, 1978.

26. Franks, L. M. Etiology and epidemiology of human prostatic disorders. In *Urologic Pathology: The Prostate*, edited by M. Tannenbaum. Lea & Febiger, Philadelphia, 1977, p. 23.

27. Breslow, N., Chan, C. W., Dhom, G., Drury, R. A. B., Franks, L. M., Gellei, B., Lee, Y. S., Lundberg, S., Sparke, B., Sternby, N. H., and Tulinius, H. Latent carcinoma of prostate at autopsy in seven areas. *Int. J. Cancer 20:* 680, 1977.

28. Kastendieck, H., Altenähr, E., Hüsselmann, H., and Bressel, M. Carcinoma and dysplastic lesions of the prostate. *Z. Krebsforsch. 38:* 33, 1976.

29. Dhom, G. Das Prostatakarzinom und die Bedeutung seiner Früherkennung. *Med. Unserer Zeit 5:* 134, 1978.

30. International Union against Cancer. *TNM Classification of Malignant Tumors*, 3rd. Ed. Springer Publ., Berlin, 1978..

31. Mostofi, F. K., and Price, E. B. Tumors of the male genital system. *Atlas of Tumor Pathology*, 2nd Ser. Fasc. 8. Armed Forces Institute of Pathology, Washington, D.C., 1973.

32. Dhom, G., and Hautumm, B. Die Morphologie des klinischen Stadiums 0 des Prostatakarzinoms (incidental carcinoma). *Urologe A 14:* 105, 1975.

33. Dias, R., Larengood, R. W., and Gaetz, H. P. Überlebenszeiten bei Patienten mit einem Prostatakarzinom, das zufällig bei der operativen Behandlung eines Prostataadenoms gefunden wurde. *Extracta Urol. 1:* 411, 1978.

34. Khalifa, N. M., and Jarman, W. D. Study of 48 cases of incidental carcinoma of prostate followed 10 years or longer. *J. Urol. 116:* 329, 1976.

35. Correa, R. J., Jr., Anderson, R. G., Gibbons, R. P., and Mason, J. T. Latent carcinoma of the prostate—why the controversy. *J. Urol. 111:* 644, 1974.

36. Golimbu, M., and Morales, P. Stage A_2 prostatic cancer. *Urology 13:* 592, 1979.

37. Montgomery, T. R., Whitlock, G. F., Nohlgren, J. E., and Lewis, A. M. What becomes of the patient with latent or occult carcinoma of the prostate. *J. Urol. 86:* 655, 1961.

38. Catalona, W. J., and Scott, W. W. Das Prostatakarzinom. *Extracta Urol. 1:* 317, 1978.

39. Hohbach, Ch., and Dhom, G. Pathology of prostate cancer. *Scand. J. Urol. Nephrol. Suppl. 55:* 37, 1980.

Editorial Comment to Chapter 6

During the preparation of this volume, a *German Pathological-Urological Study Group for Prostate Cancer* has completed a Grading System, which, in accordance with the endeavors of the WHO, combines histologic and cytologic criteria in a scoring system (Table 6.8), the latter being illustrated in Figure 6.12. This system results in *Grades I–III of malignancy*. It is hoped that, in the face of incomplete to poor reproducibility of the grading systems currently in widespread use (Murphy and Whitmore, 1979), this WHO system will gain wide application in the future.

The major problem, however, still remains that we must rely on biopsy material in the majority of cases, and that the grade obtained does not necessarily reflect that of the entire tumor (Figure 6.13).

G. H. J.
R. H.

Table 6.8
Combined Histological and Cytological Scoring System to Assess Grade of Malignancy of Prostate Cancer.[a]

Score Sum		Grade of Malignancy	
0–1		I	
2–3		II	
4–5		III	

Histological	Score	Cytological
Highly differentiated adenocarcinoma	0	
	0	Mild nuclear anaplasia
Poorly differentiated adenocarcinoma	1	
	1	Moderate nuclear anaplasia
Cribriform carcinoma	2	
	2	Marked nuclear anaplasia
Solid carcinoma	3	

[a] From H. -A. Müller *et al.*, 1980.

Grading Score

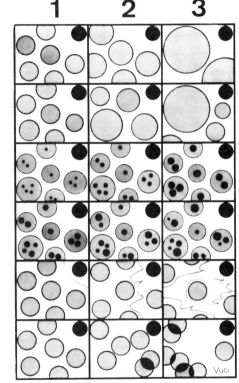

1. Nuclear Area

2. Variability
   of Nuclear Area

3. Nucleolar Size

4. Variability of
   Nucleolar Size

5. Dissociation
   of Cells

6. Regularity
   of Nuclear
   Arrangement

Figure 6.12 Cytological grading of prostate cancer: six cellular criteria of prognostic relevance are rated from 1 to 3 according to their derivation from normal; *black dot* on *right upper corner* represents size of erythrocyte for comparison; (Reproduced with permission from A. Böcking, 1981.)

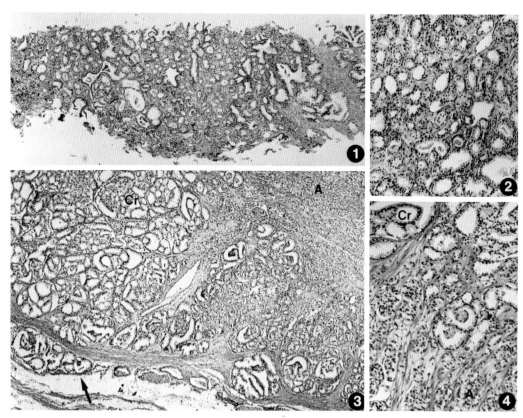

Figure 6.13 Marked discrepancy in grade of tumor differentiation in transrectal punch biopsy *versus* radical prostatectomy specimen: *1 and 2*, Uniform glandular carcinoma of high to moderate grade of differentiation in the biopsy specimen. *3 and 4*, Cribriform (*Cr*) and partially anaplastic (*A*) carcinoma in the prostatectomy specimen. (Reproduced with permission from H. Kastendieck, 1980.)

References

Böcking, A. Reproducible grading of prostatic carcinoma based on cytological criteria of malignancy. *Akt. Urol. 12:* 240, 1981.

Kastendieck, H. Morphologie des Prostatacarcinoms in Stanzbiopsien und totalen Prostatektomien. Untersuchungen zur Frage der Relevanz bioptischer Befundaussagen. *Pathologe, 2:* 31, 1980.

Müller, H.-A., Altenähr, E., Böcking, A., Dhom, G., Faul, P., Göttinger, H., Helpap, B., Hohbach, Ch., Kastendieck, H., and Leistenschneider, W. Über Klassifikation und Grading des Prostatacarcinoms. *Verh. Dtsch. Ges. Pathol. 64:* 609, 1980.

Murphy, G. P., Whitmore, W. F., Jr. A report of the workshops on the current status of histologic grading of prostate cancer. *Cancer 44:* 1490, 1979.

7

The TNM Classification of Prostatic Cancer and Activities of British Prostate Group

G. D. Chisholm, Ch.M., F.R.C.S., F.R.C.S.E.

STAGING METHODS IN PROSTATIC CANCER

Perhaps the most difficult problem that faces any oncologist is the virtual impossibility of determining the *exact* extent of either the primary tumor or the distant metastases. The difficulties are obvious: a clinical classification can never have the precision of a pathological classification, and ideally the latter requires an almost unlimited amount of tissue. A biopsy is mandatory for establishing the diagnosis and determining the cell grade, but a biopsy is usually only a piece of the tumor rather than the whole organ with the tumor. Thus, any attempt at classifying the extent of local spread from most biopsy material is limited. Even when a large piece of tissue or organ is available, the pathologist will select only certain areas to examine and only rarely examine the specimen by serial step sections.

Detecting distant metastases relies on methods that all have their limitations. Tumor markers in urological cancer such as α-fetoprotein, β-human chorionic gonadotropin, and serum acid phosphatase may all be helpful but may also be falsely negative.[1] The radioisotope bone scan is also valuable, yet no one would imply that it can detect micrometastases.[2] Invasive methods such as bone biopsies or lymph node biopsies are all liable to miss small or micrometastases.

Thus, a compromise must be made between the theoretical ideal, clinical practicality, and patient acceptance. Inevitably, several systems of tumor staging of prostatic cancer have evolved, and each has its proponents and each has certain merits. Attempts to achieve international acceptance have so far met with only limited success.

In 1956 Whitmore[3] described a system of staging which, in principle, has remained the main classification used in North America. In *stage A* the tumor is not palpable and is detected by microscopy of tissue removed for "prostatic obstruction." In *stage B* there is a palpable nodule localized within the gland and not deforming the outline of the gland. A *stage C* tumor is palpable within the gland and extends outside the gland and/or involves the seminal vesicles. In *stage D* the patient has distant metastases. This system of staging has achieved its deserved popularity because of its simplicity, but it is this very simplicity which hides problems of terminology for each stage. Thus, subdivisions have evolved and these are included in the legend to Figure 7.1.

In 1959, the *American Joint Committee for Cancer Staging and End-Results Reporting* recommended the same system of staging but advised the use of the Roman numerals I, II, III, IV.[4] This system was adopted by the *Veterans Administration Cooperative Urological Research Group* (VACURG) in their studies[5] and remains very similar to the original Whitmore recommendation.

The fact that the ABCD system has been modified illustrates the

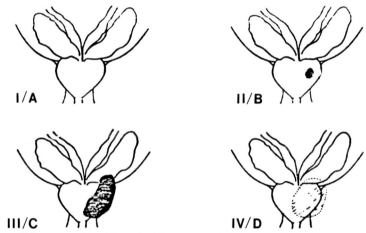

Figure 7.1 *Stage I/A*, No palpable tumor. Normal serum prostatic acid phosphatase. Bones and lymph nodes are negative, *i.e.* no distant metastases. A1$_F$, focal microscopic tumor. A1, microscopic tumor involving less than one lobe. A2, multifocal or diffuse microscopic involvement. *Stage II/B*, Palpable localized tumor "nodule". Normal serum prostatic acid phosphatase. Bones and lymph nodes are negative, *i.e.* no distant metastases. B1, tumor involving less than one lobe. B2, tumor involving all of one lobe or more. *Stage III/C*, Palpable tumor with local extension outside prostate. Normal serum prostatic acid phosphatase. Bones and lymph nodes negative, *i.e.* no distant metastases. C1, tumor less than 6 cm in diameter. C2, tumor greater than 6 cm in diameter. *Stage IV/D*, Tumor has distant dissemination to bones and/or lymph nodes, or serum prostatic acid phosphatase is raised. There may be any local findings in the prostate—from normal to extensive local spread. (Reproduced with permission from G. D. Chisholm.[2])

dilemma as to how much accuracy can be put into such a system and also recognizes that, in terms of clinical management, there are important differences between tumors of the same stage.

The *Tumor Node Metastases* (TNM) system for the classification of malignant tumors was developed by Denoix of France between the years 1943 and 1952 and subsequently adopted by the UICC (see Preface of UICC Publication, 1978). Basically, the three main symbols of the TNM system describe:

 T, the local extent of the primary tumor as determined by clinical and biopsy examination
 N, the clinical evidence of spread to the regional lymph nodes
 M, the presence of distant metastases including distant lymph nodes.

The UICC[6] concept of the TNM system was to have a tumor classification whose rules could be applied to almost all tumor sites combining accuracy with flexibility in use. Most staging systems include a variety of factors so that it is impossible to separate out those that are important in either treatment or prognosis, whereas the TNM system aimed to keep some of these factors identifiable. Wallace *et al.*[7] suggested that the TNM classification was similar to the *"appellation contrôlée"* as applied to French wines, *i.e.* a reliable description of the contents (or tumor). One further object of the TNM classification was to sharpen the distinction between a series of patients treated on the basis of a clinical assessment and a series treated by excisional surgery, where the extent of the tumor is more accurately known.

Inevitably there are some tumor sites where either parts or all of this system are difficult to apply. Thus, for example, the T category in renal carcinoma is virtually impossible to apply since determination of the primary tumor by palpation and even angiography are liable to significant errors.[8] Prostatic cancer was classified by the UICC in 1974 and revised in 1978; it is the intention of the UICC that the 1978 edition of the *"Livre de Poche"* should remain unchanged for at least 10 years unless "some major advance in diagnosis or treatment, relevant to a particular site, makes the current classification unrealistic."

TNM CLASSIFICATION FOR PROSTATE

Rules for Classification

The classification applies only to carcinoma. There should be histological verification of the disease, to permit division of cases by histological type. Any unconfirmed cases must be reported separately.

The following are the minimal requirements for assessment of the T, N, and M categories. If these cannot be met the symbol T_X, N_X, or M_X will be used.

 T categories Clinical examination, urography, endoscopy, and biopsy (if indicated), prior to definitive treatment.
 N categories Clinical examination and radiography including lymphography and urography.

M categories Clinical examination, radiography, skeletal studies, and relevant biochemical tests.

Regional and Juxtaregional Lymph Nodes

The regional lymph nodes are the pelvic nodes below the bifurcation of the common iliac arteries. The juxtaregional lymph nodes are the inguinal nodes, the common iliac nodes, and the para-aortic nodes.

TNM Pretreatment Clinical Classification

T: PRIMARY TUMOR (FIG. 7.2)

Tis Preinvasive carcinoma (carcinoma *in situ*).
T_0 No tumor palpable

Note: This category includes the incidental finding of carcinoma in an operative or biopsy specimen. Such cases should be assigned an appropriate pT category.

T_1 Tumor intracapsular surrounded by palpably normal gland
T_2 Tumor confined to the gland; smooth nodule deforming contour but lateral sulci and seminal vesicles not involved
T_3 Tumor extending beyond the capsule with or without involvement of the lateral sulci and/or seminal vesicles
T_4 Tumor fixed or infiltrating neighboring structures.

Note: The *suffix* (*m*) may be added to the appropriate T category to indicate multiple tumors, *e.g.* $T_{2(m)}$.

T_x The minimal requirements to assess the primary tumor cannot be met.

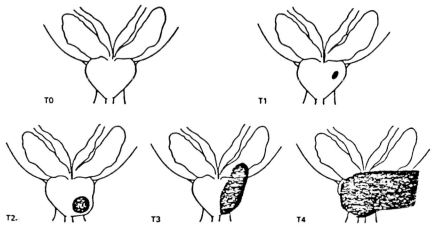

Figure 7.2 *Category T0,* No evidence of a primary tumor. *Category T1,* Tumor nodule in palpably normal gland. *Category T2,* Smooth nodule deforming contour of gland. *Category T3,* Tumor extending beyond capsule or into seminal vesicles. *Category T4,* Tumor fixed or invading neighboring structures. (Reproduced with permission from G. D. Chisholm.[2])

N: REGIONAL AND JUXTAREGIONAL LYMPH NODES

N_0 No evidence of regional lymph node involvement

N_1 Evidence of involvement of a single homolateral regional lymph node

N_2 Evidence of involvement of contralateral or bilateral or multiple regional lymph nodes

N_3 Evidence of involvement of fixed regional lymph nodes (there is a fixed mass on the pelvic wall with a free space between this and the tumor)

N_4 Evidence of involvement of juxtaregional lymph nodes

Note: If lymphography indicates extension to the juxtaregional lymph nodes, a scalene node biopsy is recommended.

N_X The minimal requirements to assess the regional and/or juxtaregional lymph nodes cannot be met.

M: DISTANT METASTASES

M_0 No evidence of distant metastases

M_1 Evidence of distant metastases

M_X The minimal requirements to assess the presence of distant metastases cannot be met.

pTNM Postsurgical Histopathological Classification

pT: PRIMARY TUMOR

pTis Preinvasive carcinoma (carcinoma *in situ*)

pT_0 No evidence of tumor found on histological examination of specimen

pT_1 Focal (single or multiple) carcinoma

pT_2 Diffuse carcinoma with or without extension to the capsule

pT_3 Carcinoma with invasion beyond the capsule and/or invasion of the seminal vesicles

pT_4 Tumor with invasion of adjacent organs

pT_X The extent of invasion cannot be assessed

G: HISTOPATHOLOGICAL GRADING

G_1 High degree of differentiation

G_2 Medium degree of differentiation

G_3 Low degree of differentiation or undifferentiated

G_X Grade cannot be assessed

pN: REGIONAL AND JUXTAREGIONAL LYMPH NODES

The pN categories correspond to the N categories.

pM: DISTANT METASTASES

The pM categories correspond to the M categories.

Stage Grouping

No stage grouping is at present recommended.

Summary for Prostate

T_0 Incidental carcinoma
T_1 Intracapsular/normal gland
T_2 Intracapsular/deformed gland
T_3 Extension beyond capsule
T_4 Extension fixed to neighboring organs
N_1 Single homolateral regional
N_2 Contra- or bilateral/multiple regional
N_3 Fixed regional
N_4 Juxtaregional.

APPRAISAL OF TNM IN PROSTATIC CANCER

T-Category

Just as there is concern over the nonuniformity of stage A[9] so there must be doubt about the range of pathology that is included in the T_0 (and pT_0) category. The lack of uniformity in the Whitmore stage A can be accommodated using $A1_F$ focal microscopic tumor, A_1, microscopic tumor involving less than one lobe, and A_2, multifocal or diffuse microscopic involvement, but the TNM system has only the sole expression of T_0. Most urologists would agree that an incidentally diagnosed low grade focal tumor must be separated from a multifocal or diffuse high grade tumor, in terms of management. Thus, T_0 will require to be subdivided in any future revision of this category.

It is of interest to note that group A or T_0 is an increasing proportion of patients presenting with carcinoma of the prostate. In a recent review of 100 patients seen by my department, 23% were T_0, 1% T_1, 13% T_2, 52% T_3, and 11% T_4. This trend has been observed by others and Donohue et al.[10] reported an incidence of 37% stage A tumors. Thus, an exact description of tumors within this group has become of even greater importance since the choice of no treatment or radical radiotherapy/surgery must be based on a more detailed description of these tumors.

The remaining T categories (as well as B and C tumors) notoriously understage the exact extent of the tumor, and most series reporting radical prostatectomy illustrate how a precise stage can only be achieved by histological examination of an adequate specimen. This statement could be challenged by those who use rectal ultrasound to delineate the prostate, and it is already evident that this technique provides a much more accurate assessment of invasion of the capsule than any other method clinically available.[11]

It might be pertinent to ask how important is it to have such precision in local tumor staging. The answer is that it is essential for those urologists who prefer radical excision for early stage disease; it is important also for the correct analysis of data in a clinical trial. It must be conceded that precision in tumor staging is not essential when the primary local treatment is external radiotherapy and is only of academic interest for the patient who already has metastatic disease (Chapter 3).

N-Category

In the TNM system metastases to lymph nodes (N) are separated from metastases elsewhere (M) to emphasize the important role that lymph node involvement has in the management and prognosis of so many tumors. The minimal requirements for N category include lymphography, but regrettably this investigation has proved so unreliable (for both false positive and false negative rates) that most clinicians would recommend abandoning this test.[2]

Surgical staging of the prostate by pelvic lymph node dissection has become increasingly popular, especially by those who advocate primary treatment using interstitial ^{125}I-treatment; the node dissection can then be carried out at the same time as the interstitial implantation.[12] Surgical staging as a preliminary to a radical prostatectomy is usually a separate procedure, since the favored approach to the prostate is via a perineal incision. As a result of these procedures there are now many reports of the strong correlation between tumor size and the incidence of positive (pelvic) lymph nodes.[2]

There remain several aspects to surgical staging which further emphasize why this procedure should remain special center-orientated and not introduced into the TNM requirements: a) The operative technique of pelvic lymphadenectomy is variable: it can range from a full dissection of all nodes associated with the iliac vessels, to a selected "plucking" of nodes that *appear* suspicious. The morbidity from the former is considerable while the inaccuracy of the latter should be self-evident and calls into question the description of this limited operation as a staging procedure. Furthermore, even pathologists are uncertain as to how many blocks should be made from these specimens and few pathologists are likely to carry out routine step sections of all material submitted. All of these problems were experienced by the author in a study of 40 patients undergoing pelvic lymphadenectomy[13] and recently emphasized by the Stanford University Group who, on the basis of their complication rate (46%), stated that "pelvic lymphadenectomy is not an entirely benign procedure."[14]

Lymph node dissection for staging can be justified only if the information will *directly* affect the choice of treatment. Thus, a radical excision of the prostate must be preceded by such a staging procedure, but if external radiotherapy is the preferred treatment, then lymph node status *per se* will have little or no influence on the treatment, though obviously the long-term results would be variable.

It must be accepted that by not assessing the lymph node status, much of the accuracy claimed for the TNM system will be lost. However, with increasing use of external radiotherapy for localized (M_0) tumors, this would seem to be an example where consideration for the patient out-weighs the ideal of maximal precision in all tumor staging.

M-Category

In contrast to the problems of obtaining a reliable N category, the M category in prostatic cancer appears to be a great deal easier, even though the reliability of the methods can generate debate.

It is the role of this category in carcinoma of the prostate that illustrates how the TNM system is more descriptive than the (Whitmore) ABCD system. For example, using T and M categories it is possible to determine the proportion of early and late tumors with metastases. In a current review of new patients attending my Prostate (cancer) Clinic, 32% of my patients with T_0-T_1, and 61% of T_2, T_3, and T_4 tumors had metastatic disease at the time of presentation.

The minimal requirements for the M category are clinical examination, radiography, skeletal studies, and relevant biochemical tests. Substantial advances have been made in the use of radioisotope bone scans for studying prostatic cancer to the extent that this test has earned the title of a tumor marker; it is a better screening test for metastases than the routine skeletal survey, and it is a better monitor of the progress of the disease than routine methods determining acid and alkaline phosphatases.[15, 16]

The phrase *"relevant biochemical tests"* in the TNM classification is used in hopeful anticipation of a more precise tumor marker than the serum acid phosphatase as measured by standard enzymatic methods. The hope that radioimmunoassay (RIA) methods will add precision to this marker must await the efforts of many centers currently evaluating this technique (see Chapter 8). It is already evident that RIA is a more sensitive method, but the exact relevance in clinical practice has yet to be determined. Other methods such as counterimmunoelectrophoresis have also been developed, but their role in clinical practice has also to be determined.

Other methods to improve the accuracy of the M category in carcinoma of the prostate (*e.g.* bone marrow acid phosphatase) have proved to be a disappointment so that, at present, this category will continue to rely on good quality bone scanning and the serum acid phosphatase. Other tumor markers such as CEA, tumor-associated antigens, polyamines, α1-acid glycoprotein and haptoglobin have all been studied, but none has been shown to be of particular use as a marker for diagnosing prostatic cancer. Hydroxyproline may be of value in monitoring the patient with metastatic carcinoma of the prostate.[17]

It must be concluded that the methods currently available for diagnosing and monitoring carcinoma of the prostate are not ideal. Nevertheless, until newer methods are fully evaluated, the clinician must continue to rely on this limited armamentarium. It is not acceptable to criticize the deficiencies of this armamentarium, instead we should aim to use those methods that are available to their best advantage. The TNM classification can only evolve into a wholly acceptable system by the determined efforts of those urologists and scientists who are making a special study of this tumor.

THE BRITISH PROSTATE GROUP

In November 1973, a group of urologists and scientists interested in both clinical and basic investigation of the prostate gland met at the *Tenovus Institute for Cancer Research*, Cardiff, to discuss their mutual problems. Since then this group has met biannually and has attracted a number of persons with a common interest in this gland. Apart from revealing that the prostate was still a little understood gland it was soon evident that urologists in the United Kingdom were not in unison over more simple matters, such as recording their clinical data on prostatic cancer. Thus, the documentation of data and the development of uniform staging and response criteria for this tumor has been a major interest of this group. This small prostate study group has now grown to become the *British Prostate Group* which, in 1980, became organized as a society for the presentation and discussion of any clinical and investigative work relating to the prostate gland.

Specific activities of this group have included:
1. The development of a standardized pro forma for the documentation of patients with carcinoma of the prostate
2. A review of bone scanning equipment and techniques available in major hospitals in the United Kingdom
3. A study of the behavior of a group of hormones in patients receiving various treatments for carcinoma of the prostate. This work has been published.[18]
4. A multicenter clinical trial to compare cyproterone acetate, diethylstilbestrol, and orchiectomy in patients presenting with metastatic carcinoma of the prostate. It is expected that the result of this trial will be reported in 1982.
5. An appraisal of the "criteria of response" in carcinoma of the prostate[16]
6. Collaboration in clinical trials sponsored by the European Organization for Research and Treatment of Cancer (EORTC) and the Medical Research Council (MRC).

As a result of these activities it is believed that there has been an important reappraisal of the diagnosis and management of carcinoma of the prostate in the United Kingdom. It is anticipated that the group will remain a national forum for discussion of all aspects of prostatic disease.

REFERENCES

1. Wahren, B. Tumour markers in urology: aids in cancer diagnosis and management. *Urol. Res. 7:* 57, 1979.
2. Chisholm, G. D. Urological malignancy: prostate. In *Tutorials in Postgraduate Medicine: Urology*, edited by G. D. Chisholm. Heinemann Medical, London, 1980, Ch. 15, p. 223.
3. Whitmore, W. F., Jr. Hormone therapy in prostatic cancer. *Am. J. Med. 21:* 697, 1956.
4. Jewett, H. J. The present status of radical prostatectomy for stages A and B prostatic cancer. *Urol. Clin. North Am. 2:* 105, 1975.

5. Byar, D. P. VACURG studies on prostatic cancer and its treatment. In *Urologic Pathology: The Prostate*, edited by M. Tannenbaum. Lea & Febiger, New York, 1977, Ch. 13, p. 241.
6. U.I.C.C. *TNM Classification of Malignant Tumors, Third edition.* International Union against Cancer, Geneva, 1978.
7. Wallace, D. M., Chisholm, G. D., and Hendry, W. F. TNM classification for urological tumors (UICC)—1974. *Br. J. Urol. 47:* 1, 1975.
8. Das, G., Chisholm, G. D., and Sherwood, T. Can angiography stage renal carcinoma? *Br. J. Urol. 49:* 611, 1977.
9. Golimbu, M., and Morales, P. Stage A₂ prostatic carcinoma: should staging system be reclassified. *Urology 13:* 592, 1979.
10. Donohue, R. E., Fauver, H. E., Whitesel, J. A., and Pfister, R. R. Staging prostatic cancer: a different distribution. *J. Urol. 122:* 327, 1979.
11. Peeling, W. B., Griffiths, G. J., Evans, K. T., and Roberts, E. D. Diagnosis and staging of prostatic cancer by transrectal ultrasonography. A preliminary study. *Br. J. Urol. 51:* 565, 1979.
12. Barzell, W., Bean, M. A., Hilaris, B. S., and Whitmore, W. F., Jr. Prostatic adenocarcinoma: relationship of grade and local extent to the pattern of metastases. *J. Urol. 118:* 278, 1977.
13. O'Donoghue, E. P. N., Shridhar, P., Sherwood, T., Williams, J. P., and Chisholm, G. D. Lymphography and pelvic lymphadenectomy in carcinoma of the prostate. *Br. J. Urol. 48:* 689, 1976.
14. Freiha, F. S., Pistenma, D. A., and Bagshaw, M. A. Pelvic lymphadenectomy for staging prostatic carcinoma: is it always necessary? *J. Urol. 122:* 176, 1979.
15. Fitzpatrick, J. M., Constable, A. R., Sherwood, T., Stephenson, J. J., Chisholm, G. D., and O'Donoghue, E. P. N. Serial bone scanning: the assessment of treatment response in carcinoma of the prostate. *Br. J. Urol. 50:* 555, 1978.
16. Chisholm, G. D. Carcinoma of the prostate: perspectives and prospects. In *Prostate Cancer—Recent Results in Cancer Research*, edited by W. Duncan. Springer Verlag, Berlin, 1981, pp. 173–184.
17. Mundy, A. R. Urinary hydroxyproline excretion in carcinoma of the prostate. A comparison of 4 different modes of assessment and its role as a marker. *Br. J. Urol. 51:* 570, 1979.
18. British Prostate Study Group. Evaluation of plasma hormone concentrations in relation to clinical staging in patients with prostatic cancer. *Br. J. Urol. 51:* 382, 1979.

Editorial Comment to Chapter 7

As mentioned in *Chapter 3*, the American staging system(s) and the TNM classification of prostate cancer are not readily interconvertible, although this is frequently done in the literature in order to compare therapy results from institution to institution. Unfortunately, nature has

Table 7.1
Opposition of the American Staging System *versus* the Newest Version of the TNM Classification of the UICC (1978)[a]

American Urological System (A–D)	Tumor-*N*odes-*M*etastases System (TNM)
Stage A: incidental finding	*Category $T_0 N_0 N_0$:* No tumor palpable
A_1 Focal	T_0 Focal or diffuse
A_2 Diffuse	
Stage B: confined to prostate	*Categories $T_{1+2} N_0 M_0$*
B_1 Small, discrete nodule	T_1 Tumor intracapsular, surrounded by normal gland
B_2 Large or multiple nodules or areas	T_2 Tumor confined to gland, smooth nodule deforming contour
Stage C: localized to periprostatic area	*Categories $T_{3+4} N_0 M_0$*
C_1 No involvement of seminal vesicles; <70 gm	T_3 Tumor beyond capsule, with or without involvement of seminal vesicles or lateral sulci or both
C_2 Involvement of seminal vesicles; >70 gm	T_4 Tumor fixed or invading adjacent structures
Stage D: metastatic disease	*Categories $T_{0-4} N_{1-4} M_0$ or $T_{0-4} N_{0-4} M_1$*
D_1 Pelvic lymph node metastases or ureteral obstruction causing hydronephrosis	N_{1-3} Regional lymph node metastases
D_2 Bone or distant lymph node or organ or soft tissue metastases	M_1 Distant metastases
	N_4 Juxtaregional lymph node metastases

[a] Modified from G. P. Murphy *et al.*, 1980.

not made things so simple that I or A = T_0, II or B = T_{1-2}, III or C = T_3, and IV or D = T_4, so that many attempts have been made to come to a consensus in the hodge podge of what some call *stages*, others *classifications*, and still others *categories*.

We feel that the proposal of Murphy and co-workers (1980) with a further slight modification by us, as given in Table 7.1, offers the best solution to the problem.

G.H.J.
R. H.

Reference

Murphy, G. P., Gaeta, J. F., Pickren, J., and Wajsman, Z. Current status of classification and staging of prostate cancer. *Cancer 45:* 1889, 1980.

8

Serum and Bone Marrow Acid Phosphatase as a Diagnostic Marker in Prostatic Carcinoma Patients

W. Prellwitz, M.D.
W. Ehrenthal, M.D.

INTRODUCTION

The acid phosphatases (orthophosphoric monoester phosphohydrolase, E.C. 3.1.3.2.) hydrolyze esters of orthophosphoric acid at acidic pH. The pH optimum varies with the source of the enzyme and the substrate used for the measurement of the enzyme activity.[7] Acid phosphatases are widely distributed in all human body fluids and tissues.[3, 46, 60, 110] Enzyme activity is present in serum, erythrocytes, platelets, leukocytes, spleen, liver, kidney, and bone, mostly in the osteoclasts.

The introduction of a lysosomal concept by de Duve[30] was a great impetus to study acid phosphatases activity in the subcellular fractions of cells and tissues. Studies with new biochemical and immunological techniques indicate that much of the acid phosphatase activity in cells is of lysosomal origin. Most of the above-mentioned tissues contain two or more molecular variants (isoenzymes) of the acid phosphatase.[7, 36, 60, 113] Some of these acid phosphatases are organ-specific, cell-specific, or subcellular organelle-specific.[1, 3, 34, 62, 96]

In prostate the enzyme activity is more than 1000 times higher than in other human organs.[45, 110] The so-called prostatic acid phosphatase is heterogenous in nature and composed of at least two isozymes both with multiple subforms.[2, 99] Much of the enzyme is localized in the glandular epithelium and in the secretions of glandular lumina.

The knowledge of the metabolic functions of the acid phosphatases is limited. In the prostatic cells they do not have a major metabolic role. Extracellulary, however, in prostatic fluid, the phosphates are concerned with the activity of spermatozoa, supplying organic phosphate and catalyzing the transfer of the phosphate group.[2, 7, 98]

ENZYME ASSAY

The activity of acid phosphatases, determined in serum or plasma of healthy subjects comes predominantly from platelets and from erythrocytes and usually not from the prostate.[7, 116, 117]

Discrimination of Tissue Acid Phosphatase Using Different Substrates and Inhibitors

Various investigators studied the importance of substrate specificity to discriminate acid phosphatase of different origin.[2, 7, 31, 33, 59, 60, 65, 89, 93, 98, 110, 113] The following substrates were used: phenylphosphate, p-nitrophenylphosphate, β-glycerophosphate, α-naphthylphosphate, β-naphthylphosphate, phenolphthalein-phosphate and thymolphthaleinphosphate. Table 8.1 shows that the selection of an appropriate substrate to discriminate different acid phosphatases is difficult. The relative activities of different human acid phosphatase isozymes measured with various substrates are demonstrated in Table 8.2.[93, 100]

Most substrates are sensitive to nonprostatic acid phosphatases in serum. Therefore, clinical testing contradicts the use of a specific substrate

Table 8.1
Substrate and Inhibitor Specificity of Acid Phosphatases of the Various Sources[a]

Substrate	Erythro-cytes	Platelets	Prostate	Spleen	Liver	Bone (Osteo-clasts)
Phenylphosphate	(+)	(+)	+	(+)	(+)	(+)
p-Nitrophenylphos-phate	+	+	+	+	+	+
β-Glycerophosphate	(+)	(+)	+	(+)	(+)	(+)
α-Naphthylphosphate	−	(+)	+	+	(+)	+
β-Naphthylphosphate	(+)	(+)	+	+	(+)	+
Phenolphthalein phosphate	(+)	(+)	+	?	?	?
Thymolphthalein phosphate	(+)	(+)	+	?	?	?
Tartrate inhibition	−	+	+	+	+	−

[a] +, determination or inhibition of the listed tissue acid phosphatase; (+), reduced determination or inhibition of the listed tissue acid phosphatase; −, no determination or no inhibition of the listed tissue acid phosphatase; ?, no investigation.

Table 8.2
Relative Activities of Various Human Acid Phosphatase Isoenzymes as Measured with Substrates[a,b]

Source	PP	PMP	NP	PNPP	GP
Prostate	2.7	1.8	3.7	2.8	3.0
Erythrocyte I	10,000	20,700	13.5	41,600	14,200
Erythrocyte II	17,300	25,300	275	30,400	12,200
Erythrocyte III	7,250	9,670	211	12,300	10,500
Liver I	8.9	1.3	4.5	11.8	14.6
Liver II	4.7	3.2	8.1	9.7	11.0
Liver III	7.0	2.8	3.5	10.1	12.6
Bone	10.2	1.9	4.0	15.2	68.2
Kidney I	8.7	1.6	2.5	12.7	16.4
Kidney II	2.9	2.1	4.1	4.0	4.4
Kidney III	3.6	2.4	4.3	4.3	5.2
Urine	3.4	1.9	4.6	3.7	4.8
Platelets	16.1	5.2	5.5	54.3	19.0

[a] From A. V. Roy et al.[93] and R. M. Townsend.[100]

[b] Values represent activities relative to sodium thymolphthalein monophosphate taken as reference. PP, phenylphosphate; PMP, phenolphthalein monophosphate; NP, α-naphthol phosphate; PNPP, p-nitrophenylphosphate; GP, β-glycerophosphate.

in the analysis of prostatic acid phosphatase. For this reason it was looked for inhibitors to achieve a more specific measurement of the prostatic acid phosphatases activity in serum. Magnesium, calcium, chromium, cobalt, manganese, nickel, zinc, copper, and formaldehyde exhibited variable inhibitory effects on both red cell and prostatic acid phosphatases. Fluoride is a powerful inhibitor of acid phosphatases, particularly of the prostatic isoenzyme. Heparin as well also inhibits the prostatic acid phosphatase.[2, 7, 33, 47, 82, 110, 112]

Today, only the L(+) form of tartrate is commonly used. L(+)-tartrate inhibits about 95% of the activity of prostatic acid phosphatase, whereas the acid phosphatase from the erythrocytes remains relatively unaffected.[33] However, acid phosphatases from platelets, kidney, liver, and spleen are also 70 to 85% tartrate-inhibitable. Therefore, it is not correct to define the tartrate-labile fraction of acid phosphatases as a specific prostatic acid phosphatase.

From the lack of specificity for both substrates and inhibitors two conclusions should be drawn concerning the interpretation of increased enzyme activities of acid phosphatases in serum:

1. False positive activities are observed if acid phosphatases from erythrocytes (hemolysis!) or platelets are released into serum during blood clotting.[62, 116, 117]
2. Beside lysis of erythrocytes and platelets falsely elevated levels may be obtained since a large number of diseases are well known with augmented activity of acid phosphatases in serum (Table 8.3).[49, 65, 98]

In spite of the mentioned difficulties to discriminate the isoenzymes, the measurement of acid phosphatase activity is still the most frequently practiced biochemical investigation in cases in which prostatic carcinoma

Table 8.3
Nonprostatic Diseases with Possible Serum Acid Phosphatase Elevation[a]

Bone
   Osteogenic sarcoma (10%)
   Metastatic carcinoma (19%)
   Paget's disease (21%)
   Osteoporosis (4%)
   Osteogenesis imperfecta
   Hyperparathyroidism (33%)
   Multiple myeloma
Reticuloendothelial system
   Gaucher's disease
   Niemann-Pick's disease
   Hodgkin's disease
   Reticulum cell sarcoma
   Eosinophilic granuloma
Liver
   Viral hepatitis
   Drug-induced hepatitis
   Extrahepatic obstruction
   Cirrhosis
   Metastatic carcinoma (2%)
Kidney
   Acute renal failure
   Chronic renal failure
Hematologic and thromboembolic diseases
   Thrombocytosis
   Polycythemia
   Chronic granulocytic leukemia
   Chronic lymphocytic leukemia
   Acute lymphoblastic or granulocytic leukemia
   Thrombosis

[a] From T. Y. Lung[65] and T. M. Sodeman and J. G. Batsakis.[98]

is suspected. Most frequently the substrate *p*-nitrophenylphosphate and the inhibitor L(+)-tartrate are used.

Stability of Serum Acid Phosphatases Activity

A standard method to determine the activity of acid phosphatase in serum does not exist.

Of all enzymes measured in the clinical laboratory, the acid phosphatases suffer the most from instability. Well known factors which cause loss of activity are pH, temperature at storage, and the acidity of the test substrates. Of these three factors pH is the most critical and temperature the least important.[7, 27, 89] Due to these variables and to various poorly defined endogenous inhibitors it has not been possible to develop a standard method to measure enzyme activity of acid phosphatases in serum. The activity is not influenced if serum samples are kept at $-20°$ for 2 or 3 months. If serum is separated from the clot and kept at room temperature (25°C) enzyme activity decreases considerably within 1 or 2 hours due to an increase of pH by loss of carbon dioxide. The activity of acid phosphatases in serum is better preserved at room temperature if clot and serum are not separated. Comparing separated serum with clot/serum samples under the same test conditions, serum manifests a 14 to 50% greater loss of activity. The reason for this phenomenon is the release of acid phosphatases from erythrocytes and platelets into serum. Therefore, hemolytic serum should not be used for enzyme activity determination, and with fresh citrate plasma the release of enzyme activity from platelets during blood clotting can be reduced.[65, 89]

The best method to preserve acid phosphatase activity is to buffer serum or plasma at pH 6.0 (1 ml serum + 20 μl 10% acetic acid or citric acid) at room temperature (25°C). The activity is then stable for about 24 hours and at 4°C for up to 3 days.

Normal Values

Enzyme activity in serum flucutates considerably with age.[57, 89] In the newborn, total enzyme activity is two to four times higher than in the adult. The activity decreased slightly in the first weeks of life, remains elevated up to the age of 14, declines gradually to normal adult activity by the age of 17, and then remains stationary throughout adulthood (Table 8.4).

Normal ranges of activity for adults depend on the substrates used (Table 8.5). Therefore, in the literature very much differing normal values are described. This fact severely compromises comparison of published data. Total and tartrate-labile activity of acid phosphatase in serum of normal adult males and females are not significantly different.[65, 89]

In plasma the activity is much lower than in serum.[89]

Plasma: Total activity, 5.08 ± 3.5 units/liter.
Serum: Total activity, 9.15 ± 4.4 units/liter.
Plasma: Tartrate-labile activity, 0.32 ± 0.65 units/liter.
Serum: Tartrate-labile activity, 1.84 ± 1.80 units/liter.

The acid phosphatase activity in serum of normal subjects does not appear to have a circadian rhythm. This is in contrast to the well-known and definite diurnal pattern exhibited by patients with prostatic carcinoma.[2, 98]

Table 8.4
Normal Ranges of Serum Activity of Acid Phosphatases in Childhood and Adolescence[a]

Age	Normal Range (units/liter)	Substrate
Newborn	10–58	*p*-Nitrophenylphosphate
Up to 6 mo	11–45	
6–12 mo	11–35	
2–9 yr	10–29	
10–14 yr	10–27	
15 yr	11–22	

[a] From E. Kraus and F. C. Sitzmann.[57]

Table 8.5
Normal Ranges of Activity of Total and Tartrate-Labile Acid Phosphatases in Serum

Total Activity	Tartrate-Labile Phosphatase Activity	Substrate	Literature
4.5–14 units/liter	0–4 units/liter	p-Nitrophenylphosphate	Own results
0.5–5.0 King-Armstrong units/dl	0–0.5 King-Armstrong units/dl	Phenylphosphate	Fishman et al.[33]
1.0–2.0 King-Armstrong units/dl	0.1–0.35 King-Armstrong units/dl	Phenylphosphate	Cook et al.[22]
1.2–2.5 King-Armstrong units/dl	0–0.6 King-Armstrong units/dl	Phenylphosphate	Murphy et al.[77]
1–2.5 units/ml		α-Naphthylphosphate	Bruce et al.[10]
0.9–1.0 Bodansky units/dl		β-Glycerophosphate	
1–2.1 units/ml		Thymolphthalein monophosphate	
0–3 units/liter		α-Naphthylphosphate	Boehme et al.[8]
0.13–0.63 units/liter		p-Nitrophenylphosphate	
0.26–0.57 units/liter		Thymolphthalein monophosphate	
0–0.8 units/liter		Thymolphthalein monophosphate	Pontes et al.[85]
1.1–1.9 Bodansky units/dl		β-Glycerophosphate	
1–3 units/liter		α-Naphthylphosphate	Khan et al.[54]
0.20–0.9 units/liter		Thymolphthalein monophosphate	Little et al.[63]

Serum Activity after Prostate Massage or Rectal Examination

An important question concerning the interpretation of elevated serum activity is whether massage of the prostate during a rectal examination leads to an increase of serum activity of acid phosphatases. Marberger[68] and Sodeman and Batsakis[98] reported an increase of activity in serum of patients with benign hyperplasia as well as with carcinoma (Table 8.6). In contrast with these findings, Johnson et al.[53] did not observe elevated activity of tartrate-labile acid phosphatases after rectal examination and massage of the prostate.

To interpret serum activity correctly, the determination in serum should be performed not before 48 hours after the manipulation.

Activity of Acid Phosphatases in Serum of Patients with Prostatic Cancer

In 1938 Gutman and Gutman[44] first described the increase of activity of acid phosphatases in serum of patients with prostatic carcinoma.

Table 8.6
**Effect of Prostatic Massage or Rectal Examination on the Serum Activity of
Acid Phosphatases 24 Hours after the Manipulation**[a]

	Patients (N = 296)		
	Normal	Prostatic Carcinoma	Prostatic Hyperplasia
Total (N)	98	25	173
No change	54%	48%	70%
Elevated	46%	48%	30%
Decreased	0	4%	0

[a] From H. Marberger[68] and T. M. Sodeman and J. G. Batsakis.[98]

Fishman et al.,[33] Mathes et al.,[77] and Murphy et al.[77] then introduced the
method to determine the tartrate-labile phosphatases, which cannot be
designated to represent true prostatic acid phosphatases.

A large number of reports have been published concerning the clinical
significance of acid phosphatase activity measurements in serum of pa-
tients with carcinoma of the prostate.[2, 5-7, 9-12, 18, 19, 22, 31, 33, 40, 41, 44, 47, 48, 52, 58-
62, 65, 70, 73, 76, 77, 79-81, 87, 88, 93-95, 98, 100, 108, 110, 113] Summarizing these results, the
ranges of increased enzyme activity of total phosphatases and the tartrate-
labile acid phosphatases are demonstrated in Table 8.7.

According to these reports the determination of tartrate-labile acid
phosphatase activity in serum seems not to be more specific or sensitive
than the determination of total activity. In Table 8.8 the data of eight
investigators are recorded. In the serum of 1504 patients without and 894
patients with metastases (soft tissue, lymphatic and bony), the activity of
the total and tartrate-labile acid phosphatases was determined in parallel.
The results vary from report to report.

Braun et al.[9] and Fishman et al.[33] did not observe a difference between
total and tartrate-labile enzyme activity. Cook et al.,[22] Mathes et al.,[70] and
Nobles et al.[81] found higher percentages of increased tartrate-labile acid
phosphatase activity compared with total activity in serum of patients
without as well as in serum of patients with metastases, while Murphy et
al.[77] published contrary results.

If patients are divided in groups with carcinoma confined to prostate,
carcinoma with metastases of soft tissue or lymph nodes, and with bony
metastases (Table 8.9), the percentage of increased activity of acid phosphatase in serum of the last group of patients is significantly higher than
in the other groups. Cook et al.,[22] London et al.,[64] and Fishman et al.[33]
described patients with prostatic cancer and normal total activity and
increased tartrate-labile enzyme activity.

Townsend[100] investigated the sensitivity, specificity, and the predictive
values to distinguish metastatic from nonmetastatic carcinoma (Table
8.10). The tartrate-labile assay for acid phosphatases provides slightly
more specific information at the cost of sensitivity.

Johnson et al.[52] and Nesbit et al.[79] observed the relationship between
elevated serum activities of total acid phosphatases and survival of patients
with prostatic carcinoma. The 3-year survival rate was 66% in patients
without metastases if on first admission the acid phosphatases in serum

Table 8.7
Elevated Serum Activity of Acid Phosphatases and Tartrate-Labile
Phosphatases (Ranges of Percentage from the Literature)

Patient Group	Total Acid Phosphatases (%)	Tartrate-Labile Phosphatases (%)
Benign prostatic hyperplasia	2–7	0
Prostate carcinoma confined to prostate	5–10	5–12
Prostate carcinoma beyond capsule	10–30	2.4–40
Prostate carcinoma with bone metastases	60–90	48–90

Table 8.8
Total or Tartrate-Labile Acid Phosphatase Activities in Serum of Patients with Prostatic Carcinoma (Metastases in Soft Tissues, Lymphatic Glands, and Bones)

Diagnosis of Metastases	Total No.	Total Acid Phosphatases Elevated		Tartrate-Labile Acid Phosphatase Elevated		Literature
		No.	%	No.	%	
Without	165	5	3	4	2.4	Braun et al.[9]
With	30	27	90	27	90	
Without	10	0	0	10	0	Cook et al.[22]
With	93	46	50	62	67	
Without	5	0	0	4	80	Fishman et al.[33]
With	7	7	100	7	100	
Without	28	7	25	10	36	Mathes, et al.[70]
With	22	11	50	19	86	
Without	104	47	45	17	16	Murphy et al.[77]
With	81	71	88	59	72	
Without	656	135	20.5			Nesbit et al.[79]
With	495	324	65.5			
Without	17	0	0	1	6	Nobles, et al.[81]
With	15	10	66	13	86	
Without	519	78	15	83	16	Jacobi and
With[b]	151	84	55.6	93	61.6	Prellwitz[a]

[a] Unpublished observations.
[b] Bone metastases only.

Table 8.9
Percentage of Elevated Activity of Acid Phosphatases in Serum of Patients with Different Stages of Prostatic Carcinoma

Stage	Total No.	Total Acid Phosphatases Elevated		Tartrate-Labile Acid Phosphatases Elevated	
		No.	%	No.	%
Carcinoma confined to prostate	65[a]	25	38	8	12
(Stages B and C)	10[b]	0	0	0	0
Carcinoma with metastases of soft	39[a]	22	57	9	23
tissue or lymph nodes	56[b]	13	23	26	47
(Stage D$_1$)					
Bone metastases	81[a]	71	88	59	72
(Stage D$_2$)	37[b]	28	76	32	87

[a] From Murphy et al.[77]
[b] From Fishman et al.[33]

were within the normal range. In contrast, this percentage decreased to 40%, when on first admission the acid phosphatase activity was elevated in serum (Table 8.11). Similar results can be observed in the group of patients with metastases. With normal serum acid phosphatases the entire group shows a 32.5% 3-year survival and 25% if elevated serum acid phosphatases were observed. The 3-year survival decreases markedly in patients refractory to endocrine therapy and is significantly better in patients who responded to endocrine therapy. Similar results were published by Johnson et al.[52] (Fig. 8.1).

The elevation of acid phosphatase activity in serum of patients with carcinoma is probably due to the greatly increased bulk of tissue in the carcinomatous prostate and metastatic foci, although in prostatic carcinoma the neoplastic glandular epithelium is poorly developed. It is known that enzyme activity of malignant prostatic tissues (8 to 280 units/mg

Table 8.10
Use of Acid Phosphatase Assay to Distinguish Metastatic from Nonmetastatic Carcinoma[a]

	Total Acid Phosphatase		Tartrate-labile Acid Phosphatase	
	No. Pos	No. Neg	No. Pos	No. Neg
Metastatic carcinoma	71	10	59	22
Nonmetastatic carcinoma	47	57	17	87
Sensitivity	88%		73%	
Specificity	55%		84%	
P.V. (+)[b]	60%		78%	
P.V. (−)[c]	85%		80%	

[a] From R. M. Townsend.[100]
[b] Predictive value of a positive test.
[c] Predictive value of a negative test.

Table 8.11
Clinical Significance of Elevated Serum Acid Phosphatase in Patients with No Evidence of Metastases[a]

	Patients without Metastases		
	Total No. of Patients	3-yr Survival	
		No.	%
Normal serum acid phosphatase on first admission	104	68	66
Elevated serum acid phosphatase on first admission	87	35	40

				Patients with Metastases			
Serum Acid Phosphatase on First Admission	Total No. of Patients	% 3-yr Survival (Entire Group)	3-yr Survival in Patients Responding to Endocrine Therapy		3-yr Survival in Patients Refractory to Endocrine Therapy		
			No.	%	No.	%	
Normal	122	32.5	22	60	40	5	
Elevated	256	25.0	122	47	134	3	

[a] From R. M. Nesbit et al.[79]

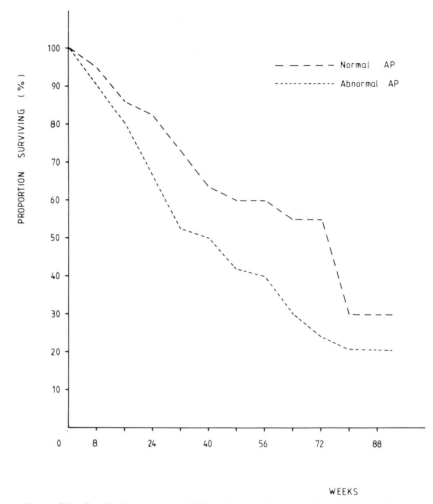

Figure 8.1 Survival protocol of 100 patients with normal and abnormal serum acid phosphatase. (Modified from D. E. Johnson *et al.*[52])

prostate) is less than in hypertrophied prostates (522 to 2284 units/ mg).[68, 77, 88, 110] On the other hand the increase of serum activity of the acid phosphatases depends to a great extent on the blood supply and lymphytic channels in the neoplastic tissue for delivery of the enzyme into blood circulation.

Why do patients with prostatic cancer and metastases (soft tissue, lymphatic and bony) frequently exhibit normal activities of total and tartrate-labile phosphatases in serum? The following explanations have to be considered:

1. The tumor cells are very poorly differentiated and have low acid phosphatase activity.
2. Small quantities of prostatic acid phosphatase are present in the serum but not detectable by our routine methods of activity determination.

3. The prostatic acid phosphatases are inactivated in the serum. London et al.[64] described many substances normally present in serum which are able to inhibit the prostatic acid phosphatase. They found an intensely active and ubiquitous inhibitor of this enzyme.
4. The invasion of vascular or lymphatic channels is not markedly pronounced.
5. In the carcinomatous prostate the rate of synthesis of the acid phosphatase is different from normal prostate.
6. There is a circadian variation of serum activity of acid phosphatases. The circadian rhythm persists in patients with prostatic cancer.[2, 98] Since peak circadian levels are not reached at the same time each day, apparent increase or decrease of serum activity may occur if only one serum sample is investigated. For this reason it is not possible to exclude carcinoma of prostate by a single measurement of acid phosphatases activity in serum.
7. Modification by prior treatment may have occurred. In serum of patients with contrasexual therapy acid phosphatase activity decreases rapidly in parallel to clinical response. The elevated activity may return to normal values during remission and may increase again when relapse occurs.[9, 50, 70, 80, 107]

In Table 8.12 the variability of elevated acid phosphatase activity in serum of patients with and without hormonal treatment is demonstrated. In serum of patients with hormone therapy the percentage of elevated activity of total or tartrate-labile acid phosphatases is significantly lower than in sera of patients without therapy.

Activity of Acid Phosphatases in Bone Marrow

The search for better and earlier staging of prostatic carcinoma led several investigators recently to the determination of the activity of acid phosphatases in bone marrow.[6, 8, 10, 21, 28, 41, 43, 48, 49, 51, 54, 56, 59, 63, 65, 73, 84, 94, 97, 98, 100, 101, 115]

In 1970 Chua and co-workers[21] were the first to introduce the deter-

Table 8.12
Increased Acid Phosphatase Activity in Serum of Patients with and without Hormone Therapy

Hormone Therapy	Metastases	Total No.	Elevated Total Acid Phosphatases		Elevated Tartrate-Labile Acid Phosphatases		Literature
			No.	%	No.	%	
Without	Neg.	165	5	3	4	2.4	Braun et al.[9]
With	Neg.	564	5	1	2	0.4	
Without	Pos.	30	27	90	27	90	
With	Pos.	144	60	41.7	60	41.7	
Without	Neg.	10	5	50	8	80	Mathes et al.[70]
With	Neg.	17	2	12	2	12	
Without	Pos.	6	4	66	6	100	
With	Pos.	16	7	43	13	80	

mination of acid phosphatase activity in bone marrow aspirates for earlier detection of metastatic carcinoma. In Table 8.13 the elevated activity of acid phosphatases in serum and bone marrow compared with positive bone scan or biopsy is demonstrated in the different stages of disease. With the exception of the results of Bruce et al.[10] in all reports the percentage of elevated acid phosphatase activity in bone marrow aspirates was higher than in serum. These results are difficult to compare because the method of measuring the activity of acid phosphatases is not standardized, neither in serum nor in bone marrow aspirates. Because of the lack of specificity of the substrates used for the various isoenzymes of the acid phosphatases the normal ranges differ markedly (Table 8.14).

Another problem is the clinical significance of the elevated activity of bone marrow acid phosphatases. Gursel et al.,[43] Chua et al.,[21] Pontes et al.,[84, 85] Veenema et al.,[101] Yarrison et al.,[114] and Yesus and Taylor[115]

Table 8.13
Elevated Activity of Acid Phosphatases in Serum and Bone Marrow of Patients with Prostatic Cancer

Stage	No.	Serum Activity Acid Phosphatases Elevated[a]		Bone Marrow Activity-Acid Phosphatases Elevated		Bone Scan or Biopsy Positive[a]		Literature
		No.	%	No.	%	No.	%	
A, B	41	10	12.2	3	6.5	—	—	Bruce et al.[10]
C	15	4	26.6	1	6.7	—	—	
D	11	9	81.8	6	54.5	—	—	
A, B	12	0	0	4	33	0	0	Chua et al.[21]
C	6	5	83	6	100	0	0	
D	10	9	90	10	100	10	100	
C	40	—	—	8	20	0[b]	0	Jacobi et al.[51]
D	31	—	—	16	52	31[b]	100	
C	14	1	7	10	71	0	0	Khan et al.[54]
D	11	8	72	8	72	5	45	
B	6	0	0	3	50	0	0	Yesus and
C	3	0	0	3	100	0	0	Taylor[115]
D	2	2	100	2	100	2	100	

[a] —, no investigation.
[b] Bone scan only.

Table 8.14
Normal Ranges of the Activity of the Bone Marrow Acid Phosphatases

Normal Range	Substrate	Literature
8–27 units/liter	p-nitrophenylphosphate	Jacobi et al.[51]
−3 units/liter	α-Naphthylphosphate	Khan et al.[54]
1.1–1.9 Bodansky units/dl	β-Glycerophosphate	Pontes et al.[85]
0.1–1.1 Bodansky units/dl	β-Glycerophosphate	Veenema et al.[101]
0.1–0.5 units/liter	Thymolphthalein mono-phosphate	Yarrison et al.[114]
0–0.8 Bodansky units/dl	Thymolphthalein mono-phosphate	Yesus and Taylor[115]

compared activity of bone marrow and serum acid phosphatases, bone biopsy, and radiological techniques. They found that bone marrow acid phosphatases were more sensitive than other measures in detecting metastases in patients with prostate carcinoma. In Table 8.15 it is shown that all patients with positive bone biopsy or skeletal survey have elevated activities of bone marrow acid phosphatases, while activity in serum was increased in only 75% of these patients.

Of 39 patients with negative bone scan and skeletal survey 16 had increased activity of bone marrow acid phosphatases. Five of these 16 patients subsequently developed metastases to the bones. Therefore the authors postulated that elevation of activity of bone marrow acid phosphatases is the earliest available indication of bone metastases and may contraindicate radical therapy of the local tumor.

On the other hand, several investigators believe that activity of bone marrow acid phosphatases is of no value in the early detection of metastases in patients with prostate carcinoma.[4, 8, 28, 49, 51, 54, 63, 94] In the bone marrow of patients with proven metastases to the bone (stage D) 52 to 100% have increased acid phosphatase activity. Jacobi and co-workers[51] observed in this group of patients an increase in tartrate-labile acid phosphatases of bone marrow in only 35% of the cases (Fig. 8.2). Belville et al.[4] studied 18 patients with bone metastases and 24 patients with benign prostatic hyperplasia by enzymatic assay. The results did not indicate a pattern that would allow discrimination between benign and metastatic disease (Fig. 8.3). The percent of false negative values with measurement of the activity of bone marrow phosphatases is accordingly too high.

A high percentage of falsely positive elevated activities in patients with nonprostatic diseases was observed by several investigators.[8, 10, 28, 49, 63, 71, 94, 114] They described about 50% increased activity of acid phosphatases in bone marrow of patients with nonprostatic diseases (Tables 8.16 and 8.17). Hematologic diseases and metastases of other carcinomas lead to increased activity of bone marrow acid phosphatases. If falsely positive elevated levels are found, the lysis of cells may be an important factor.

The high levels of acid phosphatases measured enzymatically in the bone marrow are apparently a result of the unavoidable lysis of normal

Table 8.15
Comparison of Serum and Bone Marrow Acid Phosphatase Activities in Relation to Tumor Cell Detection in Random Biopsy of Bone (Iliac Crest) and Positive Skeletal Survey[a]

	Tumor Cell-Positive Random Bone Biopsy (41 patients)		Tumor Cell-Positive Random Bone Biopsy plus Positive Skeletal Survey (32 patients)	
	Acid Phosphatase		Acid Phosphatase	
	Serum	Bone Marrow	Serum	Bone Marrow
Elevated	32	41	27	32
Normal	9	0	5	0

[a] From E. O. Gursel et al.[43]

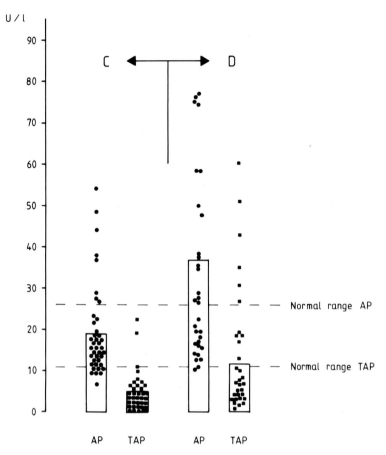

Figure 8.2   Bone marrow activity of acid phosphatase (*AP*) and tartrate-inhibited acid phosphatase (*TAP*) of patients with prostatic cancer stage C (N = 40) and D (N = 31). The values are mathematically corrected according to the free hemoglobin. (Reproduced with permission from G. H. Jacobi *et al.*[51])

cells during the process of bone marrow sampling. Thus, a number of acid phosphatases, especially from platelets and erythrocytes, are released into the bone marrow aspirate and are measured by enzymatic assay. The free hemoglobin, moreover, interferes with the enzymatic determination caused by its own high extinction.

Jacobi *et al.*[51] demonstrated a significant intraindividual correlation between the concentration of free hemoglobin and the activity of total or tartrate-labile acid phosphatases in bone marrow of patients with prostate carcinoma (Fig. 8.4).

The determination of the activity of total acid phosphatases and tartrate-labile phosphatases, in serum and in bone marrow, requires little comment as to its value as a marker for prostatic cancer confined to the prostate or with metastases in soft tissues, lymphatic glands, or bone. It has been shown that approximately 40% of patients with metastases may

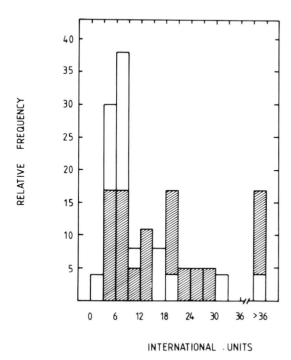

Figure 8.3   Frequency distribution of bone marrow acid phosphatase from patients with benign prostatic hyperplasia (*BPH*) or prostatic carcinoma, stage D$_2$ as determined by enzymatic analysis. (Modified from W. D. Belville *et al.*[4])

Table 8.16
Nonprostatic Diseases with Possible Elevation of Activity of Bone Marrow Acid Phosphatases

Thrombocytopenia
Acute and chronic lymphatic leukemia
Acute and chronic myelogenous leukemia
Malignant lymphoma
Hodgkin's disease
Myeloma
Anemia
Polycythemia vera
Carcinoma of the lung, breast, gastrointestinal tract
Melanoma

have a normal enzyme activity in serum and bone marrow. On the other hand, a large number of nonprostatic diseases show an elevated activity of acid phosphatases in serum as well as bone marrow.[109, 111]

SERUM AND BONE MARROW ACID PHOSPHATASES   143

Table 8.17
Elevated Activity of Bone Marrow Acid Phosphatases

Diagnosis	Total No.	Bone Marrow Acid Phosphatases Elevated	
		No.	%
All patients	104	83	80
Females only	31	26	84
Prostate cancer	19	15	79
Acute and chronic leukemia	34	24	71
Other malignancies	14	14	100
Anemia	37	30	81

^a From W. M. Boehme et al.[8]

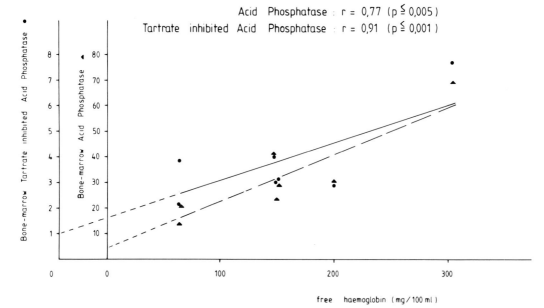

Figure 8.4 Correlation between the bone marrow activity of acid phosphatase, tartrate-inhibited acid phosphatase, and the concentration of free hemoglobin in bone marrow aspiration. (Reproduced with permission from G. H. Jacobi et al.[51])

SEPARATION OF ACID PHOSPHATASES BY ION-EXCHANGE COLUMN CHROMATOGRAPHY

Mercer[72] described a rapid ion-exchange column chromatography for separating the multiple acid phosphatases in human serum and tissues. The isoenzymes were stepwise eluted with Tris-HCl buffer containing successively 100, 200, and 300 mmol NaCl/liter. For each concentration of NaCl five 1-ml fractions were collected. In the first five fractions (100 mmol NaCl/liter) of the isoenzyme three to five (platelets, spleen, liver, and erythrocytes) were determined and identified by electrophoresis on polyacrylamide gel. The next five fractions (200 mmole NaCl/liter) contained isoenzyme-*1* of the prostate. In the last fractions (300 mmol

NaCl/liter) isoenzyme-*2* from prostate and the isoenzymes of spleen and liver were eluted.

In serum of 10 healthy persons the prostate isoenzyme-*1* activity (fraction eluted with 200 mmol NaCl/liter) ranged from 0.3 to 0.5 units/liter. In six sera of patients with prostatic cancer this prostatic isoenzyme shows activities between 3.8 and 27.6 units/liter.

IMMUNOCHEMICAL STUDIES OF PROSTATIC ACID PHOSPHATASE

In 1960 Flocks *et al.*[34] illustrated the possibility of producing antibodies against human prostatic tissue. Since only crude extracts of human prostatic tissue were applied to immunize rabbits, the obtained genuine antisera were not organ-specific. However, in further steps of the preparation common antibodies against nonprostatic tissues could be extracted by adsorption processes. Thus, the first antiserum with proved specific antiprostate activity was produced.

In the following years interest was focused on the antigenicity of human prostatic acid phosphatases, and attempts have been made to develop immunologic methods to confirm or deny the presence of prostatic cancer in patients. For the production of specific antisera in different animals in general two procedures have been used. Either immunization with a crude antigen preparation and consecutive purification of the antisera, or more or less extensively purified human prostatic acid phosphatase have been used.

Sources of the antigen have been prostatic fluid obtained by rectal massage,[11, 23, 35, 42, 96] sperm-free ejaculate,[4, 15, 16, 29, 66, 74, 75] hyperplastic prostatic tissue,[15, 20, 34, 74, 104] and carcinomatous prostatic tissue removed by surgical procedures[34] as well as at autopsy.[1] Since prostatic acid phosphatases derived from prostatic tissue are more heterogenous than those from prostatic fluid or ejaculate,[15] the choice of the source as well as the procedure to purify the antigen is of great importance. With crude extracts as antigen the genuine antisera have to be purified from the common tissue antigens by means of immunoadsorption and immunoprecipitation. However, it was found by most of the authors that this clean-up was not successful with every antiserum.[1, 34, 74] In most cases the antisera obtained from crude antigen extracts were used for gel diffusion,[1, 34, 96] immunoelectrophoresis,[1, 74, 96] and counterimmunoelectrophoresis.

When compared to the nonspecific staining for protein a more specific detection of the acid phosphatases was performed by means of staining procedures involving enzymatic, tartrate-labile cleavage of a substrate.[1, 15, 20, 29, 74, 75, 96] Since acid phosphatases are easily inactivated the staining step might be the most critical in the whole time-consuming procedure of the above-mentioned techniques. There are also hemagglutination and inhibition of hemagglutination,[1] determinations which are mainly qualitative in nature.

A more rapid enzyme immunoassay has been recently published by

Choe *et al.*[16] This assay is based on the estimation of prostatic acid phosphatase activity in resolved immune complexes which were precipitated after formation by ammonium sulfate. Purified prostatic acid phosphatase standards were used, and a good correlation with a double antibody radioimmunoassay was shown. However, a careful observation of the conditions of the assay is necessary. For example, without siliconization of the glass nonspecific binding of the acid phosphatase is observed, and different complications may occur due to high background enzymatic activity, co-precipitation of nonprostatic acid phosphatases, excess of antigen, and turbidity after resuspension. These complications are avoided with the enzyme immunoassay of the sandwich type described by Grenner and Schmidtberger.[42] In this procedure two antibodies raised in sheep and rabbit are used. One antibody is fixed to the wall of the reaction tube. After binding of the antigen via the antibody to the wall and washing, a second antibody labeled with peroxidase is bound to further binding sites on the antigen, and the excess of the peroxidase-labeled antibody is washed out. The final quantitation is done on the basis of peroxidase activity measurements in comparison to a standard curve. Highly purified prostatic acid phosphatases from prostatic fluid served as the antigen and source for the standard concentrations.

As for the enzyme immunoassay pure prostatic acid phosphatase is needed as well as radioimmunoassays for antigen production and standardization. Different purification procedures have been developed.[55, 83, 92, 105, 106] Gel filtration on Sephadex, ion exchange chromatography on different columns, affinity chromatography against a variety of fixed adsorbants, salt precipitation, and isoelectric focusing are the principal steps. The extent to which single steps have been involved during the purification of the prostatic acid phosphatases differs considerably. A generally accepted standard procedure does not exist (Table 8.18). It is reasonable to assume that differences in values reported for a normal healthy male population relate to a great extent to the purity of the antigen used and standardization procedures.[66] A small amount of cross-reactivity to other acid phosphatases is generally thought to be of minor importance. However, this factor has not been excluded in detail by many authors. Cross-reactivity to acid phosphatases of bone is questionable and examined only in one case (Table 8.18).

The basic principle of both the solid phase[35, 37] and the double antibody radioimmunoassay[4, 15, 23, 66, 104] for prostatic acid phosphatases is the competition between the radioactive and the nonradioactive antigen for a fixed number of antibody binding sites. The more unlabeled antigen from standard or sample that is present during incubation the less labeled antigen is bound to the antibody of the rabbit. In the double antibody radioimmunoassay separation of the bound from the free antigen is achieved by addition of a second antibody. This second antibody is specific against γ-globulin of the rabbit and precipitates the primary antigen-antibody complex. In the solid phase radioimmunoassay the antibody against prostatic acid phosphatases is adsorbed to the walls of a plastic tube, and separation of bound and free antigen is facilitated by discharging the content of the tube after incubation.

Double antibody radioimmunoassays currently on the market and most frequently in use are: RIANEN Prostatic Acid Phosphatase, ^{125}I RIA Kit from New England Nuclear; RIA-Quant P.A.P. Test Kit from Mallinckrodt Nuclear; P.A.P. Check RIA Kit from Serono. An enzyme immunoassay of the sandwich type from Behring-Werke is now also commercially available (see Editorial Comment to this chapter). Table 8.18 summarizes some characteristics of the above-mentioned immunochemical assays which have been reported in the literature.

Characterization of Pure Prostatic Acid Phosphatases with Respect to Their Immunologic Properties

Two isoenzymes of human prostatic acid phosphatase have been exhaustively purified.[15] They differ in enzyme activity and their isoelectric points as verified with preparative isoelectric focusing. It is suggested that the minor enzyme is a proenzyme inside the cell and that the main enzyme is for secretion. The charge heterogeneity may even be greater than proposed with the two purified enzymes since, with starch gel electrophoresis, a separation of prostatic acid phosphatase into 20 bands has been described.[99] Similar to disc electrophoresis containing 0.5% Triton X-100 in the polyacrylamide gel, at least nine subforms of prostatic acid phosphatase deriving from prostate tissues were partially resolved.[69] Recent findings support this view of charge heterogeneity.[102, 103] Prostatic acid phosphatase from purified human ejaculate exhibited a single coincident peak of protein and enzymatic activity with preparative isoelectric focusing. But when the same fraction was subjected to analytical isoelectric focusing on polyacrylamide gels in the pH range of 4 to 8, enzyme activity was resolved into 11 discrete bands.[66] The complex pattern of the native enzyme results from various amounts of sialic acid associated with this glycoprotein as can be shown by neuraminidase treatment.[66] Fortunately the neuraminic acid content does not determine the antigenic properties of the protein, and the isoenzymes are found to be immunologically cross-reactive.[15]

RESULTS OF IMMUNOLOGICAL STUDIES CONCERNING PROSTATIC ACID PHOSPHATASES IN SERUM AND BONE MARROW OF PATIENTS WITH PROSTATIC CARCINOMA

Immunodiffusion and Counterimmunoelectrophoresis

Both methods are qualitative investigations.[39, 67] The lowest detectable concentration of prostatic acid phosphatase amounts to 2.5 ng/ml. Therefore, in serum of healthy persons prostatic acid phosphatase is never found. The percentage of elevated prostatic acid phosphatase in serum of patients with prostatic cancer is demonstrated in Table 8.19. Choe et al.[15] observed in all 21 patients with metastatic carcinoma levels higher than 2.5 ng/ml; in the report of Chu and coworkers[20] this occurred in 80% of stage D patients. In stages B and C, in only 30 and 55%, respectively was prostatic acid phosphatase detectable in serum.

Table 8.18
Characterization of Antigens and Antisera Used to Develop Specific Immunochemical Assays for Prostatic Acid Phosphatases[a]

Source of Antigen (Purification,[b] Animal)	Immunochemical Assay[c]	Reactivity of the Antiserum Tested for Acid Phosphatases From:											Literature
		Serum	Erythrocytes	Platelets	Bone	Liver	Kidney	Lung	Muscle	Pancreas	Spleen	Other Specimen	
Prostatic tissue (crude extract, rabbit)	Gel diffusion	+	0	0	0	0	0	0	0	0	0		34
Prostatic fluid (supernatant, rabbit)	Gel diffusion, immunoelectrophoresis	−	−	0	0	−	−	−	0	0	0	Seminal vesicle, − Testis −	96
Prostatic tissue (crude extract, rabbit)	Gel diffusion, immunoelectrophoresis hemagglutination	−	0	0	0	−	−	−	−	0	0	Seminal vesicle −	1
Ejaculate; prostatic tissue (crude extract, goat)	Immunoelectrophoresis	0	0	0	0	0	±	0	−	±	0	Intestine ±	74
Ejaculate (B, rabbit)	Gel diffusion	−	0	−	0	−	−	−	−	−	−	Salivary gland, − Intestine, − Breast, − Lymph node −	75
Prostatic fluid (A, rabbit)	Double antibody radioimmunoassay	+	0	0	0	0	0	0	0	0	0	−	23
Prostatic fluid (A, rabbit)	Solid phase radioimmunoassay	+	0	0	0	+	0	+	+	+	+	Adrenal + Brain + Thyroid +	35 37
Ejaculate, prostatic tissue (A, C, F, I, J, monkey, rabbit)	Double antibody radioimmunoassay counterimmunoelectrophoresis, inlectrophoresis, in-	+	0	0	0	−	0	−	0	+	0	Lymphocytes − Breast carcinoma −	15

Source of enzyme or antigen (purification steps)[b]	Immunological method	direct immunofluorescent antibody technique	Uterine carcinoma	Synovia	Salivary gland	Intestine	Gastric mucosa	Lymph node	Brain	Bladder	Intestine	
Prostatic tissue (J, G, A, L, rabbit)	Double antibody radioimmunoassay	+	—	0	0	0	0	0	0	0	—	104
Ejaculate (B, rabbit)	Gel diffusion	+	—	0	—	0	—	0	0	0	—	29
Ejaculate (B, rabbit)	Double antibody radioimmunoassay	+	0	0	0	0	0	0	0	0	0	4
Prostatic tissue (H, J, E, B, A, rabbit)	Gel diffusion, counterimmunoelectrophoresis	—	0	0	0	0	0	0	0	0	0	20
Ejaculate (B, K, D, B, rabbit)	Double antibody radioimmunoassay	+	0	0	0	0	0	0	0	0	0	66
Prostatic fluid (A, B, L, rabbit, sheep)	Enzyme immunoassay of the sandwich type	+	0	0	0	0	0	0	0	0	0	42
Ejaculate	Enzyme immunoassay	+	0	0	0	0	0	0	0	0	0	16

[a] Symbols: +, activity was detected; —, activity was not detected; ±, activity detected with unpurified antisera, but not detected after purification of the antisera by immunoadsorption; 0, no investigations.

[b] Steps of purification are: A, gel filtration on Sephadex; B, ion exchange chromatography on DEAE-Sephadex A-50; C, ion exchange chromatography on DEAE-cellulose; D, ion exchange chromatography on CM-cellulose; E, ion exchange chromatography on phosphocellulose; F, affinity chromatography (concanavalin A); G, affinity chromatography on L(+)-tartrate-AH-Sepharose 4B; H, affinity chromatography on agarose: 5'-(p-nitrophenyl-phosphate)-uridine-2'(3')-phosphate; I, immunoadsorbent column chromatography; J, salt precipitation; K, acid precipitation; L, isoelectric focusing.

In serum of patients with benign prostatic hyperplasia and with non-prostatic carcinomas (colon, stomach, pancreas, kidney, lung) no elevation of prostatic acid phosphatase was found by immunoelectrophoresis. Only Drucker et al.,[29] Choe et al.,[17] and Romas et al.[91] described false positive prostatic acid phosphatase in serum of a patient with pancreatic islet cell carcinoma as well as in the serum of patients with chronic granulocytic leukemia.

The comparison between elevated prostatic acid phosphatase determined by immunodiffusion and the results of bone biopsy, skeletal surveys, and scans is shown in Table 8.20. While prostatic acid phosphatase is elevated in serum of 39 (83%) of 47 patients with stage D (metastatic cancer), only 46% of the bone biopsies, 51% of the bone surveys, and 38% of the bone scans were positive. On the other hand, one patient of eight thought to have stage C disease had a positive bone scan but lacked detectable prostatic acid phosphatase.

Radioimmunoassay: Determination of Prostatic Acid Phosphatase in Serum

Of all the immunological methods available, the radioimmunoassay is the most frequently used determination for prostatic acid phosphatase. Normal ranges of prostatic acid phosphatase from literature are compiled

Table 8.19
Percentage of Elevated Prostatic Acid Phosphatase Determined by Counterimmunoelectrophoresis in Serum of Patients with Prostatic Carcinoma

| | No. | Elevated (>2.5 ng/ml) | | Literature |
		No.	%	
Cancer				
Localized	20	0	0	Choe, et al.[15]
Metastatic	21	21	100	
Stage				
A	1	0	0	Chu et al.[20]
B	30	6	20	
C	49	27	55	
D	125	98	78	

Table 8.20
Elevated Prostatic Acid Phosphatase in Serum of Patients with Prostatic Cancer Determined by Immunodiffusion Compared with Positive Bone Marrow Biopsy, Skeletal Survey, and Bone Scan[a]

| Stage | No. | Immunodiffusion Positive | | Bone Marrow Biopsy Positive | | Bone Survey Positive | | Bone Scan Positive | |
		No.	%	No.	%	No.	%	No.	%
A	10	1	10	0	0	2	20	0	0
B	11	1	9	0	0	0	0	0	0
C	8	0	0	0	0	0	0	1	25
D	47	39	83	22	46	24	51	18	38

[a] From J. R. Drucker et al.[29]

in Table 8.21. The values differ from report to report. The reasons for these differences are as follows: the origin and the purification of the prostatic acid phosphatase are not comparable, the specificity of the antibody is not uniform, and the test procedures are not standardized.

Foti et al.[35] determined the concentration of prostatic acid phosphatase in human tissue extracts with solid phase radioimmunoassay (Table 8.22). In all investigated tissues the concentrations were lower than 1%, compared with the concentration of the prostate (100%). Other authors (Table 8.18) did not find cross-reactions with the multiple nonprostatic acid phosphatases, especially with those of platelets and erythrocytes.

The percentages of elevated concentration of prostatic acid phosphatase determined by radioimmunoassay in serum of patients with carcinoma of the prostatic are demonstrated in Table 8.23. In stage I or A (carcinoma not detectable by rectal examination) the percentage of elevated concentrations of prostatic acid phosphatase ranges from 8 to 33. In stage II or B (tumor confined to prostate) this increases from 21% to 79%. In stage III or C (periprostatic tumor extension) between 30% and 71% of the examined patients have elevated serum prostatic acid phosphatase concentrations. In stage IV or D (metastases of soft tissues, lymphatic glands,

Table 8.21
Normal Values of Prostatic Acid Phosphatase in Serum Determined by Radioimmunoassay

No. Pts.	Normal Range	Method (RIA)	Literature or Company
162	0.8–2.4 ng/0.1 ml	Double antibody	Choe, el al.[15]
200	0.5–7.2 ng/0.1 ml	Solid-phase	Cooper et al.[24]
50	1.5–6.6 ng/0.1 ml	Solid-phase	Foti et al.[37]
226	0.75–4.45 ng/ml	Double antibody	Mahan and Doctor[66]
96 (♂)	1.0–5.0 ng/ml	Double antibody	Prellwitz et al.[86]
98 (♀)	1.0–4.0 ng/ml		
53	1.0–10.0 ng/ml	Double antibody	Vihko et al.[104]
212	1.2–5.7 ng/ml	Double antibody	New England Nuclear
197	0–2.0 ng/ml	Solid-phase	Mallinckrodt

Table 8.22
Prostatic Acid Phosphatase Detected in Human Tissue Extracts by Solid-Phase Radioimmunoassay[a]

Tissue	Prostatic Acid Phosphatase (ng/100 μg Protein)	% of Prostate Value
Prostate	2700.0	100
Spleen	2.6	0.10
Liver	2.7	0.10
Adrenal	5.8	0.22
Muscle	2.1	0.07
Pancreas	4.9	0.18
Brain	23.6	0.86
Thyroid	1.6	0.06
Heart	4.3	0.16
Lung	4.8	0.17

[a] From A. G. Foti et al.[35]

Table 8.23
Percentage of Elevated Concentration of Prostatic Acid Phosphatase in Serum of Patients with Prostatic Cancer Determined by Radioimmunoassay

Stage	No.	Elevated Concentration		Literature
		No.	%	
I–II	44	20	43.5	Cooper et al.[24]
III–IV	65	62	95.4	
I	24	8	33	Foti et al.[37]
II	33	26	79	
III	31	22	71	
IV	25	23	92	
A	15	2	13	Mahan and Doctor[66]
B	34	9	26	
C	20	6	30	
D_1	16	5	31	
D_2	16	15	94	
A	26	2	8	New England Nuclear
B	34	7	21	
C	10	4	40	
D	28	24	86	

and bones) 86% of the patients have increased levels. In stage D_1 (cancer with pelvic lymph node involvement) only 30% have increased levels, whereas in stage D_2 (distant metastases) 94% of all patients show increased serum concentrations of prostatic acid phosphatases.

Choe et al.[15] and Vihko et al.[104] also described increased values of prostatic acid phosphatase in serum of patients with metastases in nearly 100%. The reported values of Vihko et al.[104] are lower than those published by Choe[15] and Foti et al.[35, 37, 38] One possible explanation discussed by Vihko is that he believes that his antigen is the one which is 100% pure. He purified his antigen directly from prostatic tissue and not from prostatic fluid.

In serum of patients with benign prostatic hyperplasia or with non-prostatic cancers (Table 8.24) the concentrations of prostatic acid phosphatase are in the normal ranges as published by Choe et al.,[15] Cooper et al.,[24] and Vihko et al.[104] Only Foti et al.[37] described elevated values in 14% of patients with benign hyperplasia and in 17% of patients with nonprostatic cancer. This percentage of false positive results can be reduced to 6% and 11%, respectively, when the cutoff limit of prostatic acid phosphatase is raised to 8.0 ng/0.1 ml serum. Most patients with false positive studies and nonprostatic cancer suffer from pulmonary tumors.

To judge the clinical significance of different methods used to determine acid phosphatases as a marker of prostatic cancer it is important to compare the percentage of elevated activities with the percentage of elevated concentrations of prostatic acid phosphatase. The respective results are shown in Table 8.25 and Fig. 8.5. Cooper et al.[24] and Foti et al.[37] proved that the percentage of elevated concentrations of prostatic acid phosphatase, determined by RIA in serum, is significantly higher

Table 8.24
Values of Prostate Acid Phosphatase in Serum of Patients with Prostatic Diseases and Nonprostatic Diseases

Diagnosis	No.	Ranges	Literature
Control	162	0.8–2.4 ng/0.1 ml	Choe, et al.[15]
Benign prostatic hyperplasia	11	0.8–2.4 ng/0.1 ml	
Nonprostatic carcinoma	10	1.2–2.4 ng/0.1 ml	
Control	200	0.5–7.2 ng/0.1 ml	Cooper et al.[24]
Benign prostatic hyperplasia	53	1.7–6.6 μg/0.1 ml	
Nonprostatic carcinoma	90	1.3–7.3 ng/0.1 ml	
Control	50	1.5–6.6 ng/0.1 ml	Foti et al.[37]
Benign prostatic hyperplasia	36	1.5–8.1 ng/0.1 ml (14% elevated)	
Nonprostatic cancer	83	1.5–9.0 ng/0.1 ml (17% elevated)	
Control	53	1–10 ng/ml	Vihko et al.[104]
Benign prostatic hyperplasia	11	1–10 ng/ml	

Table 8.25
Percentage of Patients with Elevated Prostatic Acid Phosphatase as Determined by Radioimmunoassay and by Enzymatic Assay

Stage	No.	Elevated by RIA		Elevated by Enzyme Assay		Literature
		No.	%	No.	%	
I–II	44	20	45.5	2	44.5	Cooper et al.[24]
III–IV	65	62	95.4	30	46.0	

		>6.6 ng/0.1 ml		>8.0 ng/0.1 ml				
		No.	%	No.	%			
I	24	12	50	8	33	3	12	Foti et al.[37]
II	33	26	79	26	79	5	15	
III	31	25	81	22	71	9	29	
IV	25	24	96	23	92	15	60	

than that of the activity measurement conventionally. Cooper et al.[24] are convinced that only the radioimmunoassay is sensitive enough to establish a normal range of values; it alone is specific for human prostatic acid phosphatase and does not cross-react with other nonprostatic acid phosphatases. In randomized serum samples, the radioimmunoassay detected 33% of patients with untreated prostatic carcinoma at stage I, 79% at stage II, 71% at stage III, and 92% at stage IV. The enzyme assay in contrast detected only 12% (stage I), 15% (stage II), 29% (stage III), and 60% (stage IV) of the same patients.

Based on the results of Cooper et al.,[24] Foti et al.,[37] and Carroll[13] the calculated sensitivity of the radioimmunoassay was 69% and that of the enzyme assay was 28%. The specificity of the radioimmunoassay was 62% and that of the enzyme assay was 96%. On the basis of these data it becomes apparent that the radioimmunoassay is more sensitive than the enzyme assay, but it is not more specific.

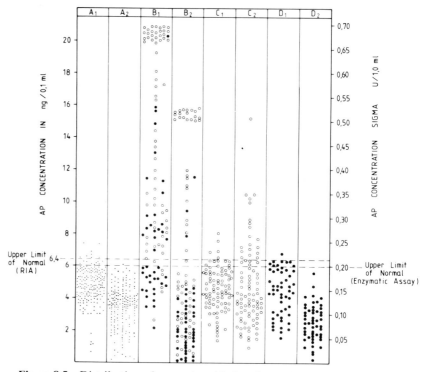

$A_1 - D_1$ = Radioimmunoassay
$A_2 - D_2$ = Enzymatic Assay

A = normal adult male sera (n = 200)
B = prostatic cancer patients • stage I, ○ stage II (n = 44)
C = miscellaneous cancers (n = 90)
D = benign prostatic hyperplasia (n = 53)

Figure 8.5 Distribution of prostatic acid phosphatase in sera of normal subjects and patients with prostatic cancer and prostatic hyperplasia. (Modified from J. F. Cooper et al.[24])

The radioimmunoassay detects more cases of prostatic cancer, but the predictive value for the radioimmunoassay is not substantially better than the enzyme assay. Mahan and Doctor[66] declare that in serum of patients with prostatic cancer and proven bony metastases, a 6% false negative result was observed. This compares favorably with the 40 to 8% false negative values observed with various enzyme assays.

A number of possible explanations may be given for the different results concerning the upper limit and the normal range of prostatic acid phosphatase concentrations in control groups, as well as for the different percentages of elevated prostatic acid phosphatase in the various stages of prostatic cancer. Different tissues and fluids have been used to purify human prostatic acid phosphatases as described above. Although there may be some differences in the sialic acid composition of the purified antigens, it is unlikely that sialic acid will be an important factor in the immunoassay of prostatic acid phosphatase. Another problem is the limited homogeneity of the prostatic acid phosphatase used as a standard of radioimmunoassay.[32, 78, 90]

Radioimmunoassay: Determination of Prostatic Acid Phosphatase in Bone Marrow

The normal ranges of prostatic acid phosphatase concentration in bone marrow are summarized in Table 8.26. Similar to serum, the values differ from report to report. In Table 8.27 and Fig. 8.6 the percentage of elevated prostatic acid phosphatase determined by radioimmunoassay in bone marrow is outlined. In metastatic carcinoma bone marrow acid phosphatase is elevated in 80% to 100% of patients. Cooper et al.[25, 26] reported that the radioimmunoassay for bone marrow prostatic acid phosphatase has shown a close correlation with bone scans. Compared with the enzyme assay the advantage of the radioimmunoassay is that the antibody used does not show a cross-reaction with acid phosphatases, especially with those from platelets and erythrocytes.[14]

Cooper and co-workers[26] described four types of results obtained with the measurement of prostatic acid phosphatase in serum and bone marrow (Table 8.28). The type I screen was found in 73% of stage A, in 50% of stage B, in 18% of stage C, and in 0% of stage D. The type II screen was observed in 27% of stage A, in 50% of stage B, in 82% of stage C, and in 19% of stage D. The type III screen was seen in three (15%) of 20 cases of stage B and in six (38%) of 16 cases of stage C. These results indicate that the three patients of stage B and the six patients of stage C obviously

Table 8.26
Normal Values of Prostatic Acid Phosphatase in Bone Marrow Determined by Radioimmunoassay

Normal Range	Method (RIA)	Literature
2–12 ng/ml	Double antibody	Belville et al.[4]
0.5–4.0 ng/0.1 ml	Double antibody	Choe et al.[15]
4.7–15.5 ng/0.1 ml	Solid phase	Cooper et al.[25]

Table 8.27
Percentage of Elevated Prostatic Acid Phosphatase Determined by Radioimmunoassay in Bone Marrow of Patients with Prostatic Cancer

Stage	No.	Elevated No.	Elevated %	Literature
A	18	1	5.5	Belville et al.[4]
B	35	0	0	
C	33	6	18	
D_1	16	4	25	
D_2	15	12	80	
Carcinoma				Choe et al.[15]
Localized	8	0	0	
Metastatic	10	10	100	

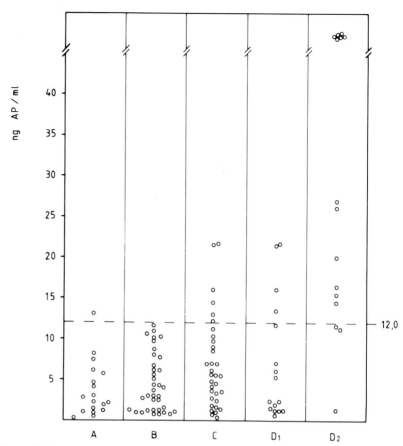

Figure 8.6 Bone marrow acid phosphatase levels determined by radioimmunoassay from patients with carcinoma of the prostate by stages (A, B, C, D_1 or D_2). (Modified from W. D. Belville et al.[4])

Table 8.28
Different Types of Concentration of Prostatic Acid Phosphatase in Serum and Bone Marrow Determined by RIA[a]

Screen	Prostatic Acid Phosphatase	
	Serum	Bone Marrow
Type I	Normal (0.5–6.5 ng/0.1 ml)	Normal (2.5–15 ng/0.1 ml)
Type II	Elevated (6.5–30 ng/0.1 ml)	Normal
Type III	Elevated (>50 ng/0.1 ml)	Elevated (>50 ng/0.1 ml)
Type IV	Normal	Elevated

[a] From J. F. Cooper et al.[26]

were clinically understaged. In fact, they represent unrecognized stage D (Table 8.29). The type IV screen was not observed in prostatic cancer, but in primary and secondary bone neoplasm, Gaucher's disease, metastatic pancreatic and pulmonary cancer.

Table 8.29
Relation of Clinical Stage of Prostatic Cancer to Serum and Bone Marrow RIA Screening Technique[a]

Screen	Stage			
	A (N = 15)	B (N = 20)	C (N = 16)	D (N = 16)
	No. (%)	No. (%)	No. (%)	No. (%)
Type I	11 (73)	10 (50)	3 (18)	0 (0)
Type II	4 (27)	10 (50)	13 (82)	3 (19)
Type III	—[b]	3 (15) (Understaged)	6 (38) (Understaged)	13 (81)
Type IV	—	—	—	—

[a] From J. F. Cooper et al.[26]
[b] —, Screen type not represented by given prostate cancer stage.

In the report of Cooper et al.,[26] 104 patients of stage C prostatic cancer were submitted for supervoltage radiation therapy. All patients showed normal activities of acid and alkaline phosphatases and normal bone survey and scan. Within 5 years 33 patients (31%) developed stage D disease with positive bone scan, 21 patients (20%) had clinical evidence of bony metastases within 3 years, and 12 patients (11%) within 5 years. There was an overall clinical staging error in 104 patients with stage C of 31%. The authors believe that a radioimmunoassay screen can detect early bone marrow metastases and thus discriminate stage C from D. On this basis they recommend that all patients with stage C prostatic cancer should have a specific determination of prostatic acid phosphatase by radioimmunoassay in serum and in bone marrow before supervoltage or ^{125}I-implantation therapy. Only these determinations would allow us to detect early bone metastases.

Enzyme Immunoassay

Choe and co-workers[16] developed a simplified enzyme immunoassay to detect prostatic acid phosphatase. The serum samples are mixed with the specific antibody, and the resulting complexes are precipitated by ammonium sulfate. The amount of precipitated prostatic acid phosphatase is then estimated by its enzymatic activity. The normal values of 40 normal males range from 0 to 37 ng/ml, those of 25 female persons from 0 to 18 ng/ml. The comparison of the values determined by radioimmunoassay and enzyme immunoassay results follow a regression line: $y = 1.02 X + 0.82$; $r = 0.9993$ (Y = double antibody radioimmunoassay; X = enzyme immunoassay).

Grenner and Schmidtberger[42] described an enzyme immunoassay (ELISA) of the sandwich type to determine acid prostatic phosphatase. The marker enzyme is peroxidase (E.C. 1.11.1.7.). Prellwitz and co-workers[86] investigated the serum of healthy female and male subjects to detect the normal range for this method. In sera of 70 female controls the normal values range from 0 to 0.70 ng/ml, those of male persons from 0 to 0.74 ng/ml. The correlations between the results determined by radioimmunoassay and enzyme immunoassay are satisfactory. In sera of

100 patients with nonprostatic cancer the values of prostatic acid phosphatase were elevated in only two cases.

Comparing all results concerning the immunological methods, especially the radioimmunoassay, it can be stated that this immunological method provides a more sensitive diagnostic marker for prostatic cancer than the various enzyme assays. Before the exact role of prostatic acid phosphatase can be defined, Mahan and Doctor[66] recommend additional standardization of the source of antigen, the purification techniques, and the staging procedures in patients with prostatic cancer. A screening test, based on serum and bone marrow concentration of prostatic acid phosphatase, would be a great benefit in detection, treatment, and study of prostatic cancer. However, further investigations and confirmation of all results are essential.

References

1. Ablin, R. J., Bronson, P., Soanes, W. A., and Witebsky, E. Tissue- and species-specific antigens of normal human prostatic tissue. *J. Immunol. 104:* 1329, 1970.
2. Batsakis, J., Briere, R. O., and Markel, S. Diagnostic enzymology. American Society of Clinical Pathologists Committee on Continuing Education, Chicago, 1970.
3. Beckmann, L. Individual and organ-specific variations of human acid phosphatase. *Biochem. Genet. 1:* 145, 1967.
4. Belville, W. D., Cox, H. D., Mahan, D. E., Olmot, J. P., Mittemeyer, B. T., and Bruce, A. W. Bone marrow acid phosphatase by radioimmunoassay. *Cancer 41:* 2286, 1978.
5. Bensley, E. H., Wood, P., Mitchell, S., and Milnes, B. Estimation of serum acid phosphatase in the diagnosis of metastasing carcinoma of the prostate. *Can. Med. Assoc. J. 58:* 261, 1948.
6. Bichler, K.-H., Harzmann, R., Heller, W., Wilms, K., Delling, G., and Schmidt, K.-H. Diagnostik ossärer Metastasen des Prostatakarzinoms. *Akt. Urol. 9:* 21, 1978.
7. Bodansky, O. Acid phosphatase. *Adv. Clin. Chem. 15:* 43, 1972.
8. Boehme, W. M., Augspurger, R. R., Wallner, S. F., and Donohue, R. E. Lack of usefulness of bone marrow enzymes and calcium in staging patients with prostatic cancer. *Cancer 41:* 1433, 1978.
9. Braun, J. S., Habig, H., and Grüsemann, D. Die diagnostische Bedeutung der sauren Phosphatase im Serum beim Prostatacarcinom. *Urologe A 13:* 236, 1974.
10. Bruce, A. W., Mahan, D. E., Morales, A., Clark, A. F., and Belville, W. D. An objective look at acid phosphatase determinations. *Br. J. Urol. 59:* 213, 1979.
11. Bruce, A. W. Carcinoma of the prostate: a critical look at staging. *J. Urol. 117:* 319, 1977.
12. Byrne, J. Acid phosphatase reappraised. *N. Engl. J. Med. 297:* 1398, 1977.
13. Carroll, B. J. Radioimmunoassay of prostatic acid phosphatase in carcinoma of the prostate. *N. Engl. J. Med. 298:* 912, 1978.
14. Catane, R. Prostatic cancer, immunochemical detection of prostatic acid phosphatase in serum and bone marrow. *NY State J. Med. 78:* 1060, 1978.
15. Choe, B. K., Pontes, E. J., McDonald, I., and Rose, N. R. Immunochemical studies of prostatic acid phosphatase. *Cancer Treat. Rep. 61:* 201, 1977.
16. Choe, B. K., Rose, N. R., Korol, M., and Pontes, E. J. Immunoenzyme assay for human prostatic phosphatase. *Proc. Soc. Exp. Biol. Med. 162:* 396, 1979.
17. Choe, B. K., Pontes, E. J., Rose, N. R., and Henderson, M. D. Expression of human prostatic acid phosphatase in a pancreatic islet cell carcinoma. *Invest. Urol. 15:* 312, 1978.
18. Chu, T. M., Shukla, S. K., Mittelman, A., and Murphy, G. P. Comparative evaluation of serum acid phosphatase, urinary cholesterol, and androgens in diagnosis of prostatic cancer. *Urology VI:* 291, 1975.
19. Chu, T. M., Wang, M. C., and Kuciel, R. Enzyme markers in human prostatic carcinoma. *Cancer Treat. Rep. 61:* 193, 1977.

20. Chu, T. M., Wang, M. C., Scott, W. W., Gibbons, R. P., Johnson, D. E., Schmidt, J. D., Loening, S. A., Prout, G. R., and Murphy, G. P. Immunochemical detection of serum prostatic acid phosphatase. Methodology and clinical evaluation. *Invest. Urol. 15:* 319, 1978.

21. Chua, D. T., Veenema, R. J., Muggia, F., and Graff, A. Acid phosphatase levels in bone marrow: value in detecting early bone metastasis from carcinoma of the prostate. *J. Urol. 103:* 462, 1970.

22. Cook, W. B., Fishman, W. H., and Clard, B. G. Serum acid phosphatase of prostatic origin in the diagnosis of prostatic carcinoma. Clinical evaluation of 2408 tests by Fishman-Lerner Method. *J. Urol. 88:* 281, 1962.

23. Cooper, J. F., and Foti, A. A radioimmunoassay for prostatic acid phosphatase. I. Methodology and range of normal male serum values. *Invest. Urol. 12:* 98, 1974.

24. Cooper, J. F., Foti, A., Herschman, H., and Finkle, W. A solid phase radioimmunoassay for prostatic acid phosphatase. *J. Urol. 119:* 388, 1978.

25. Cooper, J. F., Foti, A. G., and Shank, P. W. Radioimmunochemical measurement of bone marrow prostatic acid phosphatase. *J. Urol. 119:* 392, 1978.

26. Cooper, J. F., Foti, A., and Herschman, H. Combined serum and bone marrow radioimmunoassays for prostatic acid phosphatase. *J. Urol. 122:* 498, 1979.

27. Daniel, O. The stability of acid phosphatase in blood and other fluids. *Br. J. Urol. 26:* 152, 1954.

28. Dias, S. M., and Barnett, R. N. Elevated bone marrow acid phosphatase: the problem of false positives. *J. Urol. 117:* 749, 1977.

29. Drucker, J. R., Moncure, C. W., Johnson, C. L., Smith, M. J. V., and Koontz, W. W. Immunologic staging of prostatic carcinoma: three years of experience. *J. Urol. 119:* 94, 1978.

30. de Duve, D. The lysosome in retrospect. In *Lysosomes in Biology and Pathology,* edited by L. J. T. Dingle, and H. B. Fell. Excerpta Medica, Elsevier/North Holland, Amsterdam, 1969, p. 3.

31. Ewen, L. M., and Spitzer, R. W. Improved determination of prostatic acid phosphatase (Sodium thymolphthalein monophosphate substrate). *Clin. Chem. 25:* 627, 1976.

32. Fink, D. J., and Galen, R. S. Immunologic detection of prostatic acid phosphatase: critique II. *Hum. Pathol. 9:* 621, 1978.

33. Fishman, W. H., Dast, R. M., Bonner, C. D., Leadbetter, W. F., Lerner, F., and Homburger, F. A new method for estimating serum acid phosphatase of prostatic origin applied to the clinical investigation of cancer of the prostate. *J. Clin. Invest. 32:* 1034, 1953.

34. Flocks, R. H., Ulrich, V. C., Patel, C. A., and Opith, J. M. Studies on the antigenic properties of prostatic tissue. *J. Urol. 84:* 134, 1960.

35. Foti, A. G., Herschman, H., and Cooper, J. F. A solid-phase radioimmunoassay for human prostatic acid phosphatase. *Cancer Res. 35:* 2246, 1975.

36. Foti, A. G., Herschman, H., and Cooper, J. F. Isoenzymes of acid phosphatase in normal and cancerous human prostatic tissue. *Cancer Res. 37:* 4120, 1977.

37. Foti, A. G., Cooper, J. F., Herschman, H., and Malvaez, R. R. Detection of prostatic cancer by solid-phase radioimmunoassay of serum prostatic acid phosphatase. *N. Engl. J. Med. 297:* 1357, 1977.

38. Foti, A. G., Cooper, J. F., Herschman, H., and Sapon, S. R. The detection of prostatic cancer by radioimmunoassay: a review. *Hum. Pathol. 9:* 618, 1978.

39. Foti, A. G., Herschman, H., and Cooper, J. F. Counterimmunoelectrophoresis in determination of prostatic acid phosphatase in human serum. *Clin. Chem. 24:* 1, 1978.

40. Gittes, R. F., and Chu, T. M. Detection and diagnosis of prostate cancer. *Semin. Oncol. 3:* 123, 1976.

41. Gittes, R. F. Acid phosphatase reappraised. *N. Engl. J. Med. 297:* 1398, 1977.

42. Grenner, G., and Schmidtberger, R. Enzymimmunologische Bestimmung der sauren Prostataphosphatase. *J. Clin. Chem. Clin. Biochem. 17:* 156, 1979.

43. Gursel, E. O., Rezvan, M., Sy, F. A., and Veenema, R. J. Comparative evaluation of bone marrow acid phosphatase and bone scanning in staging of prostatic cancer. *J. Urol. 111:* 53, 1974.

44. Gutman, A. B., and Gutman, E. D. An "acid" phosphatase occurring in the serum of

patients with metastasizing carcinoma of the prostate gland. *J. Clin. Invest. 17:* 473, 1938.

45. Gutman, A. B., and Gutman, E. B. Acid phosphatase and functional activity of the prostate and preputial glands. *Proc. Soc. Exp. Biol. Med. 39:* 529, 1938.

46. Hankor, J. S., Hammarstrom, L. E., and Toolnid, S. U. Functional distribution of acid phosphatase in developing bone and teeth. *J. Dent. Res. 50:* 1502, 1971.

47. Herbert, F. K. The estimation of prostatic phosphatase in serum and its use in the diagnosis of prostatic carcinoma. *Q. J. Med. 59:* 221, 1942.

48. Herger, C. C., and Sauer, H. R. Relationship of serum acid phosphatase determination to presence of bone metastasis from carcinoma of prostate. *J. Urol. 46:* 286, 1941.

49. Hoch-Ligetti, C., and Jarsen, F. J. Enzymes in peripheral and bone marrow serum in patients with cancer. *Cancer 38:* 1336, 1976.

50. Huggins, C., and Hodges, C. V. Studies on prostatic cancer. I. The effect of castration, of estrogen, and of androgen injection on serum phosphatases in metastatic carcinoma of the prostate. *Cancer Res. 1:* 293, 1941.

51. Jacobi, G. H., Kurth, K. H., Boos, J., and Dennebaum, R. Stellenwert der Knochenmarkphosphatasen als "Staging" beim Prostatakarzinom. *Verh. Dtsch. Ges. Urol.* Springer, Berlin, 1979, pp. 395–397.

52. Johnson, E., Prout, G. R., Scott, W. W., Schmidt, J. D., Gibbons, R. P., and Murphy, G. P. Clinical significance of serum acid phosphatase levels in advanced prostatic carcinoma. *Urology VIII:* 123, 1976.

53. Johnson, C. D., Costa, D., and Castro, J. E. Acid phosphatase after examination of the prostate. *Br. J. Urol. 51:* 218, 1979.

54. Khan, R., Turner, B., Edson, M., and Dolan, M. Bone marrow acid phosphatase: another look. *J. Urol. 117:* 79, 1977.

55. Kiefer, H. C. Measurement of phosphatases in biological fluids. *Ann. Clin. Lab. Sci. 7:* 500, 1977.

56. Köllermann, M. W., Delling, D., Burchardt, P., and Klosterhalfen, H. Erfahrungen mit der Beckenkammbiopsie beim Prostatacarcinom. *Urologe 14:* 57, 1975.

57. Kraus, E., and Sitzmann, F. C. Die saure Phosphatase im Serum bei Kindern. *Pädiat. Prax. 12:* 321, 1973.

58. Kurtz, C. W., Walk, W. L. Limitation of prostatic acid phosphatase determination in carcinoma of prostate. *J. Urol. 83:* 74, 1960.

59. Ladenson, J., and McDonald, J. Acid phosphatase and prostatic carcinoma. *Clin. Chem. 24:* 129, 1978.

60. Lam, K. W., Li, O., Li, C. Y., and Yam, L. T. Biochemical properties of human prostatic acid phosphatase. *Clin. Chem. 19:* 483, 1973.

61. Leathem, A., and Dinsdale, E. Acid phosphatase as marker for carcinoma of prostate. *Lancet 2:* 1029, 1979.

62. Li, C. Y., Chuda, R. A., Lam, W. K. W., and Yam, L. T. Acid phosphatase in human plasma. *J. Lab. Clin. Med. 82:* 446, 1973.

63. Little, C., Shojania, A. M., Green, P. P., and Weinerman, B. H. Bone marrow acid phosphatase concentrations in individuals with prostatic carcinoma or other disorders. *Can. Med. Assoc. J. 119:* 259, 1978.

64. London, M., McHugh, R., and Hudson, P. B. On low acid phosphatase values of patients with known metastatic cancer of the prostate. *Cancer Res. 14:* 718, 1954.

65. Lung, T. Y. Clinical significance of the human acid phosphatases. *Am. J. Med. 56:* 604, 1974.

66. Mahan, D. E., and Doctor, B. P. A radioimmune assay for human prostatic acid phosphatase levels in prostatic disease. *Clin. Biochem. 12:* 10, 1979.

67. McDonald, I. Human prostatic acid phosphatase. III. Counterimmunoelectrophoresis for rapid identification. *Arch. Androl. 1:* 235, 1978.

68. Marberger, H. Changes in serum acid phosphatases levels consequent to prostatic manipulation or surgery. *J. Urol. 78:* 287, 1957.

69. Masood, S. Quantitative determination of endogenous acid phosphatase activity in vaginal washings. *Obstet. Gynecol. 51:* 33, 1978.

70. Mathes, G., Richmond, S. G., and Sprunt, D. S. Use of L-tartrate in determining prostatic serum acid phosphatase. Report of 514 cases. *J. Urol. 75:* 143, 1956.

71. Mercer, D. W. Acid phosphatase isoenzymes in Gaucher's disease. *Clin. Chem. 23:* 631, 1977.

72. Mercer, D. W. Separation of tissue and serum acid phosphatase isoenzymes by ion-exchange column chromotography. *Clin. Chem. 23:* 653, 1977.

73. Meißner, D., and Wehnert, J. Die saure Gesamtphosphatase und die Prostataphosphatase in der urologischen Diagnostik. *Z. Urol. Nephrol. 68:* 485, 1975.

74. Moncure, Ch. W., and Prout, G. R. Antigenicity of human prostatic acid phosphatase. *Cancer 2:* 463, 1970.

75. Moncure, Ch. W., Johnston, Ch. L., Smith, M. J. V., and Koontz, W. W. Immunological and histochemical evaluation of marrow aspirates in patients with prostatic carcinoma. *J. Urol. 108:* 609, 1972.

76. Morgan, P. Predictive value of acid phosphatase. *Br. J. Cancer 30:* 190, 1974.

77. Murphy, G. P., Reynoso, G., Kenny, G. M., and Gaeta, J. F. Comparison of total and prostatic fraction serum acid phosphatase levels in patients with differentiated and undifferentiated prostatic carcinoma. *Cancer 23:* 1309, 1969.

78. Murphy, G. P. Prostatic acid phosphatase: where are we? *Cancer J. Clin. 28:* 258, 1978.

79. Nesbit, R. M., Baum, W. C., and Mich, A. A. Serum phosphatase determination in diagnosis of prostatic cancer. A review of 1150 cases. *J.A.M.A. 145:* 1321, 1951.

80. Nilsson, T., and Müntzing, J. The prognostic value of acid phosphatase and β-glucuronidase activity in biopsy specimens from patients with reactivated prostatic cancer. *Scand. J. Urol. Nephrol. 9:* 205, 1975.

81. Nobles, E. R., Kerr, W. S., and Dutoit, Ch. H. Serum prostatic acid phosphatase levels in patients with carcinoma of the prostate. *J.A.M.A. 164:* 2020, 1957.

82. Ozar, M. B., Isaac, C. A., and Valk, W. L. Methods for the elimination of errors in serum acid phosphatase determination. *J. Urol. 74:* 150, 1955.

83. Pais, V. M., Mangold, A. W., and Mahoney, S. A. Fractionation and purification of prostatic acid phosphatase. *Invest. Urol. 12:* 13, 1974.

84. Pontes, J. E., Alcorn, S. W., Thomas, J. A., and Pierce, J. M. Bone marrow acid phosphatase in staging prostatic carcinoma. *J. Urol. 114:* 422, 1975.

85. Pontes, J. E., Choe, B. K., Rose, N. R., and Pierce, J. M. Bone marrow acid phosphatase in staging of prostatic cancer: how reliable is it? *J. Urol. 119:* 772, 1978.

86. Prellwitz, W., Ehrenthal, W., Jacobi, G. H., and Grimm, W. Methods and clinical significance of prostatic acid prosphatase (PAP) determined by RIA and ELISA. *Clin. Chem. Clin. Biochem.,* in press 1982.

87. Prout, G. J. Chemical tests in the diagnosis of prostatic carcinoma. *J.A.M.A. 209:* 1699, 1969.

88. Reif, A. E., Schlesinger, R. M., and Fish, C. A. Acid phosphatase isoenzymes in cancer of the prostate. *Cancer 31:* 689, 1973.

89. Richterich, R., Colombo, J. P., and Weber, H. Ultramikromethoden im klinischen Labor. Bestimmung der sauren Phosphatase. *Schweiz. Med. Wochenschr. 92:* 1496, 1962.

90. Romas, N. A., and Tannenbaum, M. Immunologic detection of prostatic acid phosphatase. Critique I. *Hum. Pathol. 9:* 620, 1978.

91. Romas, N. A., Hsu, K. C., Tomashefsky, Ph., and Tannenbaum, M. Counter immunoelectrophoresis for detection of human prostatic acid phosphatase. *Urology XII:* 79, 1978.

92. Romas, N. A., Rose, N. R., and Tannenbaum, M. Acid phosphatase: new developments. *Hum. Pathol. 10:* 501, 1979.

93. Roy, A. V., Brower, M. E., and Hayden, J. E. Sodium thymolphthalein monophosphate: a new acid phosphatase substrate with greater specificity for the prostatic enzyme in serum. *Clin. Chem. 17:* 1093, 1971.

94. Sadlowski, R. W. Early stage prostatic cancer investigated by pelvic lymph node biopsy and bone marrow acid phosphatase. *J. Urol. 119:* 89, 1978.

95. Shaw, L. M. An evaluation of a kinetic acid phosphatase method. *Am. J. Clin. Pathol. 68:* 57, 1977.

96. Shulman, S., Mamrod, L., Gonder, M. J., and Soanes, W. A. The detection of prostatic acid phosphatases by antibody reactions in gel diffusion. *J. Immunol. 93:* 474, 1964.

97. Seymour, E., Mandel, J. H., Schwenk, R. D., and Warfield, D. L. Diagnostic use of

bone marrow acid and alkaline phosphatases. *Am. J. Clin. Pathol. 67:* 92, 1977.

98. Sodeman, T. M., and Batsakis, J. G. Acid phosphatase. In *Urologic Pathology: The Prostate*, edited by M. Tannenbaum. Lea & Febiger, Philadelphia, 1977, p. 129.

99. Smith, J. K., and Lolutby, L. K. The heterogeneity of prostatic acid phosphatase. *Biochem. Biophys. Acta 151:* 607, 1968.

100. Townsend, R. M. Enzyme tests in diseases of the prostate. *Ann. Clin. Lab. Sci. 7:* 254, 1977.

101. Veenema, R. J., Gursel, E. O., Romas, N., Wechsler, M., and Lattimer, J. K. Bone marrow acid phosphatase: prognostic value in patients undergoing radical prostatectomy. *J. Urol. 117:* 81, 1977.

102. Vihko, P., Kontturi, M., and Korhonen, L. K. Purification of human acid phosphatase by affinity chromatography and isoelectric focusing. Part. I. *Clin. Chem. 24:* 466, 1978.

103. Vihko, P. Characterization of the principal human prostatic acid phosphatase isoenzyme, purified by affinity chromatography and isoelectric focusing. Part. II. *Clin. Chem. 24:* 1783, 1978.

104. Vihko, P., Sajanti, E., Jänne, O., Peltonen, L., and Vihko, R. Serum prostate-specific acid phosphatase: development and validation of a specific radioimmunoassay. *Clin. Chem. 24:* 1915, 1978.

105. Vihko, P. Human prostatic acid phosphatase. Purification of a minor enzyme and comparisons of the enzymes. *Invest. Urol. 16:* 349, 1979.

106. Warren, R. J., and Moss, W. D. An automated continuous monitoring procedure for the determination of acid phosphatase activity in serum. *Clin. Chim. Acta 77:* 179, 1979.

107. Watkinson, J. M., Delory, G. E., King, E. J., and Haddow, A. Plasma and serum phosphatase in carcinoma of prostate and effect of treatment with stilboestrol. *Br. Med. J. 2:* 492, 1944.

108. Wehnert, J., and Meißner, D. Die Phosphataseaktivität im Blutserum beim Prostatakarzinom in Abhängigkeit vom Tumorstadium. *Z. Urol. Nephrol. 69:* 243, 1976.

109. White, D. R., Bannayan, G., George, J., and Stears, D. Histiocytic medullary reticulosis with parallel increases in serum acid phosphatase and disease activity. *Cancer 37:* 1403, 1976.

110. Woodard, H. Q. Quantitative studies of beta-glycerophosphatase activity in normal and neoplastic tissues. *Cancer 9:* 352, 1956.

111. Woodard, H. Q. Factors leading to elevation in serum acid by glycerophosphatase. *Cancer 5:* 236, 1952.

112. Workman, P. Inhibition of human prostatic tumour acid phosphatase by N,N-p-di-2-chloroethylaminophenol, N,N-p-di-2-chloroethylaminophenylphosphate and other difunctional nitrogen mustards. *Chem. Biol. Interact. 20:* 103, 1978.

113. Yam, L. T. Clinical significance of the human acid phosphatases. *Am. J. Med. 56:* 604, 1974.

114. Yarrison, G., Mertens, B. F., and Mathies, J. C. New diagnostic use of bone marrow acid and alkaline phosphatase. *Am. J. Clin. Pathol. 66:* 667, 1976.

115. Yesus, Y. W., and Taylor, H. M. Diagnostic use of bone marrow acid and alkaline phosphatases. *Am. J. Clin. Pathol. 67:* 92, 1977.

116. Zucker, M. B., and Borelli, J. A survey of some platelet enzymes and functions: the platelets as the source of normal serum acid glycerophosphatase. *Ann. N.Y. Acad. Sci. 75:* 203, 1958.

117. Zucker, M. B., and Borelli, J. Platelets as a source of serum acid nitrophenylphosphatase. *J. Clin. Invest. 38:* 148, 1959.

Editorial Comment to Chapter 8

After the writing of this chapter the authors have, in cooperation with the Department of Urology, University of Mainz Medical School, completed a comprehensive study of a newly developed enzyme immunoassay. Patients (704) have been investigated using serum (Jacobi *et al.*, 1981) as well as bone marrow aspirates (Ehrenthal *et al.*, 1982). The following significant findings were demonstrated.

1. A laboratory accuracy comparable to that of a well established commercially available radioimmunoassay;
2. A statistically significant correlation between enzyme immunoassay and radioimmunoassay;
3. A high prostate—but considerably lower carcinoma—specificity due to a number of high phosphatase readings in patients with benign prostatic hyperplasia, prostatic infarction, and prostatic surgery;
4. A clear advantage in sensitivity for prostate cancer as compared to the conventional determination of phosphatase activity;
5. A 58% rate of elevated serum phosphatase concentrations as first indication for early, preclinical osseous spread (bone scan failures);
6. A 94% rate of elevated serum phosphatase concentration reconfirming patients with otherwise documented distant metastases;
7. An excellent correlation between phosphatase concentrations measured in serum and bone marrow aspirates, indicating that bone marrow does not represent a pool in itself for prostatic acid phosphatase in cases with osseous metastases.

On the basis of the results obtained from serum studies the conclusion was drawn that this ELISA enzyme immunoassay is reliable in identifying early osseous metastases by serum investigation. Furthermore, it has clear advantages over RIA test systems in terms of time and cost effectiveness as well as laboratory practicability.

Since the bone marrow space is continuously drained via the lymphatic system and blood circulation bone marrow does not represent a special pool for phosphatases even in case of metastatic involvement. Slightly elevated bone marrow phosphatase concentrations are influenced by the reproducibility of the test system used and by cross-reactions of enzymes and unspecific interferences within the bone marrow space.

Elevated serum phosphatase concentrations mirror those measured in bone marrow by a constant factor. Thus, bone marrow studies will not improve the predictive value for metastatic prostate cancer.

G. H. J.

References

Jacobi, G. H., Ehrenthal, W., Engelmann, U., Grimm, D., Riedmiller, H., Prellwitz, W., and Hohenfellner, R. Immunological determination of serum acid phosphatase in patients with prostate cancer. II. Serum studies with the enzyme-immunoassay ENZYGNOST®-PAP. *Akt. Urol. 12:* 283, 1981.

Ehrenthal, W., Engelmann, U., Prellwitz, W., and Jacobi, G. H. Immunological determination of acid phosphatase in patients with prostate cancer. III. Bone marrow studies of any advantage? *Akt. Urol. 13:* 127, 1982.

9

Radical Prostatectomy in Europe: Trends and Future Perspectives

H. G. W. Frohmüller, M.D.

Radical prostatectomy has been performed as a routine procedure ever since H. H. Young conceived and first carried out this operation in 1904. Its legitimate role as a curative therapeutic method for carcinoma of the prostate, however, remains controversial, in Europe even more so than in USA.

DEFINITION

The terms *"radical prostatectomy"* and *"total prostatectomy"* are used interchangeably, both referring to the surgical extirpation of the entire prostate gland and the seminal vesicles with the ampullae of the vasa deferentia together with the vesical neck. More precisely, this procedure is also named *"prostatovesiculectomy."* In the older German literature one finds occasionally the label *"radical prostatectomy"* erroneously attached to the suprapubic or retropubic removal of BPH (benign prostatic hyperplasia) in order to mark a distinctive contrast to transurethral resection (TUR-P) of BPH. This terminology obviously resulted from the erroneous opinion that the TUR-P was an inferior method as compared with one of the open methods of adenomectomy.

HISTORICAL REMARKS

H. H. Young[91] performed his first radical perineal prostatectomy, which he called prostato-seminal vesiculectomy, on April 7, 1904. He had been greatly impressed by Halsted's radical mastectomy for carcinoma of the breast and felt he should do an equally extensive procedure for carcinoma of the prostate. On this initial procedure he was assisted by Halsted.

It is of historical interest that there had been attempts to remove the prostate for primary carcinoma long before this event. In 1867 the famous German surgeon Billroth, at that time in Vienna, reported two cases, both of which were done through perineal incisions. The first of these operations was performed on a patient aged 20, who died some 14 months later. The second patient died 4 days postoperatively from peritonitis. Between 1880 and the turn of the century five other prostatectomies for cancer through the perineal route and seven other attempts suprapubically were reported. Among the surgeons were Leisrink[47] in 1883, Czerny in 1889, Küster in 1891, and Fuller in 1898. The survival times in all these relatively advanced cases were quite limited.

Young reported a preliminary series of 12 cases in 1909 in which the results were good except that all were incontinent. After careful study he concluded that this was due to disruption of nerves and vessels supplying the triangular ligament anteriorly. After avoiding this by leaving the anterolateral fascia between the prostate and these structures intact, incontinence was avoided in the next 15 cases. Other than variations in the method of perineal approach, e.g. subsphincteric by Belt et al.[8] in 1939, and changes in the method of vesicourethral anastomosis,[27, 85] there have been no significant modifications of this procedure.

The retropubic approach for radical prostatectomy was described by Millin[55] in 1945. For a number of reasons this procedure has gained in popularity in recent years, in the USA as well as in Europe. The Vest technique[85] of vesicourethral reconstruction was modified and adapted for the retropubic approach by Chute.[19] Satisfactory results with this method, comparable with those of primary anastomosis of the vesical neck and the urethra, were reported by Khan et al.[41] from the Mayo Clinic. In order to improve exposure of the apical region of the prostate and to minimize blood loss, Reiner and Walsh[65] provided an excellent description of the anatomical relationship of the dorsal vein of the penis at the prostatourethral junction and devised a method for the operative management of this troublesome venous plexus. Another technique for diminishing hemorrhage beneath the pubic arch was described by Selikowitz and Krane,[75] who suggest ligation of the deep dorsal vein of the penis distal to the penile suspensory ligament. Mittemeyer and Cox[57] advocate an antegrade approach by starting the transsection of the prostate at the vesical neck and continuing the procedure down toward the prostatourethral junction.

In order to gain better access to the retropubic area, Walker[87] first performed a symphysiotomy as an approach to radical prostatectomy. In 1965 the Japanese authors Shishito et al.[77] described their transpubic procedure which consists of resection of a segment of the pubic bone, and in 1976 Novak and co-workers[61] reintroduced this approach by doing a trapezoidal resection of the pubic bones, presenting a series of 15 cases. Notwithstanding the alleged main advantage of reconstruction of bladder neck and membranous urethra under direct vision, this variation of radical retropubic prostatectomy has not become very popular.

To most urologists another rather unfamiliar approach to radical prostatectomy is the transsacral or sacrococcygeal method, introduced in Europe in the 1940s by French urologists as well as by Übelhör[82] in Vienna (Austria) and Thiermann in Nürnberg (Germany). Marshall[50] and particularly Parry[63] in USA described the procedure in detail, and Devlesaver[23] of Bruxelles (Belgium) in 1975 reported 10 cases he had operated upon by this method.

What are the relative merits of perineal and retropubic radical prostatectomy? In general it can be said that in experienced hands the functional results of both methods are equally satisfactory. The preference for one approach or the other is usually a matter of training and experience.

A main advantage of the *perineal route* is the fact that this procedure is generally well tolerated by the patients, particularly in the poor risk and older age group. H. H. Young is supposed to have said: "The Lord intended for the prostate to be approached from the perineum, that is why he put it so close to the outside at the point." Its principal disadvantage is that it does not permit inspection and dissection of the pelvic lymph nodes. In order to perform pelvic lymphadenectomy another operative procedure is then necessary, committing patient and surgeon to two operations.

The *retropubic prostatectomy* is favored by an increasing number of urologists because of their greater familiarity with that region. The main disadvantage of this approach is the technical difficulty to rotate the prostate for obtaining an open biopsy. Since in Europe cytological and/ or histological verification of prostatic carcinoma is almost exclusively done by aspiration or punch biopsy prior to considering the indications for radical prostatectomy, this is actually no problem. The great advantage of retropubic prostatectomy is the ability to combine it with the dissection of the regional lymph nodes for staging purposes and to perform more extensive local surgery, *e.g.* cystectomy with urinary diversion, if need arises.

"RADICAL" TRANSURETHRAL PROSTATECTOMY

Since the early 1970s there have been attempts by a few German urologists (Arnholdt[6]; Sachse[68]) to perform a "radical transurethral resection" with the intention to "cure" the prostatic cancer patient. It appears conceivable to reach this objective in rare cases of a stage A ($T_0N_0M_0$) cancer with a low grade tumor, when all carcinomatous tissue is removed by TUR. Other than this, anatomical considerations alone conflict with this objective. Staging by pelvic lymphadenectomy has not been a part of the diagnostic work-up of these patients subjected to "radical transurethral prostatectomy," and there have been no reports of controlled series so far. (For more details see Chapter 12).

CLINICAL APPLICATIONS OF RADICAL PROSTATECTOMY

Because it was felt that any clinically detectable prostatic cancer is already incurable and because of the promotion of conservative endocrinologic management there were hardly any centers in Europe prior to 1970 where radical prostatectomies were performed. Übelhör in Vienna started in the 1940s to do an occasional perineal or transsacral prostatectomy. Hahn and Kubat in Prague (Czechoslovakia) reported on 15 radical prostatectomies in 1967, two of which they had performed by the transsacral route and 13 by the retropubic approach. Brosig (Berlin) began in 1962 performing radical perineal prostatectomies. At the institution of the author of this report the first radical retropubic prostatectomy was carried out in July 1969.

The situation in Germany changed dramatically since 1970 for the following two reasons:

1. In November 1969 Brosig in Berlin arranged an International Symposium on the Treatment of Carcinoma of the Prostate with the purpose "to resolve the doubts and uncertainty in the treatment of carcinoma of the prostate and formulate a new policy for treatment in the future." The causative factor for arranging this meeting was the confusion concerning the management of prostatic cancer brought about by the report of the *Veterans Administration Cooperative Urological Research Group* (VACURG[86]) in 1967. This symposium gave impetus for a thorough re-evaluation of the entire spectrum of therapeutic measures concerning carcinoma of the prostate.

2. The second stimulus originated in the introduction of the annual preventive check-up examination offered to every man over the age of 45 years in the Federal Republic of Germany by the compulsary insurance companies (see Chapter 4). This decree became legal in 1971 following a suggestion by Alken. Even though only about 17% of the male population older than 45 years participates in this preventive check-up for early detection of diseases at present,[45] this program nevertheless for the first time offered the opportunity to pick up a considerable number of patients in whom cancer of the prostate can be diagnosed at an early stage of the disease, *i.e.* in a stage in which radical prostatectomy is applicable as a potentially curative form of therapy. This is the main reason why around 1972 a number of urological centers, which have been increased in the years since, started performing radical prostatectomies.

This situation, as outlined above, is valid only in Germany and with a similar tendency, in Switzerland, and in a few centers in Austria and the Netherlands.[15, 25, 53, 70, 80, 93] In Sweden and Great Britain for instance, radical prostatectomy is at present not considered a practical method of treating cancer of the prostate.[38, 79] The latter is in obvious agreement with some American authors[10, 16] who state that "there is still doubt as to whether it is desirable to treat patients with early prostatic cancer, category T_0-T_2, and continue that "for patients with category T_3 disease, however, the choice lies between deferred treatment, radiotherapy or hormonal manipulation" without even mentioning the possibility of radical surgery as a form of treatment in such cases.

Technique

It is not within the scope of this chapter to delineate in detail the techniques of perineal or retropubic prostatectomy. Excellent descriptions of either method are abundant in the American literature and can also be found in the German literature.[14, 43]

We have recently asked a medical artist to produce a series of drawings depicting the technique of radical retropubic prostatectomy at our institution. It might be worthwhile to reproduce these sketches here with only brief legends (Figs. 9.1 and 9.2).

Complications

The operative mortality of perineal as well as retropubic radical prostatectomy is less than 1% in the hands of most experienced urologists. Intraoperative complications consist of rectal injury, which is not a problem if recognized and treated immediately, and very rarely division of a ureter, which should be reimplanted promptly.

Urinary leakage may occur as a delayed complication. It subsides within a few days after replacement of the urethral catheter. Sexual impotence is a late complication in virtually all patients. Total urinary incontinence is a sequela in 1 to 12.5% 1 year after surgery. Stress incontinence is observed more frequently, but it is usually temporary. Stricture formation can occur, usually at the urethrovesical anastomosis. It can be successfully treated by internal urethrotomy, if at all necessary.

PELVIC LYMPHADENECTOMY

Pelvic lymphadenectomy has become a well established procedure that permits a clear staging of carcinoma of the prostate. It is preferably carried out as an extraperitoneal operation removing all lymphatic and fibroareolar tissue from the obturator, internal iliac, external iliac, and at least the lower half of the common iliac lymph node areas. When a retropubic radical prostatectomy is planned, lymphadenectomy is usually performed in conjunction with, *i.e.* prior to this procedure. Histologic examination of the frozen sections ascertains the stage of the disease and determines the further progress of the procedure. In institutions without a surgical pathology department and immediate availability of frozen sections lymphadenectomy can be done as a separate operative procedure, with radical prostatectomy following 1 to 2 weeks later, after histological examination of the removed lymph nodes has shown no metastatic spread of the disease. The absence of nodal metastases indicates that the patient may be potentially curable of his cancer.

Generally, pelvic lymphadenectomy is thus considered a diagnostic staging method, with the occasional additional advantage of removing nodal metastases. Whether node dissection is of therapeutic value, affecting survival times, should be determined by controlled studies in the

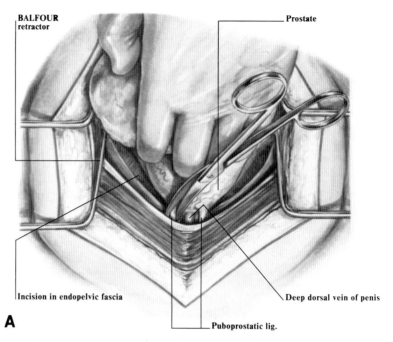

Figure 9.1 Initial part of radical retropubic prostatectomy after pelvic lymph-adenectomy has been performed. *A*, Following lower abdominal midline incision and dissection of pelvic lymph nodes the areolar tissue is removed from the posterior surface of symphysis and os pubis. The lateral endopelvic fascia is incised. Drawing shows transection of puboprostatic ligaments. There is no need to ligate these ligaments.

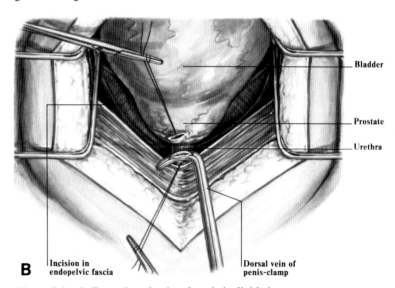

Figure 9.1 *B*, Deep dorsal vein of penis is divided.

future. There is evidence that in bladder cancer patients meticulous pelvic lymph node dissection has a positive effect on survival times with possible cure of the patient.[24] Evidence of the therapeutic value of pelvic lymph-

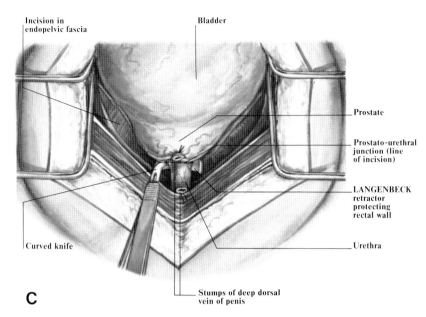

C

Figure 9.1 *C*, Small right-angle Langenbeck retractor is placed between urethra and rectum in order to protect rectal wall while transecting urethra at junction of apex of prostate and membranous urethra.

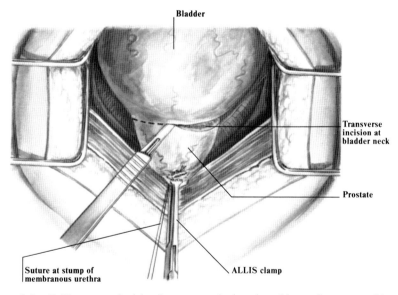

D

Figure 9.1 *D*, Transverse incision between vesical neck and base of prostate with traction of prostate toward symphysis.

adenectomy in patients with prostatic cancer was demonstrated in the Mayo Clinic series of 340 patients who underwent radical retropubic prostatectomy with pelvic lymphadenectomy for stage A,B,C, and D_1 disease. Survival of patients in which nodal metastases were found in only one lymph node was identical to patients free of lymphatic spread and

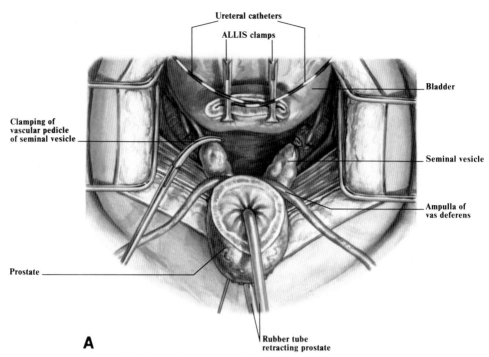

A

Figure 9.2 Second part of radical retropubic prostatectomy after prostate is dissected from bladder neck. *A*, Prostate is completely separated from bladder and retracted downward. Posterior bladder wall is grasped and bluntly mobilized superiorly. Ureteral catheters are in place. Note seminal vesicles and medially the ampullae of vasa deferentia, which are also mobilized bluntly. Prostatic pedicles are ligated.

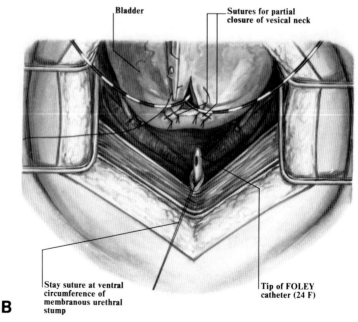

B

Figure 9.2 *B*, Closure of vesical neck to small finger-sized opening.

172   PROSTATE CANCER

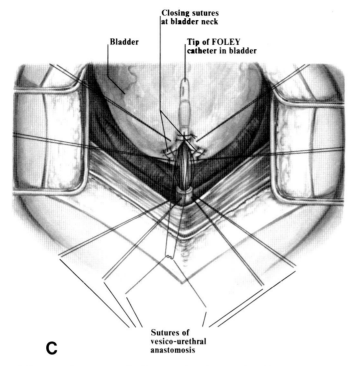

Figure 9.2 *C*, After removal of ureteral catheters tip of F 24 Foley catheter is advanced into lumen of bladder, and sutures are placed between vesical neck and membranous urethra.

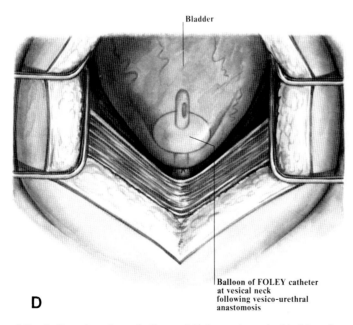

Figure 9.2 *D*, Drawing shows balloon of Foley catheter in bladder after vesico-urethral anastomosis is completed.

RADICAL PROSTATECTOMY IN EUROPE   173

superior as compared to patients with metastatic infiltration of several nodes (Table 9.1).[92]

The importance of pelvic lymphadenectomy as a staging procedure is obvious not only in conjunction with radical prostatectomy, but also when radiation therapy is intended. In the past, pelvic lymphadenectomy was frequently omitted in patients who underwent supervoltage radiotherapy, thus making an accurate staging of the tumor and treatment comparison impossible.

It should also be pointed out that the sampling of lymph nodes is a distinctly inaccurate way to determine metastatic involvement. In order to obtain exact results it is absolutely necessary to do a complete dissection of the lymphatic tissue from around the major pelvic vessels. The local extent of the carcinoma correlates well with the area and side of lymphatic involvement as well with the number of positive nodes[29a].

The operative mortality of extraperitoneal pelvic lymphadenectomy is practically zero, and the complication rate is minimal, mainly consisting of lymphocele formation in about 10% of the patients.[29b, 51] In patients undergoing radiation therapy, there is an additional significant incidence of long-lasting lymphedema of penis, scrotum, and lower extremity following pelvic lymphadenectomy.[29b]

Efforts have been made to replace surgical staging by pedal lymphangiography. Kessler and Igl[40] believe that pedal lymphography has gained widespread acceptance in staging cancer of the prostate, even though they agree with other authors that a main source of false findings is due to the fact that the primary paraprostatic, paravesical, pararectal, presacral, and hypogastric lymph nodes are not opacified by this method. The enthusiasm of these authors and others for lymphangiography as a staging tool is not justified by any objective data. On the contrary, it has been clearly demonstrated, that pedal lymphangiography is an unreliable method to evaluate accurately the status of the regional lymph nodes in carcinoma of the prostate.[48, 52, 54] Even without these statistical data it should be obvious to the unbiased observer that it is simply impossible to recognize micrometastases in the extent of 2 mm or less in diameter by lymphangiographic methods. Myers[60] sums up the discussion on this subject quite well with the following statement: "With so many false-positive and false-negative results, lymphography is almost totally useless as a diagnostic tool for the urologist." The same negative statement holds true for fine needle aspiration biopsy of retroperitoneal lymph nodes, a method ad-

Table 9.1

Influence of Pelvic Lymphadenectomy on Survival following Radical Prostatectomy in Stages C and D_1 (pT_{0-4}, pN_1M_0) Carcinoma of the Prostate[a]

Surgical Stage	No.	Survival Times (%)	
		5 yr	10 yr
C (pT_{3-4}, pN_0,M_0)	49	91	71
D_1 (pT_{0-4}, pN_1M_0)	39	89	73

[a] From H. Zincke et al.[92]

vocated for staging of urologic tumors by Rothenberger *et al.*,[67] at least as far as carcinoma of the prostate is concerned.

STAGING AND GRADING

The management of carcinoma of the prostate is regulated by a combination of the clinical stage of the disease and the classification by histological grading of the tumor (see Chapter 3).

In the United States the most widely used system of staging is that introduced by Whitmore[90] in 1956, which divides the neoplasms into the four categories A, B, C, D. This system was modified by Jewett in 1975. The use of the roman numerals I, II, III, and IV corresponding to the letters A through D was recommended by the American Joint Committee for Cancer Staging and End Results Reporting (AJC) in 1959. In Europe the prevalent staging system is that proposed by the International Union Against Cancer (UICC[83]), known as TNM system (tumor, nodes, metastases). The definition of the different stages was described in Chapter 7 of this book. Figure 9.3 shows a comparison of the different staging systems (see also Editorial Comment to Chapter 7).

Histological grading began with Broders' classification[12] in 1922. Since then a number of different systems have been developed, *e.g.* by Gleason.[32] Recently Mostofi[58] demonstrated the importance of variations in size and shape of the nucleus of the prostatic cancer cell. He considers the

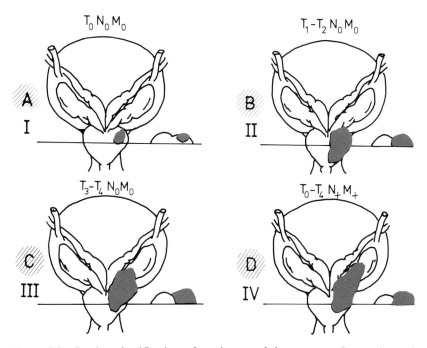

Figure 9.3 Staging classification of carcinoma of the prostate. Comparison of different staging systems, Whitmore's, AJC, UICC. (See also Editorial Comment to Chapter 7)

nuclear pleomorphism a very significant factor for the prognosis of the cancer patient. The problem of histological grading was elucidated in Chapter 6, the cytological grading criteria being outlined in Chapter 5.

DIAGNOSIS

It is well established nowadays that a diagnosis of prostatic cancer is justified only when verified by histological or cytological examination. In order to select the therapeutic method best suited to the individual patient it is further necessary to do an exact staging and grading of the tumor, as mentioned above.

For the purpose of this chapter it may suffice to cite briefly the various tools which are presently in use when the urologist is asked to establish the diagnosis of carcinoma of the prostate.

In the early stage of the disease—and only in these cases radical prostatectomy appears indicated and of value as a curative form of treatment—the patient's history usually reveals no specific symptoms, or only obstructive urinary signs caused by concomitant benign prostatic hyperplasia.

Rectal examination is the most important method to arouse suspicion of the presence of cancer of the prostate. This is the reason for the emphasis on annual rectal examination for all men over 45 years old, as it is offered to every male member of German compulsory insurance companies since 1971. By this simple and inexpensive procedure the vast majority of prostatic cancers can be detected. But rectal examination is not only important to discover the tumor, it is also still the basis for the clinical staging of the disease.

In Germany, the routine annual rectal examination is usually performed by a general practitioner. If he suspects on the ground of his rectal palpation the presence of prostatic cancer, he usually sends the patient to the urologist for confirmation of the diagnosis by biopsy. The urologist then has four different biopsy methods at his disposal, namely:

1. Transrectal fine needle aspiration biopsy which yields a cytological diagnosis. No general or local anesthesia is needed.
2. Perineal or transrectal needle biopsy ("punch biopsy"), that renders a histological diagnosis. Because the transrectal method is burdened with a higher incidence of fever and other septic symptoms, the perineal approach should be preferred.
3. Transurethral biopsy using an electro- or punch resectoscope. Since cancer of the prostate arises in 95% of cases in the peripheral part of the gland, the transurethral method is not suited to the early stage of the tumor and is therefore of minor importance.
4. Open perineal biopsy. This method has been practically eliminated by the increasing skill of urologists and thereby accuracy of diagnosis with the aspiration and punch biopsies.

A clear-cut advantage of the fine needle aspiration and the punch biopsies is the fact that these methods can be performed on an outpatient basis without any particular preparation of the patient and with a very low rate of complications. With the punch biopsy, slight injuries to the urethra and bladder with resulting bleeding, fever, etc. are known to occur.

Transrectal fine needle aspiration biopsy is considered a minor procedure with hardly any inconvenience to the patient and almost no complications and contraindications. It has been recommended, therefore, as method of choice for the morphological diagnosis of carcinoma of the prostate (Chapter 5). In order to find out whether this technique can be relied upon with the same degree of certainty as the punch biopsy, Ackermann and Müller[2] analyzed 645 simultaneous perineal punch biopsies and transrectal aspiration biopsies. Cancer of the prostate was detected in a total of 39.1% either with both procedures or with only one of them. A concordant diagnosis was obtained in only 25.1%. The tumor was found more often by perineal punch biopsy (36.1%) than by the aspiration technique (27.7%). The diagnosis was missed, however, by perineal punch biopsy in 2.6% of the cases. Unsatisfactory preparations and doubtful results were observed more frequently by the fine needle aspiration biopsy. The authors concluded that the combination of both techniques, transrectal fine needle aspiration biopsy and perineal punch biopsy, can be recommended for optimal detection of prostatic carcinoma.

It is for these reasons that the majority of urologists in Germany do not rely on a cytological diagnosis alone obtained by the fine needle aspiration technique, but do request a histological diagnosis before definite treatment, such as radical prostatectomy, is given consideration. In Scandinavia, however, the situation seems quite different (Chapter 5).

Apart from the routine laboratory tests, such as urinalysis, sedimentation rate, serum creatinine, etc., the determination of serum acid phosphatase and its "prostatic fraction" is of some diagnostic and prognostic value. However, this is true mainly in the advanced cases and not in the early stage of the cancer that is suitable for radical surgery. Improvements of this diagnostic tool can be expected from the counterimmunoelectrophoresis method, described by Chu et al.,[18] as well as the development of radioimmunoassay (RIA) techniques with their far higher sensitivity[28, 31] (see Chapter 8).

In order to improve not only the sensitivity, but in particular the specificity of RIA, investigations are being carried out at present to produce monoclonal antibodies against prostatic acid phosphatase.[1]

Bone marrow aspiration for biopsy and acid phosphatase determination seems to have been overvalued as a diagnostic test in the past. Additional diagnostic information can be obtained by radiological methods, such as excretory urography, CAT scanning, and vasoseminal vesiculography. Some centers[25] consider this last mentioned examination an essential part of their preoperative work-up for radical prostatectomy. Because of our indications for radical surgery we are not of this opinion. The low yield of lymphangiography as a diagnostic tool in the early stage of the disease has been mentioned before. Urethrocystoscopy adds little information in the early stage of the tumor, but is very useful in stage C (T_{3-4}) lesions of the carcinoma. Recent progress in sonography gives reason for hope that this technique may become a valuable aid in the diagnosis of early cancerous lesions of the prostate (Chapter 3).

Bone scanning using 99-technetium is a very useful diagnostic test always indicated before radical prostatectomy, but it is obviously not a method for early detection of the primary tumor.

In the future it is hoped that tumor markers or biological factors may become available to identify the primary tumor at an early stage. There is research in progress that may lead to a form of "immunological staging" thus eliminating the need for surgical staging.[62]

INDICATIONS FOR RADICAL PROSTATECTOMY

Reviewing the literature on the subject of indications for radical prostatectomy one must come unquestionably to the conclusion that the state of the art and science in this respect is very confused. The spectrum ranges from the innumerable "*conscientious objectors*" of radical surgery called by O. S. Culp to those intrepid urologists, who consider D_1 lesions perfectly operable. Culp and Meyer[21] listed a number of factors which apparently contribute to the widespread antipathy against radical prostatectomy. They include: (1) "failure of many surgeons to master the precise technical demands" of radical prostatectomy, be it the perineal or the retropubic approach; (2) "persistence of the thought that any clinically detectable prostatic cancer is already incurable"; (3) "promotion of conservative endocrinologic and radiologic management rather than of radical prostatic surgery", (4) "unwillingness of patients to accept the physiologic price of either postoperative impotence or stress incontinence of urine or both."

The basic dilemma in selecting the proper treatment for the individual patient with cancer of the prostate is due to the fact that so very little is known up to now about the biological potential of the cancer and the reaction of its host against the tumor. For these reasons the proposal to offer no treatment at all seems understandable for the patient with a slowly growing carcinoma, which may never overtake the particular patient. However, it is well known that the growth rate of such tumors is not predictable, and therefore, as Jewett[37] aptly remarks, "The policy of wait and see what happens to a discrete nodule of cancer in a 62 year old man with a nonobstructing prostate sounds somewhat like a game of Russian roulette."

The clinical difficulty in selecting the proper therapy for the individual patient lies in the fact that truly comparable groups of patients are not readily available. It is probably impossible to ever acquire a truly acceptable "control" series in any form of prostatic cancer.[20] Therefore, rigid criteria for the selection of candidates for radical prostatectomy, which would be acceptable universally, have not been established thus far.

Within the last decade it could be demonstrated by several investigators with reports of large series[9, 21, 37] that survival of patients with carcinoma of the prostate is mainly influenced by two factors, namely the stage and the histological grade of the tumor.

The clinical staging of the tumor lacks notoriously in accuracy, as shown by many authors. In a series of 262 patients collected by Schröder,[72] 52.3% of stage B (T_{1-2}) tumors were underestimated and pT_3 tumors were found in the surgical specimen. Belt and Schröder[9] diagnosed by rectal examination in 207 patients a stage B (T_{1-2}) cancer; histologically 114 of these patients were found to have a stage C (T_3) tumor, a false estimation of 55.1%. Kurth et al.,[46] furthermore, discovered an incidence of lymph node metastases of about 50% in stage C (T_3) carcinomas at the time of surgery. These figures make it evident that in about 50% of the cases it is not possible to differentiate carcinoma of the prostate properly preoperatively.

Combining rectal examination, bone scanning, and pelvic lymphadenectomy it is possible, however, to determine the stage of the carcinoma reasonably well. On the other hand, considerable difficulties arise with the grading of the cancerous lesion.

Kastendieck[39] examined histologically 120 prostates after radical prostatovesiculectomy by step-section technique and compared the results with the preoperative punch biopsy specimens. In 62.5% of the cases he found a complete conformity of the histological grade of the tumor between the biopsy material and the removed prostate. In 28.3% the histological classifications correlated only partially, and in 9.2% a total divergence was noted. On the basis of his findings the author concluded that the histological specimen obtained by perineal (or transrectal) punch biopsy cannot be considered typical of the entire tumor. Müller and collaborators[59] at our institution compared in 100 cases the morphology of the tumor as seen in perineal punch biopsy specimens and that observed in the total surgical specimen removed by radical prostatectomy. Forty-three of these 100 cases showed a uniform architectural pattern and 54 a pluriform morphology. Three biopsy specimens were not available for reevaluation. Uniform, well differentiated tumor in both biopsy and total prostatectomy specimens was found in only seven (33.3%) of 21 cases. In the remaining 14 cases of this group the operative specimens revealed areas of other grades of differentiation. Our collected data indicate that biopsy specimens express the complete differentiation of carcinoma of the prostate in only 20 to 25% of the cases (see Chapter 6). Figure 9.4 shows a typical example of different grades of tumor differentiation in a total prostatectomy specimen in comparison with the perineal punch biopsy specimen of the same case.

These analyses demonstrate the obvious difficulties the surgeon faces when he is asked to make a decision for or against radical prostatectomy on the basis of the morphological grading of the aspiration or punch biopsy specimen. Most authors, for instance, agree nowadays that a stage A_1 (T_0) tumor (focal incidental carcinoma), histologically classified as low grade (well differentiated), is not an indication for either radical surgery or supervoltage radiation therapy. In approximately three-fourths of these cases, however, one has to expect that remaining sections of the cancer are of higher grade and thus of more aggressive potential, and in this case some form of treatment appears indicated. The same statement holds true respectively for stage B (T_{1-2}) tumors.

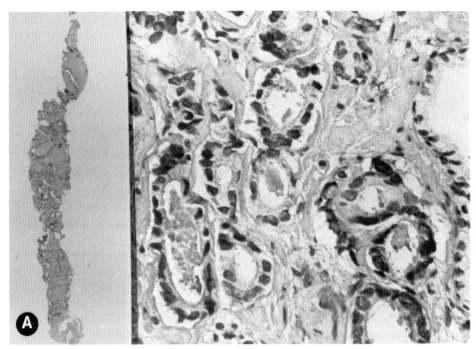

Figure 9.4 Discordance of grade of tumor differentiation in tissues obtained by biopsy and after radical prostatectomy. *A, Left,* Specimen of the prostate obtained by perineal punch biopsy. ×45. *Right,* Uniformly well differentiated adenocarcinoma. ×375.

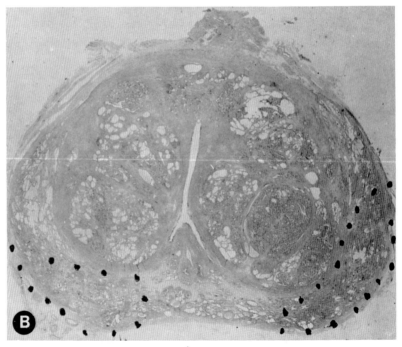

Figure 9.4 *B,* Specimen of radical prostatectomy. Gross section of the respective prostate with two malignant foci on the dorsal aspect of each lateral lobe. ×2.25.

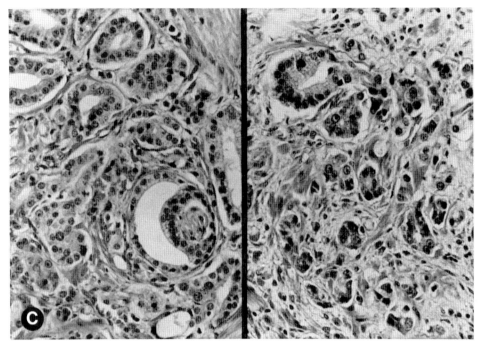

Figure 9.4 *C, Left,* Uniform, well differentiated adenocarcinoma of the right lateral lobe with perineural invasion. ×240. *Right,* Well differentiated and poorly differentiated adenocarcinoma of the left lateral lobe. ×240.

The efficacy of radical prostatectomy in properly selected patients is attested by a great number of data collected by many authors, particularly in the USA, generally on the basis of 10- and 15-year survivals.[9, 20, 21, 37, 73] Apart from these data it is a general surgical rule to excise a cancerous lesion if the condition of the patient and the localization and size of the tumor permit. No urologist, for example, would think of denying a patient with a renal carcinoma the benefit of removing the tumor if at all possible. Huggins[35] stated in this connection: "Cancer is safest when completely removed and preserved in pickle" and he added "radical prostatectomy is for the surgeon who cares."

It seems amazing, therefore, that the benefits of radical prostatectomy are still questioned by a sizable number of urologists, not to mention, of course, radiologists. Admittedly, carcinoma of the prostate is in many respects a different tumor as compared with other types of cancer in the human body, particularly as far as its biological potential is concerned. This feature has been mentioned before. But according to our present knowledge there is still no logical alternative to Jewett's following statement[37]:

> For certain types of carcinoma of the prostate the "belief in the superiority of radical prostatectomy over other single methods of treatment rests on two propositions: (1) If all the cancer cells resided in the tissue to be excised, and excision is properly accomplished, cure is assured. (2) In such a case there is no alternative treatment of equal efficacy."

The author of this chapter happens to agree with this valuation, and our choice of treatment of prostatic cancer is adjusted accordingly. Our criteria for doing or omitting a radical prostatectomy will be listed as follows, with reference to the tumor stage and its histological grade.

Stage A ($T_0N_0M_0$) ("Incidental Carcinoma" Diagnosed at Time of Transurethral Resection or Open Adenomectomy of Benign Prostatic Hyperplasia)

A_1 *Focal carcinoma, low grade (well differentiated)*: Clinical follow-up for the duration of the patient's life with rectal examination and biopsy every 6 months. If cancer becomes palpable or changing of the grade occurs, the patient is treated as in stage A_2.

A_2 *Diffuse (multifocal) carcinoma, low grade or high grade (well or poorly differentiated adenocarcinoma)*: Radical prostatectomy. If patient is in poor clinical condition or refuses the operation: external supervoltage radiotherapy or interstitial radiation.

Stage B ($T_{1-2} N_0M_0$) (B_1, Involving Less than One Lobe; B_2, Involving One Lobe or Both Lobes without Extension beyond the Capsule of the Prostate)

Low Grade (well differentiated): Transurethral prostatic resection (TUR-P), preferably with the cold punch resectoscope, which provides the pathologist with tissue that is easier to evaluate more precisely. In this way larger amounts of tissue can be sampled, and the results of the biopsy can either be confirmed or the grading will be changed. If the histological examination of the tissue obtained by TUR-P verifies a uniformly low-grade tumor, the patient is treated as in stage A_1.

High Grade (intermediate or poor differentiation): Treatment as in stage A_2.

Stage C ($T_{3-4} N_0 M_0$): Any Grade of Differentiation

In this stage the UICC classification is more precise than Whitmore's classification. Therefore we vary our indication depending on the extent of the tumor.

T_3 Tumor extends beyond the capsule and may invade the seminal vesicles: treatment as in stage A_2

T_4 Tumor is fixed and invades neighboring structures as far as the levator ani muscles: external supervoltage radiotherapy or treatment as in stage D ($T_{0-4} N_{1-4} M_1$).

Occasionally it seems possible to "downstage" a T_4 tumor by the administration of hormones (stilbestrol or cyproterone acetate), thus converting it to a T_3 tumor, which then will be treated as outlined above.

Although the results of radical prostatectomy for stage C (T_3) tumors are generally disappointing, there have been reports that radical surgery is indeed effective for some of these patients as far as mortality as well as morbidity, *i.e.* "quality of life," is concerned.[26, 73, 81]

Stage D (T_{0-4} N_{1-4} M_1), Any Grade of Differentiation

D_1 Initially diagnosed as having stage A, B, or C disease, but found at operation to have pelvic lymph node metastases[17]: If frozen sections of pelvic lymph nodes, dissected as a staging procedure, demonstrate invasion by microscopic metastases or gross involvement of no more than one or two lymph nodes, we proceed with radical retropubic prostatectomy.

D_2 Clinically metastatic carcinoma at the time of diagnosis: No radical prostatectomy or radiotherapy indicated. The treatment of these types of tumor is highly controversial at present and the discussion of the management of these patients is within the scope of Chapters 11, 13, 15, and 16.

It ought to be pointed out for the sake of objectiveness that the majority of urologists who perform radical prostatectomy stick to the classical indication of this procedure and limit it to the treatment of patients with stage A and B disease, as outlined above. Our extended indication for radical surgery is in agreement with reports by Schröder and Belt[73] and the Mayo Clinic series.[92]

After the previous remarks about pelvic lymphadenectomy it should actually not be necessary to point out that this staging operation is considered an integral part of radical prostatectomy as well as external supervoltage radiation therapy and interstitial radiation.

Observations and comparisons of operative results and survival times reported by many authors have been reviewed in excellent articles by Boxer,[11] Catalona and Scott,[17] Jewett,[37] and others, so that there is no need to repeat these data here. The interested reader is referred to these papers for very informative details.

Besides staging and grading of the tumor the selection of patients for radical prostatectomy depends on a number of further conditions:

1. The patient should have a life expectancy of about 10 years. Thus, the reasonable upper limit of age for recommendation of radical surgery is around 70 years.
2. The patient has to be free of serious unrelated diseases.
3. Serum acid phosphatase should be within normal limits.
4. Excretory urography ought to be free of obstructive signs.
5. Bone scan using radioisotopes should not demonstrate any evidence of skeletal metastases.

It is important to tell the patient the diagnosis and to discuss with him and with his family, if desired, the various methods of treatment available in his particular case. This is important not only for legal reasons but also to gain his confidence and cooperation. Although the urologist will make a proposal for definite therapy the patient should be aware of the fact that he participates in the responsibility of making the decision.

Primary transitional cell carcinoma of the prostate is an uncommon entity separate from the ordinary adenocarcinoma. These neoplasms are hormonally independent, and radiation therapy has been shown not to be successful. Radical prostatectomy, or better cystoprostatectomy, is therefore the treatment of choice in these cases, if feasible.[33, 66]

COMPARISON OF RADICAL PROSTATECTOMY VERSUS RADIATION THERAPY

Although radiotherapy of carcinoma of the prostate will be dealt with expertly and extensively in Chapter 10 of this book, it seems indicated to include a few pertinent remarks on the subject in this report.

Since Bagshaw et al.[7] in 1965 first reported on their success in treating patients with an operable carcinoma of the prostate by external supervoltage radiation, this type of therapy as well as interstitial radiation have become the main competitors of radical prostatectomy for potentially curative treatment of prostatic cancer. Whereas many authors, mainly radiologists, claim radiotherapy to be a curative method, others more cautiously circumscribe it as "potentially curative," "effective,"[88] or use formulations such as "control of the tumor by radiation," "neutralizing effect on the tumor by radiation," "sterilizing of the tumor."[36] As Jewett[37] points out, "The appeal of this treatment to most urologists is strong. It relieves them of the necessity for precise clinical staging, and of the burden of radical excision."

The usefulness of radiation treatment as a therapeutic method has to be evaluated by the local destruction of the cancer, the survival times of patients, and the complication rate. The effects of radiotherapy can only be verified by repeated biopsies and morphological examinations, as first pointed out by Sewell et al.[76] Rectal examination alone is not sufficient, as indicated by the results of Alken et al.,[5] who discovered only 71% conformity between rectal finding and the degree of regression as observed by histology (see Chapter 3).

As demonstrated in Table 9.2, which relates the biopsy data following radiotherapy of prostatic cancer, complete destruction of the tumor was detected in 13 to 86% of all cases with an average of 55%. Sewell et al.[76] were able to show that histological changes depend on the time interval following radiation therapy. Within the first year vital tumor was noticed

Table 9.2
Biopsy Findings following Radiation Therapy of Carcinoma of the Prostate[a]

Authors[b]	No. of Patients	No. of Biopsies	Positive (%)	Negative (%)	Time Interval after Therapy
Bagshaw, M.A., et al.	6	6	0	100	—[c]
George, F.W., et al.	7	7	14	86	6 mo–4½ yr
Grout, D.C., et al.	11	11	46	54	6 mo
Carlton, C.E., Jr., et al.	20	20	30	70	3 yr
Alken, C.E., et al.	16	16	87[d]	13	2–15 mo
Cosgrove, M.D., et al.	9	6	33	66	1–4 yr
Hill, D.R., et al.	68	21	24	76	1–7 yr
Mollenkamp, J.S., et al.	88	77	58	42	1 yr
Sewell, R.A., et al.	17	17	65	35	5 yr

[a] From F. H. Schröder et al.[74]
[b] Complete references given in F. H. Schröder et al.[74]
[c] —, Not specified.
[d] Sixty-three percent regressive changes.

in 87% of the cases. The final effect of radiation becomes evident only after 2 years.[36]

Alken et al.[5] observed in 38 patients, reviewed after more than 1 year following external radiation therapy, three types of regressive changes, namely: (1) the regression advances continuously (20 cases); (2) there is no significant regression (12 cases); (3) there is a transient significant regression, which is followed, however, by new tumor growth (six cases) (Fig. 9.5). Similar results were reported by Jacobi et al.[36] Alken et al.[5] could not detect any relation between the tumor type (well differentiated, low differentiated, cribriform, and solid-anaplastic) on one hand and the radiosensitive and radioresistant cases on the other hand. On the basis of these findings the authors concluded that it is not possible to prognosticate a possible therapeutic success of radiation therapy by the originally determined histological grade of the tumor.

These authors also stated on the basis of their studies that they would "of course" not claim that in their cases with very distinctive signs of regression or even complete regression of the tumor the cancer was entirely destroyed, even when several biopsies had not demonstrated any tumor tissue. This is a clear statement in view of the fact that even with multiple biopsies from both lobes of the prostate it is never possible to

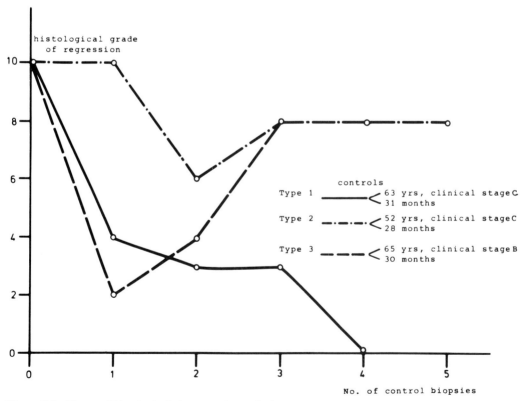

Figure 9.5 Types of histological changes after radiation therapy of carcinoma of the prostate. Histological regression is specified in Chapter 6. (Reproduced with permission from C. E. Alken et al.[5])

examine histologically the entire prostate. A few tiny nests of viable cancerous cells could remain undetected. It is indeed mainly for this reason that the authors came to the conclusion that "radical prostatectomy is the most reliable and safest method" for complete removal or destruction of prostatic cancer.

Wannenmacher et al.[89] believe that the curative potential of interstitial radiation is higher than that of external radiotherapy. However, the method is to be reserved for a more selected group of patients, e.g. incidental carcinoma is allegedly not suited for this form of therapy. Also, the safety regulations concerning the radiation hazards of the isotopes used to the environment may still be problematic.

Survival data of patients treated by radical prostatectomy or radiation therapy demonstrate almost identical results for stage B disease, but favor radical prostatectomy in stage C patients (for references see Schröder et al.[74]). An exception to this general statement are van der Werf-Messing's[84] excellent 5-year survival rates of 85% in stage C patients. The immense data available nowadays for the various therapeutic modalities make it obvious, however, that 5-year survival no longer carries weight and that attention should be directed to 10-year or better, 15-year survival rates (!).

Although a number of complications have been reported following radiotherapy, such as urethritis, cystitis, proctitis as acute manifestations, and stenoses of the ureteral orifices, urethral strictures, bladder neck contractures, strictures of the rectum, lymphedema of the lower extremities, and sexual impotence (23 to 47%) as late sequelae (for references see Schröder et al.[74]), they are usually not considered as grave as those associated with radical surgery. In addition to the operative mortality, which is less than 1%, it is particularly the sexual impotence in practically all patients treated by radical prostatectomy, as well as the complete (1 to 12.5%) and stress (11 to 27.4%) urinary incontinence (for references see Schröder et al.[74]), which require serious consideration. Incontinence, for instance, is not known after irradiation. This means that the main disadvantages of the operative procedure are impotence and the possibility of urinary incontinence.

In summary, therefore, radiation therapy seems indicated in patients who are not willing to undergo surgery, who are unwilling to accept sexual impotence, or who are poor candidates for surgery because of other reasons.

One should bear in mind, however, that radiotherapy can give a false sense of security for the following reasons (see also Editorial Comment to Chapter 10):

1. Radiation rarely can destroy all the cells in the entire cell population of the cancer.
2. Up to the present time there is no way of telling whether and for what period of time cancerous cells found in biopsy specimens following radiotherapy are capable of biological activity, i.e. to reproduce and metastasize.
3. Not all prostatic cancers are radiosensitive. Jacobi et al.[36] found no

regression of the tumor after external radiotherapy in one third of their patients.

4. Even multiple and extensive biopsies for control studies are never a substitute for histological examination of the entire prostate, and some nests of viable cancer cells could remain undetected.

Considering these circumstances it seems justified to question the following statement by Foroogh et al.[29] that "radiation therapy is a curative and acceptable alternative to radical surgery . . . in early stages (A and B) of carcinoma of the prostate."

Only a large, prospective, randomized trial can clarify the situation which at present is clouded by too many subjective evaluations, anecdotal reports, and even emotional criticism.

FUTURE PERSPECTIVES

A number of publications demonstrate convincingly[9, 21, 37, 73] that survival figures are produced by radical prostatectomy in patients with a locally confined tumor that equal the theoretical life expectancy of comparable groups of patients. These results are believed to be valid evidence for the efficacy of this type of procedure.

Recently, however, data reported by Madsen et al.[49] suggest that radical surgery does not prolong survival when compared with an untreated group of patients. These authors found no statistical difference in survival times when they compared placebo to radical prostatectomy plus placebo in a randomized study. Since their investigation is burdened with a relatively small number of patients, further reports with similar results have to be awaited before these data can be recognized as significant.

On the basis of these and other reports, Schröder[70] thinks it is possible "that the "good results" obtained by radical surgery may reflect the natural history of the disease more than the effect of the treatment". He proposed therefore, a study of radical prostatectomy in a sufficiently large prospective, randomized trial in order to clarify this situation. The investigation should compare radical prostatectomy with radiotherapy and delayed treatment. In this way a number of pertinent questions, including a valid comparison between radical surgery and radiation therapy, could possibly be answered. In spite of "strong regional and personal preferences" for various therapeutic modalities it is hoped that such a study can be undertaken with the assistance of a large number of urological centers in different European countries.

In the past 2 decades, considerable progress has been made to distinguish between high and low risk groups of tumors by more precise staging and especially by developing more informative techniques of histological grading.[32, 58] It seems that further advances in this direction can be expected less from these conventional methods than from new techniques, such as radioimmunoassays and other immunological methods. Such improvements would undoubtedly aid in further defining the usefulness as well as the limitations of radical prostatectomy.

CONCLUSIONS

1. "Local tumor requires a local attack, metastatic tumor a systemic attack" as pointed out by Hohenfellner.[34]
2. In suitable cases of carcinoma of the prostate radical prostatectomy offers a good chance of curing the patient of his disease.
3. In appropriate cases there is no alternative to radical prostatectomy of equal efficacy.
4. In experienced hands radical prostatectomy is a well outlined procedure with a low mortality (less than 1%) and acceptable morbidity.
5. Pelvic lymphadenectomy as a staging procedure is an absolute prerequisite for performing a radical prostatectomy or—for that matter—for radiotherapy with curative objective. It can in no way be replaced by pedal lymphangiography.
6. Histological evaluation of punch biopsies is capable of predicting the grade of the tumor as determined from the radical prostatectomy specimen only in a limited percentage of cases.
7. Further investigations with new techniques will be necessary in order to distinguish between various risk groups of prostatic cancer.
8. It is hoped that in the future prospective randomized studies will clarify the usefulness and the limitations of radical prostatectomy as well as the role of radiotherapy in the treatment of potentially curative cancer of the prostate.

ADDENDUM

In closing this chapter on radical prostatectomy it seems appropriate to relate a compilation of the results of this procedure at our institution. In the Urological Department of the University of Würzburg Medical School, we performed 112 radical prostatectomies up to the time of this writing, over a period of the last 11 years. The first consecutive 100 cases were evaluated for this report. From 1969 to July 1979 a total of 522 patients with carcinoma of the prostate were admitted to our institution. This means that 19.1% of these 522 patients were treated by radical prostatectomy. In each of the last 2 years that percentage was as high as 33% and in 1976 it was even 46% (Fig. 9.6).

Clinical staging of the carcinoma in these 100 patients who were treated by total prostatectomy revealed that nine belonged to stage A of Whitmore's classification, 78 were found to be in stage B, and 13 in stage C. Histopathological examination of the total prostatectomy specimen and pelvic lymphadenectomy specimens of these 100 cases, however, changed the relations. Applying the TNM system 40 patients were found to have a stage T_1 tumor, 37 stage T_2, 15 stage T_{3-4}, and eight stage $T_{1-4}N_{1-2}M_0$ carcinoma.

In approximately three-fourths of the 100 patients a radical retropubic prostatectomy was carried out, whereas in about one-fourth of the cases the perineal approach was used (Table 9.3). In 93 of the 100 patients a

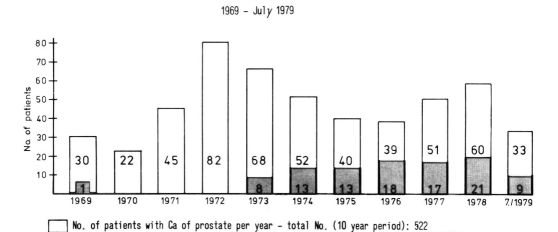

Figure 9.6 Incidence of carcinoma of prostate during 10-year period. (Department of Urology, University of Würzburg Medical School)

Table 9.3
Operative Approach in 100 Cases of Radical Prostatectomy at the Department of Urology, University of Würzburg Medical School

Operative Approach	No. of Patients
Retropubic	
With pelvic lymph node dissection, one stage operation	67
Without pelvic lymph node dissection	4
Total no.	71
Perineal	
With pelvic lymph node dissection, two stage operation	26
Without pelvic lymph node dissection	3
Total No.	29

pelvic lymph node dissection was performed as a staging procedure. This was done as a two-stage operation in the cases in which a perineal approach was utilized, and as a one-stage procedure in the retropubic prostatectomy cases.

In 91.4% of the 93 patients, in whom a pelvic lymphadenectomy had been carried out, the nodes were found to be free of metastases. In six patients (6.5%), however, one to three of the excised lymph nodes revealed metastases, and in two of the patients (2.1%) more than three nodes were involved by metastatic dissemination.

This tabulation demonstrates the apparent difficulty inherent in the frozen section technique, because in these last two cases with more than three positive nodes, as well as in three of the six cases with one to three positive nodes, the frozen sections were reported to be free of carcinoma, whereas in the final paraffin wax preparation the cancer lesions were clearly detected.

Table 9.4
Intraoperative Complications in 100 Cases of Radical Prostatectomy at the Department of Urology, University of Würzburg Medical School

Complication	No. of Patients	Approach	No.
Perforation of rectum	6	Retropubic	3
		Perineal	3
Ureteral injury	4	Retropubic	2
		Perineal	2
Mortality[a]	1	Retropubic	

[a] The death on the first postoperative day was due to a preoperatively unrecognized hematological disorder.

The mortality rate was 1% (Table 9.4). This one patient died on the first postoperative day of an uncontrollable hemorrhage because a hematological disorder had not been recognized preoperatively.

Intraoperatively the rectum was perforated in six instances, three times in 71 cases of retropubic prostatectomy, and three times in 29 cases operated upon by the perineal approach (Table 9.4). The ureter was injured in four cases, equally distributed between the perineal and retropubic procedures. As a *late complication* we found total incontinence in three patients, two of whom had been operated upon retropubically and one perineally.

This brief summary of our experiences with 100 radical retropubic and perineal prostatectomies compares satisfactorily with other reports of these procedures in the literature. Our conviction of the benefit of total prostatectomy for the individual patient as well as the low mortality and morbidity rates encourages us to continue the utilization of this operation in suitable cases of carcinoma of the prostate.

REFERENCES

1. Ackermann, R., and Köhler, J. Personal communication, 1980.
2. Ackermann, R., and Müller, H.-A. Retrospective analysis of 645 simultaneous perineal punch biopsies and transrectal aspiration biopsies for diagnosis of prostatic carcinoma. *Eur. Urol. 3:* 29, 1977.
3. Alken, C. E. Zur Radikaloperation des Prostatacarcinoms. *Urologe 1:* 120, 1962.
4. Alken, C. E. Frühdiagnose und Therapie des Prostatakarzinoms in Frage gestellt? *Dtsch. Ärztebl. 76:* 702, 1979.
5. Alken, C. E., Dhom, G., Kopper, B., Rehker, H., Dietz, R., Kopp, S., and Ziegler, M. Verlaufskontrolle nach Hochvolttherapie des Prostatacarcinoms. *Urologe A 16:* 272, 1977.
6. Arnholdt, F. Radikale, transurethrale Elektroresektion des Prostatakarzinoms. *Urol. Int. 28:* 50, 1973.
7. Bagshaw, M. A., Kaplan, H. S., and Sagerman, R. H. Linear accelerator supervoltage radiotherapy. VII. Carcinoma of the prostate. *Radiology 85:* 121, 1965.
8. Belt, E., Ebert, C. E., and Surber, A. C., Jr. A new anatomical approach in perineal prostatectomy. *J. Urol. 41:* 482, 1939.
9. Belt, E., and Schröder, F. H. Total perineal prostatectomy for carcinoma of the prostate. *J. Urol. 107:* 91, 1972.
10. Blackard, C. E., Mellinger, G. T., and Gleason, D. F. Treatment of stage I carcinoma of the prostate. A preliminary report. *J. Urol. 106:* 729, 1971.
11. Boxer, R. J. Adenocarcinoma of the prostate gland. *Urol. Surv. 27:* 75, 1977.
12. Broders, A. C. Epithelioma of genito-urinary organs. *Ann. Surg. 75:* 574, 1922.

13. Brosig, W. Introductions. In *International Symposium on the Treatment of Carcinoma of the Prostate*, edited by E. Raspé and W. Brosig. Pergamon Press, Oxford, 1971.

14. Brosig, W., and Kollwitz, A.-A. Zur Indikation und Technik der radikalen Prostatektomie. *Urologe 5:* 137, 1966.

15. Burkert, S., and Kiesswetter, H. Die radikale perineale Prostatektomie beim Prostatakarzinom. Ein Erfahrungsbericht über 30 Fälle. *Wien. Med. Wochenschr. 128:* 628, 1978.

16. Byar, D. P. Survival of patients with incidentally found microscopic cancer of the prostate. Results of a clinical trial of conservative treatment. *J. Urol. 108:* 908, 1972.

17. Catalona, W. J., and Scott, W. W. Carcinoma of the prostate: a review. *J. Urol. 119:* 1, 1978.

18. Chu, T. M., Wang, M. C., Scott, W. W., Gibbons, R. P., Johnson, D. E., Schmidt, J. D., Loening, S. A., Prout, G. R., and Murphy, G. P. Immunochemical detection of serum prostatic acid phosphatase. Methodology and clinical evaluation. *Invest. Urol. 15:* 319, 1978.

19. Chute, R. Radical retropubic prostatectomy for cancer. *J. Urol. 71:* 347, 1954.

20. Culp, O. S. Radical perineal prostatectomy: its past, present and possible future. *J. Urol. 98:* 618, 1967.

21. Culp, O. S., and Meyer, J. J. Radical prostatectomy in the treatment of prostatic cancer. *Cancer 32:* 1113, 1973.

22. Denis, L., and Declerq, G. Radical prostatectomy: choice or chance. *Eur. Urol. 4:* 18, 1978.

23. Devlesaver, P. L. J. G. Prostato-vésiculectomie totale. Voie sacro-coccygienne. *Acta Chir. Belg. 74:* 220, 1975.

24. Dretler, S. P., Ragsdale, B. D., and Leadbetter, W. F. The value of pelvic lymphadenectomy in the surgical treatment of bladder cancer. *J. Urol. 109:* 414, 1973.

25. Fiedler, U., Brosig, W., and Rost, A. Ergebnisse der radikalen perinealen Prostatektomie. *Urologe A 16:* 56, 1977.

26. Flocks, R. H. The treatment of stage C prostatic cancer with special reference to combined surgical and radiation therapy. *J. Urol. 109:* 461, 1973.

27. Flocks, R. H., and Culp, D. A. A modification of technique for anastomosing membranous urethra and bladder neck following total prostatectomy. *J. Urol. 69:* 411, 1953.

28. Foti, A. G., Cooper, J. F., Herschman, H., and Malvaez, R. R. Detection of prostatic cancer by solid-phase radioimmunoassay of serum prostatic acid phosphatase. *N. Engl. J. Med. 297:* 1357, 1977.

29. Foroogh, K. J., Aron, B., Dettmer, C. M., and Shehata, W. M. Radiation therapy as definitive treatment for localized carcinoma of prostate. *Urology 14:* 555, 1979.

29a. Fowler, J. E., and Whitmore, W. F., Jr. The incidence and extent of pelvic lymph node metastases in apparently localized prostatic cancer. *Cancer 47:* 2941, 1981.

29b. Freiha, F. S., Pistenma, D. A., and Bagshaw, M. A. Pelvic lymphadenectomy for staging prostatic carcinoma: is it always necessary? *J. Urol. 122:* 176, 1979.

30. Frohmüller, H. Radical retropubic prostatectomy. Paper presented at IX. European Surgical Congress, International College of Surgeons, Amsterdam (Netherlands), June 29–July 4, 1975.

31. Gittes, R. Acid phosphatase reappraised. *N. Engl. J. Med. 297:* 1398, 1977.

32. Gleason, D. F. Classification of prostatic carcinoma. *Cancer Chemother. Rep. 50:* 125, 1966.

33. Greene, L. F., Mulcahy, J. J., Warren, M. M., and Dockerty, M. B. Primary transitional cell carcinoma of the prostate. *J. Urol. 110:* 235, 1973.

34. Hohenfellner, R. Therapierichtlinien für das Prostatakarzinom. In *Chemotherapie urologischer Malignome*, edited by G. H. Jacobi and J. E. Altwein. S. Karger, Basel, 1979, p. 66.

35. Huggins, C. B. Commentary on the treatment of prostate cancer (Guest Editorial). *J. Urol. 102:* 119, 1969.

36. Jacobi, G. H., Kurth, K.-H., and Hohenfellner, R. Lokale Hochvolttherapie des Prostatakarzinoms unter kurativer Zielsetzung. *Akt. Urol. 10:* 291, 1979.

37. Jewett, H. J. The present status of radical prostatectomy for stages A and B prostatic cancer. *Urol. Clin. North Am. 2:* 105, 1975.

38. Jönsson, G. Bemerkungen über Diagnose und Behandlung des Prostatakarzinoms. *Verh. Ber. Dtsch. Ges. Urol.* Springer, Berlin, 1973, p. 175.

39. Kastendieck, H. Morphologie des Prostatacarcinoms in Stanzbiopsien und totalen Prostatektomien—Untersuchungen zur Frage der Relevanz bioptischer Befundaussagen. *Pathologe, 2:* 31, 1980.

40. Kessler, M., and Igl, W. Die Lymphographie und die röntgenologische Thorax–und Skelettdiagnostik beim Prostatakarzinom. In *Diagnostik und Therapie des Prostatakarzinoms,* edited by H. Göttinger. S. Karger, Basel, 1979, p. 61.

41. Khan, A. U., Tomera, F. M., and Rife, C. C. Reevaluation of Vest technique of vesicourethral reconstruction in radical retropubic prostatectomy. *Urology 13:* 149, 1979.

42. Kirchheim, D. Das Prostatakarzinom. *Dtsch. Ärztebl. 77:* 807, 1980.

43. Kirchheim, D., and McRoberts, J. W. Radikale retropubische Prostatektomie in der Behandlung des Prostatacarcinoms. *Urologe A 10:* 49, 1971.

44. Klosterhalfen, H. Derzeitiger Stand von Diagnostik und Therapie des Prostatakarzinoms. *Verh. Ber. Dtsch. Ges. Urol.* Springer, Berlin, 1974, p. 349.

45. Knipper, W. Praktische Erfahrungen mit der Vorsorgeuntersuchung in der Urologie. *Urologe B 19:* 49, 1979.

46. Kurth, K. H., Altwein, J. E., and Hohenfellner, R. Die pelvine Lymphadenektomie als Staging-Operation des Prostatakarzinoms. *Urologe A 16:* 65, 1977.

47. Leisrink, H. Beiträge zur Chirurgie der harnführenden Wege beim Manne. *Arch. Klin. Chir. 28:* 578, 1883.

48. Loening, S. A., Schmidt, J. D., Brown, R. C., Hawtrey, C. E., Fallon, B., and Culp, D. A. A comparison between lymphangiography and pelvic node dissection in the staging of prostatic cancer. *J. Urol. 117:* 752, 1977.

49. Madsen, P. O., Maigaard, S., Corle, D. K., Byar, D. P., and VACURG. Radical prostatectomy for carcinoma of the prostate, stages I and II. New results of the Veterans Administration Cooperative Urological Research Group. Presentation at the 2nd International Symposium on the Treatment of Carcinoma of the Prostate, Berlin, Dec. 1–2, 1978.

50. Marshall, D. F. Trans-coccygeal prostatectomy. *J. Maine Med. Assoc. 56:* 193, 1965.

51. McCullough, D. L., McLaughlin, A. P., and Gittes, R. F. Morbidity of pelvic lymphadenectomy and radical prostatectomy for prostatic cancer. *J. Urol. 117:* 206, 1977.

52. McLaughlin, A. P., III. Abstracter's comment. *Urol. Surv. 27:* 58, 1977.

53. Melchior, H. Tubular cystourethroneostomy after total prostatectomy. *Urol. Int. 30:* 54, 1975.

54. Middleton, R. G., Jr., Cutler, C. L., and Dahl, D. S. Further experience with pelvic lymphadenectomy for the staging of apparently localized prostatic cancer. (Experience with 203 patients.) In *A.U.A. Courses in Urology,* Vol. 1, edited by W. W. Bonney, W. L. Weems, and J. P. Donohue. Williams & Wilkins, Baltimore/London, 1979, ch. 2, p. 27.

55. Millin, T. Retropubic prostatectomy; new extravesical technique: report on 20 cases. *Lancet 2:* 693, 1945.

56. Millin, T. J. Retropubic urinary surgery. E & S. Livingstone, Edinburgh, 1947.

57. Mittemeyer, B. T., and Cox, H. D. Modified radical retropubic prostatectomy. *Urology 12:* 313, 1978.

58. Mostofi, F. K. Taken from F. H. Schröder.[70]

59. Müller, H.-A., Ackermann, R., and Frohmüller, H. G. W. The value of perineal punch biopsy in estimating the histological grade of carcinoma of the prostate. *Prostate 1:* 303, 1980.

60. Myers, R. P. Book review of *"Principles and Management of Urologic Cancer"* edited by N. Javadpour. *Mayo Clin. Proc. 55:* 61, 1980.

61. Novak, R., Rados, N., and Kraus, O. A transpubic approach to radical prostatectomy. *Eur. Urol. 2:* 300, 1976.

62. Okabe, T., Ackermann, R., Wirth, M., and Frohmüller, H. G. W. Cell-mediated cytotoxicity in patients with cancer of the prostate. *J. Urol. 122:* 628, 1979.

63. Parry, W. L. Prostate malignancies. In *Urologic Surgery, 2nd Ed.* edited by J. F. Glenn. Harper & Row, Hagerstown, Md., 1975, p. 573.

64. Ray, G. R., Pistenma, D. A., Castellino, R. A., Kempson, R. L., Meares, E., and Bagshaw, M. A. Operative staging of apparently localized adenocarcinoma of the prostate: results in fifty unselected patients. *Cancer 38:* 73, 1976.

65. Reiner, W. G., and Walsh, P. C. An anatomical approach to the surgical management of the dorsal vein and Santorini's plexus during radical retropubic surgery. *J. Urol. 121:* 198, 1979.

66. Rhamy, R. K., Buchanan, R. D., and Spalding, M. J. Intraductal carcinoma of the prostate gland. *J. Urol. 109:* 475, 1973.

67. Rothenberger, K., Hofstetter, A., Pfeifer, K. -J., and Rupp, N. Transperitoneale Fein-nadel-Biopsie retroperitonealer Lymphknoten in der Karzinomdiagnostik. *Fortschr. Med. 97:* 2218, 1978.

68. Sachse, H. Transurethrale Resektion beim Prostatakarzinom. In *Diagnostik und Therapie des Prostatakarzinoms,* edited by H. Göttinger. S. Karger, Basel, 1979, p. 137.

69. Schröder, F. H. Prostatakarzinom—totale Prostatektomie. *Med. Welt 29:* 1206, 1978.

70. Schröder, F. H. Die totale perineale Prostatektomie beim Prostatakarzinom. In *Diag-nostik und Therapie des Prostatakarzinoms,* edited by H. Göttinger. S. Karger, Basel, 1979, p. 127.

71. Schröder, F. H. A randomized prospective study of locally confined prostatic carcinoma, Personal communication.

72. Schröder, F. H. Prostatic carcinoma: comments on radical surgical treatment. *Scand. J. Urol. Nephrol. Suppl. 55:* 181, 1980.

73. Schröder, F. H., and Belt, E. Carcinoma of the prostate: a study of 213 patients with stage C tumors treated by total prostatectomy. *J. Urol. 114:* 257, 1975.

74. Schröder, F. H., Jellinghaus, W., and Frohmüller, H. G. W. Behandlung des lokal begrenzten Prostata-Carcinoms: Bestrahlung oder totale Prostatektomie? *Urologe A 15:* 67, 1976.

75. Selikowitz, S. M., and Krane, R. J. Hemostatic technique for radical pelvic survery. *Urology 12:* 354, 1978.

76. Sewell, R. A., Braren, V., Wilson, S. K., and Rhamy, R. K. Extended biopsy followup after full course radiation for resectable prostatic carcinoma. *J. Urol. 113:* 371, 1975.

77. Shishito, S., Kubo, T., Watanabe, H., Kato, H., and Kato, T. Transpubic radical prostatectomy. *Urol. Int. 20:* 347, 1965.

78. Skinner, D. G. Pelvic lymphadenectomy. In *Urologic Surgery,* 2nd Ed., edited by J. F. Glenn. Harper & Row, Hagerstown, Md., 1975, p. 589.

79. Smith, P. H. Medical management of prostatic cancer. Some current questions. *Eur. Urol. 6:* 65, 1980.

80. Sökeland, J. Erfahrungen mit der radikalen Prostatektomie in Deutschland. *Verh. Ber. Dtsch. Ges. Urol.* Springer, Berlin, 1974, p. 353.

81. Tomlinson, R. L., Currie, D. P., and Boyce, W. H. Radical prostatectomy: palliation for stage C carcinoma of the prostate. *J. Urol. 117:* 85, 1977.

82. Übelhör, R. Prostatakarzinom und radikale Prostatektomie. *Z. Urol. 53:* 205, 1960.

83. U.I.C.C. *TNM Klassifikation der malignen Tumoren,* Ed. 3. Springer-Verlag, Berlin, 1979, p. 114.

84. van der Werf-Messing, B., Sourek-Zukova, V., and Block, D. I. Localized advanced carcinoma of the prostate. Radiation therapy versus hormonal therapy. *Int. J. Radiat. Oncol. Biol. Phys. 1:* 1043, 1976.

85. Vest, S. A. Radical perineal prostatectomy, modification of closure. *Surg. Gynec. Obstet. 70:* 935, 1940.

86. Veterans Administration Cooperative Urological Research Group. Carcinoma of the prostate: treatment comparisons. *J. Urol. 98:* 516, 1967.

87. Walker, G. Transpubic removal of the prostate for carcinoma. *Ann. Surg. 78:* 795, 1923.

88. Wannenmacher, M. Die Strahlentherapie des Prostatakarzinoms. In *Diagnostik und Therapie des Prostatakarzinoms,* edited by H. Göttinger. S. Karger, Basel, 1979, p. 141.

89. Wannenmacher, M., Sommerkamp, H., Knüfermann, H., and Kuphal, K. Die intersti-tielle Strahlentherapie in der Behandlung des Prostatakarzinoms. *Dtsch. Ärztebl. 76:* 1371, 1979.

90. Whitmore, W. F., Jr. Symposium on hormones and cancer therapy. Hormone therapy in prostatic cancer. *Am. J. Med. 21:* 697, 1956.

91. Young, H. H. The early diagnosis and radical cure of carcinoma of the prostate. Being a study of 40 cases and presentation of a radical operation which was carried out in four cases. *Bull. Johns Hopkins Hosp. 16:* 315, 1905.
92. Zincke, H., Fleming, T. R., Furlow, W. L., Myers, R. P., and Utz, D.C. Radical retropubic prostatectomy and pelvic lymphadenectomy for high-stage cancer of the prostate. *Cancer 47:* 1901, 1981.
93. Zoedler, D., and Limbacher, G. Bericht über 100 totale Prostatektomien. *Urologe A 16:* 61, 1977.

10

Radiation Therapy of Carcinoma of the Prostate

B. van der Werf-Messing, M.D.

INTRODUCTION

Since the introduction of radiation therapy in the beginning of the 20th century it was well known that carcinoma of the prostate was only moderately radiosensitive. Because of the close proximity of the prostate to the bladder and the rectum, application of a tumor lethal dose to the prostate by external orthovoltage irradiation was almost impossible without severe damage to these adjacent organs. For these reasons early radiotherapists, who attempted radiotherapeutic cure of prostatic cancer, concentrated their efforts on interstitial prostatic application of radioactive sources; by these means a high dose could be delivered to the prostate, yet the surrounding tissues could be spared. Pasteau and Degrais,[1] Paschkis and Tittinger,[2] Young,[3] and Deming[4] were the precursors of modern interstitial therapy. Usually radium was applied either through cystotomy, through the perineum, or in a catheter through the urethra. With the discovery of the apparently effective hormone therapy by Huggins et al.[5] the radiotherapeutic approach was abandoned nearly all over the world. In the second half of this century when the Veterans Administration Cooperative Urological Research Group (VACURG) trials[6] made it evident that hormone therapy was not the ideal approach in nonmetastasized prostatic cancer, the interest in intraprostatic implantation of radioactive material revived. In the same era supervoltage radiation therapy became available which enabled the radiotherapist to deliver a tumor-lethal dose to the prostate with an acceptable risk of injury to the healthy tissues. A considerable number of clinical radiotherapy studies on prostatic cancer have been published, increasing our insight into appropriate radiotherapeutic possibilities with their inherent problems and at the same time broadening our knowledge about the behavior of this malignancy.

INTERSTITIAL RADIOTHERAPY WITH CURATIVE INTENT

Technique

Modern radiotherapists have introduced interstitial application of radioactive material mainly in growths limited to the prostate (category T_1 and T_2)[7] and to tumors with limited extension beyond the capsule and well defined borders (category T_3). As a radioactive source Flocks[8] used 2 cc diluent of ^{198}Au, Chan and Gutierrez[9] implanted gold grains; Hilaris et al.,[10] Fowler et al.,[11] and Schellhammer et al.[12] inserted ^{125}I seeds. These implants are permanent and deliver a dose of about 16,000 rads in 1 year to the malignancy.[10]

Court and Chassagne[13] utilize interstitial tubes with iridium; as the iridium has to be removed, it is possible to calculate the application time so as to deliver the required tumor lethal dose which is roughly the equivalent of 6,000 to 7,000 rads in about 6 days.

As with interstitial radiotherapy the radiation effect is limited to the implanted prostate; regional lymph nodes which might be involved will not be covered by this treatment modality. Hence this technique is usually combined with either surgical lymph node dissection (the majority of authors) or with additional external irradiation.[9, 12]

Results

The results of this combined modality approach are presented in Table 10.1. Prognosis is influenced by various and to some extent interrelated factors. The most important ones are T-category, lymph node involvement, and histological degree of differentiation. With increasing number of T-category (see Chapter 7) prognosis becomes worse: 5-year survival and relapse-free survival rates being, respectively, 100% and about 90% in category T_1 and T_2; the corresponding figures in category T_3 are about 70% and 45%. In cases of histologically negative regional lymph nodes 5-year survival is significantly better (about 92%) than in cases of proven positive lymph nodes (about 45%). Disregarding the T-category poor histological grade significantly reduces the chance of cure: about 80% relapse-free 5-year survival in cases of well differentiated growths *versus* about 45% in cases of poorly differentiated malignancies. As a rule local failure is not a problem after interstitial radiation therapy as long as an adequate dose has been delivered. Postradiation biopsies have shown that usually the growth disappears within 2 years after implantation. Positive biopsies prior to this period might just demonstrate slow elimination of already killed tumor cells.[10]

Complications

Reported impotence after interstitial therapy varies between 7%[11, 12] and 0%[10] in patients potent prior to treatment. As the periprostatic tissue

Table 10.1
Prognosis after Interstitial Irradiation Combined with Lymph Node Dissection or with External Irradiation of Regional Lymph Nodes

Author	Type of Treatment	Type of Growth	No. Treated	Prognosis	Free of Disease
Flocks[8]	Radical surgery + interstitial therapy 100 mCi ^{198}Au, 2 cc diluent	Category T_3M_0	147	5 yr surv.[a] 60%	
Chan and Gutierrez[9]	Gold grain implant (±4000 rads) + external megavoltage to a total dose of ±8000 rads	Stage C (Category T_3M_0, $T_4?M_0$) Normal serum acid phosphatase Abnormal serum acid phosphatase Total stage C ($T_3M_0 + T_4?M_0$)	13 3 ____ 16[b]	3 yr surv. 13 0 ____ 13/16	8 0 ____ 8/16
Hilaris et al.[10]	Bilateral lymphadenectomy + prostate implant with ^{125}I 16,000 rads/1 yr = 2023 rets	Category T_1M_0 T_2M_0 Limited T_3M_0 / T_4M_0 Lymph nodes negative histologically Lymph nodes positive histologically	65 40 23 80 102 84	Crude 5 yr surv. 100% 100% 77% 87% Actuarial 5 yr surv. 92% 46%	
Barzell et al.[44]	Series from Memorial Sloan Kettering Cancer Center (Hilaris et al.[10])	Histological grade according to Gleason Well differentiated Moderately differentiated Poorly differentiated Size of the primary <2.5 cm^3 2.5–7.9 cm^2 8–18 cm^3	 19 46 15 18 50 32	5 yr relapse-free 81% 69% 48% 89% 65% 26%	

[a] surv., survival.
[b] All controlled locally.

is almost not irradiated by interstitial techniques, complications due to irradiation are mainly limited to temporary urinary irritability and to transitional mild rectal burning or bleeding.[14] Serious urinary or rectal complications (fistulas, necrosis, ulceration) are the sequelae of the combination of surgery and implantation.[8]

Fowler et al.[11] observed in a series of 600 cases a 6% operative complication rate, mainly being prostatic or periprostatic hemorrhage and nerve injury. In the same series the postoperative complication rate rose to about 23%: pelvic complications such as lymphocele, hematoma, abscess, and cellulitis; cardiovascular accidents; wound infection and hematoma; urinary complications such as retention, fistula, epididymitis, and prostatitis. The late complications were mainly urinary, persisting voiding symptoms, such as urgency and stress incontinence; edema of the lower extremities and genitalia; rectal discomfort and bleeding; wound problems, such as persistent sinus and hernia. The total late complication rate amounted to 28%. It is evident that the more serious complications, not pertaining to micturition and defecation, are largely due to the concomitant surgical procedure.

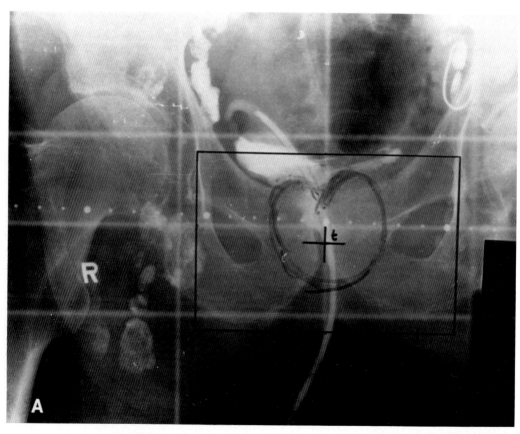

Figure 10.1 *A*, Anterior view of the irradiation field. The bladder is filled with contrast medium via a catheter in the urethra. The area of the prostatic cancer is indicated.

EXTERNAL SUPERVOLTAGE RADIATION THERAPY WITH CURATIVE INTENT

Techniques

With the use of megavoltage photons and electron beams it has become possible to deliver a tumor-lethal dose of ionizing irradiation to the prostatic cancer, yet at the same time to relatively spare the adjacent healthy tissues. However, careful assessment of the appropriate irradiation fields and meticulous dosimetry are mandatory. The majority of radio-

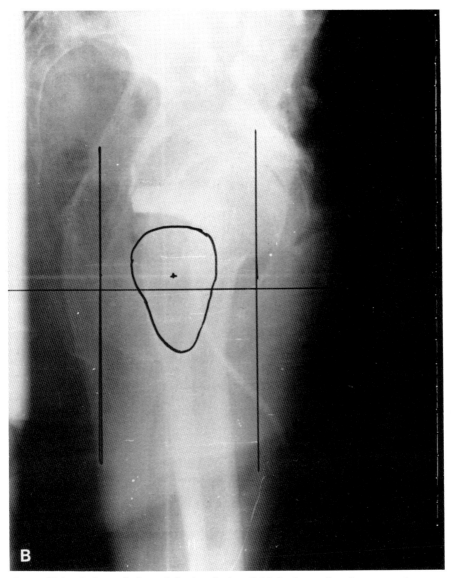

Figure 10.1 *B,* Lateral view of the irradiation field. It shows that the rectum is to a large extent excluded from exposure.

therapists consider 6,500 to 7,000 rads, five weekly fractions in 6½ to 7 weeks—or its biological equivalent—an appropriate tumor dose. A dose less than 6,500 rads in 6½ weeks—or its biological equivalent—is considered to be inadequate.[15]

The field size depends on the philosophy of the therapist. In cases of a growth limited to the prostate the majority considers irradiation of the prostate with a small margin of healthy tissue a satisfactory policy; rotation or right and left lateral arc therapy in this situation is usually applied. In cases of growths of the primary beyond the prostate some authors irradiate only the prostate with adjacent regional lymph nodes in the whole true pelvis or in part of it; this technique is based on the philosophy that in case of lymph node involvement beyond this limited area, distant micrometastases are present anyhow, which implies that radiotherapy will only postpone the need of systemic therapy. Four portals (two lateral and two opposing anteroposterior fields) ("brick technique," Figs. 10.1 and 10.2) or three fields (one posterior and two anterior wedge fields) are commonly used. Other clinicians expect that in cases of locally more advanced growths prognosis can be improved by including all regional lymph nodes and even juxtaregional nodes into the irradiation field (Fig. 10.3). These clinicians usually apply a dose varying between 2,000 and 4,000 rads in 3 to 6 weeks to the lumbar and the pelvic nodes, with a booster dose of up to 6,000 to 7,000 rads to the prostate.

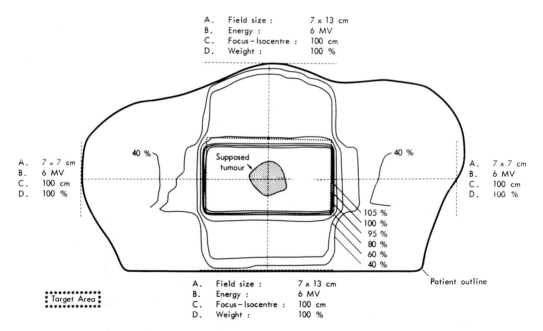

Figure 10.2 Computer planning for two lateral opposing fields and two opposing anteroposterior fields. The area of the tumor is indicated. The isodose curves from 100 to 40% of the given dose are visualized. Standard "brick technique" in the Rotterdam Radiotherapy Institute.

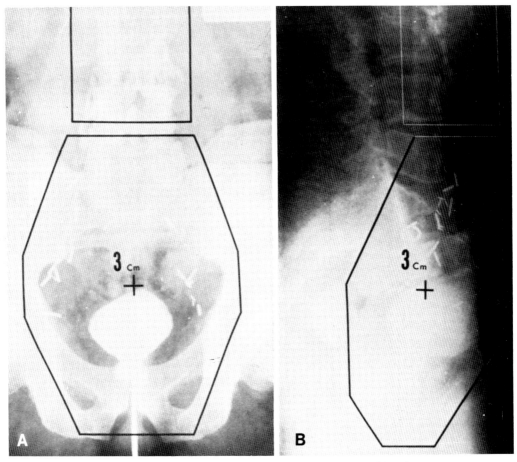

Figure 10.3 Extended field irradiation. *A*, Anterior view of the pelvic field and part of the lumbar region field. The bladder is filled with contrast medium by a urethral catheter. Clips have been placed after lymph node dissection. *B*, Lateral view of the pelvic field and of part of the lumbar regional field. (Reproduced with permission from M. A. Bagshaw *et al.*[16])

Prognosis

As after interstitial irradiation, survival rates after external irradiation are determined by T-category of the primary and even more so by histological degree of differentiation of the growth (Table 10.2). Survival rates after limited field irradiation[17-19] are not inferior to those after extended field irradiation, supporting the hypothesis that lymph node involvement beyond the most adjacent prostatic regional lymph nodes indicates a high probability of the existence of micrometastases beyond the regional and probably even beyond the juxtaregional lymph nodes. A prospective clinical trial comparing small fields with large fields might clarify this problem.[20] External irradiation in combination with hormone treatment or orchiectomy has not been proven to be more effective.[15, 19, 21-24]

Table 10.2
Prognosis after External Supervoltage Irradiation

Author	Type of Treatment and Selection	Type of Growth	No. Treated	Prognosis			
Cantril et al.[45]	25 MeV photons (40 patients: Co[60] or 4 MeV) 4 fields or rotation to prostate + periprostatic tissue 60% of patients: 7000–7500 rads/7–7.5 wk	Category T_3M_0, T_4M_0 Well differentiated Poorly differentiated	166 71	5 yr surv.[f] 60% 30%			
Edsmyr et al.[46]	6 MeV photons 5500 rads/5–7 wk 2 ant. wedge fields, 1 post. field + Hormones: Stilbestrol and/or Estradurin	Category T_3M_0, T_4M_0 Poorly differentiated	25	3 yr surv. 64%[a]			
Bagshaw et al.[47]	4 MeV photons 7000–7600 rads/7–7½ wk to prostate and periprostatic tissue (rotation or R + L lat. arc therapy)	Limited to prostate (Category T_1M_0, T_2M_0)	230	5 yr surv. 72%	10 yr surv. 44%		
		Extracapsular (Category T_3M_0, T_4M_0)	200	5 yr surv. 51%	10 yr surv. 38%		
Ray and Bagshaw[18]	4 MeV photons Small field to prostate + periprostatic tissue ± 7000–7500 rad/7–7½ wk	Limited to prostate (Category T_1M_0, T_2M_0) Extracapsular extension (Category T_3M_0, T_4M_0)	81 28 82 23	5 yr surv. Free of disease 72% 42%	With disease 2% 6%	10 yr surv. Free of disease 46% 26%	With disease 4% 5%
Bagshaw et al.[16]	4 MeV photons Patients ≤ 70 yr of age; lymph node biopsy at laparotomy	Stage A, B, C (Category T_0M_0; $T_{1-2}M_0$, $T_{3-4}M_0$)		F-u period, 1–50 mo (median, 22 mo)[f]			

		Free of disease	
A. Nodes histologically negative → randomization:			
a. 7000 rads/7 wk to prostate	17	15	
b. a + pelvic nodes 4000 rads/7 wk	18	16	
c. a + b + paraaortic nodes	2	1	
	37	32	87%
B. Pelvic nodes histologically positive → randomization:			
a. b.	9	7	
a. c.	5	3	
	14	10	72%
C. Paraaortic nodes histologically positive			
a. c.	10	3	30%
	Total 61	45	74%

				5 yr surv.	
			Free of disease	Alive with tumor	Dead with tumor
Perez et al.[24]	Stage C (Category T_3M_0, T_4M_0)	22 MeV photons			
	I 47	Total 7000 rad to prostate Total 6000 rad to true pelvis Total 5000 rad to pelvis incl. L5	97	42%	0	22%
	II 50	Idem + hormone therapy (orchiectomy + estrogens)		—b		
Taylor et al.[23]	Stage C (Category T_3M_0, T_4M_0)	10 MeV photons Whole pelvic fields + booster to prostate	221	5 yr surv. 58%c		

Table 10.2—Continued

Author	Type of Treatment and Selection	Type of Growth	No. Treated	Prognosis
Neglia et al.[19]	22 MeV photons I. 4 fields (10 × 10 cm to 12 × 15 cm) Trial: 5000 rads/± 5 wk Prostate booster 1000–2000 rads via ant. + post. field Additional hormones Randomization < DES 5 mg/day / No hormones No hormones II. Previous series (no trial): 6000–7000 rads/6–7 wk to true pelvis with or without hormones.	Stage $B_1C_1C_2$ Category T_2M_0: 4 Category T_3M_0: 97 Category T_4M_0: 53	 79 75	Mean F-u, 4 yr, 7 mo 5 yr surv. 74.7% after radiation only 61.3% after radiation + hormones No diff. between 7000 rads and ± 6000–6500 rads No difference between "small" and "large" radiation fields
McGowan[40]	^{60}Cobalt 6000 rads/6 wk, 5 fields daily Patients ≤ 75 yr Only patients with negative lymphography are included in study	Stage (Category) A ($T_0N_0M_0$) B_1 ($T_1N_0M_0$) B_2 ($T_2N_0M_0$) C ($T_{3+4}N_0,M_0$)	 21 43 30 13	5 yr surv. — Free of disease 88% — 84% 90% — 61% 66% — 43% 39% — 37%
van der Werf-Messing[48]	Trial: A. 1 mg Lynoral daily B. 1 mg Lynoral daily + 25 MeV photons 7000/7 wk by 2 opposing fields covering prostate and surroundings	Stage C (Category T_3M_0, T_4M_0)	26 30	5 yr surv. 65% 55%
van der Werf-Messing[17]	25 MeV photons 4000 rads + 2 wk split + 3000 rads 4 portals to prostate and surrounding tissue			

			n	3 yr	Free of disease	5 yr	Free of disease
		T3M0 well and moderately differentiated	40	80%	65%	80%	65%
		T3M0 poorly and undiff.	15	55%	35%	—[d]	
		T4M0 well and moderately differentiated	22	65%	65%	65%	63%
		T4M0 poorly and undiff.	7	50%	25%	—[d]	
				5 yr surv.		**10 yr surv.**	
Harisiadis et al.[15]	6 MeV photons or Cobalt[60] ± 6000–6800 rads in ± 6–7 wk	Stage A (Category T0M0)	13	±85%			
	Rotational therapy or 4 field technique	Stage B (Category T1+2M0)	21	±85%			
		Stage C (Category T3M0 + T4M0)	112	55%		±30%	
	Combination of whole pelvis with additional irradiation. With or without hormones.	Well + moderately diff.	84	±65%			
		Undifferentiated	16	±30%			
		IVP normal	128	±70%			
		IVP abnormal	18	±25%			
	Dose > 6500 rads	All T-categories M0	55	±85%			
	Dose < 6500 rads	All T-categories M0	91	±55%			
	Radiotherapy started within 6 mo after diagnosis	All T-categories M0	121	±70%			
	Radiotherapy started after ≥ 7 mo	All T-categories M0	25	±30%			
				5 yr surv.[e]		**10 yr surv.[e]**	
Taylor et al.[49]	10 MeV photons or Cobalt[60]	Stage B (Category T1+2M0)	36	59%			
	Pelvic irradiation 3 or 4 fields 6500–7000 rads/7–8 wk with or without hormones	Stage C (Category T3M0 + T4M0)	123	58%		30%	

[a] Two patients died.
[b] No difference between I and II.
[c] Additional hormone therapy had no bearing on prognosis.
[d] Follow-up too short for evaluation.
[e] No difference between radiation only and radiation plus hormones.
[f] Abbreviations used are: surv., survival; F-u, follow-up.

Slightly contradictory to these data are the findings of Green *et al.*[25] A relapse-free survival of 1.5 to 7 years was achieved in 17 of 25 patients with gross lymph node metastases (N_4 according to UICC). The patients were treated during 2 months with estrogens followed by radiation therapy to the primary, the pelvic, and the para-aortic lymph nodes. Further studies to identify the ideal indications for radiotherapy only or radiation therapy in combination with hormone therapy are desirable.

As after interstitial therapy, local failure after external irradiation is exceptional; irradiation fibrosis often makes rectal examination an unreliable tool for the assessment of a local recurrence. Transrectal aspiration and punch biopsy yield positive results up to more than 3 years. Although there are data suggesting that positive cytology after more than 2 years implies a significantly higher risk of distant metastasis than a negative cytology[26, 27] other authors[15, 17, 28–32] have not been able to support these findings. However, the hypothesis still stands that after external irradiation elimination of killed tumor cells might take at least as long as after interstitial radiotherapy.

Complications

Impotence is seen in 13 to 40% of initially potent patients.[18, 33, 34] Complications during irradiation are usually urinary frequency and diarrhea. The incidence of both can be reduced significantly by careful radiation planning, by treating concomitant urinary infection, by not starting radiation therapy until at least 4 weeks after transurethral resection, and by including a rest period of about 1 to 2 weeks after 4,000 rads.[17, 22] Late complications are urinary incontinence in about 7%,[30, 33] chronic cystitis in 4 to 8%,[31, 33] and chronic proctitis in 1 to 4%.[31, 33, 35]

More serious complications, such as ileus, requiring colostomy or ileostomy, occur usually only in patients who underwent pelvic operations prior to radiation therapy. These postoperative radiation complications might be reduced by irradiating the patient in Trendelenburg's position, thus shifting part of the bowel beyond the irradiation field.[36]

After external irradiation transurethral resection is possible for diagnostic purposes or in cases of development of severe local obstruction; however, this procedure should be limited as much as possible, since every additional trauma to the irradiated area increases the risk of permanent radiation damage.

PALLIATIVE RADIOTHERAPY

In cases of hormone-resistant metastases which cause considerable discomfort or pain, or which might lead to complications such as fractures or paralysis, and in cases of pulmonary metastases which cause severe hemoptysis or shortness of breath, external irradiation, preferably supervoltage irradiation, can be applied with palliative intent. Doses of 3,000 to 4,000 rads in 2 to 3 weeks or their biological equivalent in even shorter periods are usually effective. In case of diffuse metastases causing considerable pain, half body irradiation to the most affected half of the body, applying an approximately 600-rad midplane dose will usually alleviate pain significantly. After a 5- to 10-week interval the same radiation can be given to the other half of the body if necessary.[37, 38] Even in patients with metastases, a primary which causes complaints such as obstruction or bleeding and which is not amenable to transurethral resection and is unresponsive to hormone therapy, can effectively be controlled by palliative irradiation; the dose has to be adapted to the local situation and to the general condition of the patient.[13]

In some instances of painful diffuse skeletal metastases systemic treatment with radioactive isotopes, such as ^{32}phosphor and ^{89}strontium, can provide alleviation.[39]

POSSIBILITIES TO IMPROVE PROGNOSIS AFTER RADIATION THERAPY

All authors agree that tumor factors, which mainly influence prognosis, are the *T-category*, the degree of *differentiation* of the growth, and *lymph node involvement* beyond the most adjacent regional prostatic lymph nodes. Obstruction or nonfunctioning of a kidney might also be a poor prognosticator.[15] The prognostic value of elevated prostatic acid phosphatase has been debated. McGowan[40] and Sadlowski[41] found no correlation between an elevated value and prognosis, whereas other authors could establish such a prognostic value.[9, 17] An elevated prostatic acid phosphatase in the bone marrow aspirate showed poor prognosis in case of poorly differentiated growths.[17]

From surgical data it is evident that lymph node involvement predicts a bad prognosis; however, neither limited nor extensive lymph node dissection nor irradiation of regional and juxtaregional lymph nodes has demonstrably improved prognosis. As not only local recurrence but metastases are decisive for prognosis, the above data support the hypothesis that indicators for a bad prognosis suggest that microscopic spread has occurred beyond the regional and even beyond the juxtaregional lymph nodes (Fig. 10.4).

Improvement of prognosis of patients with bad prognosticators could be achieved by a combination of radiation therapy with adequate chemotherapy and/or immunotherapy. Another approach would be elective total body irradiation, which might kill micrometastases or at least might prolong the clinically disease-free period. Pilot studies and trials exploiting the value of various elective treatment modalities are desirable.

Although the incidence of local failure is low, improvement of local treatment might both reduce the occurrence of complications and lower the treatment burden of the patient. Shipley *et al.*[42] added a proton booster to the primary, thus reducing even more the dose to healthy tissues. In the future a *pi-meson* booster will achieve this goal equally effectively. Changes in fractionation schemes, *e.g.* 3 times a week irradiation,[43] might diminish the treatment burden without decreasing the chance of cure and without increased morbidity. The same might be achieved by

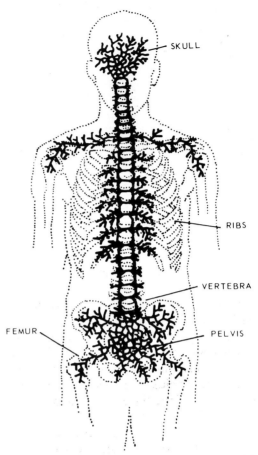

Figure 10.4. Metastatic pathways of prostatic cancer: skeletal involvement following lymphogenous and subsequent hematogenous extension. (Reproduced with permission from J. A. del Regato.[21])

the administration of radiation sensitizers or by the combination of radiation therapy with local hyperthermia. More exact adaptation of irradiation fields to the extent of the primary growth might be obtained by ultrasound examination and CT-scan evaluation.

In the series of Harisiadis *et al.*[15] patients who started radiotherapy more than 7 months after diagnosis had a significantly worse prognosis than those who started within 6 months. Yet it has not been proven that patients with a growth category T_1 or T_2, well or moderately well differentiated, have a poorer prognosis in cases of treatment delay until clinical evidence of progression than in cases of immediate treatment after diagnosis. It even cannot be excluded that a proportion of these patients might actually never require any therapy. Prospective clinical controlled trials might elucidate this problem.

Prognosis after radiation therapy—interstitial with lymphadenectomy or with additional lymph node irradiation, or external irradiation only—is comparable to prognosis after radical surgery, even disregarding the high selectivity in surgical series (see also Chapter 9). Hence only prospective clinical trials comparing optimal radiation therapy with high quality surgery in patients comparable with regard to tumor and host factors, will identify for various patient groups the therapeutic approach with the highest chance of cure and the lowest morbidity.

REFERENCES

1. Pasteau, O., and Degrais, D. De l'emploi du radium dans le traitement des cancers de la prostate. *J. Urol. Med. Chir. 4:* 341, 1913.
2. Paschkis, R., and Tittinger, W. Radiumbehandlung eines Prostatasarkoms. *Wien. Klin. Wochenschr. 23:* 1715, 1910.
3. Young, H. H. The use of radium and the punch operation in desperate cases of enlarged prostate. *Ann. Surg. 65:* 633, 1917.
4. Deming, C. L. Results in one hundred cases of cancer of prostate and seminal vesicles, treated with radium. *Surg. Gynecol. Obstet. 34:* 99, 1922.
5. Huggins, C., and Hodges, C. V. The effect of castration, of estrogen and of androgen injection on serum phosphatases in metastatic carcinoma of the prostate. *Cancer Res. 1:* 293, 1941.
6. Veterans Administration Cooperative Urological Research Group. Treatment and survival of patients with cancer of the prostate. *Surg. Gynecol. Obstet. 124:* 1011, 1967.
7. Union Internationale Contre le Cancer. *TNM Classification of Malignant Tumours*, 3rd Ed. Geneva, 1978.
8. Flocks, R. H. The treatment of stage C prostatic cancer with special reference to combined surgical and radiation therapy. *J. Urol. 109:* 461, 1973.
9. Chan, R. C., and Gutierrez, A. E. Carcinoma of the prostate. Its treatment by a combination of radioactive gold-grain implant and external irradiation. Cancer *37:* 2749, 1976.
10. Hilaris, B. S., Whitmore, W. F., Batata, M., and Barzell, W. Behavioral patterns of prostate adenocarcinoma following an ^{125}I implant and pelvic node dissection. *Int. J. Radiat. Oncol. Biol. Phys. 2:* 631, 1977.
11. Fowler, J. E., Jr., Barzell, W., Hilaris, B. S., and Whitmore, W. F., Jr. Complications of [125]Iodine implantation and pelvic lymphadenectomy in the treatment of prostatic cancer. *J. Urol. 121:* 447, 1979.
12. Schellhammer, P. F., El-Mahdi, A. M., and Wakley, J. I-125 interstitial implantation of the prostate. *Cancer Ther. Abstr. 18:* 1649, 1978.
13. Court, B., and Chassagne, D. Interstitial radiation therapy of cancer of the prostate using iridium 192 wires. *Cancer Treat. Rep. 61:* 329, 1977.
14. Hilaris, B. S., Whitmore, W. F., Batata, M. A., and Grabstald, H. Cancer of the prostate. In *Handbook of Interstitial Brachytherapy*, edited by B. S. Hilaris. Publishing Sciences Group, Acton, Mass., 1975, p. 219.
15. Harisiadis, L., Veenema, R. J., Senyszyn, J. J., Puchner, P. J., Tretter, P., Romas, N. A., Chang, C. H., Lattimer, J. K., and Tannenbaum, M. Carcinoma of the prostate: treatment with external radiotherapy. *Cancer 41:* 2131, 1978.
16. Bagshaw, M. A., Pistenma, D. A., Ray, G. R., Freiha, F. S., and Kempson, R. L. Evaluation of extended-field radiotherapy for prostatic neoplasm: 1976 progress report. *Cancer Treat. Rep. 61:* 297, 1977.
17. van der Werf-Messing, B. Prostatic cancer treated at the Rotterdam Radiotherapy Institute. Strahlentherapie, *154:* 537, 1978.
18. Ray, G. R., and Bagshaw, M. A. The role of radiation therapy in the definitive treatment of adenocarcinoma of the prostate. *Annu. Rev. Med. 26:* 567, 1975.
19. Neglia, W. J., Hussey, D. H., and Johnson, D. E. Megavoltage radiation therapy for carcinoma of the prostate. *Int. J. Radiat. Oncol. Biol. Phys. 2:* 873, 1977.
20. Aristizabal, S. A., Moore, M. J., and Boone, M. L. M. Large vs small volume irradiation in localized cancer of the prostate. *Int. J. Radiat. Oncol. Biol. Phys. 5:* 73, 1979.
21. del Regato, J. A. Long-term curative results of radiotherapy of patients with inoperable prostatic carcinoma. *Radiology 131:* 291, 1979.

22. van der Werf-Messing, B., Sourek-Zikova, V., and Blonk, D. I. Localized advanced carcinoma of the prostate: radiation therapy versus hormonal therapy. *Int. J. Radiat. Oncol. Biol. Phys. 1:* 1043, 1976.

23. Taylor, W. J., Richardson, R. G., and Hafermann, M. D. Radiation therapy of prostate cancer. *Int. J. Radiat. Oncol. Biol. Phys. 2*(Suppl. 2): abstr. 12, 13, 1977.

24. Perez, C. A., Bauer, W., Garza, R., and Royce, R. K. Radiation therapy in the definitive treatment of localized carcinoma of the prostate. *Cancer 40:* 1425, 1977.

25. Green, N., Broth, E., George, F. W., III, Goldstein, A., Melbye, R. W., Morrow, J., Onofrio, R., Polse, S., and Skaist, L. Prostate carcinoma—therapeutic considerations in the management of gross lymph node metastases. *Int. J. Radiat. Oncol. Biol. Phys. 5:* 891, 1979.

26. Kurth, K. H., Altwein, J. E., Skoluda, D., and Hohenfellner, R. Followup of irradiated prostatic carcinoma by aspiration biopsy. *J. Urol. 117:* 615, 1977.

27. Jacobi, G. H., Kurth, K. H., and Hohenfellner, R. Lokale Hochvolttherapie des Prostatakarzinoms unter kurativer Zielsetzung. *Akt. Urol. 10:* 291, 1979.

28. Sack, H., and Röttinger, E. M. Die kurative Strahlenbehandlung des Prostata-Carcinoms in den lokalisierten Stadien. *Radiologe 17:* 263, 1977.

29. Ray, G. R., Cassady, J. R., and Bagshaw, M. A. Definitive radiation therapy of carcinoma of the prostate. A report on 15 years experience. *Radiology 106:* 409, 1973.

30. Rhamy, R. K., Wilson, S. K., and Caldwell, W. L. Biopsy-proved tumor following definitive irradiation for resectable carcinoma of the prostate. *J. Urol. 107:* 627, 1972.

31. Hill, D. R., Crews, Q. E., Jr., and Walsh, P. C. Prostate carcinoma: radiation treatment of the primary and regional lymphatics. *Cancer 34:* 156, 1974.

32. Kagan, A. R., Gordon, J., Cooper, J. F., Gilbert, H., Nussbaum, H., and Chan, P. A clinical appraisal of postirradiation biopsy in prostatic cancer. *Cancer 39:* 637, 1977.

33. Perez, C. A., Ackerman, L. V., Silber, I., and Royce, R. K. Radiation therapy in the treatment of localized carcinoma of the prostate—preliminary report using 22 MeV photons. *Cancer 34:* 1059, 1974.

34. van der Werf-Messing, B. Niet gemetastaseerd prostaatcarcinoom met uitbreiding buiten de kapsel behandeld met megavoltbestraling. *Ned. Tijdschr. Geneeskd. 123:* 778, 1979.

35. Carlton, C. E., Jr., Dawoud, F., Hudgins, P., and Scott, R., Jr. Irradiation treatment of carcinoma of the prostate: a preliminary report based on 8 years of experience. *J. Urol. 108:* 924, 1972.

36. Schraub, S., Monnier, A., and Poulin, G. Prevention of late complications in the small intestine by irradiation in Trendelenburg's position. *J. Radiol. Electrol. Med. Nucl. 59:* 347, 1978.

37. Fitzpatrick, P. J., and Rider, W. D. Half body radiotherapy. *Int. J. Radiat. Oncol. Biol. Phys. 1:* 197, 1976.

38. Epstein, L. M., Stewart, B. H., Antunez, A. R., Hewitt, C. B., Straffon, R. A., Montague, D. K., Dhaliwal, R. S., and Jelden, G. Half and total body radiation for carcinoma of the prostate. *J. Urol. 122:* 330, 1979.

39. Kutzner, J., Grimm, W., and Hahn, K. Palliative Strahlentherapie mit Strontium-89 bei ausgedehnter Skelettmetastasierung. *Strahlentherapie 154:* 317, 1978.

40. McGowan, D. G. Radiation therapy in the management of localized carcinoma of the prostate. A preliminary report. *Cancer 39:* 98, 1977.

41. Sadlowski, R. W. Early stage prostatic cancer investigated by pelvic lymph node biopsy and bone marrow acid phosphatase. *J. Urol. 119:* 89, 1978.

42. Shipley, W. U., Tepper, J. E., Prout, G. R., Jr., Verhey, L. J., Mendiondo, O. A., Goitein, M., Koehler, A. M., and Suit, H. D. Proton radiation as boost therapy for localized prostatic carcinoma. *J.A.M.A. 241:* 1912, 1979.

43. DeGinder, W., Schneider, J., and Bates, B. C. Thirteen year experience with prostate carcinoma treated three times per week. *Int. J. Radiat. Oncol. Biol. Phys. 5:* 51, 1979.

44. Barzell, W., Bean, M. A., Hilaris, B. S., and Whitmore, W. F., Jr. Prostatic adenocarcinoma: relationship of grade and local extent to the pattern of metastases. *J. Urol. 118:* 278, 1977.

45. Cantril, S. T., Vaeth, J. M., Green, J. P., and Schroeder, A. F. Radiation therapy for localized carcinoma of the prostate; correlation with histopathological grading. *Front. Radiat. Ther. Oncol. 9:* 274, 1974.

46. Edsmyr, F., Esposti, P. L., Littbrand, B., and Almgard, L. E. Carcinoma of the prostate: the place of radiotherapy. In *Radiology: Proceedings of the 13th International Congress on Radiology*, Vol. 2, edited by J. Gomez Lopez, and J. Bonmati. Madrid, 15–20 October, 1973. Excerpta Medica, Amsterdam, 1974, p. 63.

47. Bagshaw, M. A., Ray, G. R., Pistenma, D. A., Castellino, R. A., and Meares, E. M., Jr. External beam radiation therapy of primary carcinoma of the prostate. *Cancer 36:* 723, 1975.

48. van der Werf-Messing, B. The experience of the Rotterdam Radiotherapy Institute (RRTI) in the treatment of urological tumours. In *The Tumours of Genito-urinary Apparatus*, edited by M. Pavone-Macaluso. Cofese Edizioni Palermo, Palermo, 1977, p. 93.

49. Taylor, W. J., Richardson, R. G., and Hafermann, M. D. Radiation therapy for localized prostate cancer. *Cancer 43:* 1123, 1979.

Editorial Comment to Chapter 10

As for all modalities in prostate cancer therapy, it sometimes takes decades of use until the initial euphoria is—step by step—replaced by a more critical and thus realistic judgement as to the efficacy of the given form of treatment (see Chapter 3).

In the last 2 years, evidence has grown from data of different comprehensive centers that the attribute *"curative"* for local external irradiation of assumed localized prostate cancer obviously places too high a demand on this modality (Alken *et al.*, 1977; Cupps *et al.*, 1980; Jacobi *et al.*, 1981; Kiesling *et al.*, 1980; Nachtsheim *et al.*, 1978; Pilepich *et al.*, 1980; Schröder *et al.*, 1976). If radiation is given with curative intent, its failure can be defined as the *failure to achieve total and persistent local eradication of the tumor or development of distant spread.*

Distant metastases clinically demonstrable after irradiation may be due to seeding from noneradicated local growth or from lymph nodes not treated appropriately. Now, what does "noneradicated local growth" mean? The frequently used term *recurrence* is misleading, since a tumor can only *recur* if it has first disappeared. The rigorous proof of the latter, however, can only be achieved at autopsy. Therefore, the carcinoma that fails to respond (totally or partially) should be termed *residual tumor* without predicting whether it will remain stable or progress. What tools are available to predict local disease? Surely rectal examination is not the only means! If we apply postirradiation biopsy, the question arises as to what is the correct time interval after treatment which would indicate success or failure of irradiation therapy.

At our Institution, repeated aspiration fine needle biopsies in a fan-shaped fashion have been repeatedly performed after local radiotherapy for 11 years (Jacobi *et al.*, 1981). After our first report (Kurth *et al.*[26]) we were unique in our assumption that biopsies persistently positive for tumor cells would indicate therapy failure. At the same time, others came to contradictory conclusions (Kagan *et al.*[32]). Currently it is still difficult not to assume that persistently positive biopsies mean treatment failure (Jacobi *et al.*, 1981). As touched on in Chapter 3, there is now strong evidence, based on a large number of patients, that a tumor-positive biopsy finding 2 years after radiotherapy indicates a tendency toward progressive tumor disease, including distant spread. As indicated in Figure 10.5, almost 90% of all tumors that respond (reproducible by biopsies) will do so within the first 2 years after irradiation. Furthermore, only 57% of all cases repeatedly biopsied (up to seven biopsies, average three) will ever experience a definitive tumor conversion (Fig. 10.6). The significance

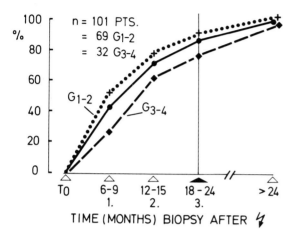

Figure 10.5 Tumor sterilization in relation to the time of biopsy and initial tumor grade. Eighty-eight percent of all prostatic carcinoma irradiated with curative intent which will become tumor-negative any time after radiotherapy will do so within 2 years after treatment. Well differentiated (G_{1-2}) adenocarcinoma do better than undifferentiated (G_{3-4}) tumors. (Modified with permission from G. H. Jacobi *et al.*, 1981.)

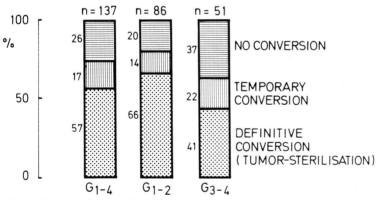

Figure 10.6 Influence of initial tumor grade on biopsy results (curative group). Overall, only 57% of tumors of all 137 patients with local irradiation of curative intent will experience a definitive conversion (repeatedly tumor-negative biopsies at the end of evaluation). Secondary positive biopsy finding after intermediate negative finding (temporary conversion) occurred in 17% of cases. Initial failure from the beginning (no conversion) was seen in 26% of cases. Well differentiated (G_{1-2}) adenocarcinoma do significantly better than undifferentiated (G_{3-4}) lesions in terms of definitive tumor conversion. (Modified with permission from G. H. Jacobi *et al.*, 1981.)

of persistent residual tumor in terms of distant spread is illustrated in Table 3.4 (page 46).

Thus, the biopsy result 2 years after radiotherapy is of paramount prognostic value and is the indication for additional systemic treatment.

The "Letterman-Group" (Nachtsheim *et al.*, 1978; Kiesling *et al.*, 1980) came to a similar conclusion based on a smaller number of patients by saying that, "Patients with residual tumor 18 months after therapy will not have resolution of the tumor at a future date and represent treatment failure" (Nachtsheim *et al.*, 1978) and that, "patients who had positive biopsies after therapy had a greater chance for disease progression ... than patients with negative biopsies" (Kiesling *et al.*, 1980). Since most high-grade tumors and massive tumors of any grade fail outside the pelvis (Pilepich *et al.*, 1980), adjuvant treatment is recommended if a biopsy from prostatic induration after radiotherapy turns out to be positive (Cupps *et al.*, 1980).

Experimental support for all these considerations derive from ultrastructural and immunohistochemical studies indicating that residual tumor formations left behind after local irradiation maintain metabolic activities necessary for further growth and metastases (Kiesling *et al.*, 1979; Mahan *et al.*, 1980). Thus, local failure after external irradiation is not "exceptional" (page 206). The obviously limited curative character of this treatment modality has to be considered when offering it to patients as an alternative to radical surgery.

R. H.
G. H. J.

REFERENCES

Alken, C. E., Dhom, G., Kopper, B., Rehker, H., Dietz, R., Kopp, S., and Ziegler, M. Prostate carcinoma: determination of progression following high-voltage therapy. *Urologe A 16:* 272, 1977.

Cupps, R. E., Utz, D. C., Fleming, T. R., Carson, C. C., Zincke, H., and Myers, R. P. Definitive radiation therapy for prostatic carcinoma: Mayo Clinic experience. *J. Urol. 124:* 855, 1980.

Jacobi, G. H., Riedmiller, H., Kurth, K. H., and Hohenfellner, R. Bioptic control is essential after external beam radiotherapy for prostate cancer: four hundred and six biopsies over eleven years. Presented at the American Urological Association, Boston, 1981.

Kiesling, V. J., Friedman, H. I., McAninch, J. W., Nachtsheim, D. A., Nemeth, T. J. The ultrastructural changes of prostate adenocarcinoma following external beam radiation therapy. *J. Urol. 122:* 633, 1979.

Kiesling, V. J., McAninch, J. W., Goebel, J. L., and Agee, R. E. External beam radiotherapy for adenocarcinoma of the prostate: a clinical followup. *J. Urol. 124:* 851, 1980.

Mahan, D. E., Bruce, A. W., Manley, P. N., and Fanchi, L. Immunhistochemical evaluation of prostatic carcinoma before and after radiotherapy. *J. Urol. 124:* 488, 1980.

Nachtsheim, D. A., Jr., McAninch, J. W., Stutzman, R. E., and Goebel, J. L. Latent residual tumor following external radiotherapy for prostate adenocarcinoma. *J. Urol. 120:* 312, 1978.

Pilepich, M. V., Perez, C. A., and Bauer, W. Prognostic parameters in radiotherapeutic management of localized carcinoma of the prostate. *J. Urol. 124:* 485, 1980.

Schröder, F. H., Jellinghaus, W., and Frohmüller, H. The treatment of locally confined prostatic carcinoma: radiotherapy versus total prostatectomy. *Urologe A 15:* 67, 1976.

11

Hormone Manipulation for Palliative Treatment of Advanced Prostatic Carcinoma

J. E. Altwein, M.D.

Rational management of prostatic carcinoma (PCA) requires accurate diagnosis, grading, and staging based on thorough examination of the patient's current status. Equally important, however, is the distinction between "virginal" PCA which has had no previous tumor-specific treatment, and pretreated PCA which is either in remission, stable, or in progression.

The *diagnosis* may be established histologically or cytologically, and must include an assessment of the *degree of differentiation*. High-grade PCAs (G_3 and anaplastic) are likely to have metastasized by the time of diagnosis (Fig. 11.1) and have a poor prognosis. This has been confirmed by Hanash *et al.*[53] in patients not subjected to any other therapy except transurethral resection. In addition, the tumor grade appears to correlate with hormone responsiveness and serves as a useful prognostic indicator when contemplating hormone administration.

While grading reflects the dynamic potential of the tumor, *stage* represents the *status quo, i.e.* tumor extension at the time of diagnosis. Once staging is completed, the appropriate treatment category is selected, which, stated simply, means that local tumors require local treatment while disseminated tumors should have systemic treatment. Unfortunately, the majority of patients already have metastases when their PCA is diagnosed. The magnitude of this problem is underlined when one realizes that metastatic spread to the skeleton ($T_{1-4}N_xM_1$) was encountered in 42.8% of a series comprising 988 patients of the third VACURG study,[25] and involvement of pelvic lymph nodes ($T_{2-3}N_1M_0$), as confirmed by lymphadenectomy of 100 consecutive PCA without distant metastases, was found in 41% of patients with alleged localized tumors.[12] Del Regato[33] pointed out that, in the absence of tumor metastases, systemic treatment is rarely, if ever, indicated. Even in PCA with extracapsular extension but negative nodes, systemic treatment is usually unwarranted.

The patient's age, performance status (Table 11.1[69]), and cardiovascular and hepatic risk factors have to be taken into account if hormone administration is being considered. Final indispensable information is related to the form of possible *previous treatment*, since active progressive carcinoma—despite previous hormone treatment—is highly resistant to most systemic measures.

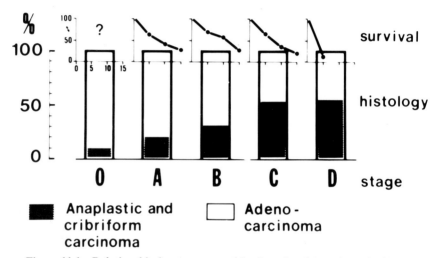

Figure 11.1 Relationship between stage, histology (grade), and survival in prostatic cancer. N = 2136 from literature survey. (Courtesy of K. H. Kurth, Rotterdam, The Netherlands)

ANDROGEN CONTROL MEASURES: INDICATION FOR HORMONE MANIPULATION

In the untreated patient with PCA, the average life-span after recognition of the first symptom was 31 months; in the presence of metastases, 66% died within 9 months and none survived 5 years.[52] Classical "androgen control" therapy (orchiectomy plus estrogens) led to a 15.5% 5-year and 3.9% 10-year survival rate.[38] Results of orchiectomy alone were somewhat inferior (5-year survival, 11.6%), and estrogens alone were slightly superior (5-year survival, 21.4%). These retrospective findings were confirmed by a prospective trial conducted in patients with locally advanced and disseminated PCA,[24] from which the following facts emerged.

1. Placebo is the worst "treatment" regarding 9-year survival.
2. Estrogens alone are superior.
3. Survival with orchiectomy plus estrogens was slightly better than

216 PROSTATE CANCER

orchiectomy plus placebo (comparable to orchiectomy alone in Emmett's retrospective study).

Thus, two independent trials demonstrated that estrogens are indeed somewhat effective in retarding the course of PCA (Table 11.2). The first VACURG study, however, indicated that lethal cardiovascular side effects more than offset the retardation of tumor growth. The second VACURG study revealed a strong influence of the estrogen dose in stage III (patients with potential longevity) and a weak influence in stage IV PCA.[24]

Considering that the action of androgen control treatment is *cancero-*

Table 11.1
Karnofsky Performance Status Index[a]

General Category	Index	Specific Criteria
Able to carry on normal activity: no special care needed.	100	Normally no evidence of disease.
	90	Normal activity; minor signs or symptoms of disease.
	80	Normal activity with effort; some signs or symptoms of disease.
Unable to work; able to live at home and care for most personal needs; varying amount of assistance needed.	70	Cares for self; unable to carry on normal activity or to do work.
	60	Requires occasional assistance from others.
	50	Requires considerable assistance from others and frequent medical care.
Unable to care for self; requires institutional or hospital care or equivalent; disease may be rapidly progressing.	40	Disabled; requires special care.
	30	Severely disabled; hospitalization indicated; death not imminent.
	20	Very sick; hospitalization necessary; active supportive treatment necessary.
	10	Moribund
	0	Dead

[a] From D. A. Karnofsky.[69]

Table 11.2
Deaths by Stage, Treatment, and Cause in Locally Advanced (Stage C) or Far Advanced (Stage D) Prostatic Carcinoma[a, b]

Cause of Death	Stage C				Stage D			
	P	E	O+P	O+E	P	E	O+P	O+E
No. patients	262	265	266	257	223	211	203	216
Carcinoma	46	18	35	25	105	82	97	82
Cardiovascular	88	112	95	108	55	76	56	59
Other causes	43	50	54	48	29	23	29	40
Total deaths	177	180	184	181	189	181	182	181

[a] From VACURG, study I.[24]
[b] Abbreviations used are: P, placebo; E, 5.0 mg diethylstilbestrol daily; O, orchiectomy.

static rather than *cancerocidal*,[19] this treatment modality cannot be qualified as curative. Therefore, those stages of PCA where a cure could be achieved should be excluded. A borderline situation is encountered in stage III or C of PCA with few positive deep and/or superficial pelvic lymph nodes, *i.e.* $T_{1-4}N_{1,2}M_0$. In the operable patient, a thorough pelvic lymphadenectomy with irradiation should precede hormone manipulation.[26] Progression despite local therapy with curative intent would render the PCA *"pseudovirginal"* and is thus still amenable to systemic treatment. Hormone manipulation is clearly indicated, however, in PCA with numerous positive lymph nodes or even distant metastases.

In cardiovascular and hepatic risk patients with advanced PCA, one should primarily rely on orchiectomy alone. Hormone application is withheld until progression occurs. In addition, inhibitors of prostaglandin synthesis (*e.g.* high dose aspirin, indomethacin) are useful in these patients.

A special situation is created by ureteral obstruction due to seminal vesical invasion or direct extension of PCA to the bladder (see Chapter 3). Michigan and Catalona[87] studied the charts of 1,065 patients and found 10% with uni- or bilateral ureteral obstruction. Orchiectomy improved upper tract dilatation in 88% of 25 patients, whereas estrogens or antiandrogens were successful in only 17% of six patients. Grade and stage did not correlate with response rate. This favorable effect of orchiectomy upon ureteral obstruction may even be encountered after long-term medical treatment (Fig. 11.2). Irradiation is far inferior in treating these patients.[87]

AIM OF HORMONE MANIPULATION

Biochemical similarity between the patient's normal and his cancerous prostatic tissue is one essential prerequisite for successful hormone manipulation basically directed at the *deprivation of androgenic influences upon the prostate*. In achieving this goal every therapeutic modality still relies on classical androgen control principles; however, new developments in the field of chemotherapeutical drugs and antihormones are being tested in multicenter phase II and III trials,[119] *e.g.* under the auspices of the National Prostatic Cancer Project (NPCP) and European Organization for Research on Treatment of Cancer (EORTC).

The aim of hormone manipulation may be achieved by the following basic mechanisms:

Androgen Withdrawal by Castration, Bilateral Adrenalectomy, or Hypophysectomy

The latter two endocrinoprival measures are not considered adequate for primary treatment of a hormone-responsive tumor. For secondary treatment, justification for this surgery rests on the premise that malignant tissue is still androgen-dependent.[128] Eradication of extratesticular sources of androgen production may be accomplished by hypophysectomy as well as adrenalectomy. The latter procedure represents an intolerable burden

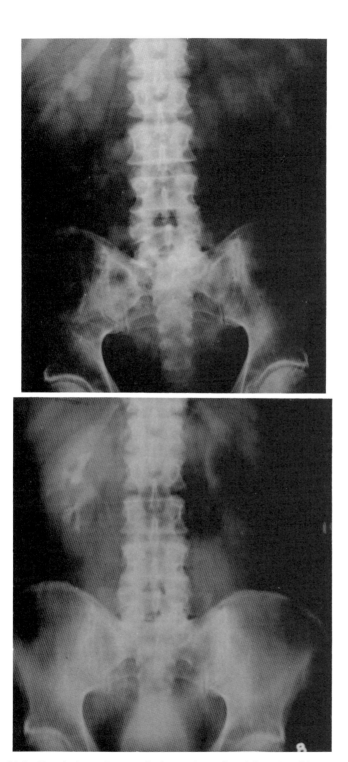

Figure 11.2 Resolution of ureteral obstruction after delayed orchiectomy. Primary treatment was instituted 1 year before with a Honvan infusion and polyestradiol phosphate maintenance treatment (80 mg/month IM).

in patients suffering from relapsing PCA, does not lower plasma testosterone in the castrated patient,[16] and even increases peripheral LH and FSH.[101] Drugs interfering with the hypothalamic dopaminergic centers (bromocriptine, lisuride, lergotrile) or suppressing the tropic hormones at the pituitary level (*e.g.* estrogens, gestagens, cyproterone acetate, and corticosteroids) and inhibitors of androgen synthesis lead to "pharmacological adrenalectomy." Thus, adrenalectomy performed for palliative purposes only may be replaced by some form of "antiadrenal" medication.[106]

Cryohypophysectomy is associated with a low morbidity and mortality (less than 10%[74]) when used for secondary treatment of PCA, but besides good temporary palliation, prolongation of life can be measured in months only. Furthermore, complete suppression of residual hormonal activity of the pituitary gland in patients with PCA progression despite orchiectomy and estrogens may be accomplished by antihormones, *e.g.* cyproterone acetate and bromocriptine.[5, 64, 65]

Even gestagens have good antigonadotropic properties and offer a desirable anabolic action.[73] However, once a PCA has escaped hormonal control, chemotherapy should be considered. Chemotherapy yields sufficient long-term responses and was found superior to either adrenalectomy or hypophysectomy[131] (see Chapter 16).

Thus, *orchiectomy* remains the preferred method of androgen withdrawal by surgical means. Castration effectively lowers the plasma testosterone level within days to approximately 10% of the preorchiectomy value: 607 ± 235 ng/100 ml to 30 ng/100 ml[102] or 620 ± 260 to 50 ± 50 ng/100 ml.[80] Plasma testosterone was suppressed for up to 2 years,[114] but in patients receiving polyestradiol phosphate monthly, a moderate increase was measured in the 2nd year following orchiectomy (Fig. 11.3).[3] Similarly, Sciarra et al.[111] found in 10 of 27 patients after castration, testosterone values of 137 ± 23 ng/100 ml and androstenedione levels of 213 ± 39 ng/100 ml. Both steroids dropped to 22 ± 20 ng/100 ml and 43 ± 11 ng/100 ml, respectively, after dexamethasone administration, indicating their adrenocortical origin. In keeping with this finding is the demonstration of an augmented adrenal androgen secretion by Robinson et al.[102] and the presence of adrenal hyperplasia as demonstrated in autopsy cases.[19, 67, 82]

In castrated males with reactivation of their tumor, however, testosterone, androstenedione, or dehydroepiandrosterone, were not elevated.[70, 125, 129] Recently, Sanford et al.[107] demonstrated testosterone secretion from the adrenals ranging from 16 to 217 mg/24 hours.

Castration modulates the action of prolactin, a peptide hormone, which directly influences the PCA as demonstrated by *in vivo* studies.[63] Asano[8] found an orchiectomy-induced elevation of prolactin activity. Following the discovery of membrane-bound prolactin-receptor sites in the liver[98] and the prostate—which possesses the highest number of binding sites as related to protein units[7]—it was shown that castration increases hepatic prolactin binding but lowers the prostatic prolactin-binding capacity (Fig. 11.4[72]; Chapters 21 and 22).

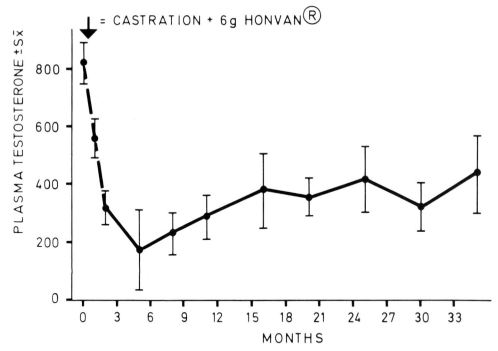

Figure 11.3 Plasma testosterone in 35 patients treated by orchiectomy, Honvan infusion, and polyestradiol phosphate plus stilbestrol. (Reproduced with permission from J. E. Altwein and K. Bandhauer.[3])

The question whether orchiectomy may be replaced by antiandrogens, especially cyproterone acetate, in virginal advanced PCA has not been tested in a phase III trial (see Chapter 15).

Extraprostatic Suppression of Hormones Relevant to the Prostate

Such an "antihormonal" action would be superfluous if selective prostatotropic hormones or their equivalents were available, but even a seemingly pure end-organ antagonist, such as flutamide, increases the testosterone plasma level and production rate.[57] The extraprostatic mode of action may become effective at the various levels of the endocrine hierarchy.

HYPOTHALAMUS

Dopamine agonists (Table 11.3) stimulate the dopaminergic neurons in the ventral nuclei which results in the release of the prolactin-inhibiting factor, dopamine (see Chapter 22). This neurotransmitter reacts with a pituitary receptor resulting in a suppression of peripheral prolactin.[63] L-dopa, a dopamine precursor, is a short-acting antiprolactin which has been used in the past for palliation in patients with stage D-PCA.[40, 96, 103] The greatest clinical experience has been gained with bromocriptine, a semisynthetic ergot derivative which possesses long-acting dopamine receptor-stimulating properties.[29, 31, 32, 64] Lergotrile is virtually equieffec-

Table 11.3
Drugs Stimulating the Release of Hypothalamic Dopamine Lowering Effectively the Peripheral Prolactin Level: Dopamine Agonists (see also Chapters 21 and 22)

Category	Drug	Clinical Signifi-cance
Dopamine precursor	L-dopa	Replaced
Ergot alkaloid	Lergotrile	Investigational
Ergot alkaloid	Bromocriptine mesilate	Demonstrated
Ergot alkaloid	Lisuride hydrogen maleate	Demonstrated

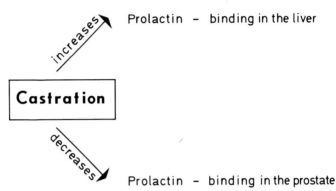

Figure 11.4   The dualistic effect of castration upon prolactin binding.

tive.[117] Having a comparable mode of action, lisuride hydrogen maleate is 10 times stronger than bromocriptine.[59]

PITUITARY GLAND

Estrogens (Table 11.4) with their main representative diethylstilbestrol, suppress LH and FSH-release.[9] Plasma testosterone decrease and testicular atrophy result primarily from central antigonadotropic action; however, a direct inhibition of testosterone formation is also involved.[132] The diethylstilbestrol-induced drop of plasma testosterone is dose-dependent: 1 mg does not cause uniform suppression, whereas 3 mg are as effective as 30 mg.[70, 102, 114] The sex hormone-binding globulin (SHBG) increment, reducing the percentage of biologically active free testosterone even further, is a therapeutic goal.[60]

Gestagens (Table 11.5) have strong antigonadotropic properties[128] with the pituitary not responding to luteinizing hormone-releasing hormone (LHRH) stimulation.[19] As a derivative of chlormadinone acetate, cyproterone acetate exerts a strong LH and FSH suppression.[35] Girard et al.[50] demonstrated a pronounced ACTH-suppression by cyproterone acetate which did not respond to 1 mg metyrapone. The recovery of ACTH-adrenal function may take several months.

In addition to their hypothalamic action, dopamine agonists (Table 11.3) bind to pituitary dopamine-receptors, directly hampering prolactin release.[32]

Table 11.4
Estrogens Used for the Treatment of Prostatic Carcinoma

Class	Drug	Dose	Remarks
Conjugated estrogens	Premarin	2.5–7.5 mg/day p.o.	Used in VACURG III[26]
Stilbene derivatives	DES	1–3 mg/day p.o.	Reference estrogen (*cf.* ref. 25)
	Dienestrol	5 mg/day p.o.	Very active
	Hexestrol	5 mg/day p.o.	Somewhat less active
	Diethylstilbestrol di-phosphate (Honvan)	360 mg/day p.o.	Active
		1.2 gm/day IV (10 days)	Excellent palliation
	Chlorotrianisene (TACE)	12–24 mg/day p.o.	Used in VACURG III,[26] no LH suppression, no PRL release
Ester of estradiol	Ethinyl estradiol	0.6 mg/day p.o.	Very active; used in combination with a long acting estrogen
	Estradiol undecylate	100 mg/month IM	Long acting
	Polyestradiol phosphate	40–80 mg/month IM	Long acting
Combination with nitrogen mustard	Estramustine phosphate	560 mg/day p.o.	Secondary treatment
Organosilicone	Cisobitane	900 mg/day p.o.	Active, rather toxic

Table 11.5
Gestagens Used for the Treatment of Prostatic Carcinoma: 17α-Hydroxyprogesterone Derivatives

Compound	Dose	Remarks
Hydroxyprogesterone caproate	1.5 gm IM/2×/wk	
Gestonorone caproate	400 mg/wk IM	Ineffective[105]
Chlormadinone acetate	0.1–2.0 gm q.i.d.	Weak
Megestrol acetate	160 mg q.i.d.	Active[47]
Medroxyprogesterone acetate (MPA)	30–500 mg/day	Active[21, 26]

ADRENAL GLAND

"Pharmacological adrenalectomy" might reasonably provide the same magnitude of response achieved by surgical adrenalectomy. The following androgen synthesis inhibitors[128] deserve mention: inhibition of the *20,21-desmolase* exerted by aminoglutethimide prevents the formation of all adrenal steroids, androgens, and corticosteroids as well. Cortisol suppression induces ACTH-release which is able to override the aminoglutethimide blockade unless cortisol is administered.[106]

Selective inhibition of *17,20-desmolase* by spironolactone lowers adrenal androgen secretion, *i.e.* testosterone, androsterone, and dehydroepiandrosterone levels decline.[129] Even though cyproterone acetate possesses the ability to interfere with the same enzyme, this action is weak as compared to its antiandrogenic properties.[85] The same applies to its inhibition of 3β-hydroxysteroid dehydrogenase and isomerase, which are equally affected by estradiol-17β, megestrol acetate, and medrogestone, to name only a few.[48]

TESTES

Although estrogen seems capable of directly inhibiting testicular steroidogenesis, this action requires particularly high concentrations.[132] The primary mechanism responsible for lowered plasma testosterone is LH suppression. Cyproterone acetate was found to inhibit testosterone synthesis in the testis[110]; however, the cyproterone acetate-induced drop of plasma testosterone may be attributed to the suppression of LH release.[35] Among the gestagens, megestrol acetate, which lowers plasma testosterone only temporarily (the so-called "*escape phenomenon*") may have a similar mode of action.[48]

Aminoglutethimide, recently studied in 16 normal men, led to an acute inhibition of testosterone synthesis in the testis.[108]

Another androgen-synthesis inhibitor is the aldosterone antagonist spironolactone which destroys the microsomal enzyme *cytochrome P-450* in the animal testis.[84] The decline in plasma testosterone with a compensatory rise of LH demonstrated in man after 400 mg spironolactone can be explained by an interference with the cytochrome P-450-dependent testicular 17-hydroxylase.[121]

Intraprostatic Suppression of Hormones (*End-Organ Antagonism*)

The *in vivo* situation does not allow for a clear determination of whether the endocrine effect on PCA is primary or secondary. However, hormone studies under certain extracorporeal conditions support the assumption of direct action at the target organ. Regarding the estrogenic hormones, Franks[43] stated that this therapy constitutes a pharmacologic modality that will consistently produce cytologic damage to malignant prostate cells. Cosgrove et al.[28] treated nine patients with stage T_{3+4}-PCA with estrogens only, who were rebiopsied after a minimal period of treatment of 12 months. In four patients with grade 1 and 2 PCA, no tumor cells were found. Histological examination of the total prostatectomy specimen in one of the four patients disclosed squamous metaplasia but no trace of tumor. In examining PCA grown in organ culture Bard and Lasnitzki[10] demonstrated that at higher concentrations estradiol decreased the production of dihydrotestosterone from testosterone and androstenedione, but at low concentrations estrogens enhanced the formation of androstanediol, androstenedione, and dihydrotestosterone from testosterone.

For competitive inhibition of intracellular dihydrotestosterone binding a much lower estrogen dosage is required.[13, 115] Certain synthetic estrogens interfere with the intranuclear polymerase system,[54] an observation which could well account for the cytotoxic effect of the *C 18*-steroids.

Progestogens compete with testosterone for the cytoplasmic 5α-reductase system.[4] Cyproterone acetate, which is the most extensively studied antiandrogen, blocks the intranuclear dihydrotestosterone binding, thus preventing cellular proliferation[127] (see Chapter 14). Spironolactone apparently acts similarly by androgen receptor blockade within the target organ.[27] In comparison to cyproterone acetate possessing a relative potency of 100, flutamide reaches 100 to 140, chlormadinone acetate 10, and medrogestone only 2.[85]

PREDICTION OF HORMONAL RESPONSIVENESS

In pursuing the therapeutic goal one faces the situation that between 10 and 40% of all virginal PCA are primarily hormone-resistant. Patients who develop symptoms from their metastases while under estrogen treatment—or who have never responded to them—represent one of the great unsolved problems of urological management. It would be desirable to predict the individual hormone responsiveness. Several methods have been investigated:

Morphological Parameters

There is now overwhelming evidence that cellular differentiation correlates strongly with estrogen responsiveness[34] (Table 11.6). Some variance in the use of diagnostic terms and particularly grades even by experienced pathologists must be anticipated when grading is employed as a prognostic indicator (Chapter 6). Kern[71] demonstrated that only 38 of 101 PCA originally designated "grade 1" were placed in this category on review, albeit these "second look" grade 1 tumors signaled an excellent prognosis with a 87% 5-year survival. Thus, the histological heterogeneity of most PCA and their metastases is reflected in their ultimate escape from control by estrogens.[58] This was recently confirmed by Müller et al.[89] who noticed a pluriform pattern in 55% of total prostatectomy specimens. These authors questioned the accuracy of biopsy samples in expressing high differentiation. Similar objections apply to DNA histograms[45] or ploidy studies by DNA measurements[123] believed to predict which PCA is hormone-responsive and which is not.

Sinha et al.[118] examined ultrastructurally the biopsy cores of 22 patients and described two distinct types of basal cells in the acini, type I (light) and type II (dark) cells. PCA which subsequently became refractory to endocrine manipulations showed more abundant type II cells than in endocrine-responsive tumors. So far, these attractive results have neither been confirmed nor used by others on a routine basis.

Biochemical Parameters

Tumor grade apparently correlates with the testosterone conversion rates of a given tumor.[88] This is in keeping with the measurement of PCA tissue dihydrotestosterone levels by Geller et al.[49] indicating a positive correlation with dihydrotestosterone content and the ultimate clinical response to hormonal treatment.

Table 11.6
Five-Year Survival of Estrogen-Treated Patients with Prostatic Carcinoma: The Influence of the Degree of Differentiation

Grade	Schirmer et al.[109] (%)	Esposti[39] (%)	Faul et al.[41] (%)
I	90	67.9	59.6
II	71	54.7	65.5
III	65	11.0	35.8
IV	52		32.1

Serum Parameters (See Chapter 8)

Among the various parameters, cholesterol, triglyceride, fibrinogen, and plasminogen were good indicators of risk of death, but were not clearly related to hormone responsiveness.[112, 113] They are, however, nonspecific for prostate cancer.

Test Systems of Hormone Sensitivity (See Chapter 17)

The prostatic 5α-reductase and arginase activity in the presence of various drugs do not represent the PCA responsiveness.[104] The clinical value of the distinction of androgen-sensitive from androgen-insensitive tumors derived from the Dunning rat adenocarcinoma is not yet clear.[61]

Prostatic Receptor Content (See Chapter 20)

In breast carcinoma estrogen and progestin receptor studies show a positive correlation between the concentration and response rate.[83] Controversial results are reported, however, in prostate cancer. Estrogen receptors have been measured by deVoogt,[126] whereas Ekman et al.[37] could not find these receptors. Walsh et al.[130] cautioned the expectation in stating that because steroidal hormones exert their major influences within the nucleus of target tissues the measurement of nuclear receptor content may provide a more accurate means to predict the hormone responsiveness of PCA.

In essence, at the present time there is no reliable method that detects with certainty which tumor is sensitive and which is not. It remains uncertain whether indicators of an ultimate grave prognosis are also indicators of hormone resistance (Chapter 3).

PRINCIPAL WAYS OF ENDOCRINE MANIPULATION

The variety of treatment actually given to patients with *distant* PCA is remarkable. Aided by the regional tumor registry at Rosewell Park Memorial Institute,[90] the following figures give an overview of patients treated within a single year:

Hormones	35.8%
Surgery, hormones	19.4%
None	18.2%
Surgery	14.9%
Radiation, hormones	2.9%
Surgery, radiation, hormones	2.9%
Surgery, chemotherapy, hormones	2.9%
Chemotherapy, hormones	1.5%
Radiation	1.5%

The situation appears to be quite similar worldwide (*cf.* the treatment varieties reported in East Germany[81]) and reflects the urologist's dilemma in trying to cope with advanced PCA.

In *categorizing* the most promising therapeutic modalities based on hormone manipulation of some kind, four controversial regimens evolve:

1. Orchiectomy plus estrogens.
2. Orchiectomy only; hormonal therapy is withheld until symptoms arise.
3. Hormones only; orchiectomy is postponed.
4. Hormones plus chemotherapy.

Orchiectomy Plus Estrogens

This treatment category is widely practiced in Germany in widespread M_1-PCA and may be considered a standard treatment.[51, 55] Once staging is completed, subcapsular orchiectomy is carried out followed by a diethylstilbestrol diphosphate (Honvan) infusion (usually 15 gm given within 10 days). Maintenance therapy consists of monthly injections of 80 mg polyestradiol phosphate (Estradurin) or 100 mg estradiol undecylate (Progynon Depot).[17] Some advise additional intake of an oral estrogen, *e.g.* TACE, ethinyl estradiol, or diethylstilbestrol (DES).[55] However, the drawback of all oral medication in chronically ill patients is the poor patient compliance.[6]

In "early" PCA, endocrine manipulation resulted in a 10-year survival of 50% (44 of 88 patients) and a 15-year survival of 30% (22 of 74 patients).[11] However, in a phase III trial, placebo was found even better than orchiectomy plus 5 mg DES regarding 5-year survival.[23] Thus, in "early" PCA the alleged cure rates after orchiectomy plus estrogen are more compatible with survival despite endocrine manipulation.

On the contrary, this treatment provides an excellent but transient palliation in advanced disease. There are some long-term survivors even with PCA of this stage. A recent retrospective study revealed 40% (17 of 43 patients) 5-year and 12% (5 of 42 patients) 10-year survival following orchiectomy and estrogens.[124] The results of the best known phase III trial, the first VACURG study, fall short of De Vere White's study (Fig. 11.5); in particular at the 5-year follow-up neither treatment arm to which the patients were randomized, *i.e.*, placebo, 5 mg DES, orchiectomy plus placebo, or orchiectomy plus 5 mg DES, was found superior. At 9 years, orchiectomy and placebo appeared to be the worst therapy (Fig. 11.5).

In analyzing the causes of death in study I for stage D PCA (Table 11.2) it is obvious that estrogens increase the noncancer deaths. Menon *et al.*[85] muse about the possibility that if these patients had lived long enough they would have succumbed to their cancer. This appears to be the case when taking into account the results of VACURG II[24] comparing placebo, 0.2, 1, and 5 mg DES. The two highest doses of estrogens slowed down the progression of stage C to D PCA.

The widely discussed data of the VACURG I have been reconsidered by Jordan *et al.*[68] who arrived at the conclusion that estrogens are more effective than orchiectomy in preventing deaths from PCA and that the *addition of orchiectomy* to estrogens does not offer any clear-cut advantage over estrogen therapy alone. If cancer symptoms necessitate treatment these authors prefer estrogens. Orchiectomy should, according to these

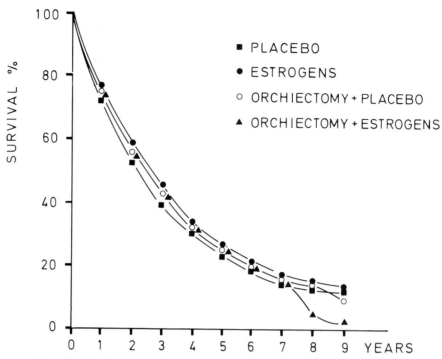

Figure 11.5 Survival after treatment of stage D prostatic cancer randomly allocated to four different regimen: orchiectomy plus placebo (N = 266), orchiectomy plus DES 5 mg (N = 254), DES 5 mg (N = 265), and placebo (N = 262). (Modified from D. P. Byar.[25])

authors, be reserved for those circumstances in which a patient is not reliable, cannot tolerate estrogens, or has severe cardiovascular disease. Similarly, the simultaneous use of *orchiectomy plus estrogen* from the beginning is rejected by Menon *et al.*,[85] but their preferred form of hormonal therapy is bilateral orchiectomy alone. This view is shared by Paulson[94] who states that there is little advantage in giving hormonal therapy prior to the onset of symptoms of bone pain or evidence of active progression, such as weakness, anemia, progressive outflow or ureteral obstruction. Furthermore the combination of orchiectomy plus estrogens is no longer recommended, since (1) two valuable (as far as palliation is concerned) therapeutic modalities are used from the beginning, leaving little to offer when the disease progresses; (2) at the very first estrogen attack on the prostatic cancer, the development of estrogen resistance commences; (3) PCA patients are unnecessarily subjected to the considerable estrogen side effects.

Orchiectomy Only, Hormones Withheld

This concept is favored by Paulson[94] in the asymptomatic patient. Likewise, at Johns Hopkins Hospital[85] orchiectomy alone is preferred with relapses treated by chemotherapy. However, two large scale retrospective studies have demonstrated the inferiority of orchiectomy *versus* estrogens[38, 91] (Fig. 11.6). At 9 years even a prospective randomized trial,

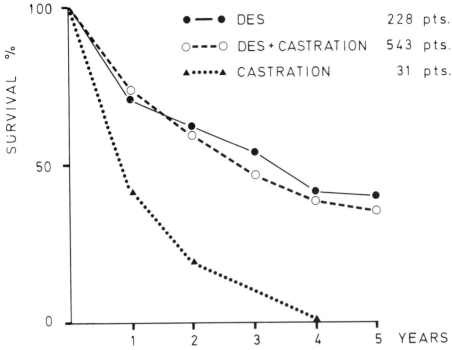

Figure 11.6 Survival of patients after three different therapeutic regimen (retrospective study. (Reproduced with permission from K. Ochiai and H. Takeuchi.[91])

VACURG I, revealed a slight, however insignificant, inferiority of castration *versus* estrogens. This trial clearly demonstrated that estrogens are more effective in preventing deaths from PCA than orchiectomy[68] (*cf.* Table 11.2).

The main advantage of orchiectomy alone for distant PCA is that it's well tolerated by the patient; this is more than offset by the observation of Brendler and Prout[22] that patients refractory to castration did not respond to estrogen application. It should be stated at this point that patients not responding anymore to estrogens as the only treatment still benefit from delayed castration[87] (*cf.* Fig. 11.2).

Hormones Only, Orchiectomy Deferred

In addition to estrogens, progestogens and certain antihormones are used.

ESTROGENS

Since the attempts of Strohm[122] to ease pain with estrogen in patients with advanced PCA, a multitude of reports dealing with a variety of estrogenic preparations have appeared in the literature (Table 11.4). Besides two large scale retrospective studies[38, 91] (*cf.* Fig. 11.6) two phase III trials (VACURG I and II; *cf.* Fig. 11.5 and Fig. 11.7) have exemplified the effectiveness of DES in comparision to orchiectomy plus placebo, placebo, and orchiectomy plus estrogens.

The use of estrogens has been discredited for the following reasons:

1. Cardiovascular toxicity (myocardial infarction, cerebrovascular accidents, arteriosclerotic heart disease, pulmonary embolism), is a phenomenon to which Blanchot et al.[18] had already directed attention in 1952. However, it required the widely discussed first VACURG study to prove that the cardiovascular death rates in the two estrogen arms reach 36 and 27% *versus* 24 and 27% in the two nonestrogen arms for stage IV PCA (Table 11.2). One should note that the differences are distinct only in the estrogen *versus* the placebo arm. Further investigation on this subject has made clear that patients with preexisting cardiovascular disease are at risk (Fig. 11.8), and that the cardiovascular side effects are dose-related. Cardiovascular toxicity was particularly distressing in patients with potential longevity (stage III PCA) where the 5 mg DES led to an excess of noncancer deaths as compared to 1 mg DES, which still produced equal survival rates (Fig. 11.8). The risk may be further reduced if those patients with elevated triglyceride and plasminogen levels[112, 113] are excluded or receive an inhibitor of platelet aggregation.[36]

2. Hyperprolactinemia. This may be overcome by administration of bromocriptine or lisuride (Chapter 22).

3. Impairment of immune response (Fig. 11.9).

4. The occurrence of hepatic toxicity[76] and salt-water retention.[77]

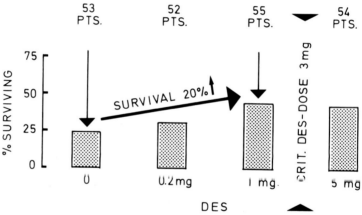

Figure 11.7 Survival of patients with stage D prostatic carcinoma after DES application: influence of the estrogen dose (prospective study of the VACURG[24]). (Modified from D. P. Byar.[24])

GESTAGENS

The availability of well tolerated 17α-hydroxyprogesterone derivatives (*cf.* Table 11.5) led Geller *et al.*[47] to practice its administration in patients with PCA. The rationale for its use was the virtual lack of serious side effects,[100] even in a phase II study employing daily injections of 1,500 mg medroxyprogesterone acetate (MPA, Depot Provera) over 30 days[93] and the *dopamine agonistic action* induced by gestagens with subsequent

CARDIOVASCULAR DEATHS

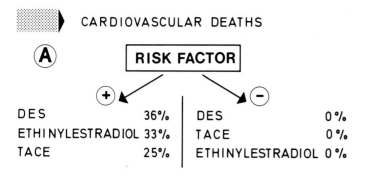

(A) RISK FACTOR

(+)   (−)

DES	36%	DES	0%
ETHINYLESTRADIOL	33%	TACE	0%
TACE	25%	ETHINYLESTRADIOL	0%

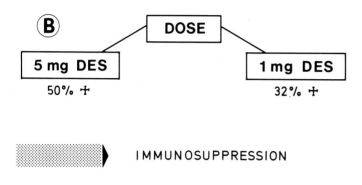

(B) DOSE

| 5 mg DES | 1 mg DES |
| 50% ✝ | 32% ✝ |

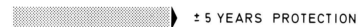

IMMUNOSUPPRESSION

± 5 YEARS PROTECTION

Figure 11.8 Sequelae of estrogen treatment. (Modified from Bennett et al.[14])

prolactin suppression.[30] A survey of the various phase II trials is provided by Bouffioux[19] showing none of the 17α-hydroxyprogesterone derivatives as being clearly effective.

Phase III Trials. Sander et al.[105] found gestonorone caproate, 400 mg IM/week, *versus* orchiectomy alone, ineffective. MPA (30 mg) was compared to 2.5 mg Premarin, 1 mg DES, and 1 mg DES plus 30 mg MPA in the third VACURG study in 424 stage IV PCA patients. With a roughly 3-year follow-up, no significant differences in survival were detected. Byar[25] concluded from the third study that none of the treatments studied provide any advantage over 1 mg DES. The EORTC compared cyproterone acetate (250 mg/day), MPA (500 mg IM twice a week; then 100 mg b.i.d. *per os*), and 3 mg DES in protocol no. 30761. Three years after activation of the study, 41% of the patients with PCA treated with MPA showed progression *versus* 19% in the DES arm, and 33% after cyproterone acetate.[95]

The most recent randomized prospective trial was conducted by Bouffioux[20] employing 500 mg MPA 2 to 4 times a week for 1 month, followed by MPA 100 mg q.i.d. *per os*. The results (Table 11.7) can be summarized in stating:

	IMMUNE RESPONSE	
	HUMORAL	CELL-MEDIATED
ESTROGEN	STIMULATED/SUPPRESSED	SUPPRESSED
TESTOSTERONE	NOT DONE	SUPPRESSED/UNAFFECTED
PROGESTERONE	UNAFFECTED	SUPPRESSED
ANTIANDROGEN	NOT DONE	SUPPRESSED/UNAFFECTED
PROLACTIN	UNAFFECTED	SUPPRESSED
ORCHIECTOMY	UNAFFECTED	STIMULATED

Figure 11.9 Hormonal influence on immunologic functions. (Courtesy of R. Ackermann.[1])

Table 11.7
Medroxyprogesterone Acetate (MPA) *versus* Diethylstilbestrol (DES): Bouffioux's Phase III Trial in Advanced Prostatic Carcinoma[20]

	No. of Patients	Survival		
		1 yr	2 yr	3 yr
DES (3–5 mg/day p.o.)	20	16/20	14/20	11/20 (55%)
MPA (1.0–2.0 gm/wk; then 0.1 gm q.i.d.)	20	19/20	15/20	6/17 (35%)

1. MPA seems less efficient than DES in the treatment of advanced PCA with shorter periods of remission.
2. MPA was well tolerated. The 60% impotence rate is reversible after discontinuation of the drug. Gynecomastia or even mastodynia does not occur.

ANTIESTROGENS

Tamoxifen was tested in drug-resistant PCA in a few patients resulting in short-term remission.[75, 92] A phase II trial is expected.

ANTIANDROGENS

Three compounds have been tested in PCA patients: cyproterone acetate, flutamide, and megestrol acetate.

1. Megestrol Acetate (Megace). This compound was employed in a phase II trial; four of nine patients with PCA experienced a 12-month partial remission.[48] Embarrassing is the "escape" of plasma testosterone suppression beginning at 2 to 6 months, possibly responsible for the development of resistance.

2. Flutamide. In a phase II trial involving 13 men with virginal stage D PCA, 750 mg flutamide was given over a period of 2 to 20 months. Seven of 13 patients showed an objective response.[99] Similarly 21 stage D PCA patients were treated by Sogani et al.[120]; eight of 10 patients with bone pain experienced analgesia lasting from 3½ to 16½ months. Remarkably, in three of four patients with measurable lymph nodes the lesion disappeared. Altogether 19 patients responded with an average duration of 10½ months. Although none of the 21 men enrolled in the trial had previous hormonal therapy, 13 had had irradiation (!).

Phase III Trials. Airhart et al.[2] compared 1.5 gm and 0.75 gm flutamide with 1 mg DES in 20 patients with virginal stage D PCA. Objective response was noted in three of six patients receiving DES *versus* six of 14 men on flutamide. Fifty percent of the patients started on flutamide survived 1 year, and 43% 2 years. A similar study comprising 15 patients is reported by Jacobo et al.,[66] who concluded that neither DES nor flutamide displayed significant superiority.

In light of the latter investigations, the side effects are crucial. Sogani et al.[120] noticed gynecomastia in 18 of his 21 patients; two had pathological liver function tests; and four suffered from cardiovascular toxicity (one death). Fukushima et al.[46] observed a markedly altered cortisol metabolism in eight patients with PCA, presumably due to intrahepatic cholestasis or hepatocellular damage. In the continuation of this study, reversible cirrhosis-like disturbances of steroid metabolism were found.[133] A positive effect of the drug is the apparent preservation of sexual potency.[120]

A critical review on the effectiveness of flutamide is given by Neumann and Jacobi.[134]

3. Cyproterone Acetate (Androcur). This antiandrogen has been investigated in more than 1000 patients with PCA.[21, 65, 134] The present estimation rests on two phase III studies which are covered in Chapter 15.

HORMONALLY UNRESPONSIVE PROSTATE CANCER

Administration of the aforementioned drugs with hormonal activity to patients with PCA which had escaped hormonal control is likely to achieve very limited success. This merely reiterates a similar statement by Walsh[128] in 1975. Patients with hormone-insensitive PCA should be examined as suggested by Berry et al.[15] to determine those factors of prognostic association. Patients with favorable prognostic factors (*e.g.* age less than 65 years, absence of severe bone pain and anemia, acceptable performance status) would still benefit from multimodal chemotherapy despite endocrine-unresponsiveness of the PCA.

Hormones Plus Chemotherapy

This treatment category is covered in Chapters 12 and 15. Primary chemotherapy would be the ideal modality for patients with PCA refractory to hormone manipulation; however, at the present time this cannot be reliably predicted (*see above*). Among the few *primary* chemotherapy trials reported, a partial objective response to *cis*-platinum was present in 22 of 34 patients (64%) with an average duration of 9.3 months[86]; however, orchiectomy and estrogens were administered at the same time (!).

RESPONSE CRITERIA

In order to evaluate the efficacy of hormonal drugs in PCA, but particularly to assess the progression of malignant growth, certain response criteria are necessary. Unfortunately PCA rarely produces easily measurable soft tissue lesions, and such patients have a poor prognosis, not representative of the majority of patients.

1. *The primary lesion.* Rectal examination and recording of the results on a standard diagram of the prostate with a square centimeter grid overlaid is useful; however, ultrasound and CAT scanning may replace the grid technique in the near future.
2. *Repeated punch and aspiration biopsies* are reliable predictive factors in determining the response to treatment (Chapters 3 and 5).
3. *Skeletal metastases* rarely disappear completely.[42] However, objective clinical remission after treatment is represented by an osteoblastic response[97] (Fig. 11.10). Serial bone scans reveal a decrease or normalization of the skeletal radioactivity distribution.[79]
4. *Acid phosphatase.* A fall of acid phosphatase without objective evidence of disease progression may indicate that the therapy is controlling the disease,[62] whereas a rise in phosphatase levels is indicative of disease progression, but levels which remain normal during treatment are of no value in the assessment of the probability of progression (see Chapter 8).
5. *Hydroxyprolin excretion* proved reliable.[56]
6. *Non-specific ancillary factors.* Kvols[78] has designed an ancillary scoring system using these parameters and levels of acid and alkaline phosphatases which he believes are indicative of tumor response. (Table 11.8). A score of 9 or less indicates a response, 10 to 14, stable disease, 15 or more, progression. Franks[44] reports that 50% of patients in Kvols[78] progressive category developed new or enlarging skeletal metastases.

In essence, if progression is most likely based on the above criteria, the primary treatment, particularly in category 2 (orchiectomy only) and 3 (hormones only), ought to be altered.

SUMMARY AND CONCLUSION

More than 80% of all newly diagnosed PCA have already metastasized (= stage N_+ and/or M_1). Their management still relies predominantly on *hormonal manipulation*, a treatment modality with the drawback of being merely cancerostatic rather than cancerocidal.

Table 11.8
Ancillary Scoring System ("Kvols Index")[a]

Ancillary Factors	Score and Changes			
	0	1	2	3
Weight	Stable or increase	Stable or increase	Stable or increase	Decrease ≥5%
Hemoglobin	Normal[b]	Increase ≥10%	Stable	Decrease ≥10%
Alkaline phosphatase	Normal[c]	Decrease ≥50%	Stable	Increase ≥50%
Acid Phosphatase	Normal[c]	Decrease ≥50%	Stable	Increase ≥50%
Pain	None	Improved	Stable	Worse
Performance status	Asymptomatic	Improved	Stable	Worse

[a] From L. Kvols et al.[78]
[b] 13 gm/100 ml or equivalent.
[c] Upper limit of individual laboratory.

The aim of hormonal manipulation may be achieved through androgen deprivation (*i.e.* orchiectomy), extraprostatic suppression of "prostatotropic" hormones (*e.g.* dopamine antagonists; estrogens, gestagens, cyproterone acetate) as well as by means of "pharmacological adrenalectomy," and also through intraprostatic suppression of hormones relevant to the prostate. Prediction of hormonal responsiveness is impossible at the present time; thus, approximately one-third of the afflicted patients are unlikely to benefit from endocrine treatment. Furthermore, due to the rate of hormone-insensitive tumors, randomized clinical trials are a desirable prerequisite before large-scale use of allegedly effective new forms of endocrine treatment is advocated.

In accordance with the latter statement, one is able to distinguish four therapeutic regimens for distant PCA:

1. Orchiectomy plus estrogens;
2. Orchiectomy first, hormonal treatment later;
3. Hormone application first, orchiectomy later; or
4. Hormones plus chemotherapy.

The employment of orchiectomy plus estrogens has been seriously questioned by the VACURG (study I), and it appears that the addition of orchiectomy to estrogen treatment does not give better results than estrogen alone. Some authors[85, 90, 95] prefer orchiectomy alone in asymptomatic patients with stage D cancer (M_1, UICC) and reserve estrogens until the disease progresses. However, evidence has been provided[22] that patients whose PCA has progressed despite castration do not respond to estrogen application. Furthermore, it has been shown that estrogens are superior to orchiectomy in preventing cancer deaths. The argument that an undue rate of lethal cardiovascular complications more than outweighs the anticancer activity has been refuted by Bennett et al.[14] and De Vere White et al.[124]

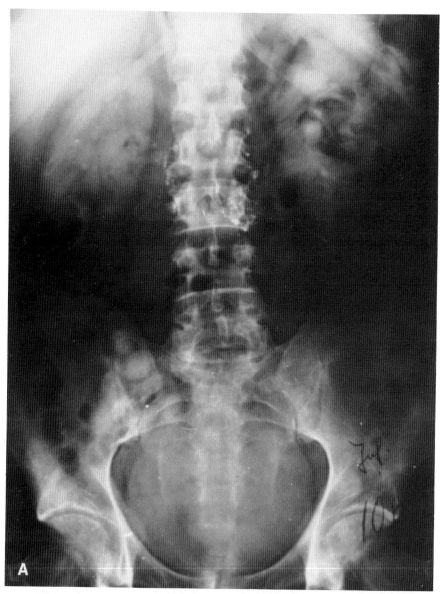

Figure 11.10 *A*, Osseous metastases of pelvic girdle and upper tract dilatation on IVP in patient with previously untreated prostate cancer. Osteoblastic response to ureteral obstruction after orchiectomy and estramustine phosphate treatment.

Thus, *hormones* evolve as the primary treatment of choice in metastatic PCA, independent of the patient's symptoms, as long as the PCA is "virginal." Taking into account the phase III trials dealing with hormonal therapy only, one is surprised to find neither estrogen nor the nonestrogen compounds superior. Among the latter, cyproterone acetate is clearly the most effective drug among the available compounds. Since the most significant estrogen side effects are lacking, one would favor cyproterone acetate as the first choice in patients with disseminated PCA and a good

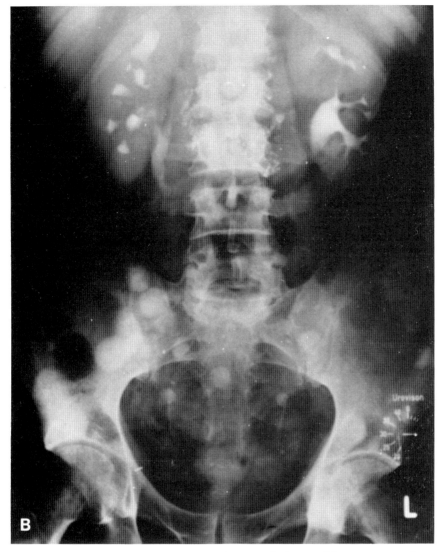

Figure 11.10 *B*, Osteoblastic response of osseous lesions and improvement of ureteral obstruction after hormonal treatment.

performance status (see Chapter 15). Progression while on cyproterone acetate requires a change of the primary treatment; it appears reasonable to use delayed orchiectomy, and possibly, as a secondary treatment, estrogens.

Adjunctive application of antiprolactins serve to suppress the estrogen and cyproterone acetate induced hyperprolactinemia. The latter phenomenon was found to be partly responsible for the development of gynecomastia, the increment of ACTH-like action upon the adrenal gland, and a rise of prolactin-binding to the prostate in the noncastrated individual.[5] It is tempting to speculate that prolactin may contribute to the development of hormone resistance in the patient suffering from metastatic carcinoma of the prostate.

REFERENCES

1. Ackermann, R. Immunologische Veränderungen unter einer Hormontherapie. In *Antihormone, Bedeutung in der Urologie*, edited by J. E. Altwein, G. Bartsch, and G. H. Jacobi. Zuckschwerdt Publ., München, 1981, pp. 259–268.

2. Airhart, R. A., Barnett, T. F., Sullivan, J. W., Levine, R. L., and Schlegel, J. U. Flutamide therapy for carcinoma of the prostate. *South. Med. J. 71:* 798, 1978.

3. Altwein, J. E., and Bandhauer, K. Langzeituntersuchungen der testikulär-hypophysären Wechselbeziehung beim Prostatakarzinom. *Akt. Urol. 7:* 101, 1976.

4. Altwein, J. E., Orestano, F., and Hohenfellner, R. Testosterone turnover in cancer of the prostate: suppression by gestagens in vitro. *Invest. Urol. 12:* 157, 1974.

5. Altwein, J. E., and Jacobi, G. H. Adjunctive bromocriptine in advanced prostatic carcinoma: a phase II study. In *II. International Symposium on the Treatment of Carcinoma of the Prostate*, Berlin, December 1978. Proceedings published by A. Rost and U. Fiedler, Berlin, 1980, p. 79.

6. Anikwe, R. M. Effect of estrogen therapy on metastatic carcinoma of the prostate. *Int. Surg. 62:* 532, 1977.

7. Aragona, C., and Friesen, H. G. Specific prolactin binding sites in the prostate and testis of rats. *Endocrinology 97:* 677, 1975.

8. Asano, M. Basic experimental studies on the pituitary prolactin-prostate interrelationships. *J. Urol. 93:* 87, 1965.

9. Baker, H. W. G., Burger, H. G., de Kretser, D. M., Hudson, B., and Straffon, W. G. Effects of synthetic oral oestrogens in normal men and patients with prostatic carcinoma: lack of gonadotrophin suppression by chlorotrianisene. *Clin. Endocrinol. 2:* 297, 1973.

10. Bard, D. R., and Lasnitzki, I. The influence of oestradiol on the metabolism of androgens by human prostatic tissue. *J. Endocrinol. 74:* 1, 1977.

11. Barnes, R. W., Bergman, R. T., Hadley, H. L., and Dick, A. L. Early prostatic cancer: long-term results with conservative treatment. *J. Urol. 102:* 88, 1969.

12. Barzell, W., Bean, M. A., Hilaris, B. S., Whitmore, W. F., Jr. Prostatic adenocarcinoma: relationship of grade and local extent to the pattern of metastases. *J. Urol. 118:* 278, 1977.

13. Belis, J., Blume, C., and Mawhinney, M. G. Androgen and estrogen binding in the male guinea pig accessory sex organs. *Endocrinology 101:* 726, 1977.

14. Bennett, A. H., Dowd, J. B., and Harrison, J. H. Estrogen and survival data in carcinoma of the prostate. *Surg. Gynecol. Obstet. 129:* 505, 1972.

15. Berry, W. R., Laszlo, J., Cox, E., Walker, A., and Paulson, D. Prognostic factors in metastatic and hormonally unresponsive carcinoma of the prostate. *Cancer 44:* 763, 1979.

16. Bhanalaph, T. Varkarakis, M. J., and Murphy, G. P.: Current status of bilateral adrenalectomy for advanced prostatic carcinoma. *Am. Surg. 179:* 17, 1974.

17. Birke, G., and Wadström, L.: Progynon™, a depot preparation with oestrogenic action in the treatment of prostate carcinoma. *Acta Chir. Scand. 130:* 388, 1965.

18. Blanchot, H., and Laporte, F.: Traitement hormonal des néoformations prostatiques. Rapport 46 e Session, AFU. Imprimerie Saints-Péres, Paris, 1952, p. 5.

19. Bouffioux, Chr. Le cancer de la prostate. *Acta Urol. Belg. 47:* 189, 1979.

20. Bouffioux, Chr. Treatment of prostatic cancer with medroxy-progesterone-acetate (MPA). In *Bladder Tumors and other Topics in Urological Oncology*, edited by M. Pavone-Macaluso, P. H. Smith, and F. Edsmyr. Plenum Publishing, New York, 1980, p. 463.

21. Bracci, U. Antiandrogens in the treatment of prostatic cancer. *Eur. Urol. 5:* 303, 1979.

22. Brendler, H., and Prout, G. A cooperative group study of prostatic cancer: stilbestrol versus placebo in advanced progressive disease. *Cancer Chemother. Rep. 16:* 323, 1962.

23. Byar, D. P. Treatment of prostatic cancer: studies by the Veterans Administration Cooperative Urological Research Group. *Bull. N.Y. Acad. Med. 48:* 751, 1972.

24. Byar, D. P. The Veterans Administration Cooperative Urological Research Group's studies of cancer of the prostate. *Cancer 32:* 1126, 1973.

25. Byar, D. P. VACURG Studies on Prostatic Cancer and its Treatment. In *Urologic Pathology: The Prostate*, edited by M. Tannenbaum. Lea & Febiger, Philadelphia, 1977, p. 241.

26. Carlton, C. E. Combined interstitial and external radiotherapy in the definitive management of carcinoma of the prostate. Presented at the II International Symposium on the Treatment of Carcinoma of the Prostate, Berlin, December 1978.

27. Corvol, P., Mahoudeau, J. A., Valcke, J. C., Menard, J., and Bricaire, H. Effets sexuels secondaires des spirolactones. Mécanismes possibles de l'action antiandrogens. *Nouv. Presse Med. 5:* 691, 1976.

28. Cosgrove, M. D., George F. W., III, and Terry, R. The effects of treatment on the local lesion of carcinoma of the prostate. *J. Urol. 109:* 861, 1973.

29. Coune, A., and Smith, P. Clinical trial of 2-bromo-α-ergocryptine (NSC-169774) in human prostatic cancer. *Cancer Chemother. Rep. 59:* 209, 1975.

30. Cramer, O. M., Parker, C. R., and Porter, J. C. Stimulation of dopamine release into hypophysial portal blood by administration of progesterone. *Endocrinology 105:* 929, 1979.

31. Del Pozo, E., Brun del Re, R., Varga, L., and Friesen, H. The inhibition of prolactin secretion in man by CB-154 (2-Br-α-ergocryptine). *J. Clin. Endocrinol. Metab. 35:* 768, 1972.

32. Del Pozo, E., and Brownell, J. Prolactin. I. Mechanism of control, peripheral actions and modification by drugs. *Horm. Res. 10:* 143, 1979.

33. Del Regato, J. A. Long-term curative results of radiotherapy of patients with inoperable prostatic carcinoma. *Radiology 131:* 291, 1979.

34. Dhom, G. Pathology and classification of prostatic carcinoma. In *Prostatic Disease. Prog. Clin. Biol. Res. 6:* 111, 1976.

35. Donald, R. A., Espiner, E. A., Cowles, R. J., and Fazackerley, J. E. The effect of cyproterone acetate on the plasma gonadotrophin response to gonadotrophin releasing hormone. *Acta Endocrinol. 81:* 680, 1976.

36. Eisen, M., Napp, H. E., and Vock, R. Inhibition of platelet aggregation caused by estrogen treatment in patients with carcinoma of the prostate. *J. Urol. 114:* 93, 1975.

37. Ekman, P., Snochowski, M., Dahlberg, E., and Gustafsson, J. A. Steroid receptors in metastatic carcinoma of the human prostate. *Eur. J. Cancer 15:* 257, 1979.

38. Emmett, J. L., Greene, L. F., and Papantoniou, A. Endocrine therapy in carcinoma of the prostate gland: 10-year survival studies. *J. Urol. 83:* 471, 1960.

39. Esposti, P. L. Cytologic malignancy grading of prostatic carcinoma by transrectal aspiration biopsy. A 5-year follow-up study of 469 hormone-treated patients. *Scand. J. Urol. Nephrol. 5:* 199, 1971.

40. Farnsworth, W. E., and Gonder, M. J. Prolactin and prostate cancer. *Urology 10:* 33, 1977.

41. Faul, P., Schmiedt, E., and Kern, R. Die prognostische Bedeutung des zytologischen Differenzierungsgrades beim östrogenbehandelten Prostata-Carcinom. *Urologe A 17:* 377, 1978.

42. Fergusson, J. D. Prostatic cancer—endocrine therapy. In *Malignant Disease,* edited by B. A. Stoll. W.B. Saunders, London, 1972, p. 237.

43. Franks, L. M. Some comments on the long-term results of endocrine treatment of prostatic cancer. *Br. J. Urol. 30:* 383, 1958.

44. Franks, C. R. Melphalan in metastatic cancer of the prostate: a pilot study. *Cancer Treat. Rep. 63:* 228, 1979.

45. Frederiksen, P., Thommesen, P., Kjyer, T. B., and Bichel, P. Flow cytometric DNA analysis in fine needle aspiration biopsies from patients with prostatic lesion. Diagnostic value and relation to clinical stages. *Acta Pathol. Microbiol. Scand.* [A] *86A:* 461 1978.

46. Fukushima, D. K., Levin, J., Kream, J., Freed, S. Z., Whitmore, W. F., Hellman, L., and Zumoff, B. Effect of flutamide on cortisol metabolism. *J. Clin. Endocrinol. Metab. 47:* 788, 1978.

47. Geller, J., Fruchtman, B., Newman, H., Roberts, T., and Silva, R. Effect of progestational agents on carcinoma of the prostate. *Cancer Chemother. Rep. 51:* 41, 1967.

48. Geller, J., Albert, J., and Yen, S. S. C. Treatment of advanced cancer of the prostate with megestrol acetate. *Urology 12:* 537, 1978.

49. Geller, J., Albert, J., De la Vega, D., Loza, D., and Stoeltzing, W. Dihydrotestosterone concentration in prostate cancer tissue as a predictor of tumor differentiation and hormonal dependency. *Cancer Res. 38:* 4349, 1978.

50. Girard, J., Baumann, J. B., Bühler, U., Zuppinger, K., Haas, H. G., Staub, J. J., and

Wyss, H. I. Cyproteronacetate and ACTH adrenal function. *J. Clin. Endocrinol. Metab. 47:* 581, 1978.

51. Göttinger, H., Schmiedt, E. Therapie des Prostatakarzinoms. *Fortschr. Med. 97:* 1881, 1979.

52. Griboff, S. I. The rationale and clinical use of steroid hormones in cancer. *Arch. Intern. Med. 89:* 635, 1952.

53. Hanash, K. A., Utz, D. C., Cook, N., Taylor, W. F., and Titus, J. L. Carcinoma of the prostate: a 15-year followup. *J. Urol. 107:* 450, 1972.

54. Harper, M. E., Fahmy, A. R., Pierrepoint, C. G., and Griffiths, K. The effect of some stilbestrol compounds on DNA polymerase from human prostatic tissues. *Steroids 15:* 89, 1970.

55. Hartung, R., and Mauermayer, W. Therapie und Nachsorge des Prostatakarzinoms. *Ther. Ggw. 118:* 162, 1979.

56. Heller, W., Harzmann, R., Bichler, K. H., and Schmidt, K. Urinary hydroxyproline in healthy patients and in prostate patients with and without bone metastases. *Curr. Probl. Clin. Biochem. 9:* 249, 1979.

57. Hellman, L., Bradlow, H. L., Freed, S., Levin, J., Rosenfield, R. S., Whitmore, W. F., and Zumoff, B. The effect of flutamide on testosterone metabolism and the plasma levels of androgens and gonadotropins. *J. Clin. Endocrinol. Metab. 45:* 1224, 1977.

58. Holland, J. M., and Grayhack, J. T. Basis of hormone treatment. In *Scientific Foundations of Urology,* edited by D. I. Williams and G. D. Chisholm. W. Heinemann, London, 1976, p. 338.

59. Horowski, R., and Wachtel, H. Direct dopaminergic action of lissuride hydrogen maleate, an ergot derivative, in mice. *Eur. J. Pharmacol. 36:* 373, 1976.

60. Houghton, A. L., Turner, R., and Cooper, E. Sex hormone binding globulin in carcinoma of the prostate. *Br. J. Urol. 49:* 227, 1977.

61. Isaacs, J. T., Isaacs, W. B., and Coffey, D. S. Models for development of non-receptor methods for distinguishing androgen-sensitive and -insensitive prostatic tumors. *Cancer Res. 39:* 2652, 1979.

62. Ishibe, T., Usui, T., and Nihira, T. Prognostic usefullness of serum acid phosphatase levels in carcinoma of the prostate. *J. Urol. 112:* 237, 1974.

63. Jacobi, G. H., Sinterhauf, K., Kurth, K. H., and Altwein, J. E. Bromocriptine and prostatic carcinoma: plasma kinetics, production and tissue uptake of ^{3}H-testosterone in vivo. *J. Urol. 119:* 240, 1978.

64. Jacobi, G. H., and Altwein, J. E. Bromocriptin als Palliativtherapie beim fortgeschrittenen Prostatakarzinom. Experimentelles und klinisches Profil eines Medikamentes. *Urol. Int. 34:* 266, 1979.

65. Jacobi, G. H., Altwein, J. E., Kurth, K. H., Basting, R., and Hohenfellner, R. Treatment of advanced prostatic cancer with parenteral cyproterone acetate: a phase III randomised trial. *Br. J. Urol. 52:* 208, 1980.

66. Jacobo, E., Schmidt, J., Weinstein, S., and Flocks, R. Comparison of flutamide (SCH-13521) and diethylstilbestrol in untreated advanced prostatic cancer. *Urology 8.* 231, 1976.

67. Jönsson, G., and Nilsson, T. Pharmacology of drug therapy. In *Scientific Foundations of Urology,* edited by D. I. Williams and G. D. Chisholm. William Heinemann Medical Books, London, 1976, p. 347.

68. Jordan, W. P., Blackard, C. E., and Byar, D. P. Reconsideration of orchiectomy in the treatment of advanced prostatic carcinoma. *South Med. J. 70:* 1411, 1977.

69. Karnofsky, D. A. Experimental cancer chemotherapy. In *Physiopathology of Cancer,* edited by C. Homburger and S. Fishman. Harper, New York, 1953, p. 783.

70. Kent, J. R., Bischoff, A. J., Arduino, L. J., Mellinger, G. T., Byar, D. P., Hill, M., and Kozbor, X. Estrogen dosage and suppression of testosterone levels in patients with prostatic carcinoma. *J. Urol. 109:* 858, 1973.

71. Kern, W. H. Well differentiated adenocarcinoma of the prostate. *Cancer 41:* 2046, 1978.

72. Kledzik, G. S., Marshall, S., Campbell, G. A., Gelato, M., and Meites, J. Effects of castration, testosterone, estradiol and prolactin on specific prolactin binding activity in ventral prostate of male rats. *Endocrinology 98:* 373, 1976.

73. Klippel, K. F., and Altwein, J. E. Palliative Therapiemöglichkeiten beim metastasierenden Hypernephrom. *Dtsch. Med. Wochenschr. 104:* 28, 1979.

74. Klosterhalfen, H., Becker, H., Lotzin, C., and Kautzky, R. Die Hypophysektomie als Behandlungsmöglichkeit beim Endstadium des Prostatakarzinoms. *Urologe A 19:* 85, 1980.

75. Kocze, A., and Szekely, J. Tamoxifen in advanced prostatic carcinoma. *Lancet 1:* 539, 1980.

76. Kontturi, M., and Sotaniemi, E. Effect of estrogen on liver function of prostatic cancer patients. *Br. Med. J. 1:* 204, 1969.

77. Kunze, U., and Orestano, F. Intra- und extrazelluläre Elektrolytkonzentration unter Östrogen-Therapie bei Prostatacarcinom-Patienten. *Urologe A 12:* 274, 1973.

78. Kvols, L., Eagan, K., and Myers, R. P. Evaluation of melphalan, ICRF-159, and hydroxyurea in metastatic prostate cancer: a preliminary report. *Cancer Treat. Rep. 61:* 311, 1977.

79. Langhammer, H., Sintermann, R., Hoer, G., and Pabst, H. W. Serial bone scintigraphy for assessing the effectiveness of treatment of osseous metastases from prostatic cancer. *Nukl. Med. (Stuttg.) 17:* 87, 1978.

80. Mackler, M. A., Liberti, J. P., Smith, M. J. V., Koontz, W. W., and Prout, G. R. The effect of orchiectomy and various doses of stilbestrol on plasma testosterone levels in patients with carcinoma of the prostate. *Invest. Urol. 9:* 423, 1972.

81. Magyar, K., Hindrof, J., and Richter, C. Prostata-Karzinom. Ein territorial epidemiologischer Beitrag. *Z. Gesamte. Hyg. 24:* 946, 1978.

82. Martz, G. Die Behandlung des Prostatacarcinoms beim Versagen der Oestrogene. *Urologe A 1:* 124, 1962.

83. McGuire, W. L., Horwitz, K. B., Pearson, O. H., and Segaloff, A. Current status of estrogen and progesterone receptors in breast cancer. *Cancer 39:* 2934, 1977.

84. Menard, R. H., Stripp, B., and Gillette, J. R. Spironolactone and testicular cytochrome p-450: decreased testosterone formation in several species and changes in hepatic drug metabolism. *Endocrinology 94:* 1628, 1974.

85. Menon, M., and Walsh, P. C. Hormonal therapy for prostatic cancer. In *Prostatic Cancer*, edited by G. P. Murphy. PSG Publishing Co., Littleton, Mass., 1979, p. 175.

86. Merrin, C. E. Treatment of previously untreated (by hormonal manipulation) stage D adenocarcinoma of prostate with combined orchiectomy, estrogen, and cis diamminodichloroplatinum. *Urology 15:* 1275, 1980.

87. Michigan, S., and Catalona, W. J. Ureteral obstruction from prostatic carcinoma: response to endocrine and radiation therapy. *J. Urol. 118:* 733, 1977.

88. Morfin, R. F., Leav, I., Chavles, J. F., Cavazis, L. F., Ofner, P., and Floch, H. H. Correlative study of the morphology and C_{19}-steroid metabolism of benign and cancerous human prostatic tissue. *Cancer 39:* 1517, 1977.

89. Müller, H.-A., Ackermann, R., and Frohmüller, H. G. W. The value of perineal punch biopsy in estimating the histological grade of carcinoma of the prostate. *Prostate 1:* 303, 1980.

90. Murphy, G. P. Current status of therapy in prostatic cancer. In *Urologic Pathology: The Prostate*, edited by M. Tannenbaum. Lea & Febiger, Philadelphia, 1977, p. 225.

91. Ochiai, K., and Takeuchi, H. Some considerations on rationale for antiandrogenic treatment of advanced prostatic carcinoma. Proceedings of the 16th Congress of the International Society of Urology, Vol. 2. Doin, Paris, 1973, p. 256.

92. Osama El-Arimi, M. Response to tamoxifen in drug-resistant prostatic carcinoma. *Lancet 2:* 588, 1979.

93. Pannuti, F., Rossi, A. P., and Piana E. Massive doses of medroxyprogesterone acetate (MPA): pilot study in the treatment of advanced prostate cancer. *IRCS Med. Sci. Libr. Compend. 5:* 375, 1977.

94. Paulson, D. F. The role of endocrine therapy in the management of prostatic cancer. In *Genitourinary Cancer*, edited by D. G. Skinner and J. B. deKernion. W.B. Saunders, Philadelphia, 1978, p. 388.

95. Pavone-Macaluso, M. Phase III studies of the EORTC: treatment of prostatic carcinoma with antihormones. Presented at the symposium *Antihormones—Current Knowledge and Prospective Clinical Relevance in Urology.* Innsbruck, Dec. 14–15, 1979.

96. Plumpton, K., and Morales, A. Levodopa in cancer of the prostate. *J. Urol. 114:* 482, 1975.

97. Pollen, J. J., and Shlaer, W. J. Osteoblastic response to successful treatment of metastatic cancer of the prostate. *Am. J. Radiol. 132:* 927, 1979.

98. Posner, B. I., Kelly, P. A., Shiu, R. P. C., and Friesen, H. G. Studies of insulin, growth hormone and prolactin binding: tissue distribution, species variation and characterization. *Endocrinology 96:* 521, 1974.

99. Prout, G. R., Irwin, R. J., Kliman, B., Daly, J. J., MacLaughlin, R. A., and Griffin, P. P. Prostatic cancer and SCH-13521: II. Histological alterations and the pituitary gonadal axis. *J. Urol. 113:* 834, 1975.

100. Rafla, S., and Johnson, R. The treatment of advanced prostatic carcinoma with medroxyprogesterone. *Curr. Ther. Res. 16:* 261, 1974.

101. Reynoso, G., and Murphy, G. P. Adrenalectomy and hypophysectomy in advanced prostatic carcinoma. *Cancer 29:* 941, 1972.

102. Robinson, M. R. G., and Thomas, B. S. Effect of hormonal therapy on plasma testosterone levels in prostate carcinoma. *Br. Med. J. 4:* 391, 1971.

103. Sadoughi, N., Razvi, M., Bush, I., Ablin, R., and Guinan, P. Cancer of the prostate, relief of bone pain with levodopa. *Urology 4:* 107, 1974.

104. Sandberg, A. A., Kirdani, R. Y., Yamanaka, H., Varkarakis, M. J., and Murphy, G. P. Potential test systems for drugs against prostatic cancer. *Cancer Chemother. Rep. 59:* 175, 1975.

105. Sander, S., Nissen-Meyer, R., and Aakvaag, A. On gestagen treatment of advanced prostatic carcinoma. *Scand. J. Urol. Nephrol. 12:* 119, 1978.

106. Sanford, E. J., Drago, J. R., Rohner, T. J., Santen, R., and Lipton, A. Aminoglutethimide medical adrenalectomy for advanced prostatic carcinoma. *J. Urol. 115:* 170, 1976.

107. Sanford, E. J., Paulson, D. F., Rohner, T. J., Santen, R. J., and Bardin, C. W. The effects of castration on adrenal testosterone secretion in men with prostatic carcinoma. *J. Urol. 118:* 1019, 1977.

108. Santen, R. J., Cohn, N., Misbin, R., Samojlik, E., and Foltz, E. Acute effects of aminoglutethimide on testicular steroidogenesis in normal men. *J. Clin. Endocrinol. Metab. 49:* 631, 1979.

109. Schirmer, H. K. A., Murphy, G. P., and Scott, W. W. Hormonal therapy of prostatic cancer—a correlation between Broders' classification (and staging) and clinical course. *Urol. Digest 3:* 15, 1965.

110. Sciarra, F., Sorcini, G., Di Silverio, F., and Gagliardi, V. Biosintesi in vitro degli androgeni nel testicolo di soggetti con cancro della prostata, trattati con estrogeni e ciproterone acetato. *Folia Endocrinol. (Roma) 23:* 264, 1970.

111. Sciarra, F., Sorcini, G., Di Silverio, F., and Gagliardi, V. Plasma testosterone and androstenedione after orchiectomy in prostatic adenocarcinoma. *Clin. Endocrinol. 2:* 102, 1973.

112. Seal, U. S., Doe, R. P., Byar, D. P., Corle, D. K., and VACURG. Response of serum cholesterol and triglycerides to hormone treatment and the relation of pretreatment values to mortality in patients with prostatic cancer. *Cancer 38:* 1095, 1976.

113. Seal, U. S., Doe, R. P., Byar, D. P., Corle, D. K., and VACURG. Response of plasma fibrinogen and plasminogen to hormone treatment and the relation of pretreatment values to mortality in patients with prostatic cancer. *Cancer 38:* 1108, 1976.

114. Shearer, R. T., Hendry, W. F., Sommerville, I. F., and Fergusson, J. D. Plasma testosterone: an accurate monitor of hormone treatment in prostatic cancer. *Br. J. Urol. 45:* 668, 1973.

115. Shimazaki, J., Jurihara, H., Ito, K., and Shida, K. Testosterone metabolism in prostate; formation of androstane-17-β-ol-3-one and natural and synthetic estrogens. *Gumna J. Med. Sci. 14:* 313, 1965.

117. Sinha, Y. N., Salocks, C. B., and Vanderlaan, W. P. A comparison of the effects of CB-154 and lergotrile mesylate on prolactin and growth hormone secretion in mice. *Horm. Metab. Res. 8:* 332, 1976.

118. Sinha, A. A., Blackard, C. E., and Seal, U. S. A critical analysis of tumor morphology and hormone treatments in the untreated and estrogen-treated responsive and refractory human prostatic carcinoma. *Cancer 40:* 2836, 1977.

119. Smith, P. H., Akdas, A., Mason, M. K., Richards, B., Robinson, M. R. G., De Pauw, M., and Sylvester, R. Hormone therapy in prostatic cancer. *Acta Urol. Belg. 48:* 98, 1980.
120. Sogani, P. C., and Whitmore, W. F. Experience with flutamide in previously untreated patients with advanced prostatic cancer. *J. Urol. 122:* 640, 1979.
121. Stripp, B., Taylor, A. A., and Bartter, F. C. Effect of spironolactone on sex hormones in man. *J. Clin. Endocrinol. Metab. 41:* 777, 1975.
122. Strohm, J. G. Carcinoma of the prostate. *Urol. Cutan. Rev. 45:* 770, 1941.
123. Tavares, A. S., Costa, J., and Maria, J. C. Correlation between ploidy and prognosis in prostatic carcinoma. *J. Urol. 109:* 676, 1973.
124. De Vere White, R., Paulson, D. F., and Glenn, J. D. The clinical spectrum of prostatic cancer. *J. Urol. 117:* 323, 1977.
125. Vermeulen, A., and Verdonck, L. Studies of the binding of the testosterone to human plasma. *Steroids 11:* 609, 1968.
126. deVoogt, H. J. Receptors in prostatic cancer. Presented at the 3rd Congress of the European Association of Urology, Monte Carlo, June 14–18, 1978.
127. Walsh, P. C., and Korenman, S. G. Mechanism of androgenic action effect of specific intracellular inhibitor. *J. Urol. 105:* 850, 1971.
128. Walsh, P. C. Physiologic basis for hormonal therapy in carcinoma of the prostate. *Urol. Clin. North. Am. 2:* 125, 1975.
129. Walsh, P. C., and Siiteri, P. K. Suppression of plasma androgens by spironolactone in castrated men with carcinoma of the prostate. *J. Urol. 114:* 254, 1975.
130. Walsh, P. C., Greco, J. M., Tananis, C. E., Hicks, L. L., McLoughlin, M. G., and Menon, M. The binding of a potent synthetic androgen—Methyltrienolone (R 1881)— to cytosol preparations of human prostatic cancer. *Trans. Am. Assoc. Genitourin. Surg. 69:* 78, 1977.
131. Welvaart, K., Merrin, C. E., and Mittelman, A. Stage D prostatic carcinoma. Survival rate in relapsed patients following new forms of palliation. *Urology 4:* 283, 1974.
132. Yanaihara, T., and Troen, P. Studies of the human testis. III. Effect of estrogen on testosterone formation in human testis in vitro. *J. Clin. Endocrinol. Metab. 34:* 968, 1972.
133. Zumoff, B., Fishman, J., Freed, S., Levin, J., Whitmore, W. F., Hellman, L., and Fukushima, D. K. Effect of flutamide on estradiol metabolism. *J. Clin. Endocrinol. Metab. 49:* 467, 1979.
134. Neumann, F., and Jacobi, G. H. Tumour treatment with antiandrogens. *Clinics in Endocrinol.*, Vol. 1, 1982.

Editorial Comment to Chapter 11

The following completely new approach to the conventional strategy of androgen withdrawal for prostatic carcinoma palliation is currently being investigated in our institution.

The gonadotropin-releasing hormone (Gn-RH), a hypothalamic decapeptide, releases both LH and FSH from the pituitary. A variety of nonapeptides have been synthesized, which exert agonistic effects comparable to the native Gn-RH. Some of these so-called gonadotropin-releasing hormone analogues (Gn-RH$_A$) require much lower doses and have a prolonged duration of action as compared to the native Gn-RH, and were initially used therapeutically with "pro-fertility" intention.

Chronic administration in supraphysiological doses, however, contributes to a paradoxical effect: Due to pituitary overstimulation, depletion of the releasable LH pool occurs with subsequent down-regulation of Gn-RH receptors and desensitization and refractoriness of the pituitary. This continuous LH depletion, which is reversible after discontinuation of Gn-RH$_A$ administration, results in a profound impairment of testicular function, steroidogenic arrest, and castrate levels of peripheral testosterone (Jacobi and Wenderoth, 1982).

We have acquired this side effect as a therapeutical approach, and were able to demonstrate with high-dose Gn-RH$_A$ treatment (*Buserelin; Hoe 766*) subjective and objective responses of metastatic prostatic carcinoma identical with those seen after orchiectomy. Within 2 to 3 weeks of Gn-RH$_A$ treatment serum testosterone is suppressed to castrate levels (Table 11.9). If long-term results confirm our up to now 6-month data, Gn-RH analogues would thus be a safe, effective, and nontoxic form of medical castration. They could gain importance to replace estrogens, to serve as reversible measure in adjunct to nonendocrine treatment strategies, and, since completely reversible, as a tool to proof the hormone dependence of a given prostate cancer initially.

Reference

Jacobi, G. H., and Wenderoth, U. K. Gonadotropin-releasing hormone analogues for prostate cancer: untoward side effects of high-dose regimens acquire a therapeutical dimension. *Eur. Urol. 8:* 129, 1982

U. K. W.
G. H. J.

Table 11.9
Serum Testosterone of Six Patients with Newly Diagnosed Metastatic Prostatic Carcinoma Initially Treated with the Gonadotropin-Releasing Hormone Analogue *Buserelin* (Hoe 766)[a]

Testosterone[b,c] (ng/ml)	Time of Treatment (days)[d]									
	0	2	4	6	8	10	12	14	28	56
Mean[e]	5.2	5.7	7.2	5.9	4.2	2.6	1.4	1.0	0.3	0.2
S.E.M.	1.0	0.8	0.9	0.7	0.5	0.3	0.1	0.1	0.1	0.0

[a] Investigational compound from *Hoechst A. G.*, Frankfurt, FRG.
[b] Determined by radioimmunoassay.
[c] Based on four serum samples per patient per time interval.
[d] Two times 200 µg/day s.c. for 14 days, and 3 × 400 µg/day via the pernasal route thereafter.
[e] Mean value of 24 individual figures.

12

Has Transurethral Resection a Place in Prostate Cancer Management?

K. Bandhauer, M.D.

"Yes—but. . . . " This is the abbreviated answer to the question posed in the title. Our intent here is to substantiate both the "yes" *and* the "but" responses.

Clinically, prostatic carcinoma is distinguished by several factors which deserve particular attention in the evaluation of transurethral resection (TUR):

1. A histologically or cytologically confirmed early diagnosis of prostatic cancer enables planning of a relatively specific stage- and grade-dependent therapy with a chance of cure.
2. Histological and cytological follow-up studies evaluate the local effect of therapy and may indicate the need for changes in therapy planning and strategy.
3. Infravesical obstruction at the bladder outlet due to prostatic carcinoma can negatively influence the course of tumor disease independent of the grade of malignancy. This may lead to micturition disturbances, with the resulting consequences for bladder, upper urinary tract, and the entire organism, possibly even achieving the status of a secondary disease.
4. Metastatic spread in prostatic carcinoma can occur extremely rapidly, sometimes even like an "explosion."

These factors raise the following questions in regard to the value of TUR in the management of prostatic carcinoma:

1. Does TUR offer the possibility of early diagnosis of prostatic carcinoma?

2. Can TUR be used for follow-up control of different forms of therapy?
3. Can TUR be employed as a radical therapeutical measure in prostatic carcinoma?
4. Is TUR a suitable measure for elimination of obstruction?
5. Can a change in the course of disease be expected by TUR?

VALUE OF TUR FOR THE DIAGNOSIS OF PROSTATIC CARCINOMA

Early Diagnosis

If we define "early diagnosis" as detection at Stage T_1 and T_2, and consider the fact that more than 80% of "early" prostatic carcinoma occur in the peripheral zones of the gland, then the transurethral "biopsy" is of no importance when compared to the perineal or transrectal biopsy taken from the peripheral zones of the gland and hence directly from the tumor. Improvements in the various perineal and transrectal biopsy modalities, in particular the increasing efficiency of cytological diagnostic methods after aspiration biopsy with the Franzén-needle, have to a large degree superseded transurethral biopsy.

The mostly highly differentiated microcarcinoma within the surgical specimen of benign prostatic hyperplasia (BPH) (incidental carcinoma/ T_0, according to UICC) can be discovered by TUR although it is usually impalpable by rectal examination. Nevertheless, this is usually of little importance for the therapeutic planning of prostatic carcinoma, as the pathological value of this defined, incidentally discovered, and usually clinically irrelevant carcinoma is so minimal that, as a rule, no consequences for therapy planning can be drawn from their diagnosis aside from strict follow-up controls (see Chapter 6).

Follow-up Diagnosis

Histological confirmation of a clinically advanced prostatic carcinoma, which has already penetrated the periurethral zones of the glands, can be done by primary transurethral biopsy if a radical operation is no longer possible and, at the same time, obstructive symptoms of micturition suggest a transurethral resection. Both procedures can be done at the same time.[6] The operation with these intents includes diagnosis *and* treatment.

The technique of "tissue separation" of TUR-material described by O'Donoghue and Pugh[11] also plays an insignificant role in the primary diagnosis of "early" prostatic carcinoma. The authors determined that the method is only able to detect locally extensive tumors, and that within the framework of their pilot study, it was not possible to improve the detection of unsuspected tumors. The question of whether histological studies of specimens taken from different zones of the prostate would actually improve stage and grade classification of the carcinoma is still unanswered at present.

TUR IN THERAPY PLANNING OF PROSTATIC CARCINOMA

The therapeutic value of transurethral resection in cases of prostatic carcinoma lies *solely* in the elimination of bladder outlet obstruction. The so-called "radical transurethral prostatectomy" described by Arnholdt[2] and Sachse[14] in Germany, cannot be considered radical when viewed anatomically and technically. Jewett[8] has pointed out the relatively frequent occurrence of microscopic invasion of the seminal vesicles and of perivascular tumor spread through the capsule in apparently clinically localized prostatic carcinoma (stage T_2) and traces the failure of radical prostatovesiculectomy to this factor. Apart from this clinically undetectable tumor spread, the transurethral resection cannot be compared to the "open" prostatovesiculectomy as a radical procedure when the technical maneuvers are taken into account. It is technically not possible to completely remove the entire prostate gland without conflicting with the rectum and prostatic plexus. In addition, no statistical data on the late results of the so-called "radical transurethral prostatectomy" have been published which could be effectively evaluated. The TUR is therefore not suitable for radical treatment of prostatic carcinoma.

The TUR is additionally of little importance as a measure to reduce the local tumor mass (debulking). While reduction of the primary tumor is of value in carcinoma of other organs, in which a therapeutic effect can be achieved by cytotoxic drugs, the prostatic carcinoma cannot be included in this group at present. The results of cytotoxic therapy are still rather modest despite the use of different combinations (see Chapter 16), so that the attempt to reduce the tumor mass surgically cannot be considered a true indication for TUR.

In contrast, transurethral resection of a prostatic carcinoma to remove obstructing tumor parts in patients with urinary retention is a recognized and valuable form of therapy. In many cases it may be the only way to remove bladder outlet obstruction, despite the fact that it is possible to reduce an infravesical obstruction with long-term hormone treatment[5] or high-voltage radiotherapy in certain cases. TUR can also be considered the treatment of choice for superficial tumors of the prostatic urethra in the rare cases of transitional cell carcinoma of the prostate (primary urothelial origin or intraductal development from prostatic urethra), which is known to grow relatively rapidly.[15]

The technical problems of TUR in obstructing prostatic carcinoma are not significantly different from those of resection of benign prostatic hyperplasia. In most cases, however, it is not possible to determine the edge of the resection by recognition of the capsule fibers. Another difference is the pronounced danger of hemorrhage in carcinoma because of increased fibrinolysis. Furthermore, there is a greater danger of postoperative incontinence due to infiltration of sphincter zone of the urethra and subsequent rigidity of the proximal urethra.

In our own prostate cancer material of 270 TURs, postoperative stress incontinence traceable to a too generous resection of the distal tumor was observed in 0.5%. Transurethral removal of these tumor portions in infiltrating prostatic carcinoma should be done with great care. True hyperfibrinolytic bleeding was only observed in one of our cases.

The question of deciding whether TUR is indicated is problematic, in particular the setting of the time of operation. In terms of indication for TUR, all the possible risks must be taken into consideration. Less important are the usually calculable operative risks; considerably more important are the possible dangers associated with primary tumor manipulation, *i.e.* possible propagation of tumor spread in terms of local progression and distant metastases. Although it is extremely difficult to provide evidence for this, and a large number of urologists believe there is no significant change in the course of prostatic cancer disease after TUR, there are nevertheless several experimental and clinical indications for possible tumor seeding, or influence of TUR on the course of tumor disease.[3, 4] As early as 1956, Marberger and co-workers[10] pointed out a significant rise in serum acid phosphatase after rectal prostate palpation. These signs of a traumatically caused passage of the enzyme into the circulatory system after TUR could be confirmed immunologically in experiments by proof of prostate antigens. These observations permit discussion of the only apparently "simple" concept of passage of malignant cell groups into the blood stream during resection when large veins are opened. Although to our knowledge no exact studies of cellular spread during TUR have been done, Gittes and McCullough[7] have pointed out the theoretical possibilities of cell seeding in prostatic carcinoma. Immunologically seen, tumor cells disseminated into the veins must be considered antigenic substances which trigger an antigen-antibody reaction, providing the immune system is intact. Under favorable conditions, *i.e.* if the defense function is sufficient, metastases formation is prevented by the protective antigen-antibody reaction, as stated by Gittes and McCullough.[7] If there is a temporary or long-standing disturbance of the defense system, this immunological barrier can be broken and metastases may occur.

In this connection, the interesting observations of Alsheik and co-workers[1] must be mentioned. On the basis of the lymphocyte transformation rate, this clinical study showed a statistically significant depression of the cellular immune response after transurethral resection of prostatic cancer. The cause of this impaired immune response is unconfirmed but corresponds to similar results observed in other surgical interventions reported by Riddle and Berenbaum[12] as well as Roth and co-workers.[13] A possible cause of the reduced cellular immune response after TUR discussed by Alsheik *et al.*[1] is a dilution hyponatremia resulting in damage to the small lymphocytes. These authors concluded—from their experience with 34 patients who died of prostatic carcinoma between 1972 and 1974 (31 deaths after TUR)—that TUR has a negative effect on the course of prostate cancer. Küss and Khoury,[9] from France, question the clinical value of this study, without, however, providing very substantial arguments against Alsheik's results, other than clinical observations.

OWN INVESTIGATIONS AND RESULTS

A retrospective study of the clinical course of 310 patients who had not undergone radical prostatectomy and who did not have any primarily established metastases, gave some indications of the possible influence of TUR on the development of disseminated cancer disease. Regardless of the mode of therapy used (estrogen treatment and/or orchiectomy—high voltage radiotherapy—or a combination of both), it was seen that of those patients requiring a TUR because of obstruction, 47% developed metastases within the first 2 years after the primary diagnosis and TUR, while in the group without TUR the rate of metastases formation within the first 2 years was 28.4% (Table 12.1). This difference in clinical course, despite the different distribution patterns of the primary histological or cytological grading in the two patient groups, is certainly noteworthy. However, in the patient group with TUR, there was primarily a clear majority of poorly differentiated and undifferentiated carcinoma, while in the patient group without obstructive symptoms a greater number of highly differentiated carcinoma were encountered.

The possible relationship indicated here between TUR and metastases formation or a more rapid progression of the cancer process—as tenuous as the relationship may be—should at least be considered when contemplating TUR for prostate cancer. A TUR should not be performed for every prostatic carcinoma with moderate obstructive micturition com-

Table 12.1
Appearance of Distant Metastases (M_1) Two Years after TUR of Initially Localized Prostate Cancer ($T_{2+3}N_XM_0$); Nonrandomized Control Group without TUR for Comparison

	Initial Stage N_XM_0 (UICC, 1978)	No.	Grading (UICC, 1978)	No.	M_1 after 2 yr No.	Total (%)
Treated by TUR	T_2	47	I	14	3	
(n = 215)			II	21	10	
			III	12	7	
	T_3	168	I	4	3	
			II	93	35	
			III	71	43	
						101/215 (46.9)
Treated without	T_2	42	I	12	2	
TUR (n = 95)			II	13	4	
			III	17	4	
	T_3	53	I	11	3	
			II	22	8	
			III	20	6	
						27/95 (28.4)

plaints, as regression of the local tumor and reduction of the obstructive symptoms can be achieved by hormone therapy or local radiotherapy.

CONCLUSIONS

The introductory question "Has TUR a place in prostate cancer management?" can be answered as follows:

1. As a diagnostic measure, TUR has no significance, either for the primary diagnosis or for follow-up controls.
2. For therapy planning, TUR cannot be considered a radical operative measure. One exception is the highly differentiated microcarcinoma found in the surgical specimen after TUR for BPH, a situation which does not require further treatment in cases of unifocal, highly differentiated lesions.
3. In unequivocal cases of infravesical obstruction due to prostatic carcinoma with urinary retention and the corresponding symptoms and dilatation of the upper tract, TUR should be the method of choice for elimination of obstruction. Its use is clearly justified in this situation.
4. *However*, as it is not possible to exclude negative influences of TUR on cancer disease with absolute certainty, whether this be due to reduction of the immune response or due to enhanced tumor dissemination, or a combination of both, the decision for TUR deserves careful thought, including the consideration of alternative measures for elimination of obstruction, such as high-voltage radiotherapy or contrasexual measures.
5. For aimed tumor reduction alone, the use of TUR in prostatic carcinoma is out of the question.

REFERENCES

1. Alsheik, H. I., Guinan, P. D., Ablin, R. J., Nourkayhan, S. H., Bruns, R. G., Sadoughi, N., and Bush, I. M. The effect of transurethral resection of the prostate on lymphocyte response in patients with prostatic cancer. *J. Urol. 118:* 1022, 1977.
2. Arnholdt, F. Radikale, transurethrale Elektroresektion des Prostatakarzinoms. *Urol. Int. 28:* 50, 1973.
3. Bandhauer, K. The possible role of transurethral resection in the dissemination of prostatic cancer. *Eur. Urol. 1:* 272, 1975.
4. Bandhauer, K. Immunreaktionen bei Fertilitätsstörungen des Mannes. *Urol. Int. 21:* 247, 1966.
5. Barnes, R. W., Bergman, R. T., Hadley, H. L., and Dick, A. L. Early prostatic cancer: long term results with conservative treatment. *J. Urol. 102:* 88, 1969.
6. Bissada, N. K. Accuracy of transurethral resection of the prostata versus transrectal needle biopsy in the diagnosis of prostatic carcinoma. *J. Urol. 118:* 61, 1977.
7. Gittes, R. F., and McCullough, D. L. Occult carcinoma of the prostate. An Oversight of immune surveillance—a working hypothesis. *J. Urol. 112:* 241, 1974.
8. Jewett, H. J. Radical perineal prostatectomy for prostatic cancer. In *Prostatic Disease.* Progress in Clinical and Biological Research, Vol. 6, edited by H. Marberger, H. Hascheck, H. K. A. Schirmer, J. A. C. Colston, and E. Witkin. Alan R. Liss, New York, 1976, pp. 205–218.
9. Küss, R., and Khoury, S. Letter to the Editor. *J. Urol. 120:* 388, 1978.

10. Marberger, H., Segal, S. J., and Flocks, R. H. Changes in serum acid phosphatase level consequent to prostatic manipulation or surgery. *J. Urol. 78:* 287, 1957.
11. O'Donoghue, E. P. N., and Pugh, R. C. B. Early diagnosis of prostatic carcinoma: the role of transurethral resection. *Br. J. Urol. 49:* 705, 1977.
12. Riddle, P. R., and Berenbaum, M. C. Postoperative depression of the lymphocyte response to phytohaemagglutinine. *Lancet 1:* 746, 1967.
13. Roth, J. A., Golub, S. H., Grimm, E. A., Eilber, F. R., and Morton, D. L. Effect of surgery on in vitro lymphocyte function. *Surg. Forum 25:* 102, 1974.
14. Sachse, H. Die radikale Prostataresektion beim Prostatakarzinom. *Therapiewoche 26:* 4208, 1976.
15. Shenasky, J. H., and Gillenwater, J. Y. Management of transitional cell carcinoma of the prostate. *J. Urol. 108:* 462, 1972.

Editorial Comment to Chapter 12

The "*yes—but. . . .* " sentence with which Professor Bandhauer begins his chapter reflects the well-aimed criticism of this authority in the field. He quips that *radical* transurethral resection does not exist, and the value of his contribution lies in the fact that he does not discredit a surgical procedure which is applied to an indication for which it was not originally designed.

R. H.
G. H. J.

13

Estramustine Phosphate (Estracyt): Experimental Studies and Clinical Experience

F. Edsmyr, M.D.
L. Andersson, M.D.
I. Könyves, M.D., Ph.D.

INTRODUCTION

In cancer chemotherapy it is desired to use, if possible, drugs displaying their action mainly in the tumor tissue. One possibility to enhance selectivity is to use agents possessing latent activity. The selective effect of such agents depends on higher levels of drug-activating enzymes in tumor cells as compared to normal tissues.[1]

The binding of cytostatic agents to cell-specific carriers is one of the possibilities to reach selectivity. The carrier can recognize the target cells and allow the drug to act either on the surface or intracellularly after uptake of the carrier drug complex. The drug, when bound to the carrier, will not only be less toxic, but also more active, if its rate of penetration and intracellular concentration is higher than if the active compound was given alone.[2]

In order to improve the selectivity of agents with antitumor properties various cytostatic agents have been linked to steroid hormones as carriers.[3] It was anticipated to reach higher drug concentration in the target organ through interaction of the hormone receptors. After hydrolysis of the hormone-cytostatic drug complex the cytostatic compound can be released from the carrier in an active form, and both the hormone moiety and the alkylating moiety can exert their effect independently. In addition, the hypothesis behind these syntheses was that the passage of the cytostatic agents across the cell membranes might be facilitated by the more lipophilic character of these hormone-linked drugs.

One possible way of creating a hormone-linked alkylating agents is to attach alkylating agents in the form of a carbamate to various steroid hormones. In this type of compound the alkylating part can be located in various positions on the steroid skeleton.[3] One of the compounds synthesized in this series is estramustine, where the *nor-nitrogen mustard* is connected in the form of a carbamate to *estradiol* in the 3-position. Estramustine phosphate, a water-soluble derivative of estramustine, was achieved through esterification of the 17β-hydroxyl group with phosphoric acid.[3] Estramustine phosphate is used as a meglumine salt for intravenous administration and as a sodium salt for oral treatment (Fig. 13.1).

EXPERIMENTAL STUDIES

In those experimental transplantable tumors, generally used in the screening of alkylating agents, the drug displayed weak cytostatic activity.[4] Estramustine inhibited the growth of dimethylbenzanthrocene (DMBA)-induced mammary tumors in the rat, which were refractory to estradiol.[5] In mice bearing levulose sarcoma, estramustine phosphate had a cytostatic effect similar to that of cyclophosphamide, in contrast to estradiol phosphate which had no influence on the growth of this tumor.[6] There was reported a higher inhibitory effect on the growth of transplantable R-3327 prostatic cancer in rats by this drug than by diethylstilbestrol, which is a compound with much stronger estrogenic properties.[7, 8]

Estramustine phosphate has an estrogenic effect about 100 times weaker than that of estradiol, as demonstrated by the uterotropic effect in juvenile mice.[9] The drug also antagonizes the uterotropic effect of estrone in juvenile mice, indicating an antiestrogenic effect.[10] Estramustine phosphate decreases the 5α-reductase activity of the prostate in several species[11] and is able to reduce the incorporation of thymidine into DNA of the rat prostate *in vitro*.[12]

Distribution studies showed that the uptake of radioactivity in the rat prostate was about 10 times higher after administration of ^{3}H-estramustine than after ^{3}H-estradiol or ^{3}H-estradiol-17β-phosphate.[13] Most of the radioactivity was found to be the dephosphorylated compound, estramustine, and its 17-dehydrogenated analogue,[14] showing that the steroid-carbamate complex was intact at the uptake into the prostate.

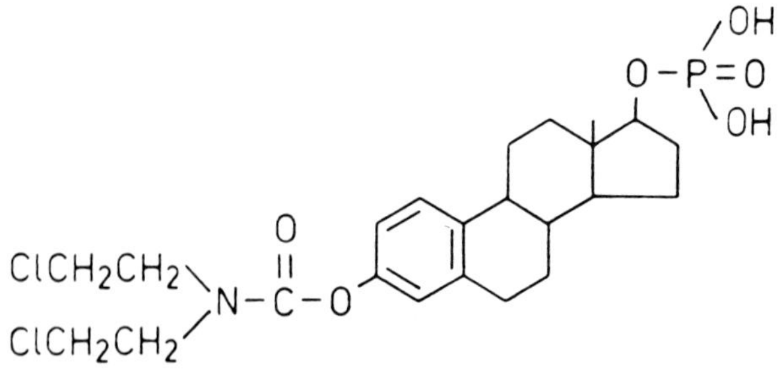

Figure 13.1 The structural formula of estramustine phosphate.

Also in man estramustine phosphate is readily dephosphorylated to estramustine, which is then oxidized to the estrone analogue.[15, 16] When estramustine phosphate was given orally in therapeutic doses over a long time, the estrone analogue was the major metabolite found in plasma with considerably lesser amounts of estramustine itself.[16] Highly elevated levels of estradiol and especially estrone were also found in plasma as a consequence of the carbamate hydrolysis. *In vitro* studies have demonstrated that this hydrolysis occurs in several human tissues including normal and cancerous prostate.[17]

Recent investigations have demonstrated that the cytosol fraction of the rat ventral prostate contains a protein of a molecular weight of approximately 50,000 which seems to be responsible for the concentration of estramustine in that organ. *In vitro* studies demonstrated that the estramustine was bound to this protein to a much higher extent than was estradiol or dihydrotestosterone.[18] This protein was found in a large amount in the rat ventral prostate and in a lower amount in other androgen-sensitive tissues. Preliminary results have indicated that a macromolecule similar to the "estramustine binding" protein is present also in the human prostate.[19]

ESTRAMUSTINE PHOSPHATE IN HORMONE REFRACTORY PROSTATIC CARCINOMA

The efficacy of Estracyt in the treatment of patients with metastatic prostate carcinoma, who were or had become unresponsive to conventional hormone treatment, was evaluated in many phase II trials during the last 10 years. In general, patients entering these trials were in progression of their disease after conventional estrogenic therapy for various periods.

The intravenous dosage used as a rule has been 300 to 600 mg/day for 2 to 3 weeks. If the patient improved, the treatment continued with the same dose once or twice weekly for about 2 months. After this initial treatment period the patients received injections once or twice weekly for periods of 4 to 8 weeks followed by treatment-free intervals of various length. Oral Estracyt is now the most common mode of therapy in our country (Sweden) and is given in a total daily dosage of 560 to 840 mg, divided into two doses. Normally the given dosage in the United States is higher.

As with all kinds of deep tissue tumors the evaluation of therapeutic response is hampered by the lack of exact measurement techniques. Criteria of tumor remission have been stated by many authors, *e.g.* the *National Prostatic Cancer Project* (NPCP) in the United States, the European Organization for Research on Treatment of Cancer (EORTC), and the WHO (see Chapters 3, 11, and 16). Objective signs of remission have been the reduction of the local tumor by at least 50%, as evaluated on rectal palpation, and disappearance or reduction of metastases. Bone scanning in correlation with skeletal x-ray, if necessary, is a sensitive technique to detect skeletal lesions but less useful to indicate tumor regression. Calcification of lytic lesions is not necessarily a healing process, as demonstrated by autopsies that revealed neoplastic tissue in these calcified lesions and because most metastases are primarily osteoplastic.[20] Reduction of ureteric obstruction is an objective criterion, indicating reduction of deep soft tissue dissemination. Reduction to normal of elevated serum acid phosphatase activity is an indirect measurement reflecting retardation of the neoplastic process. In recent years cytomorphologic and cytophotometric studies of the primary tumor have proved reliable techniques to study the disease. Up to now they have not been used in most trials. Subjective signs were disappearance or marked reduction of pain, significant improvement of the general condition, and reduction of urgency and dysuria. If only subjective criteria are monitored the evaluation is uncertain.

In the majority of publications on record the objective and subjective criteria of remission were those stated by the U.S. National Prostatic Cancer Project. In other reports there was no satisfactory description of the criteria of response. In Table 13.1 are presented a number of publications where the criteria of remission were specified. Some trials that included a relatively small number of patients have been omitted. These studies were phase II trials. The patients had a histologically or cytologically confirmed progressive, estrogen-treated, prostatic carcinoma prior to Estracyt treatment. The cytological grading has not been specified in most cases. All publications except for two, Leistenschneider and Nagel[27] and Edsmyr et al.,[22] had patients belonging to grades I, II, and III. These two series[22, 27] contain only poorly differentiated prostatic carcinomas. In most trials there were no histologic or cytologic evaluation of the prostate after the Estracyt treatment.

The variation among the different selected publications according to objective and subjective responses is notable (Table 13.2). In four publications, only pain was included in subjective response. In another five both pain, dysuria, and performance status were included. Benson et al.[30] reported on Estracyt treatment in 217 cases of disseminated carcinoma,

Table 13.1
Compilation of Adequately Documented Data on Estracyt Response

Author	Patients	Response	
		Objective	Subjective
Chisholm et al.[21]	29	8/29	10/29
Edsmyr et al.[22]	64	31/64	30/48
Jönsson et al.[23]	91	28/91	24/91
Küss et al.[24]	15	3/15	1/4
Mayer[25]	25	8/12	12/20
Mittelman et al.[26]	32	7/32	14/32
Leistenschneider and Nagel[27]	57	8/23	10/23
Nillius and Könyves[28]	20	9/16	11/20
Szendröi et al.[29]	50	22/50	32/50
Total	383	124/332 (37%)	144/317 (45%)

Table 13.2
Response to Estracyt[a]

Author	Response	
	Subjective (%)	Objective (%)[b]
Chisholm et al.[21]	34 (pain)	28
Edsmyr et al.[22]	63 (pain)	48
Jönsson et al.[23]	26	31
Küss et al.[24]	25	20
Mayer[25]	60 (pain)	67 (acid phos.)
Mittelman et al.[26]	44	22
Leistenschneider and Nagel[27]	43	35
Nillius and Könyves[28]	55 (pain)	56 (acid phos.)
Szendröi et al.[29]	53	44 (palp.)

[a] For details, see text.
[b] Abbreviations used are: acid phos., acid phosphatase; palp., palpation.

refractory to standard hormone therapy. Partial objective regression was observed in 9% and stable disease in 39%, with a median response duration of 35 weeks.

The following conclusions can be drawn from these publications: Estracyt had a beneficial effect in more than one third of the cases of estrogen refractory carcinoma of advanced stage. Soft tissue metastases seemed to respond best of all metastases, and supraclavicular conglomerates of lymph nodes regressed completely within a short period of treatment. Very few patients with skeletal metastases could be observed with definite regression. The metastases either remained unchanged or deteriorated. The most common objective response was reduction of an elevated phosphatase activity. Encouraging results were noted with respect to subjective parameters, such as pain relief and improved general condition. Nearly half the number of patients definitely improved, and there was relief in the symptoms caused by metastases (Table 13.3).

In the Stockholm area Estracyt treatment was given to 64 cases of poorly differentiated prostatic carcinoma, all of them in a progressive state during estrogen therapy. All had disseminated disease with metastases and/or elevated acid phosphatase activity. The tumors were diagnosed by fine needle aspiration biopsy, skeletal x-ray and/or scintigraphy, and serum acid phosphatase determination. All patients received Estracyt orally in a dose of 560 to 840 mg daily. The treatment used before the initiation of Estracyt was estrogens in 25 patients and estrogens plus local radiotherapy in 39 patients, where radiotherapy was given in a tumor dose of 5,400 rads in 6 weeks.

The results of the treatment outlined above were evaluated on the basis of the following criteria: Primary tumor (cytology and palpation), laboratory findings of serum acid phosphatase, possible changes in skeletal and lymph node metastases, and the subjective parameter of pain. In this series the local tumor was confirmed by fine needle aspiration biopsy before and during Estracyt therapy. The influence of Estracyt on pain was the only subjective criterion.

Forty-eight patients had pain due to skeletal lesions prior to the Estracyt therapy. In 30 patients the pain disappeared completely and in 16 the pain was unchanged or in progression (Table 13.3). The duration of the effect was on the average 11 months. No evaluation was possible in two patients, who died shortly after initiation of treatment.

In 27 patients there was a palpable pelvic mass prior to therapy and in eight of these there was a significant tumor reduction (Table 13.4). In 39 patients fine needle aspiration biopsy proved malignant cells in the prostate gland before initiation of Estracyt therapy. In 12 of these patients no cancer cells were detected by the same technique during the therapy and over an average period of 21 months.

At the start of therapy eight patients had supraclavicular lymph node metastases. In five of these the supraclavicular mass disappeared; in three it was not affected. There were only three patients of 42 with distant skeletal metastases in which definite regression could be observed. In all the other patients the metastases either remained unchanged or increased.

In 34 patients an elevated serum acid phosphatase activity was noticed before the Estracyt therapy. In 10 of these 34 patients the treatment with Estracyt caused a decrease to normal values. The duration of remission was around 10 months. Seven still had a slight elevation of their acid phosphatase. In four other patients the acid phosphatase level was unchanged and high, and in eight there was a further increase of the values. In five patients there were no evaluations performed because of the short survival time.

Summarizing the results of treatment, pain relief occurred in 63% of the patients, with an average duration of 11 months, and some objective signs of tumor remission were observed in 48%, with an average duration of 12 months.

Table 13.3
Subjective Response[a]

Prior to Estracyt	During Estracyt[b]		
	No Pain	Unchanged or Progression	Not Evaluable
48	30	16	2

[a] Before treatment all patients suffered from metastatic bone pain.
[b] Response interval average 11 months.

Table 13.4
Objective Signs of Remission

	Prior to Estracyt	During Estracyt
Local tumor	27	8
Cytology	39	12
Supraclavicular mass	8	5
Skeletal metastases	42	3
Acid phosphatase	34	10

[a] For details see text.

ESTRAMUSTINE PHOSPHATE IN THE PRIMARY TREATMENT OF PROSTATIC CARCINOMA

It appears that Estracyt has an antitumor effect in addition to its estrogenic property. The question arises whether Estracyt given from the beginning of therapy on will produce tumor remission in a higher frequency and of longer duration, or a longer survival, than conventional estrogenic regimens.

In a pilot study[31] and a subsequent publication,[23] Jönsson, Högberg, and Nilsson reported on 63 patients, all in stage IV according to the Veterans Administration Cooperative Urological Research Group (VACURG) classification system, who were given intravenous and/or oral Estracyt as the initial form of therapy. In 21 cases the tumor was poorly differentiated, in 23 moderately, and in 19 well differentiated or of unknown grading. Objective response was recorded in 46 patients (73%), and subjective response—pain relief—in a further 12 (19%). In 52 cases with elevated acid phosphatase activity, a reduction to normal occurred in 29. Regression or disappearance of metastases was observed in 23 patients, mainly soft tissue lesions. Only two patients had a clear reduction of skeletal lesions. It is noteworthy that 17 of 21 patients with high grade malignancy had an objective therapy response. Median survival for those patients dying during the observation period was 24.5 months in the objective responders, 12.4 months in the subjective responders, and 9.7 months in the nonresponders.

A few other European authors have recently reported on estramustine as the initial form of therapy in prostatic carcinoma. Leistenschneider and Nagel[27] treated 24 cases of poorly differentiated or anaplastic carcinoma, previously untreated, with oral Estracyt. In addition to the response criteria stated by the U.S. National Prostatic Cancer Project and the EORTC, Leistenschneider and Nagel relied on cytologic studies and single cell microscanning cytophotometric analyses of material from the local tumor. Objective response was observed in 87% of the patients on Estracyt as the primary therapy and subjective response in a further 6.5%. In a large proportion the smears contained aneuploid cell populations. In those patients displaying a favorable response to therapy the aneuploidy could no longer be observed, whereas persistence of aneuploid cell populations occurred in progressive cases.

Cytomorphological studies in a randomized series of 10 patients on Estracyt and 10 on conventional estrogen therapy showed cytological regression in seven of 10 Estracyt patients and in one of the 10 patients on conventional estrogens. Considering the difficulty and uncertainty inherent in the evaluation of therapy response, techniques to investigate the local tumor are an important progress.

Küss et al.[24] reported on oral Estracyt 560 mg/day as initial therapy in 15 cases of advanced carcinoma of the prostate. In nine patients reduction of the primary tumor by at least 50% occurred. A further two patients had pain relief. Disappearance of metastases occurred in none.

Edsmyr et al.[22] treated 17 patients with poorly differentiated prostatic carcinoma. In 13 of 15 patients the pain disappeared completely with an average duration of 15 months. In 13 patients a measurable local tumor was present. In seven of these a significant tumor regression was observed. A regression of lymph node metastases was reported in three of four cases, and in two of 13 patients a regression of bone metastases was observed. In 16 patients malignant cells were found in the prostate gland by aspiration biopsy. In four of these no cancer cells were detected after Estracyt treatment with a duration of 13 to 35 months.

In the above-mentioned and a few additional studies a total of 286 patients on primary Estracyt therapy has been reported, with a positive response in 84%. Even though primary Estracyt therapy had a good effect in a high percentage of the patients, Leistenschneider and Nagel,[27] like Jönsson et al.[23] previously, stated that the efficacy in a fraction of those patients refractory to ordinary hormone therapy is the most conspicuous property of the drug.

The investigations mentioned above were phase II trials. In 1976 a randomized multicenter study was started in the Stockholm area with the aim to compare Estracyt with our conventional estrogen regime in previously untreated prostatic cancer patients. Included were all cases of moderately or highly differentiated carcinoma of the prostate where therapy was deemed indicated. The cases of poorly differentiated carcinoma were excluded because they were involved in another trial. The treatment alternatives were either oral Estracyt, 840 mg/day (keyed as Estramustine in the figures) or intramuscular polyestradiol phosphate, 80 mg once per month plus oral ethinyl estradiol, 2 mg/day for 2 weeks and thereafter 150 µg/day (keyed as estrogen).

The following investigations were performed regularly: rectal palpation, fine needle biopsy of the prostate, bone scans and/or skeletal x-ray, x-ray examination of lungs, urography, and blood chemistry. For 2 years or longer 182 cases have been observed, 88 in the estramustine phosphate group and 94 in the estrogen group (Table 13.5). As seen in Tables 13.5 and 13.6 the majority of patients had moderately differentiated carcinoma, and the two groups were comparable with respect to tumor grade and stage.

Significant tumor reduction, as estimated by rectal palpation, was observed after 2 months in 64% of the patients in the estramustine phosphate group and in 53% of the estrogen group, and later on in a higher percentage (Fig. 13.2). The time in remission with respect to local tumor size is given in Fig. 13.3. There was no statistical difference between the groups either with respect to frequency of tumor reduction or with

Table 13.5
Patient Description according to Grade

	Estramustine Phosphate	Estrogen	Total
Grade 1	12	20	32
Grade 2	76	74	150
Total	88	94	182

respect to duration of the remission. The time to reach normal value of acid phosphatase activity was approximately the same in both groups (Fig. 13.4), as was the time to renewed enhancement of the phosphatase activity.

Cytological regression of the local tumor at 6 months treatment occurred in 40 of 47 patients investigated in the estramustine group and in 33 of 43 in the estrogen group. In 3 of 12 estramustine and 5 of 14 estrogen patients regression of skeletal metastases was recorded, as estimated by bone scans.

In none of the parameters investigated was there any statistical difference between the two groups. This led us to the conclusion that Estracyt has no place in the primary treatment of highly and moderately differentiated prostatic carcinoma.

Other controlled trials of Estracyt and standard hormone therapy in

Table 13.6
Patient Description according to Stage[a]

	Estramustine Phosphate	Estrogen	Total
Stage II	41	42	83
Stage III	20	21	41
Stage IV	27	31	58
Total	88	94	182

[a] According to VACURG classification.

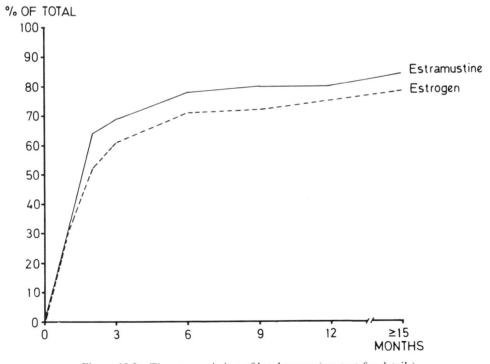

Figure 13.2   Time to remission of local tumor (see text for details).

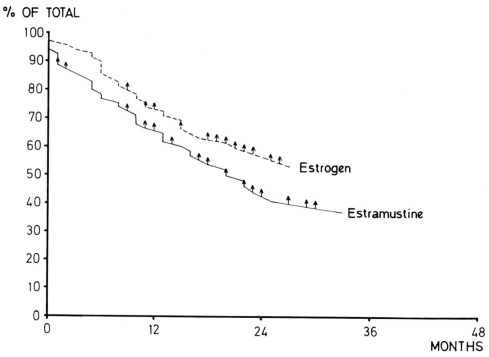

Figure 13.3   Time in remission of local tumor. *Arrows* indicate censored data.

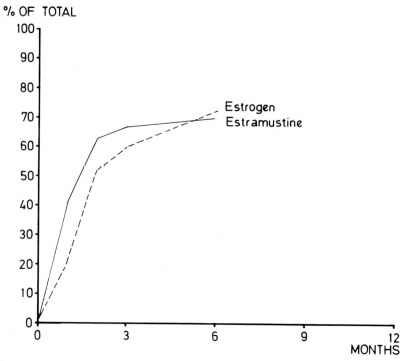

Figure 13.4   Time to reach normal value of serum acid phosphatase activity in the cases with elevated activity prior to therapy.

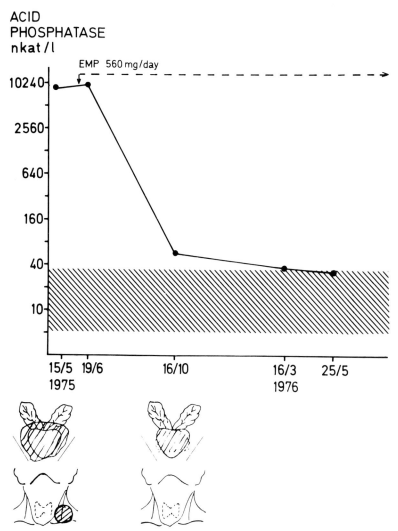

Figure 13.5 Diagram of the course in a 58-year-old patient with a supraclavicular tumor secondary to a carcinoma of the prostate. During oral estramustine phosphate therapy (EMP) the neck tumor disappeared, the prostatic tumor diminished, and acid phosphatase activity fell from very high to upper normal values. *Hatched area* indicates normal range of acid phosphatase activity.

the primary treatment of prostatic carcinoma are underway.[33, 34] A number of authors have pointed out that Estracyt has been remarkably effective in cases of disseminated poorly differentiated carcinoma which are often hormone refractory. They recommended Estracyt already from the outset for this category of patients. So far our group has at disposal only anecdotal evidence of this phenomenon.

Included in Fig. 13.5 is reported a case of poorly to moderately differentiated prostatic carcinoma where the patient presented with a supraclavicular mass. Aspiration biopsy proved the mass to be a metastasis from a symptomless carcinoma of the prostate. Following oral Estracyt,

560 mg/day, the supraclavicular mass disappeared, the prostatic tumor was reduced, and the serum acid phosphatase level fell to normal. Estracyt was given continuously. Four years later the patient died from a traffic accident. At postmortem no prostatic tumor nor metastases were found. Another patient, 73 years old, presented with widespread skeletal metastases of prostatic carcinoma and vertebral fracture due to lytic destruction. He was bedridden with severe pain. Intravenous Estracyt, 300 mg/day, was given for 3 weeks and subsequently oral medication, 560 mg/day. When the patient left hospital after 2 months he could walk and was relieved of pain. After 6 months of very good general condition he deteriorated while still on Estracyt, with periodic fever and fatigue. After 15 months of medication he died with widespread skeletal disease.

We agree with Jönsson, Nagel and other authors that estramustine appears a useful agent in highly malignant prostatic carcinoma of advanced stage. However, the definite evaluation awaits a controlled study.

UNTOWARD EFFECTS OF ESTRACYT

In patients on Estracyt therapy there was an increased morbidity in cardiovascular disease and thromboembolism in the same manner as with conventional estrogen therapy and of about the same magnitude. The majority of these complications appeared within the first 12-month period. Local thrombophlebitis sometimes occurred following intravenous administration. Bone marrow toxicity mainly in the form of thrombocytopenia, and nearly always after intravenous distribution, has been reported but was always reversible. Nausea and/or vomiting have been the most frequent adverse effects, occurring in about 40% of patients on oral therapy. The nausea often disappeared on reduction of the dosage. In about 8% the medication had to be discontinued due to gastrointestinal disturbance. Liver dysfunction with enhanced levels of serum bilirubin, SGOT, and LDH has also been observed following oral therapy, but was reversible.

Summarizing the side effects in the evaluated publications of secondary therapy six of nine authors reported that 11 of 84 patients died of cardiovascular disease. In publications containing 178 patients, 24 had

Table 13.7
Untoward Effects of Estracyt and Conventional Estrogen Therapy

Untoward Effect	Estracyt[a] (n = 88)	Estrogen[a] (n = 94)	Estracyt[b] (n = 51)	Stilbestrol[b] (n = 53)
Cardiovascular	8	10	4	4
Thromboembolic	4	7		
Gastrointestinal	2		6	1
Allergic	2			
Gynecomastia			8	16
Others	3	2	4	3

[a] From L. Andersson et al.[32]
[b] From M. Pavone-Macaluso et al.[33]

marked nausea and vomiting, and of these 13 had symptoms severe enough to discontinue treatment. In Table 13.7 are presented the adverse effects observed in two recent Estracyt trials.

CONCLUSION

In cases of previously untreated prostatic carcinoma of high to moderate differentiation, the effect of Estracyt equals that of conventional estrogenic therapy. It appears that poorly differentiated or anaplastic carcinoma of advanced stage, frequently refractory to standard hormone therapy, is often responsive to Estracyt. A phase III trial of the latter phenomenon is still needed. The most interesting effect of the drug is that about 40% of hormone refractory cases respond to Estracyt medication. The untoward reactions are relatively mild in comparison with those of other cytotoxic agents.

Acknowledgment. The authors want to express their gratitude to Mrs. Siv Diab, for her excellent help with this manuscript.

REFERENCES

1. Workman, P., and Double, J. A. Drug latentiation in cancer chemotherapy. *Biomedicine 28:* 255, 1978.
2. Trouet, A. Increased selectivity of drugs by linking to carriers. *Eur. J. Cancer 14:* 105, 1978.
3. Könyves, I., and Liljekvist, J. The steroid molecule as a carrier of cytotoxic groups. *Excerpta Med. Int. Cong. Ser. 375:* 98, 1976.
4. Könyves, I. Estracyt. In *Bladder Tumours and Other Topics in Urological Oncology,* edited by M. Pavone-Macaluso, Ph. Smith, and F. Edsmyr. Plenum Press, New York, 1980, pp. 493–499.
5. Müntzing, J., Jensen, G., and Högberg, B. Pilot study on the growth inhibition by estramustine phosphate (Estracyt) of rat mammary tumours sensitive and insensitive to oestrogen. *Acta Pharmacol. Toxicol. 44:* 1, 1979.
6. Wakisaka, M., Iwasaki, I., and Shimasaki, J. Effect of estramustine phosphate (Estracyt) on transplantable mouse tumours. *Urol. Res. 7:* 291, 1979.
7. Smolev, J. K., Coffey, D. S., and Scott, W. W. Experimental models for the study of prostatic adenocarcinoma. *J. Urol. 118:* 216, 1977.
8. Müntzing, J., Kirdani, R. Y., Saroff, J., Murphy, G. P., and Sandberg, A. A. Inhibitory effects of Estracyt on R-3327 rat prostatic carcinoma. *Urology 10:* 439, 1977.
9. Fredholm, B., Jensen, G., Lindskog, M., and Müntzing, J. Effects of estramustine phosphate (Estracyt) on growth of DMBA-induced mammary tumours in rats (abstr.) *Acta Pharmacol. Toxicol. 35(Suppl. 1):* 28, 1974.
10. Müntzing, J. Personal communication, 1967.
11. Kirdani, R. Y., Müntzing, J., Varkarakis, J. M., Murphy, G. P., and Sandberg, A. A. Studies on the antiprostatic action of Estracyt, a nitrogen mustard of estradiol. *Cancer Res. 34:* 1031, 1974.
12. Høisaeter, P. A. Incorporation of ³H-thymidine into rat ventral prostate in organ culture. *Invest. Urol. 12:* 479, 1975.
13. Plym-Forshell, G., and Nilsson, H. The distribution of radioactivity after administration of labelled estramustine phosphate (Estracyt) estradiol-17β-phosphate and estradiol to rats. *Acta Pharmacol. Toxicol. 35(Suppl. 1):* 28, 1974.
14. Høisaeter, P. A. Studies on the conversion of oestradiol linked to a cytostatic agent (Estracyt) in various rat tissues. *Acta Endocrinol. (Kbh) 82:* 661, 1976.
15. Plym-Forshell, G., Müntzing, J., Ek, A., Lindstedt, E., and Dencker, H. The absorption,

metabolism and excretion of Estracyt (NSC 89199) in patients with prostatic cancer. *Invest. Urol. 14:* 128, 1976.

16. Dixon, R., Brooks, M., and Gill, G. Estramustine phosphate: plasma concentrations of its metabolites following oral administration to man, rat and dog. *Res. Commun. Chem. Pathol. Pharmacol. 27:* 17, 1980.

17. Kadohama, N., Kirdani, R. Y., Madajewicz, S., Murphy, G. P., and Sandberg, A. A. Estramustine: metabolic pattern and possible mechanisms for its action in prostate cancer. *NY State J. Med. 79:* 1005, 1979.

18. Forsgren, B., Högberg, B., Gustafsson, J.-Å., and Pousette, Å. Binding of estramustine, a nitrogen mustard derivative of estradiol-17β, in cytosol from rat ventral prostate. *Acta Pharm. Suec. 15:* 23, 1978.

19. Högberg, B., Björk, P., Carlström, K., Forsgren, B., Gustafsson, J.-Å., Hökfelt, T., and Pousette, Å. The interaction of steroidal alkylating agents with binding components in the soluble fraction of the prostate. In *Prostate Cancer and Hormone Receptors*, edited by G. P. Murphy and A. A. Sandberg. Alan R. Liss, New York, 1979, pp. 181–199.

20. Küss, R., and Khoury, S. Estramustine-phosphate et cancer de la prostate. *Semin. Uro-Nephrol.*, Paris, 1978, p. 34.

21. Chisholm, G. D., O'Donoghue, E. P. N., and Kennedy, C. L. The treatment of oestrogen-escaped carcinoma of the prostate with estramustine phosphate. *Br. J. Urol. 49:* 717, 1977.

22. Edsmyr, F., Esposti, P.-L., and Andersson, L. Estramustine phosphate therapy in poorly differentiated carcinoma of the prostate. *Scand. J. Urol. Nephrol. Suppl. 55:* 139, 1980.

23. Jönsson, G., Högberg, B., and Nilsson, T. Treatment of advanced prostatic carcinoma with estramustine phosphate (Estracyt). *Scand. J. Urol. Nephrol. 11:* 231, 1977.

24. Küss, R., Khoury, S., Richard, F., Fourcade, F., Frantz, P., and Capelle, J. P. Estramustine phosphate in the treatment of advanced prostatic cancer. *Br. J. Urol. 52:* 29, 1980.

25. Mayer, E. J. Orale Estracyt-Behandlung beim Prostatakarzinom. *Ther. Umsch./Rev. Ther. 32:* 114, 1975.

26. Mittelman, A., Shukla, S. K., Welvaart, K., and Murphy, G. P. Oral estramustine phosphate (NSC-89199) in the treatment of advanced (stage D) carcinoma of the prostate. *Cancer Chemother. Rep. 59:* 219, 1975.

27. Leistenschneider, W., and Nagel, R. Estracyt therapy of advanced prostatic cancer with special reference to control of therapy with cytology and DNA-cytophotometry. *Eur. Urol. 6:* 111, 1980.

28. Nillius, A., and Könyves, I. Oral Estracyt (estramustine phosphate) in the treatment of advanced carcinoma of the prostate. *Chemotherapy 8:* 469, 1976.

29. Szendrői, Z., Könyves, I., Szendi, L., Eckhardt, S., and Hartay, F. Estracyt in hormone-resistant prostatic carcinoma. *Int. Urol. Nephrol. 6:* 101, 1974.

30. Benson, R. C., Jr., Wear, J. B., Jr., and Gill, G. M. Estramustine phosphate therapy for hormone-resistant prostatic carcinoma. Abstracts. 11th International Congress of Chemotherapy and 19th Interscience Conference on Antimicrobal Agents in Chemotherapy, Abstr. 230. Boston, Mass., 1–5 Oct., 1979.

31. Jönsson, G., and Högberg, B. Treatment of advanced prostatic carcinoma with Estracyt, a preliminary report. *Scand. J. Urol. Nephrol. 5:* 103, 1971.

32. Andersson, L., Berlin, T., Boman, J., Collste, L., Edsmyr, F., Esposti, P. L., Gustafsson, H., Hedlund, P. O., Hultgren, L., Leander, G., Nordle, Ö., Norlén, H., and Tillgård, P. Estramustine versus conventional estrogenic hormones in the initial treatment of highly or moderately differentiated prostatic carcinoma. A randomized study. *Scand. J. Urol. Nephrol. Suppl. 55:* 143, 1980.

33. Pavone-Macaluso, M., Lund, F., Mulder, J. H., Smith, P. H., de Pauw, M., Sylvester, R., and EORTC Urological Group. EORTC protocols in prostatic cancer. An interim report. *Scand. J. Urol. Nephrol. Suppl. 55:* 163, 1980.

34. Smith, P. H. The aims and activities of the EORTC urological group. In *Bladder Tumours and Other Topics in Urological Oncology*, edited by M. Pavone-Macaluso, P. H. Smith, and F. Edsmyr. Plenum Press, New York, 1980.

Editorial Comment to Chapter 13

The most comprehensive experience on Estracyt treatment with appropriate long-term follow-ups in Germany has been accumulated by Nagel and his associates, and their first report (Nagel and Kölln, 1977) led to the registration of this compound in Germany. Besides the questions on start of treatment and dose schedule, there is still considerable debate whether the estrogen component of the molecule is able to exert biochemical effects comparable to those of a conventional estrogen preparation.

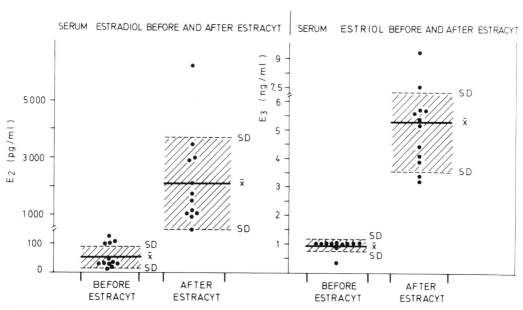

Figure 13.6 Endogenous estradiol (E_2) and estriol (E_3) serum levels of 12 patients with advanced prostatic carcinoma before and after Estracyt treatment (estramustine phosphate, 300 mg IV/day) for 5 days; determinations from an 8:00 hours blood sample by radioimmunoassay. *Solid circles* represent individual patients, *hatched area* = mean ± standard deviation: estradiol, 51.1 ± 40.8 *versus* 2102.8 ± 1636.3 pg/ml; estriol, 0.9 ± 0.2 *versus* 5.3 ± 1.8 ng/ml. (Reproduced with permission from Wenderoth *et al.*, 1982.)

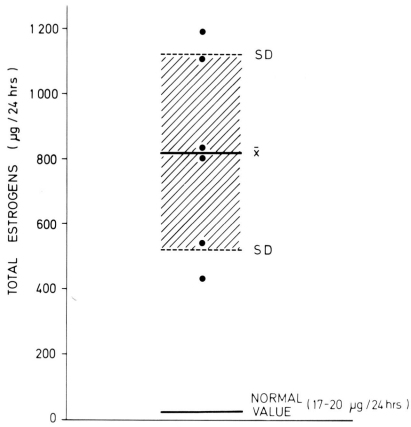

Figure 13.7 Total urinary estrogen excretion in 24-hour specimens of six patients after treatment with Estracyt (estramustine phosphate, 300 mg IV/day) for 5 days. (Same individuals as depicted in Figure 13.6). Normal value is indicated by horizontal bar at the bottom of the figure; individual values ranged from 433 to 1189 μg/24 hours (mean 819 ± SD 299 μg/24 hours). Determinations performed by gas chromatography. (Reproduced with permission from Wenderoth *et al.*, 1982.)

Although serum and urinary estrogens tremendously increase (Figs. 13.6 and 13.7), estrogen-specific side effects are rather limited. One possible explanation for this discrepancy may be the strong stimulation of sex hormone binding globulin (SHBG) (Karr *et al.*, 1980). It is conceivable that the elevation of SHBG is sufficient to bind the pharmacological concentrations of circulating estradiol.

G. H. J.

REFERENCES

Karr, J. P., Wajsman, Z., Kirdani, R. Y., Murphy, G. P., and Sandberg, A. A. Effects of diethylstilbestrol and estramustine phosphate on sex hormone binding globulin and testosterone levels in prostate cancer patients. *J. Urol. 124:* 232, 1980.

Nagel, R., and Kölln, C.-P. Treatment of advanced carcinoma of the prostate with estramustine phosphate. *Br. J. Urol. 49:* 73, 1977.

Wenderoth, U., Altwein, J. E., and Jacobi, G. H. Short-term treatment of prostatic carcinoma with estramustine phosphate: changes of endogenous steroid hormone serum levels, circulating prolactin and testosterone plasma kinetics (submitted for publication, 1982).

14

Cyproterone Acetate— Biochemical and Biological Basis for Treatment of Prostatic Cancer

F. Neumann, Vet.D.
M. Hümpel, Ph.D., Th. Senge, M.D.
B. Schenck, M.D., U. Tunn, M.D.

INTRODUCTION

Growths of the prostate—either hyperplasia or carcinoma—have never been observed in eunuchs. This suggests that androgens play an important role in the pathogenesis of prostatic tumors. The withdrawal of androgens as a therapeutic endocrine principle in the treatment of prostatic carcinoma is based on the extensive, now classical studies by Charles Huggins and co-workers [1-3] at the end of the thirties/beginning of the forties, of this century, although orchiectomy was practiced as a therapeutic principle as long ago as the last century.[4-6] The studies by Charles Huggins and co-workers, particularly those in dogs, virtually established the rational basis for the therapy of prostatic carcinoma with contrasexual hormones.[7, 8, 9] The initial euphoria following the introduction of this therapeutic principle (castration or treatment with estrogens) was, however, soon tempered when it was discovered that some patients failed to show any response at all to this therapy or developed hormone resistance (estrogen relapse).[10] Moreover, it was also demonstrated that, despite a certain therapeutic success, therapy with estrogens leads to severe side effects, primarily cardiovascular side effects. Patients were dying not from their carcinoma, but from the cardiovascular side effects of estrogens.

For theoretical reasons and because of their mechanism of action (see later), antiandrogens should offer certain advantages over surgical castration and therapy with estrogens, as regards both the therapeutic effect and the side effects. For instance, it can be assumed that, because of their mechanism of action, antiandrogens also inhibit the effect of adrenal androgens. After estrogen therapy or orchiectomy, however, the adrenal secretion of androgens tends rather to be increased (see later for details). In contrast to estrogen therapy, the phenomenon of desensitization of the gonadal-pituitary-hypothalamic axis, *i.e.* recovery of testicular androgen production despite estrogen therapy, is also unlikely during long-term treatment with an antiandrogen. This phenomenon may well be responsible for the loss of responsiveness in many patients.

This brief overview deals mainly with cyproterone acetate, although some other antiandrogens which could possibly also be of clinical interest, *e.g.* the nonsteroidal compound, *flutamide*, are also introduced in the section Chemistry of Antiandrogens. The antiandrogenic effect in the case of *spironolactone* is possibly of interest as a side effect. Mention is also made of flutamide to help clarify the interactions of antiandrogens with the gonadal (testicular)-pituitary-hypothalamic system.

DEFINITION OF THE TERM "ANTIANDROGEN"

The term "antiandrogen" was defined by Dorfman[11] as follows: "Antiandrogens are substances which prevent androgens from expressing their activity at target sites. The inhibitory effect of these substances, therefore, should be differentiated from compounds which decrease the synthesis and/or release of hypothalamic (releasing) factors, from anterior pituitary hormones (gonadotropins, particularly luteinizing hormone) and from material which acts directly on the gonads to inhibit biosynthesis and/or secretion of androgens."

According to this very restrictive definition, inhibitors of 5α-reductase, a key enzyme in androgen metabolism (*cf.* later), cannot be classified as antiandrogens. Dorfman's definition has now lost some of its validity, since even the most well known antiandrogen, cyproterone acetate, has antigonadotropic as well as antiandrogenic properties, and is therefore not a "pure" antiandrogen in the sense of Dorfman's definition. Estrogens are not counted as antiandrogens. The definition of the term "antiandrogen" is, in any case, of no great importance to the clinician.

CHEMISTRY OF ANTIANDROGENS

The first antiandrogen which was also of clinical interest–*cyproterone acetate*–was discovered at the beginning of the 1960s. A number of steroids with a very close resemblance to cyproterone acetate likewise displayed antiandrogenic properties (Fig. 14.1). Cyproterone acetate is a steroid with 21 carbon atoms or, to put it more accurately, a hydroxyprogesterone derivative. Some estrane and androstane derivatives have been found to have antiandrogenic effects, *e.g.* 17α-methyl-B-nortestosterone[12] and R 2956.[13] Even the aldosterone antagonist, spironolactone[14]–likewise a steroid hormone–has antiandrogenic properties, and attempts have in fact been made in the USA to treat hirsutism with this substance.[15]

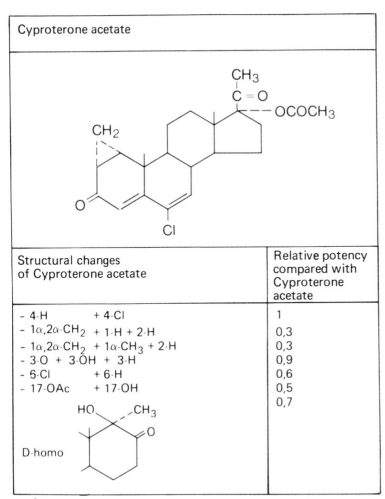

Cyproterone acetate	
Structural changes of Cyproterone acetate	**Relative potency compared with Cyproterone acetate**
- 4-H + 4-Cl	1
- 1α,2α-CH$_2$ + 1-H + 2-H	0,3
- 1α,2α-CH$_2$ + 1α-CH$_3$ + 2-H	0,3
- 3-O + 3-OH + 3-H	0,9
- 6-Cl + 6-H	0,6
- 17-OAc + 17-OH	0,5
D-homo	0,7

Figure 14.1 Relative antiandrogenic efficacy of derivatives of cyproterone acetate.

Flutamide, a toluidine derivative, was the main nonsteroidal compound to find theoretical and clinical interest.[16] Flutamide was more effective *in vivo* than *in vitro*, and it is possible that a hydroxylated metabolite (Fig. 14.2) is the effective substance. The two antiandrogens from *Uclaff Roussel* should be mentioned here, *RU 23.908* and *RU 22.930* (Fig. 14.2), both of which are structurally related to flutamide. *RU 22.930* is said to have only a local effect.

MECHANISM OF ACTION OF ANTIANDROGENS

According to the present concept of the mechanism of action of androgens, a sequence of individual mechanisms takes place in the target cell, the end product of which is the expression by the androgen-sensitive cell of its specific activity (Fig 14.3). The androgen testosterone secreted by the Leydig cell of the testis circulates in the blood bound to proteins,

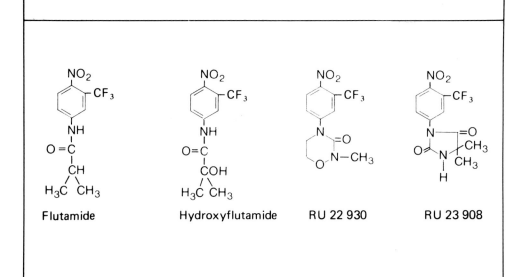

Figure 14.2 Nonsteroidal antiandrogens.

namely the specific transport protein TeBG,* and albumin. Only 1 to 3% are unbound (see Chapter 19).

Only the free hormone can enter the cell,[17, 18] and it does this not via active transport mechanisms, but presumably by means of "facilitated diffusion." After entering the cytoplasm of the prostatic cell, testosterone is reduced to 5α-dihydrotestosterone (5α-DHT) by the enzyme 5α-reductase.[19] 5α-DHT binds to specific cytosol receptors. As a result of this binding, the hormone receptor complex is activated (transformed) and then enters (translocates) into the cell nucleus, where it binds to what are called nuclear acceptors. This binding results in the synthesis of DNA and cell proliferation and/or m-RNA synthesis (transcription) with subsequent synthesis of specific proteins (translation)[20, 21] (see chapter 20).

A number of points of attack is conceivable for cyproterone acetate on the basis of the above-described mechanisms of cellular action of androgens. According to studies by Giorgi et al.,[22] cyproterone acetate inhibits the transport of testosterone into the prostatic cell. Whalen et al.,[23] on the other hand, found no inhibition of ³H-testosterone uptake in castrated rats primed with cyproterone acetate.

In vivo, cyproterone acetate also does not appear to influence the entry of testosterone into the cell to any particular extent. The 5α-reduction of testosterone to 5α-DHT is not suppressed by cyproterone acetate.[24–30] The most important mechanism of the antiandrogenic action of cyproterone acetate is probably competitive inhibition of the binding of androgens to the cytosol receptor, which prevents transformation and translocation into

---

* This is synonymous with sex hormone-binding globulin (SHBG).

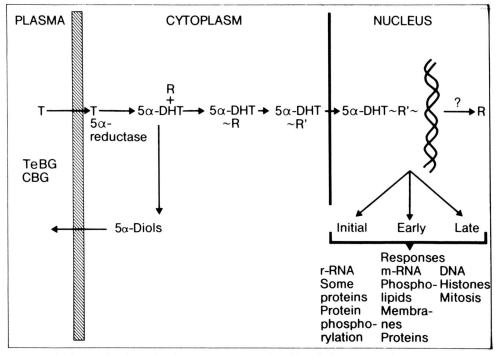

Figure 14.3 Mechanism of action of androgens (for abbreviations see text!)

the nucleus[31-38] and results in reduced concentrations of free and bound dihydrotestosterone in the nucleus.[39] All the subsequent steps, *e.g.* androgen-dependent DNA synthesis and androgen-dependent RNA polymerase, are consequently inhibited.[40-42]

PHARMACOKINETICS OF CYPROTERONE ACETATE

Since cyproterone acetate is the only commercially available antiandrogen, it seems justifiable to limit the discussion of the pharmacokinetics to this substance. As a C_{21} steroid with no free alcohol group, cyproterone acetate is a comparatively highly lipophilic substance. This physicochemical property affects several pharmacokinetic parameters, *e.g.* absorption and the distribution pattern in the organs and tissues.

Absorption and Bioavailability

Following oral administration, cyproterone acetate is completely absorbed and bioavailable from suitable galenic formulations (high adjuvant to substance ratio). This applies both to the animal species used in toxicology and pharmacology and to man. Of particular interest is the fact that, in contrast to progestogens of the 19-nortestosterone series (norethisterone, levonorgestrel), cyproterone acetate is not subject to a first-pass effect in the rat, dog, and rhesus monkey, *i.e.* the entire dose administered reaches the major circulation in unchanged form and is therefore bioavailable. Full bioavailability has also been demonstrated for man.[43]

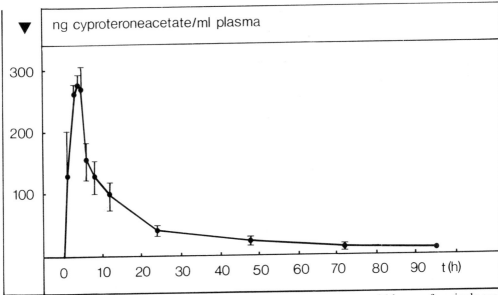

Figure 14.4 Plasma level of cyproterone acetate up to 96 hours after single oral administration of 50 mg to five male volunteers. Mean value ± standard deviation.

The absorption rate is dependent both on the solubility of the substance and on the galenic formulation. Cyproterone acetate is absorbed relatively slowly but completely from the 50 mg tablet, the half-life being about 1.5 hours. Figure 14.4 shows the substance level after a single administration of 50 mg of cyproterone acetate in five male volunteer subjects. Maximal substance levels are reached after 3 to 4 hours.[44]

Distribution

The distribution pattern of the substance can be determined directly in animal experiments (whole-body autoradiography, rat; measurement of the acute concentration in organs and tissues, rat, dog), but only indirectly in man (via the pattern of the substance concentration in plasma). In keeping with its high lipophilia, high concentrations of cyproterone acetate are found transiently in the fatty tissue and subcutis of the rat and dog. In agreement with this, an extremely high fictive distribution volume of 161 liters/kg of body weight has been estimated for man.[44]

The rate at which the distribution processes take place in the organism was calculated via the postmaximal substance level, which falls in two phases. A half-life of about 2 hours[45] was calculated for the first phase, which reflects the distribution. Similar values have also been found for other steroids,[46] so it can be assumed that the distribution phase is determined primarily by general physiological processes (blood flow). The second, or terminal, phase of the substance level describes the steady-state of the reflux of the substance from the tissues and its metabolism in the liver (see below). The concentration of cyproterone acetate in the skin following systemic administration falls from proximal to distal. Concentrations are therefore higher in the deep layers of skin than in the upper layers.

Metabolism and Excretion

The biotransformation of cyproterone acetate in man has been studied in depth.[47, 48] The greatest part of the dose was eliminated via the kidneys and bile in the form of nonconjugated metabolites. About 30% of the urinary metabolites and 50 to 60% of the metabolic products in the bile were conjugated with glucuronic acid. About 10% of the biliary and urinary metabolites were in the form of sulphates. 15β-hydroxy-cyproterone acetate was identified as the quantitatively most important metabolite in plasma and in the freely extractable portions of urine and bile. Cyproterone was found in very slight amounts only in the bile, while unchanged cyproterone acetate was found mainly in the freely extractable portion of human bile. About 30% of the metabolites of cyproterone acetate are eliminated with the urine and 70% with the bile with a half-life of 2 days.[49] The same half-life was determined for the terminal phase of the plasma substance level, so the terminal phase can also be described as an elimination phase; the concentration of the sum of substance and metabolites in plasma also fell at this rate.[46] Thus, a disproportionately high accumulation of plasma metabolites relative to the substance level is unlikely even after repeated administration.

Repeated Application: Accumulation

With a half-life of 2 days for the terminal phase of the substance level, one would expect an accumulation of the substance on daily administration. However, an equilibrium between administration and excretion becomes established after 8 to 10 days' use.[45] It is possible that this pharmacokinetic property of cyproterone acetate is one of the prerequisites of the antiandrogenic effect, since the limited accumulation of cyproterone acetate in the tissues on repeated administration probably creates a highly constant concentration, *e.g.* in the target organ prostate. In addition to the oral form (tablets), cyproterone acetate is also available for clinical use in depot form in ampoules (300 mg in oily solution). Depending on the number of treatments, the administration of 300 mg IM leads after about 2 to 3 days to maximal substance levels of about 300 to 400 ng/ml plasma. The substance levels then fall monophasically with a half-life of about 4 days.

The rate of fall of the plasma concentration of cyproterone acetate is determined by the release of the substance from the oily depot—in contrast to oral administration, where it depends on the reflux of cyproterone acetate from the tissues and on metabolism. As a lipophilic substance, cyproterone acetate is released more slowly than it is eliminated. Since the release rate has a half-life of about 4 days, accumulation must be expected with an injection interval of 7 days. This assumption is confirmed not only by the height of the maximal plasma level, but also by the *A*rea *U*nder the *C*urve level (AUC) after repeated treatment.

The time at which the equilibrium is reached between administration and excretion of cyproterone acetate with a weekly injection interval was estimated in another study in patients. The substance levels were determined before the next injection over 4 to 7 months; evaluation revealed that the equilibrium was achieved at individually different times, but never later than the fourth injection (Fig. 14.5). Once the equilibrium is established, the mean plasma concentration of cyproterone acetate is about 160 ng/ml (as measured before the next injection).

TARGET ORGANS AND FUNCTIONS AFFECTED BY ANTIANDROGENS

Antiandrogens act in all target organs for androgens and, in principle, affect all functions which are governed or influenced by androgens under physiological or pathophysiological conditions. Some of these effects are more sex specific, others less sex-specific, but the most important of them are shown in Tables 14.1 and 14.2. Of most interest in this connection is the effect of cyproterone acetate on the accessory sex glands, particularly the prostate.

ACTION OF ANTIANDROGENS ON ACCESSORY SEX GLANDS

The accessory sex glands represent classical target organs for androgens and thus also for antiandrogens. As in androgen deprivation following surgical castration, treatment with antiandrogens also leads to loss of function and atrophy. In contrast to substances such as estrogens, which exert an inhibitory effect on testicular androgen biosynthesis via inhibition of gonadotropin secretion, antiandrogens act, as already mentioned, at the cellular level by competition. Antiandrogens, unlike estrogens, are therefore also capable of inhibiting the action of exogenously administered androgens. The agonist/antagonist ratio is relatively favorable. To achieve a 50% inhibition of the stimulant action of testosterone propionate, about

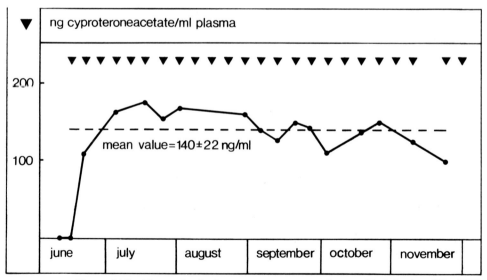

Figure 14.5 Plasma level of cyproterone acetate after weekly injection (▼) of 300 mg in oily solution.

Table 14.1
Sex-Specific Effects of Antiandrogens

Organ/Function	Effects of Antiandrogens
Accessory sexual glands	Atrophy
Epididymis, vas deferens	Atrophy
Spermatogenesis	Inhibition of maturation division[a]
Libido	Loss of libido (not all species)
Puberty	Inhibition
Male sexual differentiation	Feminization
Gonadotropin secretion	Pure antiandrogens and antiandrogens of the cyproterone acetate type behave differently

[a] Pure antiandrogens are not effective.

Table 14.2
Some Less Sex-Specific Effects of Antiandrogens

Organ/Function	Effects of Antiandrogens
Bone maturation	Ossification of epiphyseal cartilage is delayed
Sebaceous glands	Inhibition of sebaceous gland function
Sex-specific enzyme pattern (e.g. in the kidney)	Female pattern
Body weight development	Inhibition in very high doses (antianabolic effect)

3 times the equivalent amount of cyproterone acetate is required. A 10-fold preponderance of the antiandrogen produces almost 100% inhibition of the androgen effect.[50, 51] The inhibitory effect of antiandrogens and especially of cyproterone acetate on accessory sex gland function has been demonstrated in numerous animal studies as well as in man (for more details see references 50 and 51).

At this point we should like to deal briefly with the effects of cyproterone acetate on the "healthy" prostate, basing on our own recently performed studies in dogs (for more details see references 52 to 55).

Figure 14.6 shows the prostatic weights of normal dogs (first column) and of castrated dogs treated for 6 months with a dihydrotestosterone metabolite (3α, 17β-androstanediol) alone or in combination with cyproterone acetate. It can be seen that cyproterone acetate abolishes the effect of the androgen. This results in a decrease of deoxyribonucleic acid and ribonucleic acid, as Figure 14.7 shows. The content of RNA decreases to a greater extent, which is a parameter for restricted secretory activity. This can be seen in Figure 14.8, which shows the RNA to DNA ratio. Figure 14.9A shows the histological picture of a dog prostate with high secretory activity (castrated, replaced with $3\alpha,17\beta$-androstanediol), while Figure 14.9B shows the picture after additional treatment with cyproterone acetate.

Figure 14.10 shows the same in semithin sections. It can be seen that the stimulatory effect on the prostate of the androgen used for replacement is completely abolished by simultaneous administration of the antiandrogen. Under the influence of cyproterone acetate there is a loss of the

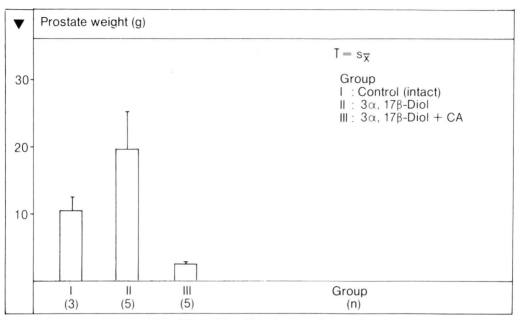

Figure 14.6 Effect of 3α,17β-androstanediol (*Diol*) and cyproterone acetate (*CA*) on prostate weight in the castrated dog. Duration of treatment: 6 months. Injections were given 3 times weekly. Weekly dose: 3α,17β-androstanediol, 25 mg; cyproterone acetate, 600 mg.

characteristic enzymes and substances of the prostate, *e.g.* acid phosphatase, aminopeptidase, and zinc. This is illustrated in the next figures, which depict the histochemical demonstration of acid phosphatase (brown-red) in a castrated animal and after replacement with the dihydrotestosterone metabolite (Fig. 14.11*A*). Figure 14.11*B* shows that this enzyme disappears completely when cyproterone acetate is administered at the same time. The same is true for the zinc content.

These experimental findings in the "healthy" prostate have been confirmed in man. The "healthy" prostate ceases its secretory activity under the antiandrogen therapy.[56] However, it is more difficult on the basis of animal expriments to determine whether antiandrogens are effective in prostatic carcinoma, since there are virtually no usable animal models (we have discussed this problem in several earlier publications, *cf.* references 57 to 60). With two possible exceptions, prostatic carcinomas, induced either experimentally by hormonal manipulations or by administration of carcinogenic hydrocarbons, have so far failed to display any androgen dependence. In fact, some paradoxical effects have even been observed— *e.g.* stimulation by estrogens. The same is true for tissue cultures of prostatic carcinomas.[57, 58] After reimplantation of a cell strain of a prostatic carcinoma (EB 33)[61] into the nude mouse, mainly dedifferentiated tumors developed. These fast-growing carcinomas had no similarities with the original tumor. Hormone dependence was not shown[62] (see Chapter 17).

We have recently heard of the successful transplantation of prostatic carcinomas into nude mice. These carcinomas are said to be androgen-

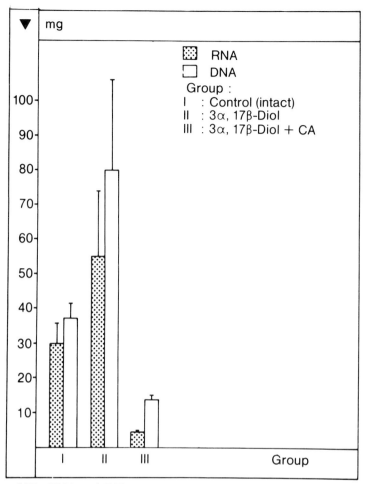

Figure 14.7 RNA and DNA content of prostate in the castrated dog after 6 months subcutaneous treatment with $3\alpha,17\beta$-androstanediol and cyproterone acetate. Weekly dose: $3\alpha,17\beta$-androstanediol, 25 mg; cyproterone acetate, 600 mg.

dependent as regards their growth, and it is also claimed that their growth can be inhibited by estrogens and cyproterone acetate.[63, 64] However, there is perhaps an animal model which gives a more indirect indication that cyproterone acetate has a direct degenerative effect at least on metaplastic carcinoma cells.

Heterotransplantation of human prostatic adenomas has proved to be a suitable model; it was at least possible to demonstrate hormone dependence (androgen dependence).[65] Naturally, the conclusions which this model allows as regards the effectiveness of a hormone or drug in prostatic carcinomas are limited. The method is based on the technique by Forsberg and Ingemanson[66] for heterotransplantation of human cervical epithelium into newborn rats. Immunosuppression is effected by treatment with antilymphocytic serum. As a rule, the duration of the experiment is 14 days to 3 weeks. The viability of the implants is checked by means of histological and enzyme-histochemical methods.[67]

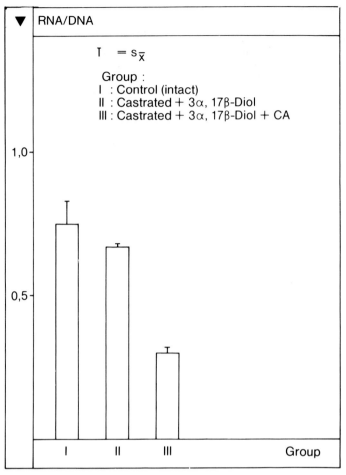

Figure 14.8 RNA/DNA ratio of prostate in the castrated dog after 6 months subcutaneous treatment with $3\alpha,17\beta$-androstanediol and cyproterone acetate. Weekly dose: $3\alpha,17\beta$-androstanediol, 25 mg; cyproterone acetate, 600 mg.

Another parameter is the demonstration of active DNA synthesis.[68] Transplants of this kind will even grow without androgen replacement, although secretory activity is very low. After replacement with testosterone propionate or dihydrotestosterone, the transplants show the typical differentiation already known from prostatic hyperplasia (Fig. 14.12). The key enzyme, such as acid phosphatase, and zinc, are also demonstrable. Metaplastic changes can be observed almost regularly in the transplants. The changes in question are of the squamous metaplasia type (Fig. 14.13). It is interesting to note that this metaplasia reacts to treatment with cyproterone acetate with hydropic degeneration (Fig. 14.14). Prostatic carcinoma patients under estrogen therapy are known to display quite similar signs of degeneration in the neoplastic areas of the carcinomatous tissue.[69–74]

To summarize, we can only assume on the basis of theoretical considerations and of the influence on the function of the healthy prostate that at least some prostatic carcinoma patients (or some of the carcinoma cells)

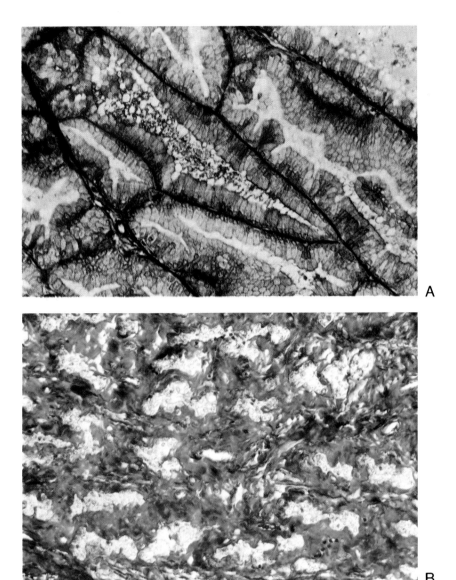

Figure 14.9 Prostate of castrated dogs. *A*, After 6 months of treatment with
3α,17β-androstanediol (25 mg weekly), (ca. ×160) and *B*, after 6 months of
treatment with 3α,17β-androstanediol (25 mg weekly) plus cyproterone acetate
(600 mg weekly). Azan stain. (*ca.* ×400).

respond to antiandrogens. Whether the responsive carcinomas display (or
still display) androgen receptors cannot be said at the present time. Strictly
speaking, *only clinical investigations can provide the proof of efficacy of
antiandrogens in the therapy of prostatic carcinoma* (see Chapter 15).

OTHER EFFECTS OF CYPROTERONE ACETATE

This brief review would not be complete without a few words on the
other pharmacological effects of cyproterone acetate. Two aspects, the

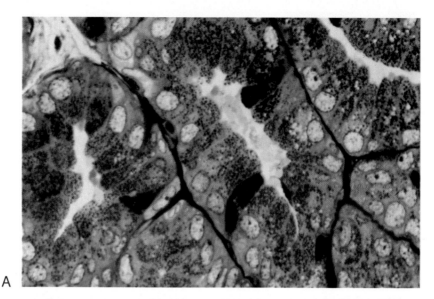

A

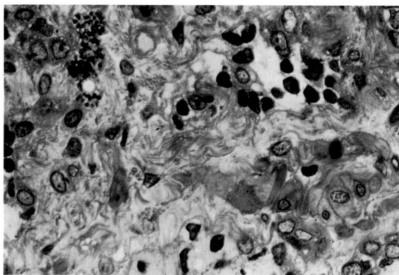

B

Figure 14.10   Prostate of castrated dogs (semithin sections). *A*, After 6 months of treatment with 3α,17β-androstanediol (25 mg weekly), (*ca.* ×1600) and *B*, after 6 months of treatment with 3α,17β-androstanediol (25 mg weekly) plus cyproterone acetate (600 mg weekly). Laczkó stain. (*ca.* ×1600).

influence on spermatogenesis and the influence on the gonadal-pituitary-hypothalamic system, are dealt with in greater detail because these effects are or could be of clinical importance in the therapy of noncastrated prostatic carcinoma patients.

Effect of the Cyproterone Acetate Type of Antiandrogen and "Pure" Antiandrogens on Testicular Function and the Gonadal-Pituitary-Hypothalamic Axis

Cyproterone acetate and similar antiandrogens not only have an antiandrogenic effect, but also progestational and therefore antigonadotropic

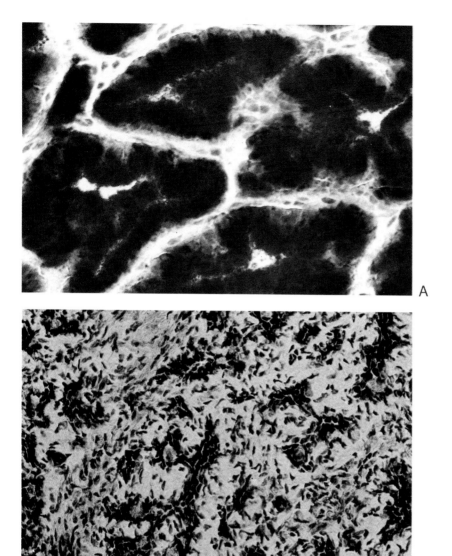

Figure 14.11 Prostate of castrated dogs (acid phosphatase stain). *A*, After 6 months of treatment with 3α,17β-androstanediol (25 mg weekly), (*ca.* ×800) and *B*, after 6 months of treatment with 3α,17β-androstanediol (25 mg weekly) and cyproterone acetate (600 mg weekly).(*ca.* ×400).

effects.[75, 76] In the case of cyproterone acetate, these latter effects are even stronger than, for example, those of chlormadinone acetate, the ovulation-inhibiting dose in the woman being about 1 mg daily p.o. In men, the progestational properties lead to a drastic fall in gonadotropin and testosterone secretion at the dosages used in the therapy of prostatic carcinoma.

This is an additional mechanism which is of importance as regards the thera-peutic effect. However, it must be stressed that the competitive inhibition of

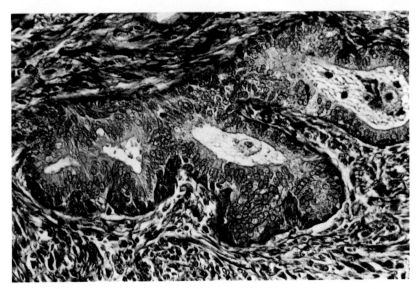

Figure 14.12 Figures 14.12 to 14.14 show prostate heterotransplants. Prostate adenoma tissue was grafted immediately after prostatectomy into newborn female Sprague-Dawley rats. Twenty-four hours after the operation, 0.07 ml of antilymphocyte serum was injected subcutaneously into the neckfolds of the rats. From the 3rd day on, the dose was increased to 0.1 ml of antilymphocyte serum once every 2nd day until day 17 after transplantation. Testosterone propionate, 1.2 mg, was given subcutaneously to the host animal in a *1:5* mixture of benzyl benzoate and castor oil between day 6 and day 18 of the experiment divided into three injections each. In this figure note fully developed glandular epithelium, which is clearly active and has pseudopapillary proliferations. *A*, Azan. ×150; *B*, Goldner. ×250.

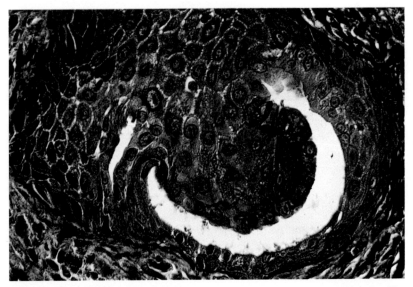

Figure 14.13 Prostate heterotransplants. For transplantation techniques see Figure 14.12. Note proliferation and metaplastic transformation of the glandular epithelium. Hematoxylin and eosin. (×100).

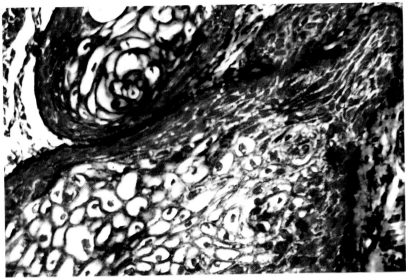

Figure 14.14 Prostate heterotransplants under combined treatment of testosterone propionate plus cyproterone acetate. Transplantation techniques the same as described in Figure 14.12. Cyproterone acetate, 36 mg, plus 0.6 mg testosterone propionate was given. Note bloated type of degeneration of the metaplastic epithelium. Azan. (×250).

androgens at the target organ is the predominant feature of the therapy, *i.e.* the clinical efficacy of the therapy of prostatic carcinoma with cyproterone acetate cannot be demonstrated by the fall in the blood levels of testosterone as occasionally happens. In this respect estrogens would be superior to cyproterone acetate because of their very much greater antigonadotropic efficacy and thus much more pronounced inhibition of testosterone synthesis.

Although spermatogenesis, Sertoli cell function, and the processes of spermatozoa maturation in the epididymis are androgen-dependent, the administration of so-called "pure" antiandrogens which display no further partial effects (progestational and antigonadotropic partial effects) leads at the most to a transient disturbance of spermatogenesis and thus only temporarily to subfertility.[77-81] This finding becomes understandable when one considers the varying (almost opposing) influence on the negative feedback system of pure antiandrogens on the one hand and of antiandrogens with additional progestational and antigonadotropic partial effects on the other.

Flutamide and *cyproterone*, the free alcohol of cyproterone acetate, for example, are pure antiandrogens. These antiandrogens apparently displace androgens even in those neural centers in which androgens exert their negative feedback and, hence, inhibitory effect on the secretion of gonadotropins. An androgen deficit is thus simulated centrally, and an increased secretion of releasing factors for gonadotropins (this has not yet been demonstrated directly) and of gonadotropins is the consequence. The biosynthesis of androgens in the Leydig cells is stimulated as a result of increased secretion of LH (for review see references 50 and 78).

CYPROTERONE ACETATE BIOCHEMISTRY   285

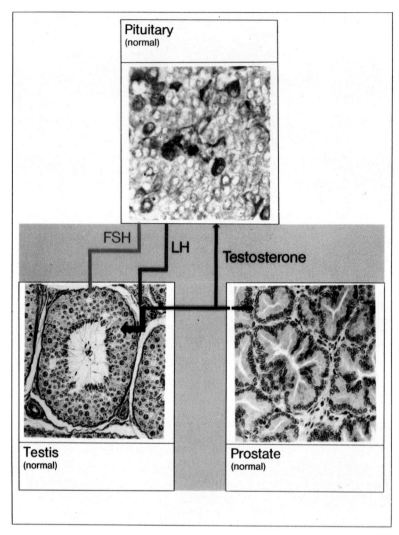

Figure 14.15 Normal feedback mechanism (Pituitary-Testis-Prostate axis).

The effects of the antiandrogen are more or less abolished because of the increased biosynthesis of testosterone, *i.e.* "pure" antiandrogens might be unsuitable for therapeutic purpose in noncastrated men because of their stimulatory effect on the negative feedback system. The concentrations of LH and testosterone increase drastically on administration of flutamide or cyproterone. Another result is hyperplasia of the interstitial cells of Leydig (compare Figs. 14.15. to 14.18). The animals are subfertile only at the start of flutamide treatment (Table 14.3); testicular function and fertility is normalized with increasing duration of treatment. The intratesticular concentrations of androgen are, in fact, so high that the antiandrogen is no longer capable of abolishing the effect of androgens in the testis itself.

Antiandrogens with progestational activities, on the other hand, inhibit

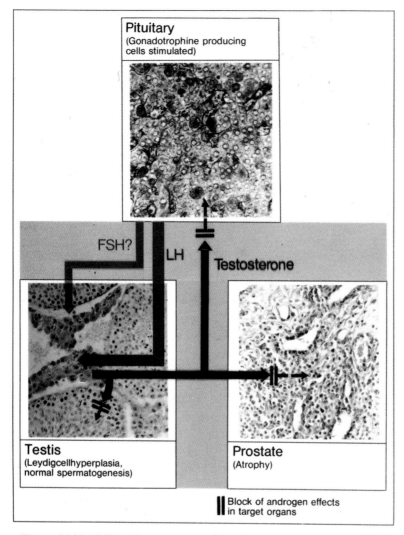

Figure 14.16 Effect of "pure" antiandrogen on the feedback mechanism.

spermatogenesis and fertility. The extent of the inhibition of spermatogenesis is dose-dependent and naturally varies from species to species. However, a consistent finding is that only spermatid maturation (spermiogenesis) is affected initially under medium doses. Meiosis fails to take place on administration of higher doses; secondary spermatocytes are the most advanced stages of spermatogenesis. Under extremely high doses the convoluted tubules are completely depopulated and, apart from Sertoli cells, only spermatogonia and early spermatocytes are recognizable (Fig. 14.19).

The extent of the disturbance of spermatogenesis—already recognizable by a decrease of testicular weights—runs parallel with a decrease of *a*ndrogen-*b*inding *p*rotein (ABP) production[82] (Table 14.4). These findings allow the conclusion that cyproterone acetate and similar antiandro-

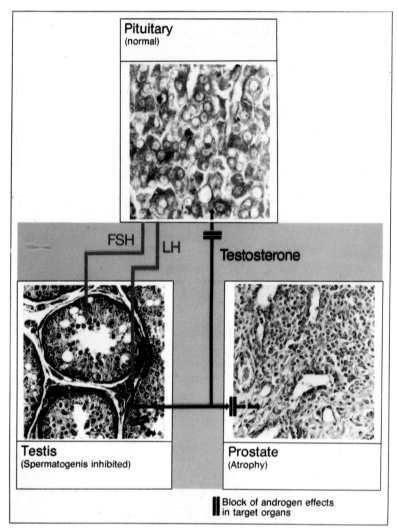

Figure 14.17 Effect of antiandrogens with progestational activities on the feedback mechanism.

gens have their point of attack primarily at the likewise functionally androgen-dependent Sertoli cells. According to this, the disturbance of spermatogenesis would be a secondary effect attributable to limited secretory activity of the Sertoli cells. This assumption is supported by the observation that the FSH-binding capacity of the Sertoli cells also decreases after treatment with cyproterone acetate.[83]

Animal studies and observations in men treated for many years with cyproterone acetate have shown that the testicular changes, *i.e.* the inhibition of spermatogenesis, are reversible (for review see reference 84).

Libido and Potentia Coeundi

Androgens are essential for the maintenance of libido and potency. Thus, it could almost be said that antiandrogens have a similar effect to

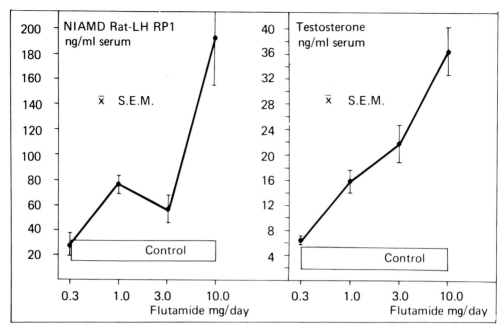

Figure 14.18 Serum LH and testosterone levels of adult male rats after 6 weeks of treatment with various doses of flutamide.

Table 14.3
Fertility of Mature Rats during the Treatment Period as Measured by the Ability to Impregnate Female Rats (± Implantation Sites)

Compound	Dose of the Antiandrogen (mg/day; 18 days)	No. of Animals	Inhibition of Fertility (%)		
			1st wk	2nd wk	3rd wk
Flutamide	10.0	8	50	25	12.5
	3.0	8	12.5	12.5	12.5
	1.0	7	50	25	12.5
	0.3	8	12.5	0	0

that of castration. Animal experiments have, surprizingly, produced controversial findings. Cyproterone acetate was unable to suppress sexual drive in the ordinary small laboratory animals, such as mice, rats, guinea-pigs, and hamsters,[85–89] whereas dogs, cats, boars, and rabbits reacted promptly to cyproterone acetate treatment with a loss of libido.[90, 91] The human male appears to react most sensitively.[84, 92–99] Decreased libido and diminished ability of penile erection are reported with 100 mg daily. The ability to reach an orgasm is generally also abolished after 3 weeks of treatment. These effects regress in the same order after discontinuation of the treatment. Libido normalizes first of all, followed by the ability to erect and to reach an orgasm.

Cyproterone acetate is used in several European countries for the treatment of pathological hypersexuality and sexual deviations. The average dose used is 100 mg given daily p.o. or 300 mg given once a week IM.

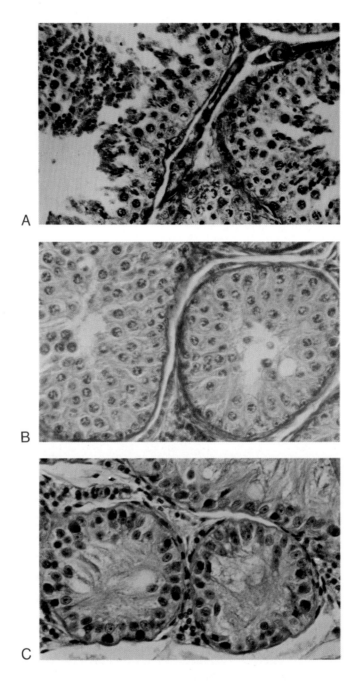

Figure 14.19 Testicular changes in the dog. *A*, Control. *B*, After 30 days intramuscular administration of 10 mg/day/kg body weight of cyproterone acetate, spermatogenesis is inhibited. *C*, After approximately 12 months oral administration of 100 mg/day/kg body weight of cyproterone acetate, meiosis is also inhibited (note the tubular atrophy and depopulation of the germinal epithelium). Hematoxylin and eosin. (×400).

Table 14.4
Effect of Cyproterone Acetate on Testis Weights and Androgen Binding Protein (ABP) Concentration in the Caput of the Epididymis[a]

Cyproterone Acetate (mg/day)[b]		Testis Wt (mg/100 gm b.w.)	ABP	
			pmoles/mg protein	pmoles/caput epididymidis
Control	(12)	759 ± 62	2.6 ± 0.3	26.3 ± 4.2
0.625	(7)	797 ± 74	2.7 ± 0.4	31.8 ± 0.4
1.25	(7)	886 ± 96	2.8 ± 0.5	30.8 ± 6.1
2.5	(8)	831 ± 65	3.2 ± 0.5	28.6 ± 7.6
5.0	(6)	743 ± 92	2.7 ± 0.4	23.4 ± 8.1
10.0	(8)	709 ± 70	2.7 ± 0.4	17.6 ± 3.6
30.0	(7)	462 ± 46[c]	1.0 ± 0.2[d]	8.4 ± 1.8[c]

[a] Organ weights and ABP concentrations are expressed as mean ± SEM.
[b] Number of animals in parentheses.
[c] $p < 0.01$ (significantly different from control).
[d] $p < 0.02$ (significantly different from control).

Puberty and Bone Maturation

The onset of puberty in male individuals can be delayed for any length of time by treatment with antiandrogens of the cyproterone acetate type.[100] Studies in rats have also shown that antiandrogens can delay bone maturation (ossification of the epiphyseal cartilages) and retard longitudinal growth.[101, 102] The treatment of precocious puberty in both sexes is one of the indications of cyproterone acetate.

Skin and Cutaneous Appendages

Androgens are of causative importance for a number of diseases of the skin and the cutaneous appendages. A particularly essential factor in the pathogenesis of acne is increased activity by the sebaceous glands. Cyproterone acetate is highly effective in inhibiting sebaceous gland function (for review see references 76, 103, 104). It is successfully employed in several European countries for the treatment of acne and seborrhoea, hirsutism, and androgenetic alopecia (for review see reference 105).

Sexual Differentiation

Some of the steps of male sexual differentiation are androgen-dependent. The same is true for the development of the so-called psychic sex in a male direction. When pregnant animals are treated with cyproterone acetate during the "critical phase" of sexual differentiation, a very special form of intersexuality is induced in the male foetuses. Differentiation of the gonads remains undisturbed; the animals, therefore, have testes. The internal genital tracts fail to develop, *i.e.* both the Müllerian and Wolffian ducts have regressed, and there is therefore no longer any communication between the gonads and the surface of the body. Accessory male glands fail to develop, and such animals display a vagina instead. The external genitalia show feminine differentiation. These changes are, of course, irreversible. This form of intersexuality corresponds to testicular feminization in man (for review see references 76, 106–109 and Table 14.5).

Influence of Cyproterone Acetate on Adrenal Function

In rats, high doses of cyproterone acetate bring about a decrease of adrenal weights and atrophy of the adrenal cortex, primarily of the zona fasciculata.[110–114] The secretion of corticosterone in rats is inhibited by cyproterone acetate.[115] No atrophy of the adrenal cortex occurred when hypophysectomized rats were treated simultaneously with ACTH and cyproterone acetate.[111] These findings suggest that inhibition of ACTH secretion is the reason for the adrenocortical atrophy under cyproterone acetate treatment.

A reduction of corticosterone secretion under stress has been demonstrated in rats and hamsters under treatment with cyproterone acetate.[115–118] Inhibition of the pituitary-adrenocortical axis has been demonstrated in rats as long as 2 weeks after discontinuation of cyproterone acetate treatment.[119] Similar findings have also been made in hamsters.[116, 120]

A glucocorticoid effect has been suggested as the cause of the ACTH-inhibitory effect of cyproterone acetate. With the exception of ACTH inhibition and a thymolytic effect, however, cyproterone acetate has no other glucocorticoid effects, *i.e.* no antiphlogistic and gluconeogenetic effects or eosinopenia have been demonstrated.[110, 111]

In addition to this indirect effect of cyproterone acetate on the adrenal cortex, a direct effect on steroid biosynthesis via inhibition of the *3β-hydroxy-steroid-dehydrogenase-5-ene-4-ene-isomerase* complex has also been demonstrated *in vitro*.[114, 121] Whether and to what extent this effect of cyproterone acetate also plays a role *in vivo* has not yet been clarified.

In man, the results regarding ACTH inhibition are controversial. Normal ACTH secretion has been demonstrated in the metyrapone test in patients being treated with cyproterone acetate for sexual deviations.[122] Treatment with cyproterone acetate likewise had no effect on the function

Table 14.5
Comparison of the Syndrome of "Testicular Feminization" with Feminized Dogs

"Testicular" Feminization	"Feminized" Dogs[a]
Chromosomal sex ♂	Chromosomal sex ♂
Gonads ♂	Gonads ♂
External genitalia ♀, development of a vagina	External genitalia ♀, development of a vagina
Absence of uterus and tubes	Absence of uterus and tubes
Absence of epididymis and ductus deferens	Absence of epididymis and ductus deferens
Absence of male accessory sexual glands	Absence of male accessory sexual glands
Incomplete testicular descent	Incomplete testicular descent (scrotal development inhibited)

[a] Treatment of mothers during pregnancy from day 23 to day 43 with daily 10 mg/kg cyproterone acetate subcutaneously.

of the pituitary-adrenocortical axis in hirsute women.[123] Reduced responsiveness of the adrenal cortex to ACTH and metyrapone has been established in children with precocious puberty under treatment with cyproterone acetate.[124, 125] Girard and Baumann[126] observed plasma cortisol concentrations of less than 1 mg/100 ml and significantly reduced ACTH concentrations in children with precocious puberty being treated with 75 mg cyproterone acetate/m^2 body surface. The elimination of free cortisol was reduced and, following administration of ACTH, the increase of plasma cortisol was suppressed.

A reduced ACTH response to metyrapone was observed in 18 of 24 healthy students after administration of a single dose of 200 mg cyproterone acetate. The response was increased in five subjects, while one subject displayed no effect. Corresponding findings have also been made in 12 hirsute women under sequential treatment with cyproterone acetate and ethinyl estradiol. Compared with the degree of stimulation at the end of the estrogen period of treatment, metyrapone stimulation of ACTH was significantly reduced at the end of the 10-day treatment with cyproterone acetate. The serum ACTH and cortisol concentrations and the cortisol response to ACTH and insulin-induced hyperglycemia were reduced in four of 11 children being treated with cyproterone acetate for precocious puberty. Suppression was doubtful in two children, while five of 11 children displayed normal function of the pituitary-adrenocortical axis. The same authors observed reduced morning ACTH levels in 10 patients with elevated endogenous ACTH levels after 10 days of treatment with 200 mg cyproterone acetate p.o. additional to the treatment with cortisone acetate.[119] In contrast, other authors found no inhibition of the pituitary-adrenocortical axis in four healthy male subjects aged 23 to 25 years during 20 days of treatment with 200 mg cyproterone acetate/day.[127]

To summarize, these findings show that, particularly in children, cyproterone acetate can suppress ACTH secretion. The effect is dose-dependent, and there appear to be distinct individual differences. A cortisol-like effect of cyproterone acetate is assumed, since stress situations during treatment with cyproterone acetate are survived without any signs of adrenocortical insufficiency both in animal experiments and in human studies. The function of the pituitary-adrenocortical axis should be supervised in children after discontinuation of therapy with cyproterone acetate, since recovery of adrenocortical function in individual cases of marked suppression can take up to several months.

Metabolic Effect of Cyproterone Acetate (Catabolism)

The anabolic effect of androgens has been well documented in a number of animal and human studies (for review see reference 128), but it does not appear to be based on the above-described mechanism of action, e.g. in the prostatic cell. Skeletal muscles display very little 5α-reductase activity.[129, 151] Furthermore, some authors have found no significant binding of androgens in skeletal muscles,[129, 130] while others have observed testosterone binding.[131, 132] The molecular mechanism of anabolic action of testosterone has not yet been definitively clarified, but it most certainly appears to be different than in the typical androgen target organs such as the prostate.[133] It is therefore not certain on the basis of these data that cyproterone acetate has no antianabolic or catabolic effect.

Distinct suppression of growth as measured by body weight has been established in male rats treated with cyproterone acetate in the peripuberal period.[100]

Eight days of treatment with 50, 100, or 200 mg cyproterone acetate/ day p.o. led to a dose-dependent negative nitrogen balance in eight healthy male volunteers. The calcium balance was not affected to any significant extent, and increased phosphate elimination was observed only occasionally. The catabolic effect in a 77-year-old patient with prostatic carcinoma being treated with 200 mg cyproterone acetate/day was less than in the young male subjects.

As long as the diet contained sufficient calories and protein, the nitrogen, calcium, and phosphate balance remained positive in hirsute women being treated continuously with 100 mg cyproterone acetate/day or with sequential therapy after Hammerstein and Cupceancu[134] of 100 mg cyproterone acetate/day and 0.05 mg ethinyl estradiol/day.[127, 135]

These findings show that the catabolic effects of cyproterone acetate are greater in younger men than in older men and women. No particular catabolic effect is likely in patients with prostatic carcinoma on the basis of these studies. Moreover, osteoporosis has never been observed under cyproterone acetate treatment.

Influence of Cyproterone Acetate on Prolactin Secretion

No animal experimental studies are as yet available on the effect of cyproterone acetate on prolactin secretion. The already increased serum prolactin concentrations in girls with precocious puberty were further increased by treatment with 50 mg cyproterone acetate/day.[136] Normal serum prolactin concentrations have been measured in women undergoing sequential therapy with cyproterone acetate after Hammerstein and Cup-ceancu[134] for idiopathic hirsutism.

Four young male subjects who were treated for 20 days with 200 mg cyproterone acetate/day displayed no increase in the serum prolactin concentration.[127] Gräf et al.[137] however, found a 2- to 3-fold increase in the serum prolactin concentration in comparison to the control period before the start of treatment in 14 young men treated with 10 or 20 mg over a period of 24 weeks and in another eight men treated with 50 or 100 mg cyproterone acetate/day for up to 2 months, although the prolactin values measured were still within the normal range. No dose dependence of the effect of cyproterone acetate on prolactin secretion could be demonstrated in these studies.

Bartsch et al.[138] found no significant change in the prolactin concentrations 2 and 4 weeks after the start of therapy in prostatic carcinoma patients being treated with 300 mg cyproterone acetate IM every 2 weeks, whereas they did observe significant increase of prolactin after 3 months of therapy in orchiectomized patients being treated with cyproterone acetate in the same dosage (see also Chapter 15).

FACTS AND CONSIDERATIONS IN SUPPORT OF THE USE OF ANTIANDROGEN THERAPY IN PROSTATIC CARCINOMA

The most commonly employed forms of endocrine therapy of prostatic carcinoma are orchiectomy and estrogen therapy. So far there are no—or only preliminary—results available from comparative studies between cyproterone acetate and the two alternative forms of therapy (Chapter 15). On the other hand, a number of good therapeutic results with cyproterone acetate in the treatment of prostatic carcinoma have already been published.[152]

There are distinct differences between the individual therapies as regards the endocrine effects. Orchiectomy and estrogen therapy bring about a rapid fall of the serum androgen concentrations to about 10 to 20% of the normal values.[139-142] The fall under estrogen therapy is not as rapid as after orchiectomy.[140, 141] The remaining androgens are produced by the adrenal cortex[143] (above all androstenedione and dehydroepiandrosterone). On the other hand, a series of studies has revealed that even adrenal hyperplasia can occur under estrogen therapy and following orchiectomy, and also that secretion of adrenal androgens is even increased.[131] The increased secretion of androgens of adrenal origin is caused by intensified secretion of adrenocorticotropic hormone (ACTH) or by greater responsiveness of the adrenal cortex to ACTH. Antiandrogens inhibit the effect of adrenal androgens as well, while ACTH secretion and the responsiveness of the adrenal cortex to ACTH are not affected in adults (Chapter 11).

The fall in the androgen concentrations following administration of cyproterone acetate is dose-dependent. While 300 mg of cyproterone acetate IM every 2 weeks does not reduce the androgen concentrations entirely to castration levels,[138] castration levels are found under 200 mg/day p.o.[127, 144]

Serum estrogen concentrations are significantly reduced after orchiectomy and cyproterone acetate treatment.[138] The prolactin concentrations remain unchanged after orchiectomy in patients with prostatic carcinoma,[138] whereas significantly increased prolactin concentrations have been demonstrated under estrogen therapy[138, 142, 145] (see Chapters 21, 22). Cyproterone acetate, on the other hand, causes only slight increases in the prolactin level (Chapter 15). The only slight effect of cyproterone acetate on serum prolactin concentrations could also be the reason why gynecomastia occurs less frequently under cyproterone acetate treatment than under estrogen therapy.

The serum SHBG concentration remains unchanged following orchiectomy,[138] whereas a distinct increase in the SHBG-binding capacity has been demonstrated under estrogen therapy.[138, 148, 149]

The results regarding the effect of cyproterone acetate on SHBG concentrations are contradictory. Both reduced[138] and unchanged SHBG-binding capacity has been observed under cyproterone acetate treatment.[150] According to the above-quoted studies, the percentage of SHBG-bound testosterone remains unchanged.[138]

The loss of responsiveness to estrogens observed under long-term therapy could be attributable to desensitization of neural centers in which estrogens exert their negative feedback in respect to gonadotropin inhibition. Because of their different mechanisms of action, however, antiandrogens are very unlikely to display this tendency on therapeutic use. Perhaps this is the reason why a number of patients who have developed resistance to estrogens have again reacted to cyproterone acetate with remissions. An alternating form of treatment with estrogens and antiandrogens might indeed be worth trying.

The direct action of estrogens on the carcinoma cells is controversial. In animal experiments, estrogens have been found to exert an antimitotic effect only at very high doses. Since the estrogen doses used clinically are relatively low, it is unlikely that estrogens can exert a direct effect on the prostate or the carcinoma cells.

The serious—particularly cardiovascular—side effects of estrogens do not occur with cyproterone acetate. In consideration of all the above-described aspects, it can be said that antiandrogens constitute at least an alternative to the commonly used methods of endocrine therapy of prostatic carcinoma.

REFERENCES

1. Huggins, C. The physiology of the prostate gland. *Physiol. Rev. 25:* 117, 1945.
2. Huggins, C., and Clark, P. J. Quantitative studies of prostatic secretion. II. The effect of castration and of estrogen injection on the normal and on the hyperplastic prostate glands of dogs. *J. Exp. Med. 72:* 747, 1940.
3. Huggins, C., and Russell, P. S. Quantitative effects of hypophysectomy on testis and prostate of dogs. *Endocrinology 39:* 1, 1946.
4. Cabot, A. T. The question of castration for enlarged prostate. *Ann. Surg. 24:* 265, 1896.
5. von Frisch, A. *Handbuch der Urologie,* edited by A. von Frisch and G. Zuckerkandl, Vol. 3. Alfred Hölder, Wien, 1906.
6. White, J. W. The results of double castration in hypertrophy of the prostate. *Trans. Am. Surg. Assoc. 22:* 103, 1895.
7. Huggins, C., and Hodges, C. V. Studies on prostatic cancer. I. The effect of castration, of estrogen and of androgen injection on the normal and on the hyperplastic prostate glands of dogs. *Cancer Res. 1:* 293, 1941.
8. Huggins, C., Stevens, R. E., Jr., and Hodges, C. V. Studies on prostatic cancer. II. Effects of castration on advanced carcinoma of prostate gland. *Arch. Surg. 43:* 209, 1941.
9. Huggins, C., Scott, W. W., and Hodges, C. V. Studies on prostatic cancer. III. The effects of fever, of desoxy-corticosterone and of estrogen on clinical patients with metastatic carcinoma of the prostate. *J. Urol. 46:* 997, 1941.
10. Huggins, C., Scott, W. W. Bilateral adrenalectomy in prostatic cancer. Clinical features and urinary excretion of 17-ketosteroids and estrogen. *Ann. Surg. 122:* 1031, 1945.
11. Dorfman, R. I. Biological activity of antiandrogens. *Br. J. Dermatol. 82*(Suppl.6)*:* 3, 1970.
12. Saunders, H. L., Holden, K., and Kerwin, J. F. The antiandrogenic activity of 17α-methyl-B-nortestosterone (SK & F 7690). *Steroids 3:* 687, 1964.
13. Raynaud, J. P., Azadian-Boulanger, G., Bonné, C., Perronet, J., and Sakiz, E. Present trends in antiandrogen research. In *Androgens and Antiandrogens,* edited by L. Martini and M. Motta. Raven Press, New York, 1977, p. 281.
14. Loriaux, D. L., Menard, R., Taylor, A., and Santen, R. Spironolactone and endocrine dysfunction. *Ann. Intern. Med. 85:* 630, 1976.
15. Ober, K. P., and Hennesy, J. F. Spironolactone therapy for hirsutism in a hyperandrogenic woman. *Ann. Intern. Med. 89:* 643, 1978.

16. Neri, R. O., Florance, K., Koziol, P., and van Cleave, S. A biological profile of a nonsteroidal antiandrogen, Sch 13521 (4'-nitro-3'-trifluoromethylisobutyranilide). *Endocrinology 91:* 427, 1972.

17. Vigersky, R. A., Loriaux, D. L., Howards, S. S., Hodgen, G. B., Lipsett, M. B., and Chrambach, A. Androgen binding proteins of testis, epididymis, and plasma in man and monkey. *J. Clin. Invest. 58:* 1061, 1976.

18. Anderson, D. C. Sex-hormone binding globulin. *Clin. Endocrinol. 3:* 69, 1974.

19. Wilson, J. D. Metabolism of testicular androgens. In *Handbook of Physiology*, edited by R. O. Greep and E. B. Astwood, Sect. 7, Vol. 5. American Physiological Society, Washington D.C., 1975, p. 491.

20. Mainwaring, W. I. P. *The Mechanism of Action of Androgens: A Survey, Monographs on Endocrinology,* Vol. 10. Springer, New York, 1977.

21. Higgins, S. J., and Gehring, U. Molecular mechanisms of steroid hormone action. *Adv. Cancer Res. 28:* 313, 1978.

22. Giorgi, E. P., Shirley, I. M., Grant, J. K., and Stewart, J. C. Androgen dynamics in vitro in the human prostate gland. Effect of cyproterone and cyproterone acetate. *Biochem. J. 132:* 465, 1973.

23. Whalen, R. E., Luttge, W. G., and Green, R. Effects of the antiandrogen cyproterone acetate on the uptake of 1,2-^{3}H-testosterone in neural and peripheral tissues of the castrate rat. *Endocrinology 84:* 217, 1969.

24. Baulieu, E.-E., Jung, I., Blondeau, J. P., and Zobel, P. C. Androgen receptors in rat ventral prostate. In *Advances in Biosciences 7*, edited by G. Raspé. Pergamon Press-Vieweg, Oxford, 1971, p. 179.

25. Orestano, F., Altwein, J. E., Knapstein, P., and Bandhauer, K. Mode of action of progesterone, gestonorone capronate (Depostat) and cyproterone acetate (Adrocur) on the metabolism of testosterone in human prostatic adenoma: in vitro and in vivo investigations. *J. Steroid. Biochem. 6:* 845, 1975.

26. Belham, J. E., and Neal, G. E. Testosterone action in rat ventral prostate. *Biochem. J. 125:* 81, 1971.

27. Massa, R., and Martini, L. Interference with the 5α-reductase system. *Gynecol. Invest. 2:* 253, 1972.

28. Stern, J. M., and Eisenfeld, A. J. Androgen accumulation and binding to macromolecules in seminal vesicles: inhibition by cyproterone. *Science 166:* 233, 1969.

29. Verhoeven, G., and de Moor, P. Nucleus associated 5α-reductase activity in the rat. *Gynecol. Invest. 2:* 290, 1971.

30. Walsh, P. C., and Korenman, S. G. Mechanism of androgenic action: effect of specific intracellular inhibitors. *J. Urol. 105:* 850, 1971.

31. Fang, S., and Liao, S. Antagonistic action of antiandrogens on the formation of a specific dihydrotestosterone receptor complex in rat ventral prostate. *Mol. Pharmacol. 5:* 420, 1969.

32. Baulieu, E.-E., and Jung, I. A prostatic cytosol receptor. *Biochem. Biophys. Res. Commun. 38:* 599, 1970.

33. Belham, J. E., Neal, G. E., and Williams, D. C. The reception of androgens in the rat ventral prostate. *Biochem. J. 114:* 32P, 1969.

34. Belham, J. E., Neal, G. E., and Williams, D. C. Testosterone metabolism in the rat ventral prostate. *Biochim. Biophys. Acta 187:* 159, 1969.

35. Fang, S., Anderson, K. M., and Liao, S. Receptor proteins for androgens. *J. Biol. Chem. 244:* 6584, 1969.

36. Fang, S., and Liao, S. Androgen receptors. *J. Biol. Chem. 246:* 16, 1971.

37. Geller, J., and McCoy, K. Correlation of biologic and biochemical effects of antiandrogens on rat ventral prostate. *Clin. Res. 20:* 177, 1972.

38. Jung, I., and Baulieu, E. E. Neo-nuclear androgen receptor in rat ventral prostate. *Biochemie, 53:* 807, 1971.

39. Bruchovsky, N. Molekulare Wirkung von Androgenen und Antiandrogenen. In *Androgenisierungserscheinungen bei der Frau*, edited by J. Hammerstein, U. Lachnit-Fixson, F. Neumann, and G. Plewig. Excerpta Medica, Amsterdam, 1979, p. 7.

40. Dahnke, H.-G., Scheuer, A., and Mosebach, K.-O. Der Einfluss von Testosteron und Cyproteronacetat auf die Mitoserate, den Nukleinsäurestoffwechsel und die Histomorphologie der Vesikulardrüsen von Ratten. 17. Symp. Dtsch. Ges. Endokrin. (abstr. 35).

Acta Endocrinol. 152: 35, 1971.

41. Jäger, E., Mosebach, K.-O., Blumenthal, H.-P., and Scheuer, A. The influence of cyproterone acetate on the uptake of testosterone and on the DNA- and RNA-amount in liver, prostate and seminal vesicles of immature male rats in vivo. *Acta Endocrinol* [Suppl.] *138:* 43, 1969.

42. Chandra, P., Orii, H., and Wacker, A. Effect of an antiandrogenic steroid on the testosterone-stimulated activity of aggregate polymerase in the prostate nuclei of rats. *Hoppe Seylers Z. Physiol. Chem. 348:* 1085, 1967.

43. Becker, H., Düsterberg, B., and Klosterhalfen, H. Bioavailability of cyproterone acetate after oral and intramuscular application in men. *Urol Int. 35:* 381, 1980.

44. Hümpel, M., Dogs, G., Wendt, H., and Speck, U. Plasmaspiegel und Pharmakokinetik von Cyproteronacetat nach oraler Applikation als 50-mg-Tablette bei 5 Männern. *Arzneim. Forsch. 28:* 319, 1978.

45. Düsterberg, B., Hümpel, M., and Wendt, H. Plasma levels of active ingredients after single and repeated administration of a new oral contraceptive containing 2 mg cyproterone acetate and 0.05 mg ethinylestradiol (Diane). *Acta Obstet. Gynecol. Scand.* [Suppl.] *88:* 27, 1979.

46. Hümpel, M., Wendt, H., Dogs, G., Weiss, C., Rietz, S., and Speck, U. Intraindividual comparison of pharmacokinetic parameters of D-norgestrel, lynestrenol and cyproterone acetate in 6 women. *Contraception 16:* 199, 1977.

47. Gerhards, E., Gutsche, H., and Riemann, J. Biodynamik von Cyproteronacetat nach oraler Verabreichung beim Menschen. *Arzneim. Forsch. 13:* 1550, 1973.

48. Bhargawa, A. S., Seeger, A., and Günzel, P. Isolation and identification of 15-β-hydroxy cyproterone acetate in dog, monkey and man. *Steroids 30:* 407, 1977.

49. Speck, U., Jentsch, D., Kühne, G., Schulze, P. E., and Wendt, H. Bioverfügbarkeit und Pharmakokinetik von Cyproteronacetat-^{14}C nach Applikation als 50-mg-Tablette. *Arzneim. Forsch. 26:* 1717, 1976.

50. Neumann, F., and Steinbeck, H. Antiandrogens. In *Handbook of Experimental Pharmacology*, Vol. 35/2, edited by O. Eichler, A. Farah, H. Herken, and A. D. Welch. Springer, Berlin, 1974, Ch. VI, p. 235.

51. Gräf, K.-J., Brotherton, J., and Neumann, F. Clinical uses of antiandrogens (other than for hypersexuality and sexual deviations). In *Handbook of Experimental Pharmacology*, Vol. 35/2, edited by O. Eichler, A. Farah, H. Herken, and A. D. Welch. Springer, Berlin, 1974, Ch. VII, p. 485.

52. Tunn, U. W., Schüring, B., Senge, Th., Neumann, F., Schweickert, H. U., and Rohr, H. P. Morphometric analysis of prostates in castrated dogs after treatment with androstanediol, estradiol and cyproterone acetate. *Invest. Urol. 18:* 289, 1981.

53. Tunn, U., Senge, Th., Schenck, B., and Neumann, F. Biochemical and histological studies on prostates in castrated dogs after treatment with androstanediol, estradiol and cyproterone acetate. *Acta Endocrinol, 91:* 373, 1979.

54. Tunn, U., Senge, Th., Schenck, B., and Neumann, F. Effects of cyproterone acetate on experimental induced canine prostate hyperplasia. A morphological and histochemical study. *Urol. Int. 35:* 125, 1980.

55. Rohr, H. P., Berchtold, C., Bergamin, A., Figilister, Ch., Oberholzer, M., Bartsch, G., Tannenbaum, M., Tunn, U., Neumann, F., and Guggenheim, R. Hormonal influences on the dog prostate—a correlation study with light electron microscopy, transmission- and scanning electron microscopy. *Scanning Electr. Microsc. 3:* 665, 1979.

56. Morse, H. C., Leach, D. R., Rowley, M. J., and Heller, C. G. Effect of cyproterone acetate on sperm concentration, seminal fluid volume, testicular cytology and levels of plasma and urinary ICSH, FSH and testosterone in normal men. *J. Reprod. Fertil. 32:* 365, 1973.

57. Neumann, F., Richter, K.-D., and Senge, Th. Animal models in the study of antiprostatic drugs. In International Symposium on Endocrine Control of the Prostate, Helsingborg/Sweden, June 1975. *Vitam. Horm. 33:* 103, 1975.

58. Neumann, F., Richter, K.-D., Schenck, B., Tunn, U., and Senge, Th. Action of antiandrogens on accessory sexual glands. In *Steriod Receptors, Metabolism and Prostatic Cancer*, edited by F. H. Schröder and H. J. de Voogt. Excerpta Medica, Amsterdam, 1980, pp. 22–40.

59. Neumann, F., Tunn, U., Funke, P. J., and Senge, Th. Male accessory sex glands—experimental basis and animal models in prostatic tumour research. In *Animal Models in Human Reproduction*, edited by M. Serio and L. Martini. Raven Press, New York, 1980, pp. 249–282.

60. Smolev, J. K., Coffey, D. S., and Scott, W. W. Experimental models for the study of prostatic adenocarcinoma. *J. Urol. 118:* 216, 1977.

61. Okada, K., and Schröder, F. H. Human prostatic carcinoma in cell culture: preliminary report on the development and characterization of an epithelial cell line (EB 33). *Urol. Res. 2:* 111, 1974.

62. Okada, K., Schroeder, F. H., Jellinghaus, W., Wullstein, H. K. and Heinemeyer, H. M. Human prostatic adenoma and carcinoma: transplantation of cultured cells and primary tissue fragments in "nude" mice. *Invest. Urol., 13:* 395, 1976.

63. Höhn, W. Personal communication, 1980.

64. Senge, Th. Personal communication, 1980.

65. Senge, Th., Richter, K.-D., and Reis, H. E. Der Einfluss von Sexualsteroiden auf Prostataadenomheterotransplantate. Verh. Dtsch. Ges. Urol. *24:* 234, 1973.

66. Forsberg, J. G., and Ingemanson, C. A. Successful growth of human columnar cervical epithelium grafted into neonatal rats. *Acta Obstet. Gynecol. Scand. 46:* 581, 1967.

67. Richter, K. D., Senge, Th., and Reis, H. E. Morphologisches und cytochemisches Verhalten von menschlichem Prostatagewebe nach Heterotransplantation. *Z. Gesamte Exp. Med. 155:* 253, 1971.

68. Senge, Th., Richter, K. D., and Lunglmayr, G. Vitality of human adenomatous prostatic tissue grafted into neonatal rats. *Invest. Urol. 10:* 115, 1972.

69. Faul, P., Klosterhalfen, H., and Schmiedt, E. Erfahrungen mit der Feinnadelbiopsie (Saug- bzw. Aspirationsbiopsie nach Franzén) der Prostata. *Urologe 10:* 120, 1971.

70. Franks, L. M. Estrogen-treated prostatic cancer. *Cancer 13:* 490, 1960.

71. Fergusson, J. D. The basis of endocrine therapy. In *Endocrine Therapy in Malignant Disease*, edited by B. Y. Stoll. W. B. Saunders, Philadelphia, 1972, p. 237.

72. Huggins, C., Scott, W. W., and Hodges, C. V. Studies on prostatic cancer. III. The effects of fever, of desoxy-corticosterone and of estrogen on clinical patients with metastatic carcinoma of the prostate. *J. Urol. 46:* 997, 1941.

73. Kahle, P. I., Schenken, I. R., and Burns, E. L. Clinical and pathological effects of diethylstilbestrol and diethylstilbestrol diprorionate on carcinoma of the prostate gland. *J. Urol. 50:* 711, 1943.

74. Ruppert, H. Zur Histopathologie der Hormonbehandlung beim Prostatakrebs. *Z. Urol. 46:* 443, 1953.

75. Neumann, F., Elger, W., Nishino, Y., and Steinbeck, H. Probleme der Dosisfindung: Sexualhormone. *Arzneim. Forsch. 27:* 296, 1977.

76. Neumann, F., Schleusener, A., and Albring, M. Pharmakologie der Antiandrogene. In *Androgenisierungserscheinungen bei der Frau—Akne, Seborrhö, androgenetische Alopezie und Hirsutismus*, edited by J. Hammerstein, U. Lachnit-Fixson, F. Neumann, and G. Plewig. Amsterdam, Excerpta Medica, 1979, p. 149.

77. Neumann, F., and Schenck, B. New antiandrogens and their mode of action. IPPF Congress of Agents Affecting Control of Fertility in the Male, New Delhi, October 1974. *J. Reprod. Fertil. [Suppl.] 24:* 129, 1976.

78. Neumann, F., Gräf, K. -J., Hasan, S. H., Schenck, B., and Steinbeck, H. Central actions of antiandrogens. In *Androgens and Antiandrogens.* International Meeting on Androgens and Antiandrogens, Milan, April 1976, edited by L. Martini and M. Motta. Raven Press, New York, 1977, p. 163.

79. Back, D. J., Glover, T. D., Shenton, J. C., and Boyd, G. P. Some effects of cyproterone acetate on the reproductive physiology of the male rat. *J. Reprod. Fertil. 49:* 237, 1977.

80. Neri, R. O., Florance, K., Koziol, P., and van Cleave, S. A biological profile of a nonsteroidal antiandrogen, Sch 13521 (4'-nitro-3'-trifluoromethylisobutyranilide). *Endocrinology 91:* 427, 1972.

81. Setty, B. S. Remark during general discussion. IPFF Congress of Agents Affecting Control of Fertility in the Male, New Delhi, October 1974.

82. Schenck, B., and Neumann, F. Influence of antiandrogens on Sertoli cell function and intratesticular androgen transport. *Int. J. Androl. 1:* 459, 1978.

83. Neumann, F., Diallo, F. A., Hasan, S. H., Schenck, B., and Traoré, I. The influence of pharmaceutical compounds on male fertility. *Andrologia 8:* 203, 1976.
84. Horn, H.-J. Administration of antiandrogens in hypersexuality and sexual deviations. In *Handbook of Experimental Pharmacology*, Vol. 35/2, edited by O. Eichler, A. Farah, H. Herken, and A. D. Welch. Berlin, Springer, 1974, p. 543.
85. Beach, F., and Westbrook, W. Morphological and behavioral effects of an "antiandrogen" in male rats. *J. Endocrinol. 42:* 379, 1968.
86. Bloch, G. J., and Davidson, J. M. Behavioral and somatic responses to the antiandrogen cyproterone (1,2α-methylene-6-chloro-; Δ⁶-17α-hydroxyprogesterone). *Horm. Behav. 2:* 11, 1971.
87. Whalen, R. E., and Edwards, D. A. Effects of the antiandrogen cyproterone acetate on mating behavior and seminal vesicle tissue in male rats. *Endocrinology 84:* 155, 1969.
88. Whalen, R. E., and Luttge, W. G. Contraceptive properties of the antiandrogen cyproterone acetate. *Nature (Lond.), 223:* 633, 1969.
89. Zucker, I. Effects of an anti-androgen on the mating behavior of male guinea-pigs and rats. *J. Endocrinol. 35:* 209, 1966.
90. Horst, P., and Bader, J. Untersuchungen zur Bedeutung der Jungebermast. 2. Mitteilung: Versuche zur Unterdrückung des Sexualgeruches. *Züchtungskunde 41:* 248, 1969.
91. Schmidtke, D., and Schmidtke, H. O. Ein neues Antiandrogen beim Hund. *Kleintierpraxis 13:* 146, 1968.
92. Laschet, U., and Laschet, L. Psychopharmacotherapy of sex offenders with cyproterone acetate. *Pharmakopsychiatr. Neuro-Psychopharmakol. 4:* 99, 1971.
93. Laschet, U., and Laschet, L. Einfluss von Cyproteronacetat auf das neuroendokrine System des Menschen. *Life Sci. Monogr. 2:* 89, 1972.
94. Laschet, U., and Laschet, L. Antiandrogens in the treatment of sexual deviations. *J. Steroid Biochem. 6:* 821, 1975.
95. Horn, H. -J. Somatische Behandlungsmethode im Strafvollzug. *Kriminol. Gegenwartsfragen 10:* 144, 1972.
96. Horn, H. -J., Luthe, R., and Schneider-Jonietz, B. Die medizinische und soziale Indikation der Antiandrogen-Behandlung. *Int. Pharmakopsychiatry 5:* 23, 1970.
97. Ott, F. Hypersexualität, Antiandrogene und Hodenfunktion. *Praxis 57:* 218, 1968.
98. Ott, F., and Hoffet, H. Beeinflussung von Libido, Potenz and Hodenfunktion durch Antiandrogene. *Schweiz. Med. Wochenschr. 98:* 1812, 1968.
99. Ott, F., Hoffet, H., and Hodel, H. Über die Erholung der Spermiogenese nach Behandlung mit Cyproteronacetat. *Schweiz. Med. Wochenschr. 102:* 1124, 1972.
100. Steinbeck, H., and Neumann, F. Effect of cyproterone acetate on puberty. *J. Reprod. Fertil. 26:* 59, 1971.
101. Hertel, P., Kramer, M., and Neumann, F. Einfluss eines Antiandrogens (Cyproteronacetat) auf Knochenwachstum und Knochenreifung männlicher Ratten. *Arzneim. Forsch. 19:* 1777, 1969.
102. Schenck, B., and Neumann, F. Einfluss von Sexualhormonen auf Knochenreifung und Knochenwachstum weiblicher Ratten. *Arzneim. Forsch. 23:* 887, 1973.
103. Neumann, F. Antiandrogene—Grundlagen und experimentelle Befunde an der Haut. In *Haar und Haarkrankheiten*, edited by C. E. Orfanos. Gustav Fischer, Stuttgart, 1979, Ch. 40, p. 961.
104. Neumann, F., Schleusener, A., and Hümpel, M. Antiandrogene—pharmakologische Grundlagen. *Gynäkologe 12:* 228, 1979.
105. Hammerstein, J., Lachnit-Fixson, U., Neumann, F., and Plewig, G. Androgenisierungserscheinungen bei der Frau—Akne, Seborrhö, androgenetische Alopezie und Hirsutismus. Vorträge und Diskussionen eines Symposiums, Berlin, February 23–24, 1979. Excerpta Medica, Amsterdam, 1979, p. 306.
106. Neumann, F., Elger, W., and Steinbeck, H. Antiandrogens and reproductive development. *Philos. Trans. R. Soc., Lond. [Biol. Sci.] 259:* 179, 1970.
107. Neumann, F., Steinbeck, H., and Elger, W. Sexualdifferenzierung. 16. Symp. Dtsch. Ges. Endokrinol., Ulm, "Endokrinologie der Entwicklung und Reifung." Springer, Berlin, 1970, p. 58.
108. Neumann, F., von Berswordt-Wallrabe, R., Elger, W., Steinbeck, H., Hahn, J. D., and Kramer, M. Aspects of androgen-dependent events as studied by antiandrogens. *Recent Prog. Horm. Res. 26:* 337, 1970.

109. Neumann, F. Endokrinologische Aspekte der Geschlechts-differenzierung. *Gynäkologe* *9:* 16, 1976.

110. Hamada, H., Neumann, F., and Junkmann, K. Intrauterine antimaskuline Beeinflussung von Rattenfeten durch ein stark gestagen wirksames Steroid. *Acta Endocrinol 44:* 380, 1963.

111. Doménico, A., and Neumann, F. Wirkung von antiandrogen wirksamen Steroiden auf die Funktion und Morphologie der Nebennierenrinden von Ratten. 12. Symp. Deutsch. Ges. Endokrinol., Wiesbaden 1966. Springer, Berlin, 1966, p. 312.

112. Denef, C., Vendeputte, M., and de Moor, P. Paradoxical effect of the androgen antagonist cyproterone acetate on steroid metabolism in the rat. *Endocrinology 83:* 945, 1968.

113. Starka, L., Motlik, K., and Schreiber, U. Effect of the antiandrogen cyproterone and cyproterone acetate on male rat adrenals. *Physiol. Bohemoslov. 21:* 233, 1972.

114. Panesar, N. S., Herries, D. G., and Stitch, S. R. Effects of cyproterone and cyproterone acetate on the adrenal gland of the rat: studies in vivo and in vitro. *J. Endocrinol. 80:* 229, 1979.

115. Neri, R. O., Monahan, M. D., Meyer, J. G., Alfonso, B. A., and Tabachnik, I. A. Biological studies on an antiandrogen (SH 714). *Eur. J. Pharmacol. 1:* 438, 1967.

116. Ziegler, B., Lux, B., and Kubatsch, B. The effect of cyproterone acetate on the adrenal of the male hamster. *Acta Endocrinol. 82:* 127, 1976.

117. Girard, J., and Baumann, J. B. Secondary adrenal insufficiency due to cyproterone acetate. *Pediatr. Res. 9:* 669, 1975.

118. Girard, J., and Baumann, J. B. Corticotropin releasing hormone and corticotropin suppression by an antiandrogenic drug (cyproterone acetate), a therapeutic possibility for congenital adrenal hyperplasia. In *Congenital Adrenal Hyperplasia,* edited by P. A. Lee, L. P. Plotnick, A. A. Kowarski, and C. J. Migeon. University Park Press, Baltimore, 1977, p. 217.

119. Girard, J., Baumann, J. B., Bühler, U., Zuppinger, K., Haas, H. G., Staub, J. J., and Wyss, H. I. Cyproterone acetate and ACTH adrenal function. *J. Clin. Endocrinol. Metab. 47:* 581, 1978.

120. Winkler, G. K., and Harkness, R. A. The effect of a strongly progestational steroid on adrenal function in the guinea pig. *J. Endocrinol. 30:* 111, 1964.

121. Ewald, W. Inhibierung von Enzymen der Steroidhormon-Biosynthese aus Nebennieren und Testes durch Cyproteron und einige anabole Steroide. In Endokrinologie der Entwicklung und Reifung. *Symp. Dtsch. Ges. Endokrinologie. 16:* 426, 1970.

122. Laschet, U., and Laschet, I. Adrenocortical function, corticotrophic responsiveness and fertility of men during long-term treatment with cyproterone acetate. In Abstract Papers 3rd Int. Congr. Hormonal Steroids, Hamburg, September 1970, edited by L. Martini. Excerpta Medica, Amsterdam, I.C.S. 210, Abstr. 415, 1970.

123. Smals, A. G. H., Kloppenburg, D. W. C., Goverde, H. J. M., and Benraad, T. J. The effect of cyproterone acetate on the pituitary-adrenal axis of hirsute women. *Acta Endocrinol. 87:* 352, 1978.

124. Bossi, E., Zurbrügg, R. P., and Joss, E. E. Cyproteronacetat und Pubertas praecox. *Med. Mitt. Schering Nr. 2:* 19, 1973.

125. Helge, H. Frühreife. *Mschr. Kinderheilk. 121:* 636, 1973.

126. Girard, J., and Baumann, J. B. Secondary adrenal insufficiency due to cyproterone acetate. *J. Endocrinol. 69:* 13P, 1976.

127. von Wayen, R. G. A., and van den Enden, A. Metabolic effects of cyproterone acetate. In *Androgenization in Women. Acne, Seborrhoe, Androgenetic Alopecia and Hirsutism,* edited by J. Hammerstein, U. Lachnit-Fixson, F. Neumann, and G. Plewig. Excerpta Medica, Amsterdam, 1980, pp. 246–258.

128. Kochakian, C. D. Anabolic-androgenic steroids. In *Handbook of Experimental Pharmacology,* Vol. 43, edited by G. V. R. Born, O. Eichler, A. Farah, H. Herken, and A. D. Welch. Springer, Berlin, 1976.

129. Mainwaring, W. I. P., and Mangan, F. R. A study of the androgen receptors in a variety of androgen-sensitive tissues. *J. Endocrinol. 59:* 121, 1973.

130. Krieg, M., Szalay, R., and Voigt, K. D. Binding and metabolism of testosterone and 5α-dihydrotestosterone in bulbo-cavernosus levator ani (BCLA) of male rats in vivo and in vitro. *J. Steroid. Biochem. 5:* 453, 1974.

131. Jung, I., and Baulieu, E. -E. Testosterone cytosol "receptor" in the rat levator ani muscle. *Nature [New Biol.] 237:* 24, 1972.

132. Michel, M. G., and Baulieu, E.-E. Receptor cytosoluble des androgènes dans un muscle strié squelettique. *C. R. Acad. Sci. [D] (Paris) 279:* 421, 1974.

133. Kochakian, C. D. Definition of androgens and protein anabolic steroids. *Pharmacol. Ther. Biol. 1:* 149, 1975.

134. Hammerstein, J., and Cupceancu, B. Behandlung des Hirsutismus mit Cyproterona-cetat. *Dtsch. Med. Wochenschr. 94:* 829, 1969.

135. van Wayen, R. G. A., and van den Enden, A. Clinical-pharmacological investigation of cyproterone acetate. *Gynecol. Invest. 2:* 282, 1972.

136. Fonzo D., Angeli, A., Sivieri, R., Andriola, S., Frajria, R., and Ceresa, F. Hyperpro-lactinemia in girls with idiopathic precocious puberty under prolonged treatment with cyproterone acetate. *J. Clin. Endocrinol. Metab. 45:* 164, 1977.

137. Gräf, K. -J., Schmidt-Gollwitzer, M., Koch, U. J., Lorenz, F., and Hammerstein, J. Hyperprolactinaemia induced by cyproterone acetate in human subjects. *Acta Endo-crinol. 87*(Suppl. 215): 96, 1978.

138. Bartsch, W., Horst, H. -J., Becker, H., and Nehse, G. Sex hormone binding globulin binding capacity, testosterone, 5α-dihydrotestosterone, oestradiol and prolactin in plasma of patients with prostatic carcinoma under various types of hormonal treatment. *Acta Endocrinol. 85:* 650, 1977.

139. Young, H. H., and Kent, J. R. Plasma testosterone levels in patients with prostatic carcinoma before and after treatment. *J. Urol. 99:* 788, 1968.

140. Boyns, A. R., Cole, E. N., Phillips, M. E. A., Hillier, S. G., Cameron, E. H. D., Griffiths, K., Shahmanesh, M., Feneley, R. C. L., and Hartog, M. Plasma prolactin, GH, LH, FSH, TSH and testosterone during treatment of prostatic carcinoma with oestrogens. *Eur. J. Cancer 10:* 445, 1974.

141. Jönsson, G., Olsson, A. M., Luttrop, W., Cekan, Z., Purvis, K., and Diczfalusy, E. Treatment of prostatic carcinoma with various types of estrogen derivatives. *Vitam. Horm. 33:* 351, 1975.

142. Harper, M. E., Peeling, W. B., Cowley, T., Brownsey, B. G., Phillips, M. E., Groom, G., Fahmy, D. R., and Griffiths, K. Plasma steroid and protein hormone concentrations in patients with prostatic carcinoma, before and during oestrogen therapy. *Acta Endocrinol. 81:* 409, 1976.

143. Cowley, T. H., Brownsey, B. G., Harper, M. E., Peeling, W. B., and Griffiths, K. The effect of ACTH on plasma testosterone and androstenedione concentrations in patients with prostatic carcinoma. *Acta Endocrinol. 81:* 310, 1976.

144. Schoones, R., Schalch, D. S., and Murphy, G. P. The hormonal effects of antiandrogen (SH 714) treatment in man. *Invest. Urol. 8:* 635, 1971.

145. Mortimer, C. H., Besser, G. M., Goldie, D. J., Hook, J., and McNeilly, A. S. The TSH, FSH and prolactin responses to continuous infusions of TRH and the effects of oestrogen administration in normal males. *Clin. Endocrinol. 3:* 97, 1974.

146. Thomas, J. A., and Manandhar, M. Effects of prolactin and/or testosterone on nucleic acid levels in prostate glands of normal and castrated rats. *J. Endocrinol. 65:* 149, 1975.

147. Johansson, R. Effect of some synandrogens and antiandrogens on the conversion of testosterone to dihydrotestosterone in the cultured rat ventral prostate. *Acta Endocrinol. 81:* 398, 1976.

148. Vermeulen, A., Verdonck, L., van der Straeten, M., and Orie, N. Capacity of the testosterone-binding globulin in human plasma and influence of specific binding of testosterone on its metabolic clearance rate. *J. Clin. Endocrinol. 29:* 1470, 1969.

149. Stahl, F., Dörner, G., Knappe, G., and Schnorr, D. Total and free testosterone in plasma of hypo- and agonadal men. *Endokrinologie 66:* 152, 1975.

150. Murray, M. A. F., Bancroft, J. H. J., Anderson, D. C., Tennent, T. G., and Carr, P. J. Endocrine changes in male sexual deviants after treatment with anti-androgens, oestrogens or tranquillizers. *J. Endocrinol. 67:* 179, 1975.

151. Wilson, J. D., and Gloyna, R. E. The intranuclear metabolism of testosterone in the accessory organs of reproduction. *Recent Prog. Horm. Res. 26:* 309, 1970.

152. Jacobi, G. H., Altwein, J. E., Kurth, K. H., Basting, R., and Hohenfellner, R. Treatment of advanced prostatic cancer with parenteral cyproterone acetate: a phase III random-ised trial. *Br. J. Urol. 52:* 208, 1980.

Editorial Comment to Chapter 14

This chapter nicely reflects the lengthy and extensive experience Prof. Neumann has accumulated, making him an authority in the field of antiandrogens. For his pioneer work, he was awarded the Schoeller-Junkmann-Price Award in 1965. A scientific generation later, his associates (Th. S. and U. T.), co-authors of this chapter, were also given this high-ranking scientific distinction by the German Society of Endocrinology in 1973 and 1980, respectively, for their work incorporated in this chapter (references 52 to 54). This is a reflection of the continuing excellence of the purposeful efforts of this group.

G. H. J.
R. H.

15

Clinical Experience with Cyproterone Acetate for Palliation of Inoperable Prostate Cancer

G. H. Jacobi, M.D.
U. Tunn, M.D.
Th. Senge, M.D.

The aim of this chapter is to summarize the current knowledge of the clinical use of cyproterone acetate for the treatment of prostatic carcinoma on the basis of the biological properties of this antiandrogen outlined in Chapter 14.

The interpretation of previous studies using cyproterone acetate for prostatic cancer has been limited by several factors:

1. The inconsistent route of application, either orally or by intramuscular injection
2. The variety of dose regimens
3. Inconsistent and therefore noncomparable evaluation of tumor stage
4. Mixed data on either previously treated or newly diagnosed cases
5. Some patients included with secondary hormone unresponsiveness (hormone autonomy)
6. Cyproterone acetate only rarely given as monotherapy, usually in combination with castration
7. Inconsistent criteria of treatment response
8. Inconsistent therapeutical intentions (usually palliative intent in either asymptomatic, symptomatic or terminal stages)
9. Lack of controls under randomized conditions.

RECENT DATA ON ORAL APPLICATION

Until 1977, cyproterone acetate was only available in the oral form of 50-mg tablets. Therefore, the current data almost exclusively cover oral treatment of cyproterone acetate. In previous reviews[9, 12] we have analyzed more than 300 patients treated with oral doses of 100 to 300 mg (in most cases with an average daily dose of 200 mg). With the exception of Bracci and Di Silverio's report,[3] according to which cyproterone acetate was initially combined with orchiectomy, more than half of the patients had before been unsuccessfully treated with other contrasexual measures, whereas about 40% of patients had had no previous treatment. Most striking was the effect of cyproterone acetate on the local tumor mass in the group of patients previously untreated. Scott and Schirmer[18] reported a marked reduction of the size of the local tumor in seven of 10, Wein and Murphy[20] in 16 of 25 cases, Tveter et al.[19] in seven of 16, Isurugi et al.[8] in even 14 of 15 patients. In an excellently defined group of 15 patients followed for 2 months during oral treatment with 200 mg/day, Varenhorst[20] reported a regression of primary tumor mass in 15 patients, a moderately to marked cytological regression upon rebiopsy in eight cases, and an overall objective response in 10 patients. Further favorable therapy effects include the improvement of bone pain due to osseous metastases, decrease of serum acid phosphatase, improvement of general condition and performance as well as micturition symptoms. Except for the limited study by Varenhorst,[20] in which oral cyproterone acetate treatment was compared with orchiectomy and estrogens in a randomized fashion, and proved to be essentially as effective as the other forms of treatment, only one other randomized trial has been reported to date.[6] In this latter study the oral dose of 250 mg cyproterone acetate is compared with 200 mg medroxyprogesterone acetate and with 3 mg stilbestrol per day. By March 1980, cyproterone acetate had proved to be equally as effective as the other treatment arms with fewer side effects.[2]

Simultaneous Combination of Cyproterone Acetate with Other Contrasexual Measures

CYPROTERONE ACETATE PLUS CASTRATION

Reports on this simultaneous combination of operative and medical castration derive exclusively from Italy. On this strategy, data on hundreds of cases are available from Bracci and Di Silverio,[3] Bracci,[4] and Giuliani and co-workers.[7, 16] Bracci[4] reports on only 10 cases with cyproterone acetate as the single treatment, and in these cases, the response to this agent was used as an indicator for hormone dependence and as a selection criterion for further hormone manipulation. Giuliani and co-workers[7] articulated the presumption that cyproterone acetate given additionally after orchiectomy would result in a further depression of the remaining plasma testosterone. These authors therefore treated their patients with a minimal dose of 150 mg and a maximal one of 300 mg, depending on the amount of residual testosterone. We feel, however, that the only additional beneficial effect of cyproterone acetate along with castration might be the lowering of adrenal androgen formation and the direct intraprostatic mode of action of cyproterone acetate *along with* the residual amount of postcastration testosterone supplied to the prostate. With respect to the effects specific to cyproterone acetate, the reported Italian results are not interpretable, because the effect of castration *versus* cyproterone acetate cannot be differentiated. Controlled trials applying cyproterone acetate alone *versus* castration alone *versus* the combination of both are not yet available.

CYPROTERONE ACETATE PLUS ANTIPROLACTINS

We have administered the antiprolactin *bromocriptine* together with weekly intramuscular doses of 300 mg of cyproterone acetate to seven patients with previous antiandrogen treatment to suppress the therapy-induced hyperprolactinemia. In six patients, a significant improvement of general performance was observed.[10] Klosterhalfen and co-workers[14] have used *lisuride*, another prolactin suppressor, in combination with oral cyproterone acetate treatment in 10 hormonally relapsed cases and observed a significant relief of bone pain due to metastases in five; objective remissions did not occur. Favorable results in five patients using the combination of intramuscular cyproterone acetate along with high doses of antiprolactins have also been observed by Altwein[1] with respect to objective remission of soft tissue metastases or renal failure due to extensive lymphatic tumor disease. However, no controlled trials on this type of combination treatment are available to date.

SIMULTANEOUS COMBINATION OF CYPROTERONE ACETATE AND ESTROGENS

Nothing is known about this type of combination treatment and according to a recent *European Organization for Research on Treatment of Cancer* (EORTC) proposal, oral doses of 150 mg cyproterone acetate per day plus 1 mg diethylstilbestrol per day will be investigated in a pilot study. The main objectives of this study will be *first*, to see whether the combination of the two drugs with contrasexual activity has a therapeutic effect on patients with advanced prostatic cancer that is equal to or better than either of the two, and *second*, to see whether this combination is well-tolerated and whether the side effects are less apparent because of the lower dosages of both components.[5]

INTRAMUSCULAR ADMINISTRATION OF CYPROTERONE ACETATE

Since 1977, cyproterone acetate has been available in intramuscular form of 300-mg ampules in Germany, and since 1980 prostatic carcinoma has also been registered as an indication. In 1977, a multicentric prospective randomized study was initiated in Europe now including 191 evaluable patients from eight centers in West Germany, two centers in West Berlin, and one institution in Austria and the Netherlands each. The goal of this study was to compare short-term effect and toxicity of cyproterone acetate *versus* conventional estrogen treatment in previously untreated patients with inoperable, far advanced prostatic carcinoma (88% = stage C, 27% = stage D_2).

The following treatment protocol was used:

1. Cyproterone acetate, 300 mg IM/week for 6 months (95 patients)
2. Estradiol undecylate, 100 mg IM/month for 6 months (96 patients).

Criteria for exclusion were any pretreatment specific for prostatic carcinoma, pre-existing cardiovascular or hepatic disease, urinary obstruction requiring catheter drainage, a life expectancy of less than 6 months, and additional primary malignancy.

The patients were followed for at least 6 months according to the protocol given in Figure 15.1. Since it was felt that in advanced disease, short-term treatment would allow a valid comparison, the study was limited to 6 months. Treatment was stopped if, at any time, tumor progression required other forms of treatment, or cardiovascular or hepatic side effects occurred and necessitated such a change. Estradiol undecylate was chosen because it is a long-acting estrogen: a dose of 100 mg of this estrogen preparation is equivalent to 80 mg of polyestradiol phosphate, and both of these applications are considered "low-dose" estrogens. Patients of both groups were statistically comparable in terms of age, tumor stage, and grade of tumor differentiation. Some essential data of this study[13] are briefly summarized herein.

With respect to the subjective and objective criteria listed in Figure 15.1, cyproterone acetate was equally effective as compared to the standard estrogen treatment. However, a varying degree of side effects became evident in the two groups (Fig. 15.2). While lower extremity thrombosis was seen in an equal percentage in both groups, edema was encountered in 4% of the patients treated with cyproterone acetate *versus* 18% in the estrogen group. Furthermore, painful gynecomastia was seen in only 13%

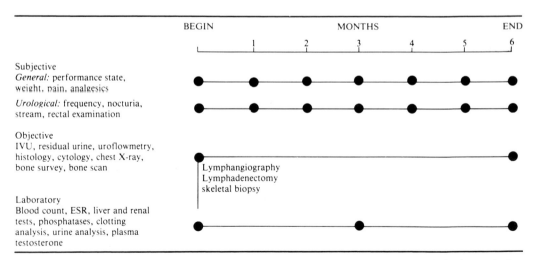

Figure 15.1 Follow-up protocol of the randomized control study analyzing parenteral cyproterone acetate *versus* standard estrogen IM medication in previously untreated patients; for the detection of lymph node metastases, lymphangiography was obligatory, surgical lymphostaging being optional.

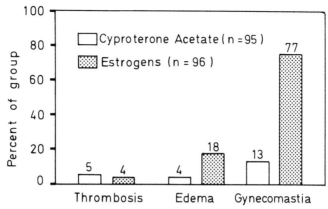

Figure 15.2 Comparison of side effects after short-term treatment with either cyproterone acetate (300 mg/week IM) or estradiol undecylate (100 mg/months IM) during the first 6 months of single treatment of 191 patients with advanced and previously untreated prostatic carcinoma. Sexual impotence occurred in essentially all patients of both groups. Differences for leg edema and gynecomastia were statistically significant.

Table 15.1
Effect of Cyproterone Acetate (300 mg IM/week) on Local Tumor Lesion in 51 Patients[a]

Parameter	6 mo Treatment		24–50 mo Treatment	Total	
	Jacobi et al.[9] (n = 21)	Rost et al.[17] (n = 10)	Tunn et al.[b] n = 20	No.	%
Local tumor mass					
Regressed	16	10	8	34	66.7
Stable	2	0	5	7	13.7
Progressed	3	0	7	10	19.6
Histological regression					
Tumor still present	10	7	8	25	49.0
No tumor upon rebiopsy	9	3	3	15	29.4

[a] In 31 patients, parameters were assessed after a 6-month IM treatment. Twenty patients received further oral treatment of 100 mg/day, and parameters were assessed after an average follow-up of 33 months (24 to 50 months).
[b] Unpublished data.

of the patients treated with the antiandrogen *versus* 77% in the estrogen-treated individuals. Sexual impotence occurred in essentially all patients of both groups.

As already summarized from the data on the oral route of administration of cyproterone acetate, there was also a marked effect of this agent when given intramuscularly, on the reduction of local tumor mass in this study. Table 15.1 summarizes the effect of cyproterone acetate on the local tumor lesion in 51 patients, 31 of them having already been published preliminarily.[9, 17] Regression of the local tumor was objectified in 66.7%; progression of the local mass occurred in only 19.6%. In 15 of 51 cases (29.4%), no residual tumor could be detected upon rebiopsy (Table 15.1).

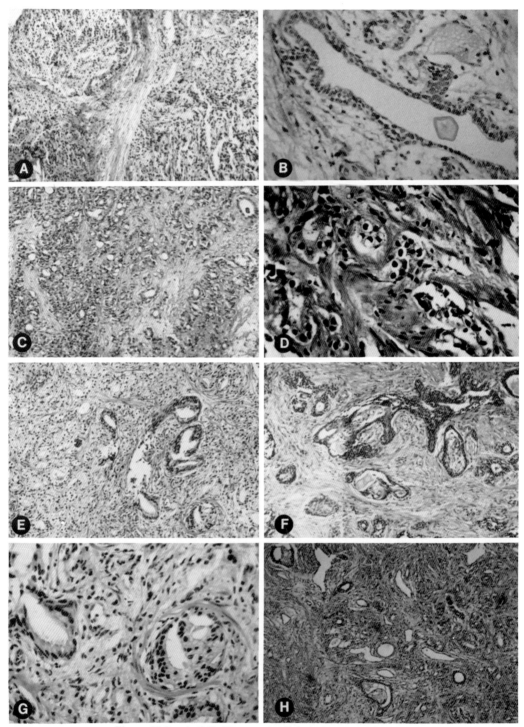

Figure 15.3 *A*, Cribriform and solid carcinoma of the prostate prior to cyproterone acetate treatment. *B*, Atrophic glandular and stromal structures without carcinoma 6 months after cyproterone acetate (pT$_0$; UICC); rectal palpation = T$_0$. *C*, Solid anaplastic and poorly differentiated adenocarcinoma of the prostate prior

Table 15.2
Histological-Cytological Regression of Local Tumor, Assessed Six Months after Cyproterone Acetate Monotreatment (300 mg IM/week) in 59 Patients with Advanced Prostatic Carcinoma[a]

Regression Grading	Initial Grade of Malignancy			Total
	I	II	III	
10–8	5	6	14	25 (42.4%)
6–4	5	5	7	17 (28.8%)
2–0	4	5	8	17 (28.8%)
Total	14 (23.7%)	16 (27.1%)	29 (49.2%)	59 (100%)

[a] Regression grading was applied as given in Chapter 6 (Table 6.3). The three grades of malignancy are characterized in the Editorial Comment to Chapter 6.

In 59 cyproterone acetate-treated cases, Professor Dhom from the *German Prostate Cancer Registry* (see Chapter 6) determined the degree of morphological regression according to a regression grading system outlined in Chapter 6. The initial grade of malignancy of the individual tumor was determined according to the system given in the Editorial Comment to Chapter 6.

Initial *Grade I* was encountered in 14 of 59 cases (23.7%), *Grade II* in 16 (27.1%), and *Grade III* in 29 cases (49.2%). As outlined in Table 15.2, the overall rate of unfavorable regression was 42.4%, moderate regression 28.8%, and excellent regression 28.8% as well. It is obvious that even in the group of initial *Grade III*, at least half of the carcinoma did respond to cyproterone acetate with a moderate to excellent regression (Table 15.2). Some morphological examples for such regressions are illustrated in Figure 15.3.

The Department of Urology, University of Bochum Medical School, contributed 37 patients to the multicenter study, 20 of whom were treated with cyproterone acetate. In addition to the initial study protocol, all 20 patients *further* received *oral* cyproterone acetate medication (100 mg/day), beginning at termination of the 6-month intramuscular regimen. Treatment was continued until objective progression requiring treatment modification or until death, respectively. Initial tumor criteria, duration of treatment, objective response, and the period after which death occurred are summarized in Table 15.3. The advanced character of the

---

to cyproterone acetate treatment. *D*, Carcinoma with pronounced regression seen as shrunken nuclei, vacuolized cytoplasm and stromal reaction 6 months after cyproterone acetate treatment. *E*, Pluriform prostatic carcinoma with glandular, poorly differentiated, cribriform and solid elements prior to estrogen treatment. *F*, Prostatic atrophy with squamous metaplasia and absent carcinoma 6 months after estrogen treatment; rectal palpation = T_0. *G*, Cribriform and solid carcinoma prior to estrogen treatment. *H*, Carcinoma still present admixed with atrophy and metaplasia (moderate regression). Staining was performed using hematoxylin-eosin with standard technique. Magnifications are (*A*) ×24; (*B*) ×152; (*C*) ×24; (*D*) ×152; (*E*) ×24; (*F*) ×24; (*G*) ×152; (*H*) ×24. (Reproduced with permission from G. H. Jacobi *et al.*[9])

Table 15.3
Objective Response Data on 20 Patients Initially Treated with Cyproterone Acetate Intramuscularly for Six Months (300 mg/week) and Maintained on a Daily Oral Dose of 200 mg for up to 50 Months

Patients	Age	Tumor Stage (UICC, 1978)	Histological Grading[a]	Duration of Treatment (mo)	Regression	Stable Disease	Progression (Mo after Beginning of Treatment)	Deaths (Mo after Beginning of Treatment)	Adjunctive Therapy at Progression[b]
K.F.	62	$T_3N_4M_0$	G_1	50	X				
W.F.	70	$T_3N_0M_0$	G_2	44	X				
W.B.	67	$T_3N_0M_0$	G_1	43	X				
A.W.	68	$T_4N_0M_0$	G_3	43	X				Pall. TUR-P (6 mo)
F.L.	70	$T_3N_4M_0$	G_3	36		X		36^c	Pall. TUR-P
B.P.	74	$T_4N_4M_1$	G_2	34		X			
A.M.	69	$T_4N_4M_0$	G_3	32	X				
J.T.	76	$T_4N_4M_0$	G_2	30			X (24) M_1	30^d	Chemotherapy (6 mo)
O.V.	75	$T_4N_4M_0$	G_3	29			X (24)		Chemotherapy (6 mo)
J.E.	71	$T_3N_4M_0$	G_2	28	X				
W.U.	72	$T_4N_4M_1$	G_1	26		X			Orchiectomy (6 mo)
F.W.	70	$T_4N_4M_1$	G_3	25			X (18)	25^d	TUR (20 mo), chemotherapy
K.Z.	63	$T_4N_4M_0$	G_3	24	X				
E.B.	63	$T_3N_4M_0$	G_3	24	X				
F.G.	74	$T_3N_4M_0$	G_2	23			X (21) M_1	23^d	
O.Q.	78	$T_3N_0M_0$	G_3	22	X			22^c	
A.R.	65	$T_4N_xM_0$	G_3	24	X				Pall. TUR-P
Ch.W.	79	$T_4N_4M_1$	G_3	11			X	11^d	Orchiect. + TUR-P + Chemother. (6 mo)
F.A.	68	$T_4N_4M_1$	G_3	8			X	8^d	
J.K.	76	$T_3N_4M_1$	G_2	8			X	8^d	

[a] According to page 121.
[b] Pall. TUR-P, palliative transurethral resection of prostate cancer.
[c] Death unrelated to tumor.
[d] Death from tumor disease.

tumors is reflected by the fact that all tumors were locally far advanced (T_{3-4} = C or D_1), six patients had widespread disease (M_1), 17 tumors were poorly undifferentiated or anaplastic, and 15 patients had juxtaregional lymph node metastases (N_4 according to UICC). Eight tumor regressions occurred, all in the M_0-category, seven progressions occurred, and stable disease was seen in five patients. In two patients with cancer initially limited to the prostate, distant metastases occurred. During the follow-up of 24 to 50 months (mean, 33 months), three patients died of their cancer within the first year. An additional two patients died during the second year of follow-up, one due to progressive widespread tumor disease. Thus, the overall cancer death rate was 6 of 20; no patient died of drug toxicity. No significant cardiovascular or hepatic side effects occurred that would have required discontinuation of treatment. It should be pointed out that this patient group constitutes the first well-documented report on the long-term effects of cyproterone acetate as a single treatment modality in advanced cases.

UNTOWARD REACTIONS AFTER CYPROTERONE ACETATE

Due to differing dose regimens, occasional pretreatment with estrogens, and incomparable patient selection with respect to pre-existing cardiovascular risk factors, the reported side effects widely range from author to author.

Due to the gestagenic component of action of cyproterone acetate (see Chapter 14), appropriate untoward reactions should be expected in males. Bracci and Di Silverio[3] observed gynecomastia in only 1.8% of a large group of patients partially even pretreated by other contrasexual measures. Under treatment with 100 mg of cyproterone acetate orally, a deterioration of coronary heart disease with subsequent myocardial infarction occurred in only two patients. Isurugi and co-workers[8] treated 15 patients with the same oral dose, observed disturbances of sexual life in all cases, and stated that, "other side effects, including easy fatigability and mild breast pain also were noted." In a later report from Italy, Bracci did not give interpretable information on side effects but stated: "CPA (cyproterone acetate) is, in general, very well-tolerated and treatment, even if continuous and prolonged, does not lead to untoward effects. A slight feeling of asthenia and lack of concentration has been observed. . . . "[4] With respect to untoward reactions, only the following statement is found in the report of Giuliani and co-workers:[7] "Such treatment differs from the estrogen therapy in that it does not bring about a substantial increase in the death risk caused by myocardial disease or cerebrovascular accident and its side effects are less than those described for estrogenic therapy alone or with orchiectomy."

However, Tveter et al.[19] reported on a high rate of side effects after an oral daily dose of 200 mg of cyproterone acetate: Serious cardiovascular complications in six of 16 patients with myocardial infarction, and one case each of cerebrovascular accident and sudden cardiac death. Consequently, these authors concluded that cyproterone acetate in the oral dose of 200 mg daily may not be recommended. The pretreatment cardiovascular status, however, is not outlined in this study.

Based on the large number of cases of our randomized prospective study described above, toxicity due to cyproterone acetate was significantly lower than after standard estrogen treatment. If gynecomastia, edema, thrombophlebitis, leg thrombosis, deterioration of coronary heart disease, gastrointestinal symptoms, pruritus and dermatitis are taken together, and sexual impotence is excluded, an overall rate of side effects of about 20% can be expected.[12] As in other treatment regimens, side effects can only be judged correctly if the evaluation is based on a thorough *prospective* analysis. There is no question that it is this limitation which results in the widely differing judgements of this issue. Only rarely have objective laboratory parameters of cardiovascular risk been investigated under cyproterone acetate treatment. In a comprehensive Swedish study, the effect of cyproterone acetate on antithrombin-III, tissue fibrinolysis, and serum lipoprotein were studied.[20-22] These results are summarized in Table 15.4.

Table 15.4
Summary of the Effect of Treatment with *Estrogens* (Long-Term Polyestradiol Phosphate, 80 mg IM/month plus Ethinyl Estradiol 0.5 mg p.o./day), Bilateral Subcapsular *Orchiectomy* or *Cyproterone Acetate* (200 mg p.o./day) on Plasma Hormones and on Variables Associated with Cardiovascular Risk in 46 Patients with Previously Untreated Prostatic Carcinoma[a, b]

	Testosterone	LH	FSH	Plasma Vol.	AT III	Fibrin. Activity	LDL	HDL	HDL/LDL
Estrogens	⇓⇓	⇓	⇓	⇑	⇓⇓	⇓	⇓⇓	⇑⇑	⇑⇑
Castration	⇓⇓	⇑	⇑⇑⇑	∅	∅	∅	∅	∅	∅
Cyproterone acetate	⇓⇓	⇓	⇓	∅	↑	↑	⇓	⇓⇓	↓

[a] From E. Varenhorst.[20]

[b] Abbreviations used are: AT III, antithrombin III; LDL, low density lipoprotein; HDL, high density lipoprotein.

After a critical judgement of all that has been reported about side effects of cyproterone acetate, it can be stated that in a daily oral dose of 100 mg or a weekly IM dose of 300 mg, cyproterone acetate is associated with significantly fewer cardiovascular side effects as compared to standard estrogen treatment, and that other untoward reactions are usually mild and do not require discontinuation of medication.

PLASMA HORMONE CHANGES

Along with the prospective clinical trial mentioned above, a number of biochemical investigations on the effect of cyproterone acetate on hormone parameters have been performed. It was shown that there was a more pronounced suppression of testosterone in the estrogen arm than in the cyproterone acetate arm, the mean value being 29.7 ng/100 ml for the first and 102 ng/100 ml for the latter treatment group.[9] Other findings included a moderate increase of serum prolactin[12] and no effect on the plasma sex hormone-binding globulin level. In the patients constituting the initial report on clinical response,[9] serum levels of testosterone, dihydrotestosterone, androstanediol, 17β-estradiol, prolactin, and luteinizing hormone (LH) were measured before treatment as well as after 3 and 6 months of medication.

The most significant biochemical ratios of these parameters are summarized in Figure 15.4. The probably most important parameter is the *testosterone to LH* ratio, showing a rapid decrease and maintenance at a less than 50% level of that computed before treatment. Due to an only moderate prolactin increase and the aforementioned marked testosterone drop, the *testosterone to prolactin* ratio decreased to about one-sixth of its pretreatment figure, the same being true if the sum of potent androgens in serum (testosterone plus dihydrotestosterone plus androstanediol) was rated to serum prolactin (Fig. 15.4). The strong androgen depletion effect of cyproterone acetate is also demonstrated in Figure 15.5. The intramuscular dose of 300 mg/week is as effective as castration and is only surpassed by high-dose estrogen treatment or castration plus cyproterone acetate.

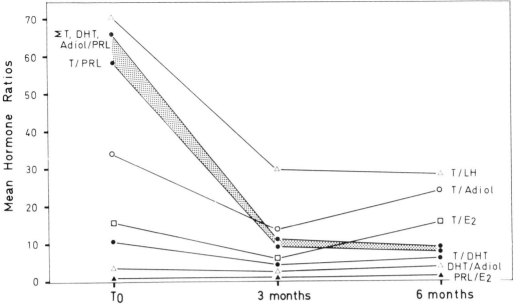

Figure 15.4 Hormone ratios from plasma (mean value of 20 patients) before (T_0) and 3 and 6 months after monotreatment with cyproterone acetate 300 mg IM/week. No patient had had any previous treatment. Testosterone (T), dihydrotestosterone (DHT), 3 α-androstanediol (Adiol), 17β-estradiol (E_2), luteinizing hormone (LH), and prolactin (PRL) were determined by radioimmunoassay. Except for T/Adiol and T/E_2, ratios did not differ significantly at 6 months as compared to the 3-month values.

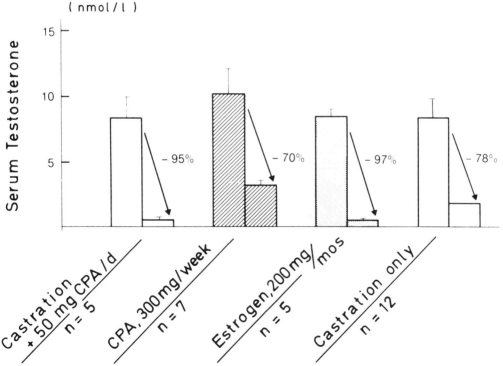

Figure 15.5 Comparative data on testosterone suppression by various contrasexual means. CPA = cyproterone acetate (50 mg oral; 300 mg IM). As estrogen preparation, high monthly dose estradiol undecylate (200 mg IM) was used. *Left bar* represents pretreatment, *right bar* the 6-month posttreatment value plus standard deviation; testosterone decrease is given as percent reduction from initial value.

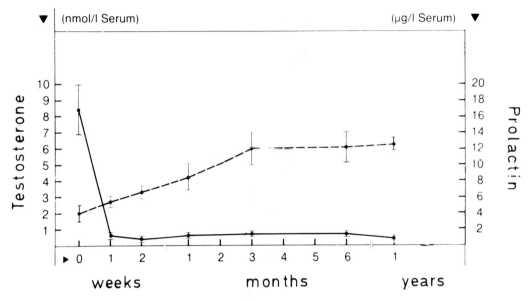

Figure 15.6 Serum testosterone (•———•) and prolactin (•– – –•) monitoring of five patients with prostatic carcinoma treated by orchiectomy plus "low-dose" oral cyproterone acetate (50 mg/day) up to 1 year. Mean ± standard deviation. Drop of testosterone was significantly different at 1 week, the increase of prolactin at 1 month.

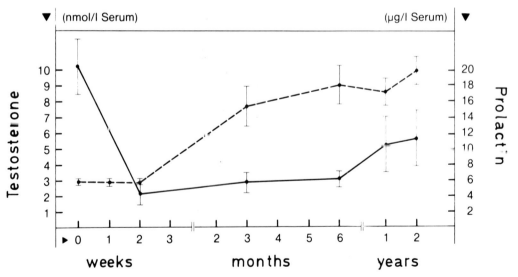

Figure 15.7 Serum testosterone (•———•) and prolactin (•– – –•) monitoring of seven patients with prostatic carcinoma treated by "norm dose" cyproterone acetate with 300 mg IM/week for 6 months and 100 mg p.o./day for up to 2 years. Mean ± standard deviation. Drop of testosterone was significantly different at 2 weeks, the increase of prolactin at 3 months.

In Figure 15.6, the effect of combination treatment of orchiectomy plus the low oral dose of 50 mg of cyproterone acetate/day on serum levels of testosterone and prolactin is illustrated. Besides the rapid and marked drop of testosterone, a steady increase of prolactin is encountered, which is due to the antiandrogen component of this treatment regimen. This moderate, but statistically significant prolactin stimulation seems to be dose-dependent, since the double oral dose of cyproterone acetate further increases prolactin levels in time (Fig. 15.7). Certain stimulatory effects of cyproterone acetate on prolactin release have previously been reported.[8, 12, 15] It is tempting to consider that the moderate prolactin increase as compared to the marked increase after estrogen treatment, is responsible for the low rate of gynecomastia after cyproterone acetate treatment.

When the plasma levels of cyproterone acetate were measured by radioimmunoassay in the patients characterized in Figure 15.7, the mean cyproterone acetate concentration was 348 ng/ml, values favorably comparable with those of Rost et al.[17] for intramuscular administration. There was a statistically significant negative correlation between the height of plasma cyproterone acetate and testosterone in those patients experiencing tumor regression or stable disease during treatment. In contrast, in patients with tumor progression under treatment, this correlation between cyproterone acetate and testosterone in plasma was not present. If cyproterone acetate is administered intramuscularly in weekly doses of 300 mg, a plasma peak of the compound of around 270 ng/ml is already reached at the third day.[17] Up to the third weekly injection, cyproterone acetate levels increase to up to 400 ng/ml, the biological half-life being 4 days on the average. From the currently available data, the optimal oral or intramuscular dose of cyproterone acetate cannot yet be defined for the treatment of prostatic carcinoma.

PROSPECTIVES OF FUTURE THERAPY STRATEGIES INCLUDING CYPROTERONE ACETATE

Cyproterone Acetate as Monotreatment

Based on the testicular and intraprostatic mode of action, cyproterone acetate should exceed or at least be equal to orchiectomy alone. Limited data on a prospective trial are indicative of this assumption.[20]

Cyproterone Acetate in the Status of Hormone Autonomy

Since additional androgen depletion after conventional estrogen treatment and/or castration cannot be expected by cyproterone acetate, an additional clinical effect can only be expected if specifically considered as located within the prostatic carcinoma cell.

Cyproterone Acetate plus Simultaneous Orchiectomy

Since orchiectomy almost completely depletes endogenous testosterone, additional cyproterone acetate may only affect the interprostatic utilization of the remaining small amounts of testosterone from other sources.

Cyproterone Acetate plus Antiprolactins

Cyproterone acetate, in contrast to estrogens, only moderately induces serum prolactin. Since the influence of such moderate prolactin increase on the growth behavior of prostatic carcinoma is still unknown, there seems to date to be no clear-cut evidence to justify this treatment combination.

Cyproterone Acetate plus Chemotherapy

This combination has not yet been investigated.

Cyproterone Acetate as an Alternative to Standard Estrogen Treatment

On the basis of our own data summarized in this chapter and on numerous reports reviewed herein, it can be stated that cyproterone acetate must be considered as a valuable alternative to conventional estrogen regimens. Side effects are comparably lower, the effectiveness in terms of objectifiable regression is comparable, and the value of cyproterone acetate in estrogen-relapsed cases is documented. However, the optimal dose regimen and the exact indication with respect to tumor stage and grade of differentiation has still to be assessed. Further prospective randomized trials are thus warranted to put this valuable alternative into its correct clinical perspective.

REFERENCES

1. Altwein, J. E. Unpublished observations.
2. Altwein, J. E. Aktuelle Aspekte der Hormontherapie des Prostatakarzinoms. *Helv. Chir. Acta 48:* 391, 1981.
3. Bracci, U., Di Silverio, F. Role of cyproterone acetate in urology. In *Androgens and Antiandrogens,* edited by L. Martini and M. Motta. Raven Press, New York, 1977, pp. 333–339.
4. Bracci, U. Antiandrogens in the treatment of prostatic cancer. *Eur. Urol. 5:* 303, 1979.
5. de Voogt, H. J. Pilot study of the combination of DES (diaethylstilboestrol) and CPA (cyproterone acetate) in the treatment of advanced prostatic cancer. EORTC Study Proposal, 1981.
6. EORTC Urological Group. Protocol for a randomized prospective study on the treatment of patients with advanced prostatic cancer category T_3 and T_4 to compare the effect of cyproterone acetate, medroxyprogesterone and stilbestrol. Protocol No. 30761, 1977.
7. Giuliani, L., Pescatore, D., Giberti, C., Martorana, G., and Natta, G. Treatment of advanced prostatic carcinoma with cyproterone acetate and orchiectomy—5 year follow-up. *Eur. Urol. 6:* 145, 1980.
8. Isurugi, K., Fukutani, K., Ishida, H., and Hosoi, Y. Endocrine effects of cyproterone acetate in patients with prostatic cancer. *J. Urol. 123:* 180, 1980.
9. Jacobi, G. H., Altwein, J. E., Kurth, K. H., Basting, R., and Hohenfellner, R. Treatment of advanced prostatic cancer with parenteral cyproterone acetate: a phase III randomised trial. *Br. J. Urol. 52:* 208, 1980.
10. Jacobi, G. H., Altwein, J. E., and Hohenfellner, R. Adjunct bromocriptine treatment as palliation for prostate cancer: experimental and clinical evaluation. *Scand. J. Urol. Nephrol. Suppl. 55:* 107, 1980.
11. Jacobi, G. H., Senge, Th., and Ackermann, R. Östrogene oder Antiandrogene beim Prostatakarzinom? Ein randomisierter Therapievergleich bei bisher unbehandelten Patienten, eine Kooperative Therapiestudie 12 urologischer Zentren. Presented at the XXXII Annual Congress of the Germany Society of Urology, Berlin, 1980.

12. Jacobi, G. H. Therapie des Prostatakarzinoms mit Antiandrogenen. In *Antihormone, Bedeutung in der Urologie*, edited by J. E. Altwein, G. Bartsch, and G. H. Jacobi. Zuckschwerdt, München, 1981, pp. 277–289.

13. Jacobi, G. H., Senge, Th., and Dhom, G. Ergebnisse einer multizentrischen Therapiestudie über die Effektivität von Cyproteronazetat beim fortgeschrittenen Prostatakarzinom. *Akt. Urol.*, in press 1982.

14. Klosterhalfen, H., Becker, H., and Krieg, M. Antiprolactin treatment in metastasizing prostatic cancer. First International Congress on Hormones and Cancer, Rome, 1979.

15. Lunglmayr, G., and Spona, J. Prolaktin-Serumspiegel unter Behandlung des Prostatakarzinoms mit Östradiol-17beta-Undezylat und Cyproteronacetat. *Verh. Ber. Dtsch. Ges. Urol.* Springer, Berlin, 1981, pp. 413–415.

16. Pescatore, D., Gilberti, C., Martorana, G., Natta, G., and Giuliani, L. The effect of cyproterone acetate and orchiectomy on metastases from prostatic cancer. *Eur. Urol. 6:* 149, 1980.

17. Rost, A., Hantelmann, W., and Fiedler, U. Cyproteroneacetate and testosterone levels in serum and first clinical results after intramuscular application of cyproterone acetate in the treatment of prostatic cancer. *Proceedings of the II. International Symposium on the Treatment of Carcinoma of the Prostate.* A. Rost & U. Fiedler, Berlin, 1978, pp. 84–88.

18. Scott, W. W., and Schirmer, H. K. A. A new progestational steroid effective in the treatment of prostatic cancer. *Trans. Am. Assoc. Genito-Urin. Surg. 58:* 54, 1966.

19. Tveter, K. J., Otnes, B., and Hannestad, R. Treatment of prostatic carcinoma with cyproterone actetate. *Scand. J. Urol. Nephrol. 12:* 115, 1978.

20. Varenhorst, E. Metabolic changes during endocrine treatment in carcinoma of the prostate. A prospective study in man with special reference to cardiovascular complications during treatment with oestrogens or cyproterone acetate or after orchiectomy. Linköping University Med., Diss. no. 103, 1980.

21. Varenhorst, E., Wallentin, L., and Risberg, B. The effects of orchiectomy, oestrogens and cyproterone-acetate on the antithrombin-III concentration in carcinoma of the prostate. *Urol. Res. 9:* 25, 1981.

22. Varenhorst, E., and Risberg, B. Effects of estrogen, orchidectomy, and cyproterone acetate on tissue fibrinolysis in patients with carcinoma of the prostate. *Invest. Urol. 18:* 355, 1981.

23. Wein, A. J., and Murphy, J. J. Experience in the treatment of prostatic carcinoma with cyproterone acetate. *J. Urol. 109:* 68, 1973.

16

Value of Chemotherapy in Prostate Cancer Management and Present Data on EORTC Therapy Trials

M. Pavone-Macaluso, M.D.

INTRODUCTION

Cytotoxic chemotherapy is still rarely employed in prostatic cancer. Some recent results indicate, however, that its use deserves a thorough evaluation not only in advanced disease relapsing after hormonal treatment but perhaps also in earlier stages as the only treatment. It can also be employed in association with estrogens or with other forms of hormonal treatment. Only well-designed trials will eventually solve this problem.

INDICATIONS

The faith in hormonal therapy has reserved a secondary role to cytotoxic chemotherapy. It is usually quoted that 80% of patients with prostatic cancer respond to one or another form of hormonal manipulation, although the number of cases where measurable objective regression can be demonstrated is considerably lower. On the other hand, chemotherapy is considered to be a more toxic and dangerous form of treatment than the administration of hormones.

This has led to limiting the use of chemotherapy to the following indications:

1. Advanced, metastatic cancer no longer responding to hormonal therapy

2. Relapse after irradiation

3. Anaplastic tumors.

Alternative forms of treatment, however, can be found for each of these indications and their relative roles still need to be defined.

REVIEW OF THE LITERATURE

Personal Contributions

The earliest data were reviewed in 1972.[1] The experience was almost uniformly bad, including our own. In our report[3] to the 16th Congress of the International Society of Urology, in 1973, we discussed the results obtained in 55 patients, as shown in Table 16.1. The objective responses were reported as "good" and "fair." "Fair" was equivalent to category *1 A* according to Karnofsky's classification (significant regression in all measurable parameters, with subjective improvement having a duration of at least 1 month); "good" corresponded to categories *1 B* (greater than 50% objective regression in all palpable lesions, persistent for at least 1 month, in a relatively asymptomatic patient) and *1 C* (complete regression

Table 16.1
Results of Systemic Treatment of Estrogen-Resistant Advanced Prostatic Carcinoma with Chemotherapeutic Agents[a]

Treatment		No. of Cases	Objective Regression		Subjective Improvement with or without Objective Regression	Regression of Acid Phosphatase	Regression of Distant Metastases	Deceased
Class	Drug		Good	Fair				
Alkylating agents	Cyclophosphamide	17	1	4	10	4	2	12
	Peptichemio	12	1	4	8	4	2	8
	Others	2	0	2	1	0	0	2
	Total	31	2	10	19	8	4	22
Antimetabolites	5-fluorouracil	3	0	1	1	1	0	1
	Methotrexate	1	0	1	0	0	0	0
	Total	4	0	2	1	1	0	1
Antibiotics	Adriamycin	7	0	2	5	2	1	6
	Daunorubicin	2	0	1	2	1	1	0
	Mitomycin	2	0	1	1	1	0	2
	Total	11	0	4	8	4	2	8
Various[b]		5	0	1	3	1	0	2
Associations		4	0	1	3	1	0	2
Total		55	2 (3.6%)	18 (32.7%)	34 (61.8%)	15/40 (37.5%)	6/26 (23%)	35 (63.6%)

[a] Modified from M. Pavone-Macaluso.[3]
[b] VM 26, hydroxyurea, procarbazine.

lasting at least 1 year). No distinction was made between stable and progressive disease. Decrease in acid phosphatase was evaluated in 40 patients in whom the values were elevated at the beginning of treatment. Likewise, the effects of treatment on distant metastases were investigated in 26 patients in whom secondary deposits were present before the onset of chemotherapy.

Our conclusion was that life was not significantly prolonged as a result of chemotherapy and that toxicity was rather severe in patient with reduced bone marrow reserve due to extensive bony metastases. It should be noted that, prior to 1973, most therapeutic regimens consisted of daily administration of chemotherapeutic agents. This regimen is more toxic than the administration of a larger dose at intervals of 3 to 4 weeks, which allows recovery of bone marrow between cycles. Furthermore, mainly patients with very advanced disease and poor performance status were subjected to chemotherapy. For these and other reasons, our older results cannot be compared to subsequent studies, employing more appropriate criteria of evaluation and different treatment schedules and indications.

The significance of a poor performance status, as an ominous prognostic factor, was suspected but not yet fully appreciated. The poor results coincided with the theoretical assumption that a slowly growing tumor, with a low mitotic index and a long doubling time, would likely be insensitive to the effect of drugs acting during the proliferative cell cycle. The reader is referred to our reviews[1-3] for a list of references of work prior to 1973.

Further Contributions

Subsequent reviews by Yagoda,[4] Carter and Wasserman,[5] and Schmidt[6] led to a similar conclusion. Recently more data were analyzed in various chapters in books or review articles.[7-14] These data and more detailed information can be summarized in Tables 16.2 and 16.3. In general, it appears that cytotoxic chemotherapy in the treatment of prostatic cancer cannot be adequately evaluated. Criteria for response, staging, grading, and other important prognostic factors are often poorly defined. In most studies only few patients were included. Some investigations belong to "drug-orientated" rather than to "disease-orientated" research.

According to Carter and Wasserman[5] only three drugs, *i.e.* cyclophosphamide, nitrogen mustard, and 5-fluorouracil, had been submitted up to 1975 to adequate evaluation, although drug activity could not be clearly established. The vast majority of potentially useful drugs had never been evaluated.

Lack of uniformity in response criteria is a very critical point. Data from different investigators cannot be compared, in view of the fact that some authors consider "remission" or "response" only objective regression greater than 50% in the product of the two largest diameters of an evaluable lesion, whereas other authors include stabilization of disease in the category of "responses."

If merely randomized trials are taken into consideration, as recommended by Coune[9] according to the policy of EORTC, only the data

Table 16.2
Chemotherapy of Prostatic Cancer with Single Agents

Drug	No. of Patients	Complete Regression	Partial Regression	Stable Disease	"Responses" (%)	Progression (%)	Author(s) and Reference(s)
Alkylating agents							
Cyclophosphamide	7	0	2		28.5		Bonetti et al.[15]
	7		6				Sinclair et al.[16]
	17		5 (29. 4%)		29.4		Pavone-Maca-luso[3]
	88	0	3 (3. 4%)	31 (35.2%)	38.6	61.3	Beckley et al.[17]
	14				21		Scott et al.[18, 19]
	15	0		8 (53%)	53		Chlebowski et al.[20]
Peptichemio	12	0	5 (41.6%)		41.6	58.4	Pavone-Maca-luso[3]
	16	0	8 (50%)	3 (18.7%)	68.7	31.3	Aliffi and De Grande[21]
Busulfan	12	0	0	0	0	100	Arduino and Mellinger[22]
Melphalan	12	0	4 (33.3%)	4 (33.3%)	66.6	33.3	Franks[23]
	15	0	0	1 (6.6%)	6.6	93.3	Houghton et al.[24]
Mechloretamine	31		12 (39%)		39		Carter and Wasserman[5]
Antimetabolites							
5-Fluorouracil	33	0	4 (12%)	8 (24%)	36	64	Beckley et al.[17]
	9				11		Scott et al.[18, 19]
	14		5 (35.7%)	7 (50%)	85.7	14.2	De Wys[25, 26]
Methotrexate	8		2	1	37.5		Wright et al.[27]
Hydroxyurea	13	0	0	0	0	100	Beckley et al.[17]
	35				51	49	Kvols et al.[28] Lerner and Malloy[29]
Antibiotics							
Adriamycin	4		1		25		Eagan et al.[30]
	4		2		50		Pavone-Maca-luso[3]
	26				27		De Wys et al.[27, 28]
Mithramycin	8			6			Persky et al.[31]
Mitomycin C	8		1		12.5		Carter and Wasserman[5]
Mitotic inhibitors							
Vincristine	14	0	0	1 (7%)	7	93	Beckley et al.[17]
Demecolcine	3		2				Zbinden[32]
Nitrosoureas							
Lomustine (CCNU)	10				40		Johnson et al.[33]
Methyl-CCNU	14	0	1	4 (29%)	36	64	Beckley et al.[17]
Streptozotocin	38	0	0	12 (31.6%)	31.6	55.3	Beckley et al.[17]
1,3-bis-2-chlore-thylnitrosourea (BCNU)	15		2		14		Carter and Wasserman[5]

Table 16.2—*Continued*

Drug	No. of Patients	Complete Regression	Partial Regression	Stable Disease	"Responses" (%)	Progression (%)	Author(s) and Reference(s)
Others							
Dacarbazine (DTIC)	55	0	2 (4%)	13 (24%)	27.3	72.7	Schmidt et al.[34]
Procarbazine	39	0	0	5 (13%)	13	87	Schmidt et al.[34]
Cis-platinum	21	0	9 (43%)	2 (9.5%)	52.5		Merrin[35]
	100				24		Merrin,[36] Yagoda,[37] and Rossof et al.[38]
Hexamethylene-melamine	6	2			33.3		Carter and Wasserman[5]

Table 16.3
Combination of Chemotherapy of Prostatic Cancer

Drugs[a]	No. of Patients	Complete Regression	Partial Regression	Stable Disease	"Responses" (%)	Progression (%)	Author(s) and Reference
ADM + CTX	21	0	15%	25%	40	60	Izbicki et al.[39]
	20				65		Merrin et al.[40]
	18				33		Inde et al.[41]
ADM + DDP	21				42.8		Perloff et al.[42]
ADM + CTX + 5-FU	17	0	2	11	76.5	23.5	Collier and Soloway[43]
	12			6	50		Chlebowski et al.[20]
ADM + CTX + MTX	12				75		Straus et al.[44]
CTX + 5-FU	13				69.3		Merrin et al.[40]
	4				0		Eagan et al.[30]
NH₂ + 5-FU	12			11			Flocks and Cheng[45]
CTX + MTX + 5-FU + VCR + P	16	2	3	1	69		Buell et al.[46]
VCR + MTX + L-PAM + 5-FU + P	25				20		Kane et al.[47]
ADM + VCR + 5-FU + CTX	30				30–40		Lachand et al.[48]
5-FU + DGR + RCM + P	59				33		Chauvin[49]

[a] Abbreviations used are: ADM, doxorubicin (adriamycin); CTX, cyclophosphamide; 5-FU, 5-fluorouracil; DDP, *cis*-platinum; MTX, methotrexate; VCR, vincristine; NH₂, nitrogen mustard (mechloretamine); P, prednisone; DGR, degranol; RCM, rufochromomycin; L-PAM, melphalan.

given in Table 16.4 can be presented, besides the more recent work of the *National Prostatic Cancer Project (NPCP)*.

The Experience of NPCP

The matter was investigated in a more systematic fashion by the *National Prostatic Cancer Project* group. The first studies were instituted

Table 16.4
Randomized Trials in Prostatic Cancer, besides the NPCP[a] Studies

Author(s)	Year	Reference		Drug[b]	Response
Scott et al.	1975	18,19	I	5-FU	36%
			II	CTX	46%
			III	Standard therapy	20%
Sinclair et al.	1975	16	I	Honvan[c]	6/7
			II	CTX	7/7
Eagan et al.	1975	30	I	ADM	26%
			II	5-FU + CTX	11%
De Wys and ECOG	1975	25	I	ADM	12,5%
			II	5-FU	36%
Eagan et al.	1975	30	I	ADM	30%
			II	5-FU	11%
Merrin et al.	1976	40	I	5-FU + CTX	69%
			II	ADM + CTX	65%
Chlebowski et al.	1978	20	I	CTX	53%
			II	CTX + 5-FU + ADM	50%

[a] National Prostatic Cancer Project.
[b] Abbreviations are the same as those used in Table 16.3.
[c] Diethylstilbestrol diphosphate.

in patients no longer responding to hormonal therapy in order to achieve the following goals: (1) to alleviate signs and symptoms of disease; (2) to prolong survival, if possible; and (3) to compare the course of the tumor in patients receiving new forms of treatment with the natural history of the disease in untreated individuals and with the results obtained in patients receiving conventional forms of treatment. The first results of these early multicentric randomized trials were given by Scott et al.[19] in 1975.

The criteria for response (including objective complete response, objective partial regression, and objectively stable disease) and for objective progression were clearly defined. A distinction was made between patients who had been irradiated and thus compromised their bone marrow reserves and patients who had received no irradiation.

The most recent review of the NPCP results published is, to our knowledge, that of Murphy.[50] However, Beckley et al.[17], from the same group, have presented an updated report to the WHO meeting held in Stockholm in 1979. Table 16.5 shows the general design of the NPCP protocols.

The NPCP preliminary data are presented in Table 16.6.

ANTINEOPLASTIC AGENTS WITH HORMONES AS BIOLOGICAL CARRIERS (SEE ALSO CHAPTER 13)

Estramustine phosphate (Estracyt) and prednimustine phosphate belong to this newer class of drugs. The working hypothesis is to utilize cellular tropism—or even specificity—of various hormones, because of the presence of steroid receptors in some malignant cells. In addition, it was postulated that the passage of the chemotherapeutic agents across the

Table 16.5
Chemotherapy in the Treatment of Metastatic (Stage D; M_1, Respectively) Prostatic Carcinoma. National Prostatic Cancer Project: Distribution of the Various Protocols in Separate Groups, according to the Previous Treatment[a]

Group I	Group II	Group III	Group IV
Failure to hormonal therapy (orchiectomy or estrogens)	Failure to hormonal treatment and irradiation (more than 2000 rads to pelvis)	Stable with current hormonal treatment	No previous hormonal therapy (newly diagnosed)
Protocol	Protocol	Protocol	Protocol
100 5-FU *vs.* CTX *vs.* Standard hormonal therapy	200 Estracyt *vs.* streptozotocin *vs.* standard therapy	600 DES *vs.* DES + CTX *vs.* DES + Estracyt	500 DES (or orchiectomy) *vs.* CTX + DES *vs.* CTX + Estracyt
300 CTX *vs.* DTIC *vs.* PCB	400 Prednimustine *vs.* prednimustine + estracyt		
700 CTX *vs.* Methyl-CCNU *vs.* Hydroxyurea	800 Estracyt *vs.* VCR *vs.* Estracyt + VCR		

[a] Abbreviations are the same as those used in Table 16.3. DES, diethylstilbestrol; PCB, procarbazine.

Table 16.6
Results of NPCP Protocols[a, b]

Group	Protocol	Treatment	No. of Patients	Partial Regression (%)	Stable Disease (%)	Progression (%)
I	100	5-FU	33	12	24	64
		CTX	41	7	39	54
		Standard	36	0	19	81
	300	CTX	35	0	26	74
		DTIC	55	4	24	72
		PCB	39	0	13	87
	700	CTX	12	0	50	50
		Methyl-CCNU	14	7	29	64
		Hydroxyurea	13	0	0	100
II	200	Estracyt	46	6	24	70
		Streptozotocin	38	0	32	68
		Standard	21	0	19	81
	400	Prednimustine	62	0	13	87
		Predn.+Estracyt	54	2	11	87
	800	Estracyt	15	7	13	80
		VCR	14	0	7	93
		Estracyt + VCR	15	7	7	86
III	600	DES	—[c]			
		DES + CTX				
		DES + Estracyt				
IV	500	DES or orchiectomy	23	22	43	35
		CTX + DES	18	17	78	6
		CTX + Estracyt	20	10	60	30

[a] Abbreviations are the same as those used in Tables 16.3 and 16.5.
[b] Compiled from data taken from Beckley *et al.*[17]
[c] —, No results available.

cell membranes might be facilitated by the increased lipophilic properties of such compounds.

Estracyt has been dealt with in another chapter of this book, apart from a brief account of the EORTC experience that will be given in this chapter. The use of Estracyt together with antimetabolites (5-FU) is only preliminary.[51]

The experience with prednimustine (a chlorambucil ester of prednisolone) in prostatic cancer is much more limited. Only preliminary results of two studies conducted in USA are available at the present time. Catane et al.[52, 53] found, in a pilot study, 13% objective and 35% subjective responses in a heterogenous group of 23 patients. Almost identical results were obtained in a National Prostatic Cancer Project study, where prednimustine was employed alone or in association with Estracyt in previously irradiated patients.[50] Discontinuation of the treatment with prednimustine was necessary in 8% of patients because of nausea and vomiting, whereas reversible myelotoxicity was observed in 20% of cases. According to Könyves,[54] reduction in toxicity and improvement of results may be obtained using intermittent, instead of continuous therapy. A wider experience with prednimustine, alone or in combination of another, nonalkylating chemotherapeutic agent is advocated.

ACTIVITY OF THE EORTC UROLOGICAL GROUP

The EORTC Urological Group has been active since 1969 in clinical research on the treatment of prostatic cancer, including various forms of hormonal treatment, as well as chemotherapy. Preliminary data with the use of l-asparaginase were not published, due to lack of clinical response. Coune and Smith[55] reported, in 1977, an EORTC clinical trial of 2-bromo-α-ergocriptine in 24 patients with advanced prostatic cancer. No objective responses were observed. In 13 of these patients, evidence of progression was apparent during the first 8 weeks of drug administration, in spite of the reduction of prolactin levels that appeared during drug treatment. In this study bromocriptine was not used in conjunction with estrogens. When two already existing groups merged together in 1976 to set up the present EORTC Urological Group, it was made clear that the services of a Data Center were available and that the Group was ready to develop controlled clinical trials.

Accordingly, three different randomized studies were activated by the EORTC Urological Group. The first two protocols (30761 and 30762) compare various forms of hormonal treatment for the therapy of newly diagnosed and previously untreated advanced prostatic cancer. Both studies are still in progress. The third protocol (30763) was designed in order to compare two different chemotherapeutic agents in the treatment of far advanced prostatic carcinoma.

Protocol 30763

It was terminated in 1978. As of 18th October 1978, nine institutions had entered a total of 46 patients; 22 were randomized to receive adriamycin (ADM) and 24 to receive procarbazine (PCB). Only 39 were evaluable, as shown in Table 16.7. Twelve patients died shortly after the beginning of their treatment. Some of these early deaths may be attributable to cancer, but toxicity was an apparent cause in others. Early death was twice as common in PCB- as in ADM-treated patients. On the other hand, as only one patient treated with PCB had a partial regression, whereas all the others progressed, the toxicity of PCB in these patients was considered too high, especially if compared with the scarcity of useful results. It was decided therefore to stop the trail as originally designed and to treat further eligible patients with ADM, so that at least an evaluation of the efficacy of the latter drug could be achieved. However, only stabilization but no clear-cut regression was observed in the patients treated with ADM.

A preliminary analysis of protocols 30761 and 30762 was already presented in 1980 (Pavone-Macaluso and EORTC Urological Group, unpublished data). Some relevant data are given in Tables 16.8 to 16.10.

Protocol 30761

Only previously untreated patients with histologically proven category T_3 or T_4 carcinoma of the prostate, or any category with distant metastases (M_1), could be entered into this trial. The dosage schedule was the following:

Arm I: Cyproterone acetate (CPA), 250 mg/day;
Arm II: Medroxyprogesterone acetate (MPA). Loading dose, 500 mg

Table 16.7
EORTC Protocol 30763: Preliminary Analysis of Response[a]

Response	Adriamycin (25 Patients)	Procarbazine (14 Patients)
Too early to assess	8	
Complete remission	0	0
Partial remission	0	1
No change	7	0
Progression	6	5
Early death	4	8
Total	25	14

[a] From M. Pavone-Macaluso and EORTC Urological Group (1980).

Table 16.8
EORTC Protocol 30761: Causes of Death by Treatment during Study Period[a,b,c]

Cause of Death	CPA	MPA	DES	Total
Malignant disease	1 (2%)	5 (9%)	2 (3%)	8 (5%)
Cardiovascular	2 (4%)	2 (4%)	2 (3%)	6 (4%)
Other		2	1	3
Unknown		2	1	3
Assoc. Chronic Disease			1	1
Total	3/55	11/54	7/58	21/167

[a] From M. Pavone-Macaluso and EORTC Urological Group (1980).
[b] Patients showing progression at the 3 months evaluation were put off study.
[c] Abbreviations used are: CPA, cyproterone acetate; MPA, medroxyprogesterone acetate; DES, diethylstilbestrol.

Table 16.9
EORTC Protocol 30761: Response of Local Lesion to Treatment at 8 Weeks[a]

Treatment[b]	Complete Regression	Partial Regression	Stable Disease	Progressive Disease	Total
CPA	0	10 (33.3%)	16 (53.3%)	4 (13.3%)	30
MPA	0	8 (26.7%)	18 (60.0%)	4 (13.3%)	30
DES	3 (10.0%)	11 (36.7%)	15 (50.0%)	1 (3.3%)	30
Total	3 (3.3%)	29 (32.2%)	59 (54.4%)	9 (10.0%)	90

% complete or partial regression[c]
CPA *vs.* MPA *vs.* DES

33.3, 26.7, 46.7

[a] From M. Pavone-Macaluso and EORTC Urological Group (1980).
[b] Abbreviations are the same as those used in Table 16.8.
[c] $p = 0.26$.

Table 16.10
EORTC Protocol 30762: Advanced Prostatic Cancer Treated with Estracyt or Stilbestrol—Causes of Death by Treatment as of 22 October, 1979[a]

Cause of Death	Estracyt	Stilbestrol	Total
Malignant disease	16 (15%)	11 (11%)	27 (13%)
Cardiovascular	5 (5%)	8 (8%)	13 (6%)
Associated chronic disease	3	1	4
Infection	1		1
Other		1	1
Total	25/107	21/97	46/204

[a] From: Pavone-Macaluso and EORTC Urological Group (1980).

IM 3 times a week for 8 weeks. Maintenance period, 100 mg orally twice daily;

Arm III: Diethylstilbestrol (DES), 3 mg/day orally.

Treatment was continued whenever possible for a minimum of 8 weeks, at which time patients were evaluated. Therapy for complete and partial responders was continued until progression. Treatment was continued in patients with stable disease at the investigator's discretion and patients with progression went off study.

As of October 1979, 203 patients had been entered, 36 were considered nonevaluable, and 75 were off study. The main reason for going off study was progression, which occurred in about one third of the evaluable patients. Progression rate was higher in patients treated with MPA and CPA than in those given DES, but the difference was not significant. However, the patients have not yet been on study long enough to see whether there is a difference in survival. The number of cardiovascular deaths, as shown in Table 16.8, was similar in the three groups. The local response was evaluated in 90 patients (Table 16.9). It appears that a higher response rate follows treatment with DES (47%), as compared to CPA (33%) and MPA (27%). The difference is, however, not significant. The response of distant metastases and ancillary factors have yet to be analyzed, and the trial will be continued until more meaningful data are obtained.

Protocol 30762

The outline of the protocol and the forms are identical with study 30761, apart from the fact that crossover is contemplated for nonresponders. The dosage schedule is as follows: DES, 1 mg three times daily; Estracyt, orally, 280 mg twice daily for 8 weeks and 140 mg b.d. thereafter. As of October 1979, 278 patients had been entered, 204 being evaluable. Of 74 patients eliminated from the study, 35 were in progression (21% on Estracyt and 12% on DES). Cardiovascular disease was the cause of death in five patients on Estracyt and eight on DES (Table 16.10). Gastrointestinal side effects were more frequently reported on Estracyt than on DES, whereas cardiovascular toxicity and symptoms from gynecomastia were slightly more frequent in the DES-treated patients.

From a preliminary analysis of both studies it was apparent that the number of evaluable patients was too small and the follow-up too short to warrant any valid conclusion. Neither MPA, CPA, or Estracyt showed a superiority over DES in previously untreated cancer of the prostate. DES appeared to be associated with a lower progression rate in both trials, but the data must be confirmed.

An important observation emerges from analysis of the EORTC studies. It was clear that the previously adopted criteria of evaluation were scarcely reliable and that the whole subject required a thorough re-evaluation. The EORTC Urological Group is now engaged in the effort of producing more reliable response criteria. A detailed discussion of this topic will be presented elsewhere. It should be emphasized that different criteria must be adopted for phase II and for phase III trials. Only measurable lesions will be evaluated in the on-going EORTC study of vindesine.

The Combined Modality of Anticancer Drugs and Hormones

This is a very interesting approach, which is based on the principle that prostatic cancer might consist of different clones of cells, some of which are sensitive and some of which are resistant to hormonal manipulation. This principle has been developed with regard to breast cancer, where cellular heterogeneity has been demonstrated. Nenci[56] has elegantly shown, by ultraviolet electron microscopy using immunoreactive steroids, that most human breast cancers appear to be composed of hormone-dependent and autonomous mixed cell populations. The partial or complete unresponsiveness of breast cancer to endocrine management could depend on the presence of cells that lack cytoplasmic hormone receptors or display abnormal nuclear transfer of hormone-receptor complexes. According to these findings, it is stated that the existence of cellular heterogeneity must be taken into account in establishing the optimal therapeutic approach to hormone-dependent cancer. Many workers have suggested that a combined endocrine and cytotoxic treatment should be envisaged in most cases of breast cancer.[57, 58]

Heterogeneity of neoplastic prostatic cells has been suggested but not clearly demonstrated, although it has been shown that metastases in rapidly progressive cases are usually composed of receptor-negative cells. The use of immunofluorescence in prostatic cancer is however only initial, and the results are more difficult to interpret. On the other hand, despite extensive research with contradictory results, the practical role of receptor determinations in human prostatic tissues still needs to be defined.[59]

The association of hormones and cytotoxic agents has been put into practice only to a very limited extent. The preliminary results of the

NPCP group, as shown in Table 16.6, seem to indicate that, in previously untreated patients, only 6% undergo progression if estrogens (DES) are combined with cyclophosphamide, whereas 35% progress on standard hormonal treatment alone. On the other hand, progression rate is not modified if Estracyt is added to standard therapy with DES or orchiectomy (30% *versus* 35%). The addition of vincristine to Estracyt, in patients relapsing after hormonal treatment and irradiation, does not improve the results that can be obtained by Estracyt alone. The combination of cyclophosphamide and diethylstilbestrol appears to be of better effectiveness in advanced but previously untreated disease, since only 6% underwent progression (Protocol 500).

A recent report by Merrin[60] reaches the conclusion that "the combination of *cis*-platinum, orchiectomy and estrogens appears to be the most effective method of treatment for previously untreated (by hormonal manipulation) stage D adenocarcinoma of the prostate." This treatment was given to 34 patients with metastatic disease, consisting of secondary bony deposits in most cases. A partial objective response was observed in 64.7% of cases, lasting 3 to 29 months with an average of 9.3 months. Only 3% showed progression. The results do indeed appear very encouraging. It should be noted, however, that superiority over other methods of treatment is assumed from historical controls.

Merrin[60] claims that the present results are much better than those he had previously obtained using *cis*-platinum alone, which had produced objective remission only in 29% of cases, with an average duration of 6 months. He also quotes that in Yagoda's experience the only patients who responded were those submitted to castration, whereas those who did not respond had not been castrated. This is given by Merrin[60] as a clear indication of a synergistic effect of orchiectomy and *cis*-platinum treatment. This may well be true, but no valid comparison can be made between patients in relapse after failure of hormonal treatment and the present study, where only previously untreated patients were entered. These are clearly two different groups of patients. After Merrin's speculation on a possible synergism between chemotherapy and hormonal treatment,[60] Tannock[63] questioned seriously, in a Letter to the Editor, such a mechanism, the most likely mode of action being an additive one. Furthermore, the evidence for objective regression, in 15 of 22 patients, was based on a decrease of bony lesions on scintiscans. The EORTC Urological Group, however, has shown this to be a very unreliable criterion for a therapeutic response. It is believed, in particular, that any chemotherapy, *per se*, may have an antiproliferative response upon osteoblasts and that the resultant reduction of hydroxyapatite deposition in bone, reflected in the appearance of scans, is not necessarily an index of therapeutic response. This issue is nevertheless still controversial. All such data seem to indicate that the combination of hormones and cytotoxic drugs is advantageous only in the treatment of virgin cases. The available evidence is based, however, on a small number of patients, and it cannot be accepted unless significant data are reported in the future.

CONCLUSIONS

A thorough analysis of the various data presented in Tables 16.1 to 16.4 and 16.6 and 16.7 would be tedious and excessively lengthy. Only few considerations are of interest.

Despite Merrin's claim[35, 36] that *cis*-platinum is the drug of choice in prostatic carcinoma where chemotherapy is indicated, no clear superiority of one drug over the others has been demonstrated.[61] Historical controls cannot be accepted as a valid proof, unless confirmed by prospective randomized trials. We can only say that a few drugs, including *cis*-platinum, adriamycin, 5-FU, lomustine, and various alkylating agents, such as cyclophophamide and Peptichemio, appear to have some degree of activity against prostatic cancer.

The effectiveness of other drugs can hardly be evaluated, since the number of treated patients is insufficient. Conflicting results have been presented with regard to melphalan and hydroxyurea. The latter was reported to be effective in 51% of 35 patients in two series[28, 29] but did not produce any response in another series, where 100% of patients progressed.[17] Procarbazine in the dosage employed by the EORTC Urological Group is clearly too toxic, and its use should be discouraged. Very little practical information can be gained from an analysis of Table 16.3, in which various regimes of combination chemotherapy are listed. It should be stressed again that the various results cannot be compared and that the category of "responses" includes, in some studies, only patients with objective regression of measurable lesions, whereas it also comprises stabilization of disease and/or subjective remission in other reports. It appears, however, that objective results and palliation can be obtained at least in some patients treated with various combinations, such as COMP-F[46] and with the association of adriamycin and cyclophosphamide,[39-41] or with *cis*-DDP,[42] and with other drugs. From the presently available data, however, it is absolutely impossible to say that polychemotherapy yields better results than single drug treatment. Even if we decide to totally disregard this heterogeneous collection of noncomparable results and consider only the randomized trials summarized in Tables 16..4 and 16.6, it is very difficult to reach any conclusion. The various studies cannot be compared, but we can limit our comments to the groups given different treatments within each study. The levels of significance are rarely, if ever, reported. It seems to evolve that:

1. In metastatic patients, relapsing after failure of endocrine manipulation, chemotherapy with cytotoxic drugs is superior to standard hormonal treatment.[18, 19]
2. The best single agent or combination of agents is yet to be identified.
3. There is no evidence that treatment with multiple drug associations is better than therapy with a single drug. On the contrary, randomized trials have suggested that cyclophosphamide alone is at least as effective as the combination of the same drug with adriamycin and 5-FU.[20] Adriamycin alone is superior to the association of cyclophosphamide and 5-FU.[30]
4. The multiple drug cocktails may show an increased toxicity. Chlebowski *et al.*[20] did indeed demonstrate that the survival of patients responding to cyclophosphamide was significantly longer than that of patients responding to adriamycin plus 5-fluorouracil (median 18.6 months *versus* 8.1 months; $p < 0.05$).
5. Clinical response to cytotoxic chemotherapy is associated with an

increased survival. This appears to be true even if different criteria are adopted in order to define a "response." In a study where a combination of adriamycin and 5-fluorouracil was administered in 21 patients with distant metastases,[39] patients who showed either a partial objective regression or stable disease were considered as responders. The median survival was 40 weeks for responders *versus* 17 weeks for nonresponders. Similar results were obtained in another study[23] using criteria of response to treatment based on Kvols' scoring system[28] that takes into consideration ancillary factors, such as symptomatic improvement, quality of life, performance status, changes in body weight, hemoglobin, and phosphatases (see Chapter 11 for details).

6. Patients with progressive disease, who have received irradiation (more than 2000 rads to the pelvis), should be treated with drugs having little myelotoxicity. Initial results indicate that streptozotocin, vincristine, estramustine, and prednimustine are relatively well tolerated. Their efficacy needs to be confirmed, although Estracyt and streptozotocin appear to be slightly better than the standard hormonal treatment.

7. Antineoplastic agents bound to hormones, such as estramustine and prednimustine, are still in the investigational stage. Many reports, including some randomized trials, suggest that Estracyt may be of help in the treatment of advanced disease. Patients may show dramatic symptomatic relief even after failure of conventional hormonal therapy and/or irradiation. A lower number of such patients undergo progression on estramustine than on standard hormonal treatment: 70% *versus* 81%.[17] The EORTC studies indicate that estramustine, MPA, and CPA do not appear to be superior to DES, 1 mg t.i.d., if employed as the initial therapy in previously untreated patients.

8. The association of estrogens and cyclophosphamide as the first treatment in "virgin" cases rests on sound theoretical grounds. The first results appear to be promising but the experience is too short. There is an urgent need for further controlled studies and for an international agreement on uniform response criteria.

9. Not only the size of the local lesion, but also the response of bony metastases are very difficult to evaluate. Acid phosphatase changes have prognostic value, but cannot be adopted as valid response criteria. In many reports, decrease of acid phosphatase levels is not uniformly related to clinical response. Changes in carcinoembryonic antigen may probably be more accurate than acid phosphatase fluctuations in monitoring the response to chemotherapy.[62] Only patients with exactly measurable lesions should be entered in phase II trials, if the actual value of various chemotherapeutic agent or combinations in prostatic cancer is to be clearly established.

10. Systemic chemotherapy has not been shown to cure any patient, and no permanent and complete objective regression has been described so far.

11. The aim of therapy is thus merely that of obtaining an objective

and/or subjective response leading to palliation for a significant length of time and hopefully also to the prolongation of acceptable life. If this is the goal to be achieved, it is imperative, in my view, that the treatment must not lead to side effects that are more distressing for the patient than the disease itself. The anticipated benefits should be carefully weighed against the possible toxic effects due to the treatment. Highly aggressive chemotherapy, which is legitimate in malignancies where a real cure can be expected, should be withheld. Complicated and toxic treatment regimens should be avoided unless a clear-cut improvement in survival and a highly significant remission rate can be consistently shown, both in objective and subjective parameters. The *quality of life* should be given priority in the planning of treatment, and the patient with advanced prostatic cancer who is not suffering from severe pain should usually be spared the added inconvenience of prolonged hospitalization and the side effects from overenthusiastic chemotherapy. In other words, it is too early for chemotherapy of prostatic cancer to become a routine. Progress will be achieved only if the treatments can be accurately followed and monitored under the responsibility of a urologist with a wide experience of the various problems inherent in this particular disease. Advice from a competent chemotherapist is also essential.

OUTLOOK

At the present state of our knowledge, chemotherapy has an established indication in the attempt to achieve palliation in relapsing cases or in patients with undifferentiated tumors. It is too early, however, to recommend its routine use as the initial form of treatment in all cases of prostatic cancer, either as the only therapy or in association with the conventional measures (orchiectomy and/or administration of hormones). The actual value of chemotherapy under the latter circumstances has not yet been established with regard to its side effects and therapeutic rationale. The treatment schedules are still too imprecise. Many single drugs and their associations have not yet been tested. The use of chemotherapy appears to be ethically acceptable in "virgin" cases only if the treatment can be strictly conducted and followed under the form of a controlled, comparative, prospective trial. Such studies are absolutely necessary if the value of a new form of treatment is to be clearly defined. This point of view has been adopted among others by the *National Prostatic Cancer Project* (*NPCP*) in USA and by the *European Organization for Research on the Treatment of Cancer* (*EORTC*).

SUMMARY

The current literature is reviewed, regarding cytotoxic chemotherapy of prostatic cancer. The results of single drugs and of various drug combinations are presented and discussed. The studies of the EORTC Urological Group were aimed to compare standard treatment with DES to other hormones (MPA) or to antihormones (cyproterone acetate), as well as to estrogens and cytotoxic drugs bound in the same molecule (estramustine). Treatment with adriamycin and procarbazine were also investigated by the same group. The results, their analysis and the indications of cytotoxic chemotherapy are discussed, and some conclusions are anticipated. Emphasis is laid upon the need for further randomized trials and uniformity in defining response criteria.

Acknowledgements. The following members of the *EORTC Urological Group* participated in the trials mentioned in the text.

Protocol 30761

Italy:	M. Pavone-Macaluso, *Palermo* (study coordinator); R. Zolfanelli, *Vercelli*; A. Nasta, *Mestre*; E. Visentini, *Mantova*; F. Merlo, *Biella*; P. Carbone, *Torino*; V. Nadalini, *Genova*; M. Laudi, *Torino*; G. Castaldi, *Genova*; M. Porena, *Teramo*; S. Leoni, *Reggio Emilia.*
The Netherlands:	H. J. De Voogt, *Leiden*; J. Alexieva, *Rotterdam.*
France:	B. Lardennois, *Reims*; J. Guerrin, *Dijon.*
Belgium:	D. Goovaerts, *Antwerp.*
Spain:	J. A. Martinez-Pineiro, E. A. Barrilero, L. Resell-Esteve, *Madrid.*
Austria:	J. Frick, *Salzburg.*

Protocol 30762

Denmark:	F. L. Lund, *Copenhagen* (study coordinator); H. Wolf, *Hvidovre*; P. A. Gammelgaard, *Herlev*; B. E. Jacobsen, *Aarhus.*
United Kingdom:	M. Robinson, *Pontefract*; B. Richards, *York*; P. H. Smith, *Leeds*; R. E. Williams, *Leeds*; R. W. Glashan, *Huddersfield*; G. McVie, *Glasgow.*
Spain:	J. A. De Torres Mateos, *Barcelona.*
Belgium:	C. Bouffioux, *Liège*; L. Denis, *Antwerp.*

Protocol 30763

The Netherlands:	J. H. Mulder, *Rotterdam* (study coordinator); A. Van Oosterom, *Leiden*; J. Alexieva, *Rotterdam.*
United Kingdom:	M. Robinson, *Pontefract*; B. Richards, *York*; P. H. Smith, *Leeds*; Campbell Robson, *Cookridge*; J. F. Shepheard, *Oldham.*
Spain:	J. A. Martinez-Pineiro, *Madrid*; A. Escudero Barrilero, *Madrid.*

The statistical analysis was performed by R. Sylvester and M. de Pauw, EORTC Data Center, Institut J. Bordet, Brussels, Belgium.

REFERENCES

1. Pavone-Macaluso, M., Caramia, G., and Vecchioni, M. La chimiothérapie antiblastique dans le traitement du cancer de la prostate. *J. Urol. Nephrol. 78:* 621, 1972.
2. Pavone-Macaluso, M. Chemotherapy of vesical and prostatic tumours. *Br. J. Urol. 43:* 701, 1971.
3. Pavone-Macaluso, M. Chemotherapy in advanced prostatic cancer. In *XVI Congrés de la Societé Internationale d'Urologie*, Vol. 2, Part 2. Doin, Paris, 1973, p. 501.
4. Yagoda, A. Non hormonal cytotoxic agents in the treatment of prostatic adenocarcinoma. *Cancer 32:* 1131, 1973.

5. Carter, S. K., and Wasserman, T. H. The chemotherapy of urologic cancer. *Cancer 36:* 729, 1975.

6. Schmidt, J. D. Chemotherapy of prostatic cancer. *Urol. Clin. North Am. 2:* 185, 1975.

7. Paulson, D. F., Berry, W. R., Cox, E. B., and Laszlo, J. Chemotherapy of prostatic cancer. In *Cancer of the Genitourinary Tract*, edited by D. E. Johnson and M. L. Samuels. Raven Press, New York, 1979, p. 261.

8. Anderson, T. Chemotherapy of urologic cancer: principles and practices. In *Principles and Management of Urologic Cancer*, edited by N. Javadpour. Williams & Wilkins, Baltimore, 1979, Ch. 8, p. 233.

9. Coune, A. Carcinoma of the prostate. In *Randomized Trials in Cancer: A Critical Review by Sites*, edited by M. J. Staquet. Raven Press, New York, 1978, pp. 389–409.

10. Murphy, G. P. Management of advanced cancer of the prostate. In *Genitourinary Cancer*, edited by D. G. Skinner and J. B. de Kernion. W.B. Saunders, Philadelphia, 1978, p. 397.

11. Bouffioux, C. Le cancer de la prostate. *Acta Urol. Belg. 47:* 189, 1979.

12. Jacobi, G. H. Chemotherapie des Prostatakarzinoms. In *Chemotherapie Urologischer Malignome*, edited by G. H. Jacobi and J. E. Altwein. S. Karger, Basel, 1979, p. 91.

13. Nagel, R., and Leistenschneider, W. Hormonelle und zytostatische Therapie des Prostatakarzinoms. In *Diagnostik und Therapie des Prostatakarzinomas*, edited by H. Göttinger. S. Karger, Basel, 1979, p. 149.

14. Stoter, G., Rozencweig, M., and Pinedo, H. M. Genito-urinary tumours. In *Cancer Chemotherapy 1979. The EORTC Cancer Chemotherapy Annual I*, Edited by H. M. Pinedo, Excerpta Medica, Amsterdam, 1979, p. 317.

15. Bonetti, C., Pasini, G., and Missiroli, G. F. Terapia antiblastica delle neoplasie avanzate o recidivanti. *Romagna med. 15:* 21, 1963.

16. Sinclair, G., Lupu, A., and de Kernion, J. Management of adenocarcinoma of the prostate with diethylstilbestrol diphosphate and cyclophosphamide. *Urology 5:* 665, 1975.

17. Beckley, S., Wajsman, Z., Slack, N., Mittelman, A., and Murphy, G. The chemotherapy of prostatic carcinoma. *Scand. J. Urol. Nephrol. Suppl. 55:* 151, 1980.

18. Scott, W. W., Gibbons, R. P., Johnson, D. E., Prout, G. R., Schmidt, J. D., Saroff, J., and Murphy, G. P. The continued evaluation of the effect of chemotherapy in patients with advanced carcinoma of the prostate. *Trans. Am. Assoc. Genitourin. Surg. 68:* 24, 1977.

19. Scott, W. W., Gibbons, R. P., Johnson, D. E., Prout, G. R., Schmidt, J. D., Chu, T. M., Gaeta, J. F., Joiner, J., Saroff, J., and Murphy, G. P. Comparison of 5-fluorouracil (NSC-19893) and cyclophosphamide (NSC-26271) in patients with advanced carcinoma of the prostate. *Cancer Chemother. Rep. 59:* 195, 1975.

20. Chlebowski, R. T., Hestorff, R., Sardoff, L., Weiner, J., and Bateman, J. R. Cyclophosphamide (NSC 26271) versus the combination of adriamycin (NSC 19893) and cyclophosphamide in the treatment of metastatic prostatic cancer. A randomized trial. *Cancer 42:* 2546, 1978.

21. Aliffi, E., and De Grande, G. L'impiego del Peptichemio nelle neoplasie dell'apparato uro-genitale. *Minerva Urol. 28:* 247, 1976.

22. Arduino, L. J., and Mellinger, G. T. Clinical trial of busulfan (NSC-750) in advanced carcinoma of the prostate. *Cancer Chemother. Rep. 40:* 47, 1964.

23. Franks, C. R. Melphalan in metastatic cancer of the prostate. *Cancer Treat. Rep. 6* (Suppl.): 121, 1979.

24. Houghton, A. L., Robinson, M. R. G., and Smith, P. H. Melphalan in advanced prostatic cancer: a pilot study. *Cancer Treat. Rep. 61:* 923, 1977.

25. De Wys, W. D. Comparison of adriamycin (NSC-123-127) and 5-FU (NSC-19893) in advanced prostatic cancer. *Cancer Chemother. Rep. 59:* 215, 1975.

26. De Wys, W. D., Bauer, M., Colsky, J., Cooper, R. A., Creech, R., and Carbone, P. P. Comparative trial of adriamycin and 5-fluorouracil in advanced prostate cancer. Progress report. *Cancer Treat. Rep. 61:* 325, 1977.

27. Wright, J. C., Prigot, A., Wright, B. P., and Weintraub, S. An evaluation of folic acid antagonists in adults with incurable neoplasms. *J Natl. Med. Assoc. 43:* 211, 1951.

28. Kvols, L. K., Eagan, R. T., and Myers, R. P. Evaluation of melphalan, ICRF-159 and

hydroxyurea in metastatic prostate cancer: a preliminary report. *Cancer Treat. Rep. 61:* 311, 1977.

29. Lerner, H. J., and Malloy, T. R. Hydroxyurea in stage D carcinoma of the prostate. *Urology 10:* 35, 1977.

30. Eagan, R. T., Utz, D. C., Myers, R. P., and Furlow, W. L. Comparison of adriamycin (NSC-123127) and the combination of 5-fluorouracil (NSC-19893) and cyclophosphamide (NSC-26271) in advanced prostatic cancer: a pilot study. *Cancer Chemother. Rep. 59:* 203, 1975.

31. Persky, L., Guerrier, K., Rabin, R., and Albert, D. J. Mythramycin and metastatic carcinoma of the prostate. *J. Urol. 104:* 884, 1970.

32. Zbinden, F. Neue Erfahrungen mit Demecolcin (Colcemid CIBA) in der Behandlung von Leukosen und Tumoren. *Schweiz. Med. Wochenschr. 85:* 994, 1955.

33. Johnson, D. E., Scott, W. W., Gibbons, R. P., Prout, G. R. Schmidt, J. D., Ming Chu, T. Gaeta, J., Saroff, J., and Murphy, G. P. National randomized study of chemotherapeutic agents in advanced prostatic carcinoma. A progress report. *Cancer Treat. Rep. 61:* 317, 1977.

34. Schmidt, J. D., Scott, W. W., Gibbons, R. P., Johnson, D. E., Prout, G. R., Loening, S. A., Soloway, M. S., Chu, T. M., Gaeta, G. F., Slack, N. H., Saroff, J., and Murphy, G. F. Comparison of procarbazine, imidazole-carboxamide and cyclophosphamide in relapsing patients with advanced carcinoma of prostate. *J. Urol. 121:* 185, 1979.

35. Merrin C. Treatment of advanced carcinoma of the prostate (stage D) with infusion of cisdiamminedichloroplatinum II (NSC 119875): a pilot study. *J. Urol 119:* 522, 1978.

36. Merrin, C. Treatment of genitourinary tumours with cis-diamminedichloroplatinum. Experience in 250 patients. *Cancer Treat. Rep. 63:* 1579, 1979.

37. Yagoda, A. Phase II trials with cis-diamminedichloroplatinum II in the treatment of urothelial tumours. *Cancer Treat. Rep. 63:* 1565, 1979.

38. Rossof, A. H., Talley, R. W., Stephens, R., Thigpen, T., Samson, M. K., Groppe, C., Eyre, H. J., and Fisher, R. Phase II evaluation of cis-diamminedichloroplatinum (II) in advanced malignancies of the genitourinary and gynecologic organs. *Cancer Treat. Rep. 63:* 1557, 1979.

39. Izbicki, R. M., Amer, M. H., and Al Sarraf, M. Combination of adriamycin and cyclophosphamide in the treatment of metastatic prostatic carcinoma: a phase II study. *Cancer Treat. Rep. 63:* 999, 1979.

40. Merrin, C., Etra, W., Waisman, Z., Baumgartner, G., and Murphy, G. Chemotherapy of advanced carcinoma of the prostate with 5-fluorouracil, cyclophosphamide and adriamycin. *J. Urol. 115:* 86, 1976.

41. Ihde, D. C., Bunn, P. A., Cohen, M. H., *et al.* Combination chemotherapy in metastatic carcinoma of the prostate: methods of detecting tumour response and progression. *Proc. Am. Soc. Clin. Oncol. 19:* 339, 1978.

42. Perloff, M., Ohnyma, T., Holland, J. F., Kennedy, B. J., and Curtis Mills, R. Adriamycin (ADM) and diamminedichloroplatinum (DDP) in advanced prostate carcinoma. *Proc. Am. Soc. Clin. Oncol. 18:* 333, 1977.

43. Collier, D., and Soloway, M. S. Doxorubicin hydrochloride, cyclophosphamide and 5-fluorouracil combination in advanced prostate and transitional cell carcinoma. *Urology 8:* 459, 1976.

44. Straus, J. M., Parmelee, J., Olsson, C., and De Vere White, R. Cytoxan, adriamycin, methotrexate (CAM) therapy of stage D prostate cancer. *Proc. Am. Soc. Clin. Oncol. 19:* 314, 1978.

45. Flocks, R. H., and Cheng, S. F. Combination therapy for prostatic carcinoma, with special emphasis on the role of chemotherapy. *J. Iowa Med. Soc. 58:* 125, 1968.

46. Buell, G. V., Saiers, J. H., Saiki, J. H., and Bergreen, P. W. Chemotherapy trial with COMP-F regimen in advanced adenocarcinoma of the prostate. *Urology 11:* 247, 1978.

47. Kane, R. D., Stocks, L. H., and Paulson, D. F. Multiple drug chemotherapy regimen for patients with hormonally unresponsive carcinoma of the prostate: a preliminary report. *J. Urol. 117:* 467, 1977.

48. Lachand, A., Carcia-Giralt, E., Pallangie, T., *et al.* Polychimiothérapie sequentielle, comme traitement du cancer de prostate avec métastases. Abstract, 3rd Congress European Urological Association, Monte Carlo, 1978, p. 135.

49. Chauvin F. Essai de chimiothérapie associée discontinue dans les cancers de la prostate. *J. Urol. Nephrol. 79:* 397, 1973.

50. Murphy, G. P. Chemotherapeutic treatment on a national randomized trial basis by the National Prostatic Cancer Project. In *Cancer of the Genitourinary Tract,* edited by D. E. Johnson and M. L. Samuels. Raven Press, New York, 1979, p. 249.

51. Welch, D. A., *et al.* Treatment of advanced carcinoma of the prostate with estramustine and 5-fluorouracil. *Proc. Am. Assoc. Cancer Rep. 19:* 325, 1978.

52. Catane, R., Kaufman, J. H., Mittleman, A., and Murphy, G. Combined therapy of advanced prostatic carcinoma with estramustine and prednimustine. *J. Urol. 117:* 332, 1977.

53. Catane, R., Kaufman, J. H., Madajewicz, S., Mittelman, A., and Murphy, G. P. Predmustine therapy for advanced prostatic cancer. *Br. J. Urol. 50:* 29, 1978.

54. Könyves, I. Prednimustine. In *Bladder Tumours and Other Topics in Urological Oncology,* edited by M. Pavone-Macaluso, P. H. Smith, and F. Edsmyr. Plenum Press, New York, 1980, p. 13.

55. Coune, A., and Smith, P. H. Clinical trial of 2-bromo-α-ergocryptine (NSC-169774) in human prostatic cancer. *Cancer Chemother. Rep. 119:* 240, 1977.

56. Nenci, I. Receptor and centriole pathways of steroid action in normal and neoplastic cells. *Cancer Res. 38:* 4204, 1978.

57. Leclercq, G., and Heuson, J. C. Therapeutic significance of sex-steroid hormone receptors in the treatment of breast cancer. *Eur. J. Cancer 13:* 1205, 1977.

58. Tormey, D. C., and Carbone, P. P. Changing concepts in therapy of breast cancer. *Methods Cancer Res. 13:* 1, 1976.

59. De Voogt, H. J. Steroid receptors in human prostatic tissue. In *Bladder Tumours and Other Topics in Urological Oncology,* edited by M. Pavone-Macaluso, P. H. Smith, and F. Edsmyr. Plenum Press, New York, 1980, p. 443.

60. Merrin, C. E. Treatment of previously untreated (by hormonal manipulation) stage D adenocarcinoma of prostate with combined orchiectomy, estrogen, and cis-diammine-dichloroplatinum. *Urology 15:* 123, 1980.

61. Smith, P. H. Medical management of prostatic cancer. Some current questions. *Eur. Urol. 6:* 65, 1980.

62. Kane, R. D., Mickey D. D., and Paulson, D. F. Serial carcinoembryonic antigen assays in patients with metastatic carcinoma of the prostate being treated with chemotherapy. *Urology 8:* 559, 1976.

63. Tannock, I. Cis-platinum and hormones in cancer of prostate (Letter to the Editor). *Urology 16:* 331, 1980.

2
Section

Experimental

17

Experimental Models in the Study of Prostatic Cancer

F. H. Schröder, M.D.

From the very beginning experimental studies have strongly influenced clinical management of prostatic cancer. Knowledge obtained by urologists with an experimental mind about the endocrine dependence of growth and function of the dog prostate lead to the discovery of endocrine treatment of prostatic carcinoma.[14, 15] This treatment, still the most effective palliation known for most patients with this frequent disease, has changed the urological management of these patients drastically since 1940. Before this event nothing could be offered but symptomatic help. Acid phosphatase, introduced as a serum marker for prostatic carcinoma as early as 1936,[9] is another example of the direct benefit patients with prostatic cancer had from clinically applied basic experimental research in this field.

Some of the problems of prostatic carcinoma may be solved by results obtained in cancer research in general. It would, however, not make any sense to wait for solutions obtained in other fields which may or may not be applicable to prostatic cancer. Present knowledge about this tumor offers insight into very specific problems which should be solved. Their solution should be a contribution to the solution of the cancer problem in general.

Prostatic cancer is different from other human cancers because in most instances mechanisms of control of growth and function resemble those known physiologically for the tissue of origin, the prostate. Theoretically, this offers a unique opportunity to study one of the mechanisms of control of malignant growth, provided suitable models become available for such studies. It is hardly imaginable that *one* model will ever satisfy the needs of all different branches of experimental research and cover all facets which require further exploration. Some studies, such as gene manipulation, hybridization, and tumor cell genetics can only be done in *in vitro* systems. Besides the mechanisms involved in endocrine control of growth and function of the prostatic carcinoma cell, hormone-independent growth, and the mechanisms involved in the process of becoming hormone-independent, need further investigation. Models should also become available which are suitable to search for other mechanisms of host-tumor interaction such as immunological surveillance and environmental and dietary factors. Furthermore, models should allow the search for more markers, and, finally, models have to become available for experimental screening for other modalities of treatment and even prophylaxis.

CHARACTERIZATION OF MODELS

The ideal model for human prostatic carcinoma would be a human tumor growing in some long-living and quickly reproducing laboratory animal *and, in vitro*, which would reflect all known characteristics of human prostatic carcinoma. Some of these characteristics, for example, endocrine dependence and autonomous growth, exclude each other. This makes it unlikely that one model will satisfy all requirements. The ideal model does not exist, and it is doubtful whether it ever will exist. In spite of the fact that some good models have been developed in recent years more are needed.

The usefulness of a model system will depend on and will be restricted to the study of such properties which are identical with, or strongly similar to, known characteristics of human prostatic carcinoma in its natural human host. Therefore "characterization" of models is an absolute prerequisite for relevant experimental studies with prostatic cancer models. In practice this means that once a model system is established the whole catalog of known properties of the tissue of origin needs to be checked against the model system. From the results obtained it will then become evident to what degree similarity exists between the tumor of origin and the new system. These data will be relevant for the usefulness of further studies. A transplantable tumor containing no stroma can hardly be used for the study of interrelation between stromal and epithelial elements, and so on.

It is obvious that for characterization of tumor models there is a great need for well defined and easily reproducible characteristics of the original tumor, the host-tumor interrelationship. Such data are available from the current literature; they will have to be kept up to date and can serve as guidelines and checklists for investigators. They should contain morphological biochemical, endocrine, kinetic, genetic, immunologic, and all other parameters known for host and tumor. A list of "some idealized properties of animal models of prostatic cancer" is available in.[17] Further development of such parameters is obligatory and essential for the development of good model systems for prostatic cancer.

An attempt will be made to review the currently available model systems in the field of animal models, tissue culture, and heterotransplantation into immunodeficient animals.

ANIMAL MODELS

Excellent recent reviews of this subject are available.[4, 10, 17, 24] No complete review will therefore be attempted.

The Dunning *R 3327* Prostatic Carcinoma in Rats

This important line resulted from a spontaneously occurring prostatic carcinoma in a Copenhagen rat found by Dunning in 1961.[7] Since that time at least 10 sublines with different properties have been developed by Dunning and others.[17] A short summary of their characteristics is given in Table 17.1. The results of this work have most recently been summarized by Isaacs and Coffey.[17] There is little doubt that this model of all available ones satisfies the greatest number of requirements and has many similarities with the different types of human prostatic cancer. This is especially true for the sublines *R 3327 H, HI,* and *AT*. These represent hormone-dependent adenocarcinoma (*H*), hormone-insensitive adenocarcinoma (*HI*), and anaplastic carcinoma (*AT*), which is not squamous carcinoma as the older subline *R 3327A*. The lines can be transferred by injecting single cell suspensions without losing their original characteristics.

At least for this model it has been proven that the process of a tumor becoming hormone-independent is a selection phenomenon. About 20% hormone-insensitive cells are present in the *R 3327 H* tumors. They lead to hormone-insensitive tumors by selective overgrowth if the hormone-dependent population is inhibited by castration or estrogen treatment. Autonomous growth does not occur in the intact animal because under normal endocrine conditions the doubling times of both subpopulations are equal (15 to 20 days). A different mechanism of origin must be

Table 17.1
Sublines of the *Dunning R 3327* Prostatic Carcinoma Line and Some of Their Basic Characteristics

Subline	Characteristics
R 3327 A	Squamous cell carcinoma, no DHT receptor, no 5α-reductase, doubling time ± 2 days.
R 3327 B-F	Five poorly characterized sublines described by Dunning.
R 3327 G	Undifferentiated, androgen-dependent, fast growing.
R 3327 H	Well differentiated adenocarcinoma, secretion, DHT and E receptors, androgen-dependent, enzyme pattern similar to dorsolateral prostate, doubling time 15 to 20 days, hormone-independent subpopulation with identical growth rate has been hormone-dependent for 19 years.[17]
R 3327 HI	Well differentiated adenocarcinoma, subline of R 3327 H; E and progesteron receptor equal to R 3327 H; DHT receptor low, hormone-insensitive (HI), 5α-reductase and all other enzymes lower than in R 3327 H; doubling time 15 to 20 days.[17]
R 3327 AT	Anaplastic tumor (AT), subline of R 3327 H; DHT receptor absent, hormone-insensitive, enzymes low, doubling time 2 days.

postulated for the subline *R 3327 AT*, which also originated from the *H* line. If the *AT* population were present in the *H line* normally, it would lead to the loss of the *H line* because of selective overgrowth of the *AT cells*, which have a doubling time of only 2 days. Maybe several mechanisms can cause changes of the tumor characteristics.

For obvious reasons, the *Dunning R 3327 H* tumor cannot be cured by hormonal treatment. Relapse occurs as a result of continued growth of the hormone-insensitive subpopulation. If *R 3327 H* would precisely reflect the mechanisms involved in human prostatic adenocarcinoma becoming hormone-independent, then it would be mandatory to treat patients with some adjuvant regimen capable of killing hormone-insensitive cells right after the diagnosis is made. It makes little sense to wait until these populations form a large tumor mass which is more difficult to attack with other forms of therapy.

Another interesting aspect is that survival of animals bearing the *R 3327 H* tumor is *longer* if castration is carried out when the tumor is small. This contradicts the finding of the Veterans Administration Cooperative Urological Research Group (VACURG) trials,[61] that delay of hormonal treatment until metastases are present does not negatively influence survival (see Chapter 11). The Dunning lines rarely or never metastasize. Therefore they are not a suitable model for the study of this important event, which commonly occurs in human prostatic carcinoma.

Other Animal Models of Human Prostatic Cancer

The other important, currently known animal models for prostatic cancer and some of their properties are listed in Table 17.2.

Table 17.2
Other Animal Models Currently Available for Human Prostatic Carcinoma and Some of Their Characteristics

Name of Tumor Model	Characteristics
Lobund rat, tumor lines[33-37]	*All lines:* poorly differentiated adenocarcinoma with solid parts, partially hormone-dependent, endocrinologically not completely characterized, grows in females, transplantable in cell suspension *only* on Lobund Wistar rats, grows in culture, infiltrates locally, metastasizes to lymph nodes and lungs; fast growth rate; doubling time 18 to 20 hours. Extent of metastases reduced by cyclophosphamide, aspirin, and corynebacterium parvum; increased by inspiration anesthesia. *Line II:* better differentiation, different pattern of metastases.
A × C rat tumor[53, 54]	Originated from ventral prostate of old, virgin A × C rats. Cribriform adenocarcinomas, incidence increased with testosterone, 3 transplantable lines, characterization in progress.
Nb rat tumor[27-29]	Originated from dorsolateral lobe of Nb rats after prolonged testosterone and estrone treatment; estrogen- and androgen-dependent, hormone dependency can be manipulated, independent growth can be induced, characterization in progress.[3]

Three transplantable prostatic carcinoma lines have been developed from spontaneous tumors found in old, *germ-free Lobund Wistar rats* by Pollard and his associates.[33-37] They are named I, II, and III and are derived from three of the nine animals which were found to have prostatic carcinomas besides other tumors. Line II shows less aggressive local infiltration and a different pattern of metastatic growth combined with a better histological differentiation. Otherwise the lines are very similar.

Morphologically they consist of poorly differentiated adenocarcinomatous solid formations. The tumors are of questionable hormone dependence. Transplants grow and metastasize in female hosts. Treatment of some animals with estrogens for 8 weeks is reported to have resulted in a volume decrease of about 50%. Endocrinological characterization has not been carried out. The original tumors were grown in cell culture with success. When inoculated back into Lobund Wistar rats the tumors formed were histologically identical with the tumor of origin but exhibited a very fast rate of growth. Transplantation into rat strains other than Lobund Wistar was unsuccessful. Virus particles could not be detected.

The tumor lines metastasize into lymph nodes and lungs. The extent of metastases is markedly reduced by cyclophosphamide, aspirin, and corynebacterium parvum. Inhalation anesthesia increases the extent of metastases. This effect seems to be especially directed against the metastases because the primary tumor is not affected by these modalities of treatment.

Shain and co-workers[53, 54] detected *spontaneous adenocarcinomas in the ventral lobes of the prostate of A × C rats*. This species was previously thought to be free of this disease. The tumors were found in seven of 41 virgin male *A × C rats* which were kept alive longer than 34 months. Attempts to increase this spontaneous tumor incidence by exogenous testosterone administration lead to induction of tumors in 70% of the treated animals. Three of the tumors have been transplanted successfully. The available data on characterization are too preliminary to determine the usefulness of this model.

More than 20 years ago Noble initiated *prostatic carcinomas in Nb rats*[26-28] by prolonged exposure of these animals to testosterone propionate pellets alone or in combination with estrone. Prostatic carcinomas occur in this species spontaneously at a rate of 0.45%. With pellet implantation the incidence rises to 18 to 20%. The induction time varies between 37 and 70 weeks. The tumors originate from the dorsolateral prostate. A number of transplantable lines have been developed which include an autonomous one, an androgen-dependent one, and an estrogen-dependent one. The morphology of the autonomous line is that of a solid undifferentiated malignoma. The histological appearance of the androgen- and estrogen-dependent lines is clearly different and consists of solid sheets of carcinoma cells with occasional gland formation which are surrounded by stroma.[6]

The known characteristics of this model have recently been summarized and compared with those of other models.[3] The tumor lines metastasize to the lungs; androgen receptors were found, but the endocrinological characteristics are unknown. The volume doubling time of the dependent lines is about 15 days in the exponential phase of growth; the autonomous line seems to grow slower. There is slow growth in castrated males and in females, and partial regression was reported after castration. Complete deprivation of the hormone or the hormone combination used for the induction of a given line leads to partial regression followed by autonomous growth in all tumors studied so far. Withdrawal of the pellets and substitution of the animals with 20 to 25% of the induction doses of the same hormone prevented the event of autonomous growth in 60 to 100% of the animals. Noble concluded from these data that the change from hormone-dependent to autonomous growth can be promoted by radical withdrawal of the growth-stimulating hormone and that a low maintenance dose of this hormone preserves hormone dependence while still slowing down tumor growth.[28]

This interesting finding is at variance with the hypothesis based on the *Dunning R 3327 H line* that the step from hormone dependence to autonomous growth is a selection phenomenon. Noble's findings suggest that hormone dependence and independence are induced processes which can be manipulated and are result of adaptation of tumor cell populations to changes in the endocrine environment. For present endocrine therapy of prostatic carcinoma this would mean that, for example, castration followed by low doses of testosterone is a better treatment than castration alone. It is obvious that this hypothesis needs to be checked. The findings could be of greatest practical importance.

Some other animals such as the dog, the mastomys, the Syrian golden hamster, and the lion are known to develop prostatic cancer. None of these possible models is well explored, and none has practical importance at this moment. The available evidence has recently been reviewed.[17]

TISSUE CULTURE

Organ culture and cell culture (monolayer) techniques have been frequently applied to the study of human prostatic tissues, especially to benign hyperplasia (BPH). However, relevant results have been scarce. In spite of the urgent need of *in vitro* models for genetic, immunologic, endocrinologic, and other studies of prostatic carcinoma, no good model systems are available at present. Again, complete recent reviews were published and are recommended for more in depth information.[25, 46, 48]

Organ Culture

Theoretical advantages of organ culture techniques can be seen in the preservation of intact tissue structures (not so in cell culture). By incubating many explants from the same tissue of origin, different experimental conditions can be applied to parts of the same specimen, time course studies can easily be accomplished. The environment can easily be manipulated, systemic effects can be excluded. The technique can be applied to *human* tissues. Some of these advantages may become disadvantages. The major disadvantage, however, is that there is no proof that prostatic carcinoma tissue can be maintained in a vital state longer than 2 hours.

Short-term incubation of tissue from 147 prostatic carcinomas was carried out in autologous plasma under hyperbaric conditions to study kinetic parameters, such as the labeling index, per cent of labelled cells, and mitoses by the use of ^{3}H-thymidine.[13] The labeling index was low in all types of carcinomas but was lower in well differentiated tumors (0.69%) than in cribriform (1.5%) and anaplastic carcinomas (2.4%). Only in one case of solid, anaplastic carcinoma labelled mitoses were seen and a kinetic study could be carried out. For this tumor the labeling index was 7.0%, the mitotic index 0.6%. The generation time of the whole population was 96 hours, the durations of cell-cycle phases were $S = 9.3$ hours, $G_2 = 2$ hours, $G_1 = 83.9$ hours, and $M = 0.8$ hours, respectively. These data demonstrate the extremely slow growth rate of prostatic cancer and discourage cell-kinetic studies. Other interesting results of this study were that hormonal treatment seemed to decrease labeling of the carcinomatous part of the specimens. The percentage of labeled epithelial cells in BPH nodules was 0.53% but was significantly increased to 1.2% in BPH areas adjacent to carcinoma. To the best of our knowledge DNA labeling of prostatic carcinoma cells kept *in vitro* longer than 2 hours has not been demonstrated.

The fate of prostatic carcinoma tissue in organ culture was studied on more than 200 explants from 19 carcinomas by 6500 histological sections after time course incubation over 3 weeks.[12] In no case was vital looking tissue found after more than 6 days. Labeling of carcinoma cells with ^{3}H-thymidine could not be demonstrated. Only proliferation of metaplastic benign cells was seen.

Androgen metabolism and the effect of estradiol on it were studied in 11 cases of BPH and in 12 cases of prostatic cancer in organ culture[1] in 20-hour incubation experiments. The results showed that dihydrotestosterone (DHT) was the main metabolite of testosterone in all specimens but one. The proportion of DHT formed in seven of the carcinomas was lower than in BPH ($p < 0.05$). In the older carcinoma patients a greater proportion of *17-oxo*-metabolites was formed. Estradiol increased the uptake of ^{3}H-DHT in absence of carrier but had no effect on the uptake of 5α-androstenedione and testosterone. Estradiol decreased the formation of DHT in BPH and carcinoma in absence of carrier by about 20%. A number of interesting conclusions are drawn. The authors suggest that estradiol treatment *in vivo* and *in vitro* produces a shift from 5α-reduction to 17β-dehydrogenation. Inhibition of 5α-reductase as a cause of these events is considered. It remains unknown, in which tissue compartments (stroma, tumor, epithelium) these reactions occur.

The effect of testosterone and stilbestrol on prostatic explants in organ culture were studied by Mc Mahon *et al.*[23] First attempts to study drug treatment of prostatic carcinoma in organ culture were reported by Coffey and Isaacs.[46]

Cell Culture

Cell culture allows study of tumor cells in a dispersed form, free of stroma and host influences. Theoretical advantages of this technique are that growth can easily be monitored by cell counts, and the environment, the culture medium, can easily be manipulated. Only single cells can be used as immunological targets, and for virological studies, stroma-epithelial and host-tumor interactions can be studied. In spite of the well recognized necessity to develop useful *in vitro* models, not much success has been achieved in spite of the intense efforts of a number of investigators.[2, 21, 30–32 41, 45, 47, 49, 57–59, 62] There are several evident reasons for failure which have not been overcome: there is lack of a good reliable marker which allows one to differentiate normal prostatic epithelium from prostatic carcinoma cells. It is still doubtful as to whether currently used techniques produce cultures of carcinoma cells. Attempts to characterize cultures from prostatic epithelial cells have revealed a remarkable loss of functional properties of the tissue of origin. Reviews on this subject have been published recently.[25, 48]

Cell culture could be useful to maintain prostatic cells for short periods of time ranging from hours to several weeks (*short-term culture*), or the goal could be to develop cell lines which continue to grow for longer periods of time or permanently (*long-term culture*).

SHORT-TERM CULTURES

Initiation of cultures can be achieved in several ways. The most commonly used is the explant technique. Small pieces of tissue are suspended in suitable culture medium. Histological time course studies[12] have revealed that at least under standard culture conditions prostatic carcinoma does not survive longer than 6 days. In explants of carcinoma and adenoma an identical process takes place: within 1 to 3 days metaplasia and proliferation of the basal cells of normal acini occur. This leads to the epithelialization of the cut surface of the explants and to outgrowth of cells on the surface of the culture vessel (*primary culture*). The observation that carcinoma cells do not take part in this process is at variance with data reported.[60] Stonington et al.[60] have shown outgrowth of cells from metastatic lymph nodes which contain acid phosphatase. The observation that epithelial cells grown from prostatic carcinoma tissue were always diploid like the ones grown from BPH seems to confirm the hypothesis that prostatic carcinoma cells do not grow in primary culture under standard conditions.[18]

Another method of initiating cultures of prostatic carcinoma and other tissues consists of the preparation of cell suspensions by the use of proteolytic enzymes, such as pronase and collagenase, or by mechanical dispersion of prostatic tissue. This technique has lead to the cell line *DU 145*, which originated from a brain metastasis of an undifferentiated, hormone-insensitive prostatic carcinoma.[58] Such cell suspensions resulting from *tissue and cell separation* have been produced and characterized preliminarily.[29, 39] Viability of cells depends strongly on the quality of the separation technique. This technique produces separate populations of fresh stroma and epithelial elements. It has been used in BPH and carcinoma for the study of androgen metabolism and androgen receptor in stroma and epithelium separately.[5, 42] The results obtained suggest that most of the 5α-reductase activity is localized in the stroma, whereas most of the androgen receptor is located in the epithelium. These interesting findings, suggesting very specific stromal-epithelial interactions, require further confirmation and quantification.

Short-term cultures of fibroblasts, stromal cells which can easily be grown from prostatic explants of normal and tumorous tissue, have also been used to study androgen metabolism.[51] 5α-Reductase, the prevalent enzyme in fibroblasts from all prostatic tissues, was found in fibroblasts from prostatic carcinoma only at much lower activities. Time course experiments show that much of the testosterone is initially metabolized to 5α-androstenedione and later to DHT. All enzyme activities were lower in fibroblasts from prostatic carcinoma. In this system the presence of aromatase and the synthesis of estrone from testosterone via androstenedione was shown.[52] The significance of these findings is not yet known. They indicate, however, possible specific characteristics of tumor stroma which may influence epithelial growth and function in some way. Studies in this field should be strongly encouraged.

LONG-TERM CULTURES

A total of four long-term cell lines originating from prostatic carcinoma have been reported.[20, 22, 30, 58] A detailed review was carried out recently.[48] Two lines have been well characterized, the *line DU 145*[58] and *EB 33*.[30] The latter is of questioned prostatic origin on genetic grounds, but repeated studies in different laboratories have identified *EB 33* as a prostatic line immunologically. All lines have in common the fact that they are not hormone-dependent. A possible exception are some clones of *EB 33*[32] which have also shown slower growth in castrated nude mice.[50] The line has been used for immunological studies as target and as a source of antigen. It contains prostatic acid phosphatase.[48]

In summary, it seems that long-term cell lines have up to now contributed little to prostatic cancer research. It is questionable whether without a major change in culture techniques efforts in this direction of research should be continued. However, it requires little effort to carry on attempts to develop permanent lines as a side line of research involving short-term cell cultures and tissue separation techniques, which have produced very promising results recently. The suggestions of Sato and his co-workers[11] to approach the problem by first defining the growth requirements of prostatic cells should be followed and may indicate the most promising direction of future work in this field.

HETEROTRANSPLANTATION OF HUMAN PROSTATIC CARCINOMA

With the event of the thymous aplastic "nude" mice in 1966[8, 38] transplantation of human tumor tissues into these immunodeficient animals seemed to be within close reach and a solution to all "model problems." Also in the field of prostate tumors investigators began to use the nude mouse with great enthusiasm, but with little success. Attempts to originate serially transferable tumor lines failed except for a few instances. In our own laboratory the 82nd transplanted carcinoma could be serially passaged and surprisingly the 93rd as well. Up to now a total of more than 100 transplantations have not resulted in further "takes."

Okada et al.[31] studied 19 different human prostatic carcinomas as subcutaneous transplants in 84 male nude mice to establish whether the tissues remain vital and grow. The result was disappointing: all grafts had lost weight during the transplant periods varying from 33 to 157 days. Vital prostatic tissue was found in most grafts by means of histological examination, but vital appearing prostatic carcinoma tissue was found only in eight mice. The tumors were all adenocarcinomas. No increase of graft size was found during the observation periods.

In the literature only very few reports on successful heterotransplantation of human prostatic carcinoma were found. Two prostatic tumors grew in the series of Shimosato.[55, 56] One of these (PR 1) was transferred three times. Histologically this tumor is undifferentiated; growth does not depend on hormones. More recently a successful transplantation of a moderately differentiated human prostatic adenocarcinoma was described by Reid et al.[40] This tumor can be serially passaged. Its growth rate is slow, it contains tartrate-inhibitable acid phosphatase, and it is moderately dependent on androgens.

The transplantable line PC 82 was developed in 1977 in our own laboratory from the radical prostectomy specimen of a moderately differentiated, cribriform adenocarcinoma.[16, 43, 44] At this moment the tumor grows in its 7th animal passage. Some properties of this model are summarized in Table 17.3.

Its histological appearance is very similar to the tissue of origin and has not changed during serial transplantation. The tumors contain stroma which is derived from the host animal. This has been confirmed by genetic studies. Preliminary electron microscopical studies show all characteristics of human prostatic cancer. Immunohistochemistry and immunofluorescence studies have confirmed the presence of large amounts of prostatic acid phosphatase.

The tumor does not "take" in female nude mice and in previously castrated males. In intact males the volume doubling time is 18 ± 5 days. Castration leads to a regression of about 50% of the volume within 2 weeks in preliminary studies. Estradiol has a similar effect and leads to atrophy of the tumor cells and arrest of the normally present secretional activity. More quantitative studies are presently being undertaken.

Preliminary biochemical studies were carried out. The tumor and the tumor secretion contain excessively high amounts of acid phosphatase. Serum acid phosphatase of tumor-bearing animals is elevated. Human LDH isoenzymes were recovered from the serum of the tumor-bearing nude mice. Androgen receptor was found in the tumor tissue.

Primary cultures can be initiated from the tumor transplants and have been used for genetic studies. The data are unpublished but show hypotriploidy, evidence that the culture cells are indeed human carcinoma cells.

Table 17.3
Some Characteristics of the Transplantable Human Prostatic Carcinoma Line in Nude Mice (*PC 82*)

PC 82	Characteristics of Transplantable Line
Morphological	Cribriform, moderately differentiated adenocarcinoma, mouse stroma with electron microscopical characteristics of human prostatic cancer.
Functional	Secretion present (pseudocysts); human prostatic acid phosphatase present in tumor, secretion, and mouse serum. Human LDH isoenzyme pattern in tumor extract and mouse serum.
Growth	Doubling time in male mouse, exponential phase 18 ± 5 days.
Endocrine	No growth in female mice, partial regression after castration or estradiol treatment; androgen receptor present.
Tissue culture	Grows in short-term culture.
Genetics	Hypotriploid.

In spite of all difficulties these results encourage further efforts in this field. A serious difficulty is the high cost of maintaining large colonies of nude mice. Serious drawbacks in this work can result from animal room epidemics and conditions which tend to decrease the life span of the animals.

The slow growth rate of the tumor line reflects one important property of human prostatic cancer and is therefore desirable. On the other hand growth experiments have to extend over 3 to 6 months, and this is only possible with stable, healthy populations of animals.

Obvious advantages of models using nude mice or other immunodeficient animals lie in the fact that *human* prostatic cancer can be studied. Characterization must concentrate on similarities with the tumors of origin but also on the possibility of changes which may reflect the specific relationship with the new host. Up to now such changes have not been found. The model could be used for endocrinologic studies, kinetic studies, the study of ideal tissue culture conditions for human prostatic carcinoma, the search for new chemotherapeutic agents, the effect of combined forms of treatment and could help to solve many other open questions.

REFERENCES

1. Bard, D. R., and Lasnitzki, I. The influence of oestradiol on the metabolism of androgen by human prostatic tissue. *J. Endocrinol. 74:* 1, 1977.
2. Brehmer, B., Marquardt, H., and Madsen, P. O. Growth and hormonal response of cells derived from carcinoma and hyperplasia of the prostate in monolayer cell-culture. A possible in vitro model for clinical chemotherapy. *J. Urol. 108:* 890, 1972.
3. Bruchowsky, N., and Rennie, P. S. New considerations in the hormonal induction and regulation of animal tumors. In *Prostate Cancer*, edited by D. S. Coffey and J. T. Isaacs, *UICC Tech. Rep. Ser. 48*. Geneva, 1979, pp. 134–144.
4. Coffey, D. S., Isaacs, J. T., and Weisman, R. M.: Animal models for the study of prostatic cancer. In *Prostatic Cancer*, edited by G. P. Murphy. P. S. G. Publishing Company, Littleton, Mass., 1979, pp. 89–109.
5. Cowan, R. A., Cowan, S. K., Grant, J. K., and Elder, H. Y. Biochemical investigations of separated epithelium and stroma from benign hyperplastic prostatic tissue. *J. Endocrinol. 74:* 111, 1977.

6. Drago, J. R., Ikeda, R. M., Maurer, R. E., Goldman, L. B., and Tesluk, H. The Nb rat prostatic carcinoma model. *Invest. Urol. 16:* 353, 1979.
7. Dunning, W. F. Prostate cancer in the rat. *Natl. Cancer Inst. Monogr. 12:* 351, 1963.
8. Flanagan, S. P. "Nude," a new hairless gene with pleiotrophic effects in the mouse. *Genet. Res. 8:* 295, 1966.
9. Gutman, E. B., Sproul, E. E., and Gutman, A. B. Significance of increased phosphatase activity of bone at the site of osteoplastic metastases secondary to carcinoma of prostate gland. *Am. J. Cancer 28:* 485, 1936.
10. Handelman, H. The initiations of model systems in prostatic cancer. *Oncology 34:* 96, 1977.
11. Hayashi, I., Larner, J., and Sato, G. Hormonal growth control of cells in culture. *In Vitro 14:* 23, 1978.
12. Heinemeyer, H. M. Prostata-Tumoren in Organkultur und Heterotransplantation. Dissertation, Universität Würzburg, 1978.
13. Helpap, B., Stiens, R., and Brühl, P. The proliferative pattern of untreated and treated prostatic carcinoma. *Z. Krebsforsch. 87:* 311, 1979.
14. Huggins, C., and Hodges, C. V. Studies on prostatic cancer. I. The effect of castration, of estrogen and of androgen on serum phosphatases in metastatic carcinoma of the prostate. *Cancer Res. 1:* 293, 1941.
15. Huggins, C. Endocrine-induced regression of cancers. Les Prix Nobel, Stockholm, 1966, p. 172.
16. Hoehn, W., Schroeder, F. H., Riemann, J. F., Joebsis, A. C., and Hermanek, P. Human prostatic adenocarcinoma: some characteristics of a serially transplantable line on nude mice. *Prostate 1:* 95, 1980.
17. Isaacs, J. T., and Coffey, D. S. Spontaneous animal models for prostatic cancer. In *Prostate Cancer*, edited by D. S. Coffey and J. T. Isaacs. *UICC Tech. Rep. Ser. 48.* Geneva, 1979, pp. 195–219.
18. Jellinghaus, W., Okada, K., Ragg, C., Gerhardt, H., and Schroeder, F. H. Chromosomal studies of human prostatic tumors in vitro. *Invest. Urol. 14:* 16, 1976.
19. Kaighn, M. E., and Babcock, M. S. Monolayer cultures of human prostatic cells. *Cancer Chemother. Rep. 59:* 1975.
20. Kaighn, M. E. Characteristics of human prostatic cells cultures. *Cancer Treat. Rep. 61:* 147, 1977.
21. Lerch, V. L., Rodd, J., Lattimer, J. K., and Tannenbaum, M. A technique for the study of human prostatic epithelial cells in vitro by time-lapse cinematography. *J. Urol. 104:* 564, 1970.
22. Lubaroff, D. M. Development of an epithelial tissue culture line from a human prostatic adenocarcinoma. *J. Urol. 118:* 612, 1977.
23. McMahon, M. J., Butler, A. V. J., and Thomas, G. H. Morphological responses of prostatic carcinoma to testosterone in organ culture. *Br. J. Cancer 26:* 388, 1972.
24. Merchant, D. J. Model systems for the study of prostatic cancer. *Oncology 34:* 100, 1977.
25. Merchant, D. J. Cell and organ culture in prostatic cancer. In *Prostatic Cancer*, edited by G. P. Murphy. P.S.G. Publishing Company, Littleton, Mass., 1979, pp. 75–88.
26. Noble, R. L. The development of prostatic adenocarcinoma in Nb rats following prolonged sex hormone administration. *Cancer Res. 37:* 1929, 1977.
27. Noble, R. Sex steroids as a cause of adenocarcinoma of the dorsal prostate in Nb rats, and their influence on the growth of the transplants. *Oncology 34:* 138, 1977.
28. Noble, R., and Hoover, L. A classification of transplantable tumors in Nb rats controlled by estrogen from dormancy to autonomy. *Cancer Res. 35:* 2935, 1975.
29. Oishi, K., Romijn, J. C., and Schroeder, F. H. Cell-separation and characterization of epithelial cells from human benign prostatic hyperplasia. *Prostate 2:* 281, 1981.
30. Okada, K., and Schroeder, F. H. Human prostatic carcinoma in cell culture: preliminary report on the development and characterization of an epithelial cell-line (EB 33). *Urol. Res. 2:* 111, 1974.
31. Okada, K., Schroeder, F. H., Jellinghaus, W., Wullstein, H. K., and Heinemeyer, H. M. Human prostatic adenoma and carcinoma: transplantation of cultured cells and primary tissue fragments in "nude mice." *Invest. Urol. 13:* 395, 1976.
32. Okada, K., Laudenbach, I., and Schroeder, F. H. Human prostatic epithelial cells in

culture: clonal selection and androgen dependence of cell-line EB 33. *J. Urol. 115:* 164, 1976.

33. Pollard, M. Spontaneous prostate adenocarcinoma in aged germ free Wistar rats. *J. Natl. Cancer Inst. 51:* 1235, 1973.

34. Pollard, M., Chang, C. Fe., and Luckert, P. H. Investigations on prostatic adenocarcinomas in rats. *Oncology 34:* 129, 1977.

35. Pollard, M., and Luckert, P. H. Transplantable metastasizing prostate adenocarcinomas in rats. *J. Natl. Cancer Inst. 54:* 643, 1975.

36. Pollard, M., and Luckert, P. H. Chemotherapy of metastatic prostate adenocarcinoma in germ free rats. *Cancer Treat. Rep. 60:* 619, 1976.

37. Pollard, M. Prostate adenocarcinomas in Wistar rats. *Rush Presbyt. St. Luke's Med. Bull. 14:* 12, 1975.

38. Poulson, C. O., and Rygaard, J. Heterotransplantation of human adenocarcinomas of the colon and rectum to the mouse mutant "nude." A study of nine consecutive transplantations. *Acta Pathol. Microbiol. Scand. 79:* 159, 1971.

39. Pretlow, T. G., II. Disaggregation of prostates and purification of epithelial cells from normal and cancerous prostates using sedimentation in an isokinetic density gradient of ficol in tissue culture medium. *Cancer Chemother. Rep. 59:* 143, 1975

40. Reid, L., Leav, I., Mark, F., Albert, J., and Gellner, J. Androgen-dependent human prostatic carcinoma in nude mice. Proceedings of AACR and ASCO, *AACR abstracts 19:* 151, 1978.

41. Roehl, L. Prostatic hyperplasia and prostatic carcinoma studies with tissue culture technique. *Acta Chir. Scand.* [Suppl.] *33:* 240, 1959.

42. Romijn, J. C., Oishi, K., Bolt- de Vries, J., Schweikert, H. U., Mulder, E., and Schröder, F. H. Androgen metabolism and androgen receptors in separated epithelium and stroma of the human prostate. In *Steroid Receptors, Metabolism and Prostatic Cancer*, edited by F. H. Schröder and H. J. de Voogt. Excerpta Medica, Amsterdam, 1980, pp. 134–143.

43. Romijn, J. C., van Steenbrugge, G. J., Oishi, K., Bolt- de Vries, J., Hoehn, W., and Schroeder, F. H. Characterization of a transplantable androgen-dependent human prostatic carcinoma (PC 82). *J. Steroid Biochem. 11:* XXIV, 1979.

44. Romijn, J. C., van Steenbrugge, G. J., Oishi, K., Bolt- de Vries, J., Hoehn, W., and Schroeder, F. H. Characterization of a transplantable androgen-dependent human prostatic carcinoma (PC 82). *Proceedings of the 3rd Workshop on Nude Mice*, Montana, 1979. *Gustav Fischer Verlag*, Stuttgart, in press 1982.

45. Rose, N. R., Choe, B. K., and Pontes, J. E. Cultivation of epithelial cells from the prostate. *Cancer Chemother. Rep. 59:* 143, 1975.

46. Sandberg, A. A. Regulation of prostate growth in organ culture. In *Prostate Cancer*, edited by D. S. Coffey and J. T. Isaacs. *UICC Tech. Rep. Ser. 48*. Geneva, 1979, pp. 165–194.

47. Sanford, E. J., Geder, L., Jones, R. E., Rohner, T. J., and Rapp, F. In vitro culture of human prostatic tissue. *Urol. Res. 5:* 207, 1977.

48. Schroeder, F. H., Oishi, K., and Schweikert, H. U. Application of cell culture techniques to human prostatic carcinoma. In *Prostate Cancer*, edited by D. S. Coffey and J. T. Isaacs. *UICC Tech. Rep. Ser. 48*. Geneva, 1979, pp. 145–164.

49. Schroeder, F. H., Sato, G., and Gittes, R. F. Human prostatic adenocarcinoma: growth in monolayer tissue culture. *J. Urol. 106:* 734, 1971.

50. Schroeder, F. H., and Jellinghaus W. EB 33, an epithelial cell line from human prostate carcinoma: a review. *Natl. Cancer Inst. Monogr. 49:* 41, 1978.

51. Schweikert, H. U., Hein, H. J., Romijn, J. C., and Schroeder, F. H. Testosterone metabolism of fibroblasts grown from prostatic carcinoma, benign prostatic hyperplasia and non genital skin. *Invest. Urol.*, in press 1982.

52. Schweikert, H. U. Conversion of androstenedione to estrone in human fibroblasts cultured from prostate, genital and non genital skin. *Horm. Metab. Res. 11:* 635, 1979.

53. Shain, S. A., McCullough, B., Nitchuk, M., and Boesel, R. W. Prostate carcinogenesis in the AXC rat. *Oncology 34:* 114, 1977.

54. Shain, S. A., McCullough, B., and Segaloff, A. Spontaneous adenocarcinomas of the ventral prostate of aged AXC rats. *J. Natl. Cancer Inst. 55:* 177, 1975.

55. Shimosato, Y., Kameya, T., Nagai, K., Hirohashi, S., Koide, T., Hayashi, H., and Nomura, T. Transplantation of human tumors in nude mice. *J. Natl. Cancer Inst. 56:*

1251, 1976.

56. Shimosato, Y., Kameya, J., Kobuta, T., Hirohashi, S., Hayashi, H., Ikeuchi, S., and Nagai, K. Experimental chemo-radio- and endocrine therapy for human cancers transplanted in nude mice. *Proceedings 2nd International Workshop on Nude Mice. Gustav Fischer Verlag*, Stuttgart, 1977, p. 499.

57. Stone, K. R., Paulson, D. F., Bonar, R. A., and Reich, C. F., III. In vitro culture of epithelial cells derived from urogenital tissues. *Urol. Res. 2:* 149, 1975.

58. Stone, K. R., Mickey, D. D., Wunderli, H., Mickey, G. H., and Paulson, D. F. Isolation of human prostate carcinoma cell line (DU 145). *Int. J. Cancer 21:* 274, 1978.

59. Stonington, O. G., and Hemmingsen, H. Culture of cells as a monolayer derived from the epithelium of the human prostate: a new cell growth technique. *J. Urol. 106:* 393, 1971.

60. Stonington, O. G., Szwec, N., and Webber, M. Isolation and identification of the human malignant prostatic epithelial cell in pure monolayer culture. *J. Urol. 114:* 903, 1975.

61. Weissman, R. M., Coffey, D. S., and Scott, W. W. Cell kinetic studies of prostatic cancer: adjuvant therapy in animal models. *Oncology 34:* 133, 1977.

62. Wojewski, A., and Przeworska-Kaniewicz, D. The influence of stilbestrol and testosterone on the growth of prostatic adenocarcinoma in tissue culture. *J. Urol. 93:* 721, 1965.

Editorial Comment to Chapter 17

The most comprehensive summary on the subject emerged from a Planning Meeting of the *National Prostatic Cancer Project* (NPCP) held in 1979 in Buffalo and recently published by Murphy (1980). In their compilation Coffey and Isaacs (1980) gave a summary of the spontaneous prostatic carcinomas observed in animals which is reproduced in Table 17.4.

Three additional papers recently reviewed critically prostatic carcinoma cell lines currently under investigation (Ackermann, 1981; Kaighn, 1980; Williams, 1980). A phenomenon occasionally underestimated is the contamination of a considerable number of the reported cell lines by other cell lines, particularly *HeLa* ! Williams (1980) states that there are at

Table 17.4
Spontaneous Prostatic Adenocarcinomas in Animals[a]

Species	Year	Investigator	Tumor
Rat	1961	W.F. Dunning	From dorsal prostate of aged (22 mo) Copenhagen rat, syngeneic; androgen-dependent; transplantable
	1973	M. Pollard P.H. Luckert	Aged, germ-free Lobund Wistar; ?lobe, prostate; hormone-sensitive; transplantable
	1975	S.A. Shain B. McCullough A. Segaloff	Aged A × C rats; ventral prostate; no metastases; not transplanted
Hamster	1960	J.G. Fortner J.W. Funkhauser M.R. Cullen	Aged Syrian golden hamster; transplantable; tumor has been lost
Dog	1968	I. Leav G.V. Ling	Aged (>8 yr) mongrels; metastases; no occult tumor
Mastomy	1965	K.C. Snell H.L. Stewart	Aged female African rodent prostate
	1970	J. Holland	
Monkey	1940	E.T. Engle A.P. Stout	Aged Macaca mulatta

[a] From D. S. Coffey and J. T. Isaacs, 1980.

present only four characterized and *un*contaminated cell lines of prostatic cancer available for study, two originating from primary lesions (lines *HPC-36* and *1013 L*) and two from distant metastases (*DU-145* and *PC-3*).

Furthermore the transfer of data obtained from animal tumors or human prostatic carcinoma tissue kept in culture to the human *in vivo* condition is problematic (Ackermann, 1981). Dahlberg *et al.* (1980) reported pronounced differences between *R-3327H* rat prostatic carcinoma and metastatic prostate cancer from man when the biochemical hormone receptor properties of both tissues were compared. Animal data must thus be interpreted with due caution in applying such information to the human pathological situation. This is even true for tumor lines which, after transplantation, spontaneously induce lymphatic or hematogenous metastases (Pollard and Luckert, 1980). However, with human tumor tissue transplanted into appropriately conditioned animals we have vital and metabolically functioning cancer tissue *plus stroma* (in contrast to the situation in cell culture) available for morphological, histochemical, and biochemical studies (Fig. 17.1). This malignant growth is, although developing in an xenogenic host, not withdrawn from its physiological (or pathophysiological), and pharmacological influences.

With regard to cell culture studies we should cite Kaighn (1980), who

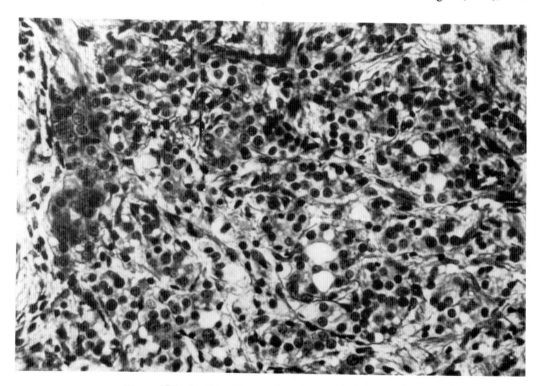

Figure 17.1 Proliferative carcinoma transplant into *nude mouse* (nu/nu, BALB/c) from human adenocarcinoma 18 days after heterotransplantation. The xenograft shows cribriform tumor patterns with mitoses (×153). (Courtesy of Th. Senge, Herne, Federal Republic of Germany)

stated that "There is no guarantee that a cultured cell, regardless of its authenticity, will behave the same in culture as it does in the intact organism."

G. H. J.
R. H.

REFERENCES

Ackermann, R. Model systems of human urogenital tumors—theoretical and experimental aspects of its use in tumor-biological research. *Akt. Urol. 12:* 52, 1981.

Coffey, D. S., and Isaacs, J. T. Requirements for an analyzed animal model of prostatic cancer. In *Models for Prostate Cancer. Prog. Clin. Biol. Res. 37.* Alan Liss, New York, 1980, pp. 379–391.

Dahlberg, E, Snochowski, M., and Gustafsson, J.-Å. Comparison of the R-3327H rat prostatic adenocarcinoma to human benign prostatic hyperplasia and metastatic carcinoma of the prostate with regard to steroid hormone receptors. *Prostate 1:* 61, 1980.

Kaighn, M. E. Human prostatic epithelial cell culture models. *Invest. Urol. 17:* 382, 1980.

Murphy, G. P. *Models for Prostate Cancer. Prog. Clin. Biol. Res. 37.* Alan Liss, New York, 1980.

Pollard, M. and Luckert, P. Patterns of spontaneous metastases manifested by three rat prostate adenocarcinomas. J. Surg. Oncol. 17: 359, 1980.

Williams, R. D. Human urologic cancer cell lines. *Invest. Urol. 17:* 359, 1980.

18

Immunological Approaches to Prostate Cancer

K. F. Klippel, M.D.

As early as 1909, Paul Ehrlich[15] attributed not only antimicrobiological defense to the immune system, but also the killing and elimination of pathologically altered cells. Later it became evident that cancer cells were likewise pathologically altered cells which present different antigens to the immune system. Thomas et al.,[43] Burnet,[7] and Good[24] in particular popularized this idea: according to their theory the normal functioning immune machinery controls the organism and prevents the growth of neoplastic "degenerated" cells by destruction (immune surveillance).

Numerous clinical observations suggest that tumor cells are able to evoke an immune response such as spontaneous remission of tumors, a well-known but rare phenomenon in renal cell carcinoma.

The theory of immune surveillance is supported by the fact that as immunologic competence decreases with age, an increase of tumor incidence can be observed; 5 to 6% of patients under immunosuppressive therapy develop de novo malignancies. Since prostatic carcinoma primarily develop in the elderly man, and every second to third 80-year-old man bears malignant cells in his prostate, one could suggest that, especially in the prostate, cancer development is in positive correlation to the loss of immunocompetence.

In the late 1920's Piccaluga[34] demonstrated the diminished "oncolytic" potency of splenic and thymic organ extracts in elderly people. When he compared the "oncolytic" effect of various organic cell extracts, the prostate cells always revealed a very low index: they were not able to kill cells from a cell culture line, whereas splenic cells killed about 80%. The conclusion of his studies concerning prostatic carcinoma were: (immunologic) resistance is in reverse relation to age; the physiological balance between the growth and killing of cancer cells becomes displaced in favor of growth.

Not only aging, but also exogenous influences were known at that time to disturb the immune competence. Peracchia[33] found a diminished "oncolytic potency" of the combined immune system (serum + spleen extracts) of prostatic carcinoma patients after radiotherapy. But when he injected tumor cells with allogenic human cells other than prostatic tissue to improve the stimulatory effect, he described a clinical reduction of metastatic lesions and improvement of "oncolytic" potency of the serum. Nevertheless Fichera[18] wrote at that time (1934): "We are still far away from achieving a real specific immunity." Sad to say, this is still true today, although we now know considerably more about the immune system and how it works.

Basically, the organism can react to foreign antigens with the humoral and the cellular systems, each of which can be divided in a specific and unspecific part (Table 18.1). In addition to the categories "specific" and "unspecific," the immune system can be divided into a cellular and a humoral branch. These four systems are not isolated but work together to potentiate the defense function. In most cases antibodies can be produced only with the help of T-lymphocytes. On the other hand, the effectiveness of antibodies is amplified by complement, while monocytes and macrophages are activated by antibodies and T-lymphocytes.

HUMORAL IMMUNE SYSTEM

Humoral specific immunity is mediated by the antibodies, which are composed of two heavy and two light polypeptide chains (*H*-chain, *L*-chain) connected by disulfide chains. Full antibody activity is achieved by additional activation of the complement system, a multifactorial system activated by single enzyme-substrate steps.

CELLULAR IMMUNE SYSTEM

T-Lymphocytes

Specific immunity is mediated by the T-lymphocytes. Subpopulations of the T-cells are: T-helper cells, T-suppressor cells, mediator substances-producing cells, and cytotoxic cells. As T-helper cells are necessary for producing antibodies (against so-called thymus-dependent antigens), T-suppressor cells are able to intercept the antibody-synthesis (Figs. 18.1 and 18.2.)

Table 18.1
Immune Defense: Basic Possibilities

	Humoral	Cellular
Specific	Antibodies	T-lymphocytes
Unspecific	Complement Properdin	Monocytes Macrophages

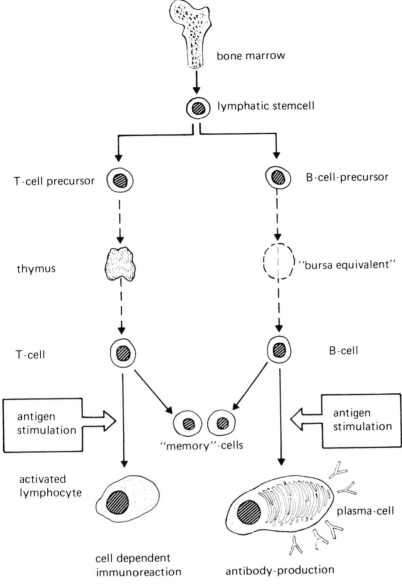

Figure 18.1 The origin of the cellular and humoral immune system.

Activated T-lymphocytes can produce mediator substances, the lymphokines:

1. Immuninterferon stimulates the production of a virus-inhibitory protein (VIP), which blocks the intracellular virus reduplication.
2. Cytotoxic factors are able to kill antigenic "foreign" cells.
3. Lymphocyte-activating factors lead to activation and co-reaction of other, unspecific lymphocytes.
4. Chemotactic factors attract phagocytes. After the invasion of these

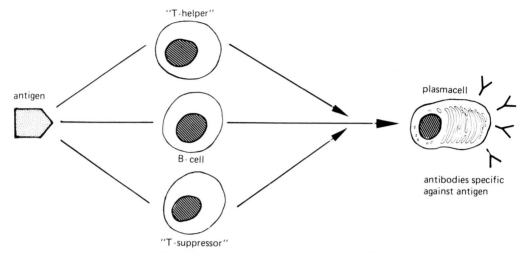

Figure 18.2 "T-helper" and "T-suppressor" cells' influence on the production of immunoglobulins. After antigenic stimulation "T-helper cells" or "T-suppressor cells" can intercept antibody synthesis by plasma cells.

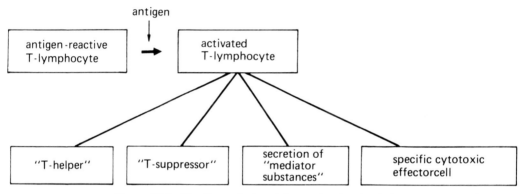

Figure 18.3 T-cell population. After antigenic stimulation "activated T-lymphocytes" divide into several functional subpopulations.

cells into the region of antigen cognition the histological feature of inflammation develops.

5. The macrophage-inhibition and macrophage-activation factors hinder the exmigration of initially attracted cells. Simultaneously, cell metabolism is intensified so that foreign antigens can be eliminated more rapidly and aggressively (Figs. 18.3 and 18.4).

The cytotoxic effector cells—the fourth of the T-cell subpopulations— are responsible for graft rejection and tumor cell elimination, but also need the help of the T-helper cells, as do the B-cells.

There is another population of lymphocytes: the K-cells (killer cells), which belong neither to the B nor to the T-cells. K-cells are able to destroy foreign cells, which are recognized and loaded by specific antibodies. K-cells link to the *Fc*-fragment of the adherent antibody and induce cytolysis (ADCC, *a*ntibody-*d*ependent *c*ell-mediated *c*ytotoxicity).

Monocyte-Macrophage System

Sessile monocytes convert to macrophages. For instance, they appear in connective tissue as histiocytes, in the liver as Kupffer's cells, in the lymph nodes as free and fixed macrophages. Besides the function of phagocytosis, macrophages are necessary for the induction of a specific immune reaction.

Tumor-Specific Antigens

Immunological tumor surveillance is only possible when a specific antigen is present on the surface of tumor cells. Actually, tumor cells contain a large number of antigens. Unfortunately, tumor cell antigenicity varies considerably from cell to cell. Generally speaking, experimentally induced tumors show strong antigenicity, whereas spontaneous tumors are of weak immunogenicity (Fig. 18.5).

MECHANISMS OF CELL DESTRUCTION

1. Specific antibodies recognize the surface antigens of a tumor cell. By activation of complement, cell death is achieved.[26] These immunoglobulins are called "cytotoxic antibodies" (Fig. 18.6).

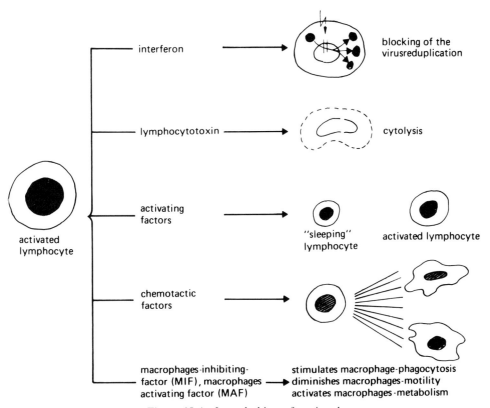

Figure 18.4 Lymphokines: functional aspects.

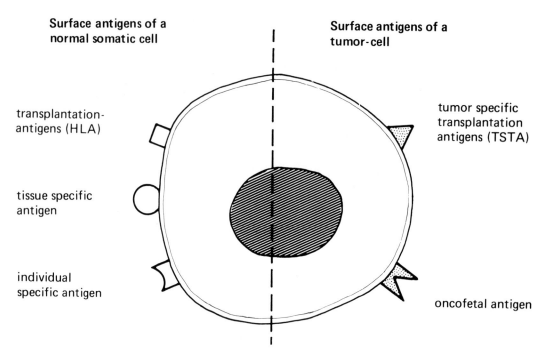

Figure 18.5 Surface-antigens of a normal and a tumor cell.

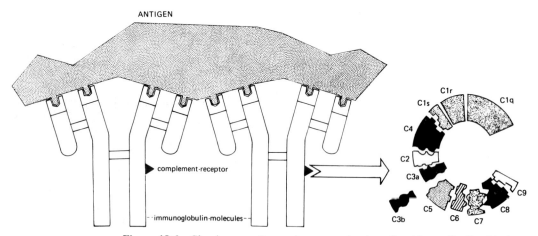

Figure 18.6 Classic way of complement activation. Specific antibodies bind to the tumor cell antigens. By complement-activation (C_3) cell death is achieved (cytotoxic antibodies).

2. Specific cytotoxic T-lymphocytes recognize foreign ("nonself") antigens on a tumor cell and destroy this target cell after activation.[49]

3. Specific T-lymphocytes capable of producing lymphokines activate macrophages ("armed macrophages"[16,17]) which destroy the tumor cells.

4. Specific, noncytotoxic antibodies linked to the tumor surface antigen are recognized by K-cells. The K-cells are activated and induce tumor cell destruction (Figs. 18.6 and 18.7).

TUMOR CELL AVOIDANCE OF IMMUNE DESTRUCTION

Sneaking Through

Several authors have described the "sneaking through phenomenon" (dilution escape) observed in animal experiments, in which a small number of tumor cells are able to escape the immune defense in a syngenetic or allogenetic system, while a large inoculum of tumor cells is destroyed.[8] The exact mechanism is not known, but perhaps the antigenic strength of a small inoculum is not able to evoke an immune response.

Antigen Modulation

Within a tumor cell population, cells with different, distinctive, tumor-specific antigens can be found. Since the immune system eliminates the cells with strong antigens, the cells with weak antigens survive, proliferate, and change the antigenic pattern of the original tumor cell population.

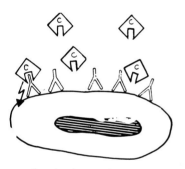

antibody dependent
activation of complement

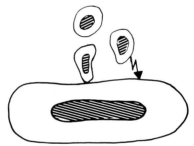

sensibilized T-lymphocytes

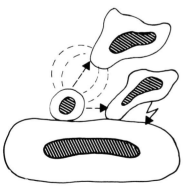

activation of macrophages
by lymphokines

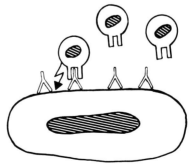

activation of killer-lympho-
cytes by tumorspecific
antibodies

Figure 18.7   Mechanisms of tumor cell killing.

Immune Suppression by the Tumor

Many authors were able to show a diminished immune function in prostatic cancer patients. Immunosuppressive factors were analyzed in the serum of cancer patients as well as in the medium of tumor cell cultures. How these factors interact with the immune system is not known; possibly they suppress the function of the macrophages.[41]

Enhancement

Several studies have suggested that the immune system is able to support neoplastic growth.[29,39] This phenomenon, known as immunologic enhancement, can be explained by the masking of superficial tumor cell antigens by noncytotoxic antitumor antibodies. Therefore, effective mechanisms like cytotoxic T-lymphocytes or cytotoxic, complement-activating antibodies cannot work. Rapid tumor progression is the consequence (Fig. 18.8).

Central Blocking

Besides blocking by masking the tumor antigens directly on the target cell, there is also the possibility of central blockade. Free, shedded tumor antigens are able to intercept the cytotoxic antibodies by forming antigen-antibody complexes.[38] Additionally, free tumor antigens and complexes appear to be able to paralyze lymphocyte activity probably by transmittance of a tolerance signal.

Immune Stimulation

Not only humoral but also cellular mechanisms may enhance tumor growth. While the injection of a great number of antitumor lymphocytes

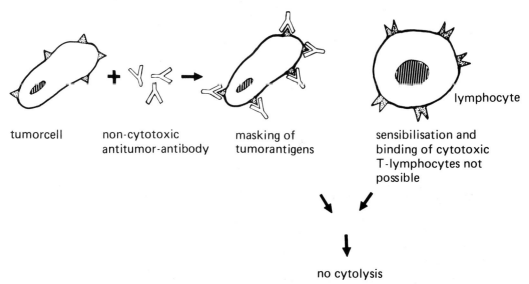

| tumorcell | non-cytotoxic antitumor-antibody | masking of tumorantigens | sensibilisation and binding of cytotoxic T-lymphocytes not possible |

no cytolysis

Figure 18.8 Possible way of "enhancement" by masking the tumor antigens.

restrains tumor growth significantly, a small inoculation of antitumor lymphocytes enhances proliferation.[19,28,45] The mechanism of this so-called immune stimulation phenomenon is still unknown.

Particularly the latter mechanisms show that one should be very reluctant to consider the immune system as an effective tumor antagonist. In the very beginning of tumor development there are only a small number of specific lymphocytes which may stimulate and not suppress tumor cell proliferation. Even the fact that most tumors *in vivo* and *in vitro* may induce an immune response should not lead to the assumption that the immune system is the only responsible, effective force in tumor cell elimination. The data presented above show that immune response may have an adverse effect. This must be considered in so-called clinical "immunotherapy."

CLINICAL IMMUNODIAGNOSTIC PROCEDURES

Acute Phase Proteins (APP)

Acute phase proteins are represented by acid α_1-glycoprotein (AGP), haptoglobin (HP), α_1-antitrypsin (AAT), C-reactive protein (CRP), ceruloplasmin (CP), and α_1-antichymotrypsin (ACT). It seems as if there is a general correlation between APP-concentration and tumor stage (Table 18.2). In normal healthy persons there is no correlation between the concentration of the single APPs.

In the U.S. Veterans Administration Cooperative Urological Research Group (VACURG) study[37] of more than 1,300 patients with prostatic carcinoma, the haptoglobin concentrations were correlated with survival time and reflected stage and seriousness of the disease. A significant correlation also existed between the HP-concentration and metastases as well as between fibrinogen and cortisol.

Estrogen therapy diminishes acid α_1-glycoprotein and haptoglobin concentration, whereas ceruloplasmin and α_1-antityrpsin are increased. This effect suppresses totally the acute phase response toward the tumor, but CRP is not affected.

In summary, the determination of acute phase proteins by immunological methods may give useful information about the prostate cancer patient, but an APP-profile is not applicable for cancer screening.

Table 18.2
The Comparison of the Concentration of Acid α_1-Glycoprotein, Haptoglobin, and C-Reactive Protein between Patients with BPH, Localized, and Metastasized Cancer of the Prostate[a]

	No.	Acid α_1-Glycoprotein	Haptoglobin	C-Reactive Protein (% > 10 mg/liter)
BPH	22	0.83 ± 0.21	2.5 ± 1.01	4
Cancer				
M_0, N_x	28[b]	0.88 ± 2.6	2.66 ± 1.22	26
M_1, N_x	28	1.26 ± 0.50	4.06 ± 1.96	56

[a] From J. F. Cooper, 1980.
[b] This comparison is insignificant, whereas metastatic lesions ($M_1 N_x$) give significant differences.

Tissue Polypeptide Antigen

Björklund et al.[4] have identified a polypeptide with antigenic properties, found to be common for several malignant tumors. It was called *tissue polypeptide antigen* (TPA) and is released by malignant cells *in vitro* as well as *in vivo*.

TPA is a component of the endoplasmatic reticulum and the cell membrane. The structuring main amino acids are aspartic acid, glutamic acid, and leucine. Since the molecular weight does not exceed 20,000, it is filtered through the kidney and excreted in the urine. Special notation should be made of urinary TPA-determinations in bladder cancer patients.

In a small series of patients with prostatic cancer, nine of 17 (53%) showed elevated TPA-titers in the serum, whereas normal control persons were positive for TPA only in two of 67 (3%).

Serum Globulins

Ablin et al.[3] reported a progressive increase in the level of α_2- and β-globulins in patients with prostatic cancer. A progression from localized (stage I) to metastatic (stage IV) disease was accompanied by significant increases in the level of α_2-globulin. Levels of albumin, α_1-globulin and γ-globulin were within the normal range. After cryoprostatectomy, a decrease in albumin, α_2- and β-globulin and increase in γ_1 and γ-globulin from the preoperative levels were observed.

Gursel et al.[23] found the mean values of IgG higher in stage III than in stage IV prostate cancer, although no remarkable changes were observed in the mean values of immunoglobulin-A (IgA) and IgM. In a higher percentage, they found a decreased IgM in stage IV (12 of 20) than in stage III (3 of 16).

In the analysis of Deture et al.,[14] all patients with prostatic carcinoma revealed a decrease of IgM-concentration; in stage I and II, IgG was lowered, and in stage III and IV they observed an increase of IgA. Despite statistical "significance," the mean values were within normal range.

In our own study[47] of 44 patients with prostatic carcinoma, we found no useful correlation between tumor stage, immunoglobulins, and prognosis. There was a trend toward lowered albumin, α_2-globulin and β-globulin concentrations, but it was insignificant and cannot be considered a useful clinical tool. Only the metastatic tumor patients showed an increase in IgA which is consistent with the observations of Gursel et al.[23]

The value of immunoelectrophoresis as a means of determination of immunologic competency in patients with prostatic carcinoma has not been confirmed. As only a small fraction of the immunoglobulins react specifically against the tumor antigens, a hypo- or hypergammaglobulinemia gives no information about the specific reactivity. However, we believe the determination of the serum proteins and immunoglobulins is a small "puzzle piece" in researching patients' immunocompetence by a so-called "immunoprofile" or "immunostaging" program.

"Specific" Humoral Response

To investigate the presence of prostatic tumor-associated antigens and the humoral mediated immunity to these antigens, Ablin et al.[2] evaluated the presence of antibodies in the serum of prostatic cancer patients by indirect immunofluorescence. Thirteen of 24 patients (54%) were staining positive, whereas only 12% of patients with benign prostatic hyperplasia (BPH) showed positive immunofluorescence. Whether such observations represent the existence of specific tumor-associated antigens or whether an immunologic response against normal tissue components may occur during malignant development is still to be elucidated.

Cell-Mediated Immunity (CMI)

SKIN TEST

The skin tests are generally used to assess the ability of a patient to express CMI. They are designed (1) to detect immune deficiency in cancer patients; (2) to correlate tumor stages with immune competency; (3) to obtain more information for prognosis; and (4) to monitor influences of therapy, *e.g.* immune therapy.

Basically there are two types of tests in use:

1. With *recall antigens* the patient expresses delayed hypersensitivity to previously encountered antigens (*e.g.*, mumps, measles, candida, varidase, etc.)
2. With *de novo synthesized antigens*, for instance: DNCB (2,4-dinitro-chlorobenzene), KLH (*k*eyhole *l*impet *h*emocyanine) etc., primary recognition of an antigen by the immune system is tested additionally.

Usually a battery of skin tests is performed in one patient to exclude variations in test procedure.

DNCB

DNCB is a contact sensitizer which is able to build up covalent bindings to the lysin groups of the epidermal proteins thus forming a foreign antigen. The antigen is recognized and this leads to stimulation of the specifically determinated T-lymphocyte clones. After 5 to 28 days, a DNCB-specific cellular response will be seen on the skin by local lymphocytic infiltration. The advantage of DNCB over common skin test antigens is that one need not rely upon previous exposure to the antigen. DNCB tests the current ability of an individual to manifest a complete immunologic response to a newly encountered antigen.[35] Moreover, the DNCB reaction represents an *in vivo* immunologic inflammation which develops over several days, whereas the cellular tests with serum lymphocytes or monocytes merely reflect the momentary status of the cells, which normally show a circadiane rhythm of reagibility.

When related to the tumor stage, patients with metastatic prostatic cancer revealed up to 73% impaired immunity[5] compared to 30% in patients with localized tumors. The study of Huus and co-workers[25] indicated that there was no correlation between DNCB test and stage of disease, but rather a coincidence between tumor presence and depressed immunological reactivity.

Generally, healthy volunteers show positive DNCB reactions in more than 94%.[5,12,30]

In our own study, 26 of 33 (79%) patients with localized tumors and two of 11 (18%) with metastatic tumors showed a normal reaction to DNCB[47] (Fig. 18.9).

Patients with well-differentiated tumors (GI and GII) were positive for DNCB in 95%, whereas poorly differentiated carcinomas (GIII to GIV) revealed a normal response in only 40%.

To sum up, skin tests for delayed hypersensitivity are a reliable and convenient means of testing CMI in prostatic cancer patients. Anergic patients have a poorer prognosis as shown in bladder cancer patients,[30] but one should be aware that this test is totally unspecific for tumor antigens. Since no easy-to-perform *in vitro* tests for CMI are available which correlate with the existence of cancer as well as prognosis, skin tests for CMI will continue to play a role in the evaluation of cancer patients.[35]

In Vitro Tests

T-ROSETTE ASSAY

Catalona *et al.*[11] tried to determine whether impaired cellular immunoresponsiveness is related to a reduction in the number of T-lymphocytes. The results showed that T-lymphocytes are reduced but do not correlate with tumor stage. The observation that shifting proportions of the T-cell subpopulation may indicate malignant processing suggests that more sophisticated rosette procedures will probably be used for serial monitoring.[48]

LYMPHOCYTE TRANSFORMATION TESTS

Separated lymphocytes are stimulated by various mitogens, such as PHA (phytohemagglutinin), ConA (Concanavalin A), or PWM (Pokeweed-Mitogen), stimulated meaning transformed into lymphoblasts. The intracellular uptake of radiolabelled thymidine into DNA measures the ratio of blastogenesis. In most studies, prostate cancer patients revealed a significantly diminished stimulatory response of the lymphocytes.[2,31,43] In plasma exchange experiments, several authors[31,43] incriminated a serum factor as the cause of the depressed response. Catalona *et al.*[10] were able to show depressed lymphocyte-intrinsic activity in addition to the serum-mediated depression.

The mitogens used are very powerful immune stimulators; about 30% of a normal lymphocyte population will respond to *e.g.* PHA, whereas only about 2% do so after rechallenge with a tumor antigen. This amplification will help to detect low level immune defects, but will also multiply any technical mistakes.

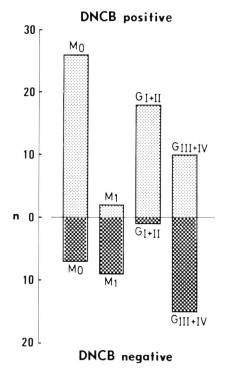

Figure 18.9 Skin tests in prostate cancer patients. DNCB test was most discrim-inative between localized tumor (79% DNCB- positive) and metastatic tumor (18% DNCB-positive). (Modified from P. H. Walz et al.[47])

There is still a need for more standardized assay conditions, since most of the tests in use lack comparability and reproducibility.

Immunologic Responses to Tumor-Associated Antigens

To investigate the presence of prostatic tumor-associated antigens, the cell-mediated immunity to these antigens was evaluated by Ablin and co-workers.[2] They measured the reactivity of leucocytes from prostatic cancer patients toward malignant prostatic tissue collected at the time of TUR. KCl-extracts were prepared from autologous and allogenic tissue. In several tissue/serum exchange tests, the team found a specific reactivity of patients' lymphocytes toward their tumors, a "block factor" in the serum which suppresses the lymphocytes reactivity and a cross-reactive immunity of lymphocytes toward allogenic tumor cells was described. Fifty-six of 73 patients (77%) showed a significant reactivity of leucocytes sensitized to extracts of prostatic cancer.

"While certainly not definitive" as Ablin wrote, the relevance of their results will need to be determined.

Hormone Effect on Immunity

While Thomas and co-workers[43] found no significant difference of the immune status between patients receiving hormonal therapy and those

Table 18.3
Immunotherapy in Prostate Carcinoma

Author(s)	Year	Technique
Peracchia[33]	1925	Cell extraction
Johnston[27]	1962	Coley's toxin
Villasor[46]	1965	BCG
Czajowski et al.[13]	1967	Gamma-globulin plus autologous tumor cell extract
Soanes et al.[40]	1969	Cryotherapy
Flocks et al.[20]	1972	Perineal cryotherapy
Merrin et al.[32]	1973	Intraprostatic BCG (Connaught)
Guinan et al.[21]	1973	Intradermal BCG (Tice)
Brosman and Hausman[6]	1975	Intradermal BCG
Robinson et al.[36]	1976	Intraprostatic BCG (Glaxo)
Tramoyeres et al.[44]	1976	Transperineal cryotherapy plus orchiectomy
Robinson et al.[36]	1978	Intraprostatic BCG
Guinan et al.[22]	1978	Intradermal BCG

not on medication, Castro and co-workers[9] showed the opposite effect in animal studies. Orchiectomized mice revealed an increased response to sheep red blood cells, potentiations of graft *versus* host disease, and accelerated rejection of skin allografts which was lost after androgen replacement. After orchiectomy the immunological potential of the individual lymphocyte was not increased; immunopotentiation was due to quantitative changes in the lymphocyte population. Humoral immune response remained unchanged. Interestingly, the rate and number of tumors induced by subcutaneous methylcholantrene were reduced in mice without testes. The results of this animal model suggest that after orchiectomy a nonspecific active immunopotentiation may occur. In our own study there was a trend in favor of improved CMI after 6 months of estrogen therapy.[47]

A very interesting aspect was given by Ablin and co-workers.[1] They hypothesized the normal human seminal plasma as contributory to the natural history of prostatic cancer. They observed a significant suppression of immunity to malignant prostatic cells by incubating patients' leucocytes with human seminal plasma.

IMMUNOTHERAPY

There are only a few studies in the literature which can be considered serious attempts to approach the aim of immunotherapy. At present there is no tumor-specific effective therapy which can be considered immunotherapy (Table 18.3).

Robinson and co-workers[36] administered BCG (Bacillus Calmette-Guérin = unspecific immune stimulator) intratumorally in patients with advanced metastatic tumor. In a postmortem examination, areas of cellular necrosis were found in the prostate, but no evidence of marked tumor destruction was noted. However, four of six patients showed an objective clinical improvement in micturition (!). Guinan et al.[22] reported on 33 patients with cancer of the prostate who received adjuvant BCG-immunotherapy. The treatment group lived 4 months longer than the control group (26 *versus* 22 months).

Our increasing knowledge of the immunological mechanisms operating in the tumor-bearing individual gives cause for hope that it may eventually be manipulated for clinical benefit. But it is clear that much more knowledge about the immunological mechanisms between host and tumor, as well as better controlled prospective studies are necessary.

REFERENCES

1. Ablin, R. J., Bhathi, R. A., Bush, J. M., and Guinan, P.D. Suppression of tumor-associated immunity by human seminal plasma and its possible role in the natural history of prostate cancer. *Eur. Urol. 6:* 225, 1980.
2. Ablin, R. J., Bhathi, R. A., and Guinan, P. D. Tumor-associated antigens and immunity in prostatic carcinoma. In *Immunodiagnosis and Immunotherapy of Malignant Tumors*, edited by D. F. Flad, G. Herfarth, and F. R. L. Belzer. Springer Verlag, Berlin, 1979.
3. Ablin, R. J., Soanes, W. A., and Gonder, M. J. Serum proteins in prostatic cancer. *Urol. Int. 34:* 339, 1979.
4. Björklund, B., Björklund, V., and Wilklund, B., III. Clinical studies of 1483 individuals with cancer and other conditions. Immunological techniques for detection of cancer. Proceedings of the Folksam Symposium, Bonniers Publ., Stockholm, 1973, p. 164.
5. Brosman, S., Hausman, M., and Shacks, S. Immunologic alterations in patients with prostatic carcinoma. *J. Urol. 113:* 841, 1975.
6. Brosman, S., and Hausman, M. BCG effect in GU tumors. *Am. Urol. Assoc. (West. Sect.) Urol. News 2:* 3, 1974.
7. Burnet, F. M. Somatic mutation and chronic disease. *Br. Med. J. i:* 338, 1965.
8. Bonmassar, E., Hencom, L., Goldin, A., and Cudkowicz, G. Escape of small numbers of allogenetic lymphoma cells from immune surveillance. *J. Natl. Cancer Inst. 53:* 475, 1974.
9. Castro, J. E., Medawar, P. B., and Hamilton, D. N. H. Orchiectomy as a method of immunopotentiation in mice. In *Immunopotentiation Ciba Foundation Symposium* 18. Elsevier, North-Holland, 1973.
10. Catalona, W. J., Tarpley, J. L., Chretien, P. B., and Castle, J. R. Lymphocyte stimulation in urologic cancer patients. *J. Urol. 112:* 373, 1974.
11. Catalona, W. J., Potwin, C., and Chretien, P. B. T Lymphocytes in bladder and prostatic cancer patients. *J. Urol. 112:* 378, 1974.
12. Catalona, W. J., Chretien, P. B., and Tiahan, E. E. Abnormalities of cell mediated immunocompetence in genitourinary cancer. *J. Urol. 111:* 229, 1974.
13. Czajowski, N. P., Rosenblatt, M., and Wolf, P. I. A new method of active immunization to autologous tumor tissue. *Lancet ii:* 905, 1967.
14. Deture, F. A., Beardourff, S. L., Kaufmann, H. E., and Centifano, Y. M. A comparison of serum immunoglobulins from patients with non neoplastic prostates and prostatic carcinoma. *J. Urol. 120:* 435, 1978.
15. Ehrlich, P. Über den jetzigen Stand der Karzinomforschung. *Ned. Tijdschr. Geneeskd. 1:* 273, 1909.
16. Evans, R. Macrophages in syngeneic animal tumors. *Transplantation 14:* 468, 1972.
17. Evans, R., and Alexander P. Cooperation of immune lymphoid cells with macrophages in tumor immunity. *Nature 228:* 620, 1972.
18. Fichera, G. *Endogene Faktoren in der Tumorgenese und der heutige Stand des Versuchs einer biologischen Therapie*. Springer Verlag, Berlin, 1934.
19. Fidler, I. J. In vitro studies of cellular-mediated immunostimulation of tumor growth. *J. Natl. Cancer Inst. 50:* 1307, 1973.
20. Flocks, R. H., Nelson, C. M., and Boatman, D. L. Perineal cryosurgery for prostatic carcinoma. *J. Urol. 108:* 928, 1972.
21. Guinan, P. T., John, R. G., Crispen *et al.* Immunotherapy in carcinoma of the prostate. In *Neoplasm Immunity*. Evanston, Ill., Schori Press, 1974.

22. Guinan, P. D., John, T., Sahadevan, V., Crispen, R., Nagale, V., McKiel, C., and Ablin, R. J. Prostate carcinoma: immunostaging and adjuvant immunotherapy with BCG. In *Workshop on Genitourinary Cancer Immunology.* NCI, 49, U.S. Dept. of Health, 1978.
23. Gursel, E. O., Megalli, M. R., and Veenema, R. J. Serum immunoglobulins in patients with prostate cancer. *Urol. Res. 1:* 145, 1973.
24. Good, R. In *Immune Surveillance*, edited by Smith and Lendy, Academic Press, New York, 1970, p. 437.
25. Huus, J. C., Kush, D., Poor, P., and Persky, L. Delayed cutaneous hypersensitivity in patients with prostatic adenocarcinoma. *J. Urol. 114:* 86, 1975.
26. Irie, K., Irie, R., and Morton, D. L. Evidence for in vivo reaction of antibody and complement to surface antigens of human cancer cells. *Science 186:* 454, 1974.
27. Johnston, B. J. Clinical effects of Coley's toxin: a controlled study. *Cancer Chemother. Rep. 21:* 19, 1962.
28. Kall, M. A., and Hellström, I. Specific stimulatory and cytotoxic effects of lymphocytes sensitized in vitro to either alloantigens or tumor antigens. *J. Immunol. 114:* 1083, 1975.
29. Kaliss, N. Immunological enhancement of tumor homografts in mice: a review. *Cancer Res. 18:* 992, 1958.
30. Klippel, K. F., Walz, H. P., Kreutz, G., and Moltke, T. V. DNCB-Test und Immuno-kompetenz. *Münch. Med. Wochenschr. 120:* 1027, 1978.
31. McLaughlin, A. P., Kessler, W. O., and Gittes, R. F. Immunologic competence in patients with urologic cancer. *J. Urol. 111:* 233, 1974.
32. Merrin, C., Hau, T., Klein, E. *et al.* Immunotherapy of prostatic carcinoma with Bacillus Calmette-Guérin. *Cancer Chemother. Rep. 59:* 157, 1975.
33. Peracchia, F. Oszillazioni nel potere oncolitico dei cancerosi in rapporto a cura chirur-gica. *Ann. Ital. Chir. IV*, 1925.
34. Piccaluga, M. Contributo allo studio dell' azione biologica dei vaggi Röntgen sui Aessuti normali e neoplastici. *Boll. Soc. Med. Chir. Pavia*, 1924, pp. 126–131.
35. Pinsky, C. M. Skin tests. In *Immunodiagnosis of Cancer*, Part 2. Edited by R. B. Herberman and K. B. McIntire. Marcel Dekker, New York, 1979.
36. Robinson, M. R. G., Rigby, C. O., Pugh, R. C. B., and Dumonde, D. C. Prostate carcinoma: intratumor BCG immunotherapy. In *Workshop on Genitourinary Cancer Immunology*, No. 49. NCI, U.S. Dept. of Health, 1978.
37. Seal, U. S., Doe, R. P., Byar, D. P., Corle, D. K., and the Veterans Administration Cooperative Urological Research Group. Response of serum haptoglobin to hormone treatment and the relation of pretreatment values to mortality in patients with prostatic cancer. *Cancer 42:* 1720, 1978.
38. Sjögren, H. O., Hellström, I., and Bansal, S. C. Suggestive evidence that the "blocking antibodies" of tumor-bearing individuals may be antigen-antibody complexes. *Proc. Natl. Acad. Sci. 68:* 1372, 1971.
39. Snell, G. D., Cloudmann, A. M., Failor, E., and Douglas, P. Inhibition and stimulation of tumor homoiotransplants by prior injections of lyophilized tumor tissue. *J. Natl. Cancer. Inst. 6:* 303, 1946.
40. Soanes, W. A., Gonder, M. J., and Ablin, R. J. Clinical and experimental aspects of prostatic cryosurgery. *J. Cryosurg. 2:* 23, 1969.
41. Synderman, R., and Pike, M. C. An inhibitor of macrophage chemotaxis produced by neoplasms. *Science 192:* 370, 1976.
42. Thomas, L. In *Cellular and Humoral Aspects of the Hypersensitive-States*, edited by G. H. Lawrence. Harper & Row, New York, 1959, p. 529.
43. Thomas, J. W., Jerkins, G., Cox, C., and Lieberman, P. Defective cell-mediated immunity in carcinoma of the prostate. *Invest. Urol. 14:* 72, 1976.
44. Tramoyeres, C. A., Sanchez-Guenca, J. M., *et al.* A lacriociururgia transperineal en el tratamiento del cancer prostatico. *Arch. Espan. Urol. 29:* 119, 1976.
45. Treves, A. H., Carnaud, C., Trainin, N., Feldman, M., and Cohen, I. R. Enhancing T lymphocytes from tumor-bearing mice suppress host resistance to a syngeneic tumor. *Eur. J. Immunol. 4:* 723, 1974.
46. Villasor, R. P. The clinical use of BCG vaccine in stimulating host resistance to cancer. *J. Phil. Med. Assoc. 41:* 619, 1965.

47. Walz, P. H., Jacobi, G. H., and Klippel, K. F. Prostatic carcinoma: the place of DNCB-testing and serum protein and immunoglobulin determination in routine diagnosis. *Akt. Urol. 11:* 379, 1980.
48. West, W. H. E-rosette formation in immunodiagnosis. In *Immunodiagnosis of Cancer*, edited by R. B. Herberman and R. McIntire. M. Dekker, New York, 1979.
49. Wybran, J., Hellström, I., Hellström, K. E., and Fudenberg, H. H. Cytotoxicity of human rosette-forming blood lymphocytes on cultivated human tumor cells. *Int. J. Cancer 13:* 515, 1974.

19

Prostate Cancer: Hormone Profiles

D. Gupta, F.R.C. Path.

INTRODUCTION

There is a wealth of information that the prostate is an androgen-dependent organ[1, 2] and benign prostatic hyperplasia (BPH) does not occur in castrated men.[3] The canine prostate model of Huggins[4] and a large number of studies conducted in other experimental animals also indicate a profound dependence on testosterone for growth and development of the normal prostate. Recently concepts regarding the metabolic events related to the action of testosterone in normal prostatic tissue have been postulated. The major step in the action of testosterone on its target tissues is mediated not through the hormone itself but by its 5α-reduced metabolite, 5α-dihydrotestosterone (DHT) formed *in situ*[5-8] the potency of which often exceeds that of the parent compound.[8] This postulation is supported by recent evidence of the association of DHT with the intracellular androgen receptor protein and its concentration in the nuclei either after the administration of testosterone *in vivo* or after the exposure of the target tissues to testosterone (Chapter 20).[7, 10-13]

For the sake of brevity and to simplify the presentation I assume that the following concepts can be agreed upon:

1. Testosterone crosses the prostatic cell membrane and is reduced by the enzyme, 5α-reductase, to DHT. Between the endoplasmic reticulum and nuclear binding sites, the enzyme is equally distributed.

2. Dihydrotestosterone gets bound to specific high affinity cytoplasmic proteins and this steroid-protein complex undergoes translocation to the nuclear membrane and enters the nucleus. Here it becomes bound to chromatin. Dihydrotestosterone acts as the major nuclear androgen. This process initiates transcription of messenger-ribonucleic acid.

3. Dihydrotestosterone is further metabolized to other steroids that pass from the cell.

The purpose of this chapter is to review the state of our present knowledge with respect to the following three questions:

1. The peripheral and tissue concentrations of androgens in BPH and cancer patients.
2. The biotransformation of androgens by BPH and carcinomatous tissues.
3. The androgen-binding proteins and androgen receptors in the BPH and cancerous prostatic tissues.

PERIPHERAL AND TISSUE CONCENTRATIONS

One of the most paradoxical findings in the complex course of the pathogenesis of prostatic disease is that although the level of peripheral testosterone is diminished in old age,[14-16] prostatic tumors are very frequent in this age group.[17]

Androgen Concentrations in Tissues

Figure 19.1 shows in a schematic way the metabolism of testosterone to various metabolites. Siiteri and Wilson[18] observed that the level of DHT, the 5α-reduced metabolite of testosterone, was higher in the periurethral region, while the outer gland region contained a higher concentration of testosterone. Hammond,[19] however, failed to observe any difference in the steroid composition of these histologically distinct regions. In BPH tissue an almost five-fold increase in the level of DHT has been observed by various investigators,[18-22] and the relative concentration of DHT has been seen to greatly exceed that of its 17-oxo counterpart. This observation demonstrates the occurrence of this specific bias toward the accumulation of DHT as opposed to 5α-androstanedione in BPH. Hammond[19] also found a striking difference in the concentrations of 3α-androstanediol (3α-diol) and androsterone in BPH and normal tissues which agreed with the observations of Geller et al.[23] that the concentrations of androstanediols are lower in BPH. This probably indicates a change in 3α-hydroxysteroid dehydrogenase activity in the BPH tissue. In the untreated carcinomatous tissue, however, high levels of testosterone and androstenedione were found by various investigators.[19, 24] Together with this there may be accumulation of DHT and especially 3α-androstanediol. This is perhaps at the expense of a depletion of the corresponding 17-oxo-metabolites in untreated carcinomatous tissue. The accumulation of DHT rather than 5α-androstanedione in adenomatous and especially carcino-

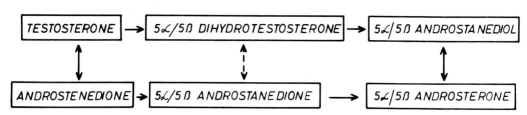

Figure 19.1 Pathways for testosterone and androstenedione metabolism.

matous tissue suggests an alteration in 17β-hydroxysteroid dehydrogenase activity when compared with normal tissue. Thus, it seems that in the normal prostate 3α-androstanediol and androsterone are major metabolites of testosterone and 5α-androstanedione via the formation of DHT and androstenedione, whereas in the BPH tissue, although the formation of 3α-androstanediol and androsterone may proceed via DHT and 5α-androstanedione, the relative accumulation of 3α-hydroxylated androgens is much reduced. According to Geller et al.[23] DHT is significantly higher and androstanediol significantly lower in the BPH patients, when compared to the controls, suggesting a decrease in 3-hydroxysteroid oxido-reductase in BPH.

Androgen Concentrations in Plasma

Habib et al.[24] were able to demonstrate the absence of significant difference in the plasma testosterone levels of patients with either type of prostatic disease in agreement with other investigators.[25, 26] They also detected raised DHT concentration in normal elderly men in agreement with Horton et al.,[27] although for hyperplastic and neoplastic prostates a great increment of DHT, without any significant difference between the groups, was observed. The mean value for peripheral androstenedione in BPH and carcinoma were also of the same order.[24, 28]

This alteration in the relationship between DHT and testosterone has also been confirmed by other investigators.[30–32] Vermeulen and De Sy[32] have also reported that DHT levels are even higher after prostate surgery in their patients, indicating some extraprostatic tissues as a major source of this metabolite.

According to Habib et al.[24] the concentrations of testosterone and DHT in the two types of tissues differed considerably, levels of testosterone being significantly higher in the carcinomatous tissue while the DHT to T ratio is greater in hyperplastic prostate. This accumulation of testosterone may be related to the development of carcinoma of the prostate, and it is possible as suggested by Yamaguchi et al.[29] that the androgen dependency may be more closely related to a high degree of testosterone binding in the cytosol and nucleus than to a relatively high activity of 5α-reductase.

The kinetic studies[30] reveal a number of interesting changes in BPH prostate. The MCR^T (metabolic clearance rate of testosterone) has been found to be larger than MCR^{DHT} (metabolic clearance rate of DHT) in both young and elderly men. Both the MCR^T and MCR^{DHT} in elderly men are significantly lower than in young men. However, while MCR^{DHT} in elderly men with prostatic carcinoma is lower than in normal young men, MCR^T does not have any difference between the two groups.[33]

When production rates (PR) of testosterone and DHT are examined, it is found that while PR^T in elderly men is about 50% of PR^T in young men, PR^{DHT} in elderly men is similar to that in young men.[30] This means that DHT production is maintained in elderly men despite reduction of testosterone production. When the conversion rate (CR) of testosterone to its metabolites is determined it is found that CR^{T-DHT} is somewhat elevated in elderly men,[30] and $CR^{T-3\alpha\text{-diol}}$ and $CR^{DHT-3\alpha\text{-diol}}$ are less than one-half of those in normal men.[25]

When the transfer constants (fraction of a precursor converted to a product per unit time) for various metabolites are calculated[30], it is seen that although in young men about three-fourths of plasma DHT is derived from peripheral conversion of testosterone, in elderly men only one-half of blood DHT is derived from testosterone conversion. The remaining blood DHT may be derived from direct secretion of sex accessory tissue such as the prostate[25] or testis.[34] Similarly, Ishimaru *et al.*[30] concluded tentatively that in elderly men about 50% of blood 3α-diol is derived from DHT conversion and the contribution to blood 3α-diol of testosterone is about 20%, while in young men over 70% of blood 3α-diol is from testosterone. The calculations suggest that the relatively increased PR^{DHT} contributes to production of 3α-diol more than PR^T in elderly men.

In a very important observation Bird and Clark[33] recorded the metabolic clearance rate of DHT being significantly higher in normal young men than in normal young women, whereas this MCR for men with prostatic carcinoma in the untreated state is similar to that for normal young women.

In our own studies[16, 36, 37] age-matched subjects who did not have any symptoms of urological diseases, malignancies, or endocrinopathies, were taken as "true" controls. Our results showed that despite a decreased testosterone level in the elderly men as compared to young individuals, there is no significant change during the 6th through the 8th decade of life. In patients with prostatic carcinoma and BPH testosterone, DHT and androstanediol levels were found to be higher than in the aged controls (Table 19.1). These findings clearly demonstrate that in individuals with prostatic adenocarcinoma, high levels of testosterone and its androgenically potent metabolites, DHT and androstanediol, are maintained. Testosterone to DHT ratio was unchanged in carcinoma *versus* aged control patients and almost identical with the results from Vermeulen.[38] Since the DHT to androstanediol ratio was higher in the cancer patients, it is conceivable that in these individuals the normally predominant reductive[35] pathway changes in favor of oxidative reverse reaction from androstanediol to DHT, resulting in a diminishing adiol concentration and a DHT increment.

Free Androgens

It is now generally accepted that the expression of biological activity of steroid hormone is influenced by the extent of binding to plasma proteins. Rosenfield[39] demonstrated that the fraction of plasma androgens not bound to the specific binding globulin, which could be determined in plasma[40] correlated best with androgenic effects. A number of reports have already appeared regarding the concentrations of active androgens in BPH and prostatic carcinoma.[32, 37, 41] Vermeulen and De Sy[32] observed that the free testosterone concentration was significantly higher in BPH patients than in the control group of similar age. In our own investigation[16, 37] it was observed that *sex hormone binding globulin* (SHBG)

Table 19.1
Active Androgens in Plasma of 86 Elderly Men (50 to 80 Years) Related to Age and Prostate Pathology[a, b]

Patients	50–60 years (n=22)				61–70 years (n=35)				71–80 years (n=29)			
	T[c]	DHT[d]	ADIOL[e]/Sum		T	DHT	ADIOL/Sum		T	DHT	ADIOL/Sum	
Benign prostatic hyperplasia[f] (n=26)	415	36.7	18.0	470	383	49.3	19.2	452	431	51.4	18.5	501
Prostatic carcinoma[f] (n=41)	411	42.2	16.1	469	505	41.8	15.2	562	376	42.8	14.8	434
Age-matched controls (n=19)	401	35.4	28.2	465	352	41.6	32.6	426	334	34.7	28.2	397
Total (n=86)	405	38.5	20.9	464	442	44.4	18.6	505	381	43.2	18.3	443

[a] Data compiled from Jacobi et al.[36]
[b] All values given in nanograms/100 ml, mean values.
[c] Testosterone.
[d] 5α-dihydrotestosterone.
[e] 5α-androstane-3α, 17β-diol.
[f] Blood sampling prior to any treatment.

increased progressively with age for the older group of controls as well as for the carcinoma patients. No significant correlation could be found between various age-matched groups of subjects and free hormone constellations (Table 19.2); the concentrations of the free androgens were found to be related to tumor grade and stage. Testosterone was somewhat lower in poorly differentiated or stage D tumors than in highly differentiated and stage B/C lesions. Free fractions of DHT and androstanediol were, however, essentially similar regardless of staging or grading (Table 19.3). When total free androgens were considered 16 of 20 carcinoma having high free androgens were well differentiated, whereas 12 of 20 tumors in patients with a low level of free androgens were poorly differentiated or stage D carcinoma. A number of investigators,[42, 43] however, did not find any significant difference in the plasma concentrations of SHBG in patients with prostatic carcinoma when compared to normal men of similar age.

BIOCONVERSION OF ANDROGENS

Recently biopsy materials of normal, benign hyperplastic, neoplastic, and metastatic prostatic tissues have been used by various groups of workers to study the uptake of [^{3}H]-testosterone by these tissues and their ability to convert testosterone to DHT. Wotiz and Lemon,[44] the first to investigate steroid metabolism by the human prostate, found rapid breakdown of testosterone to androstenedione by slices of benign hypertrophic and carcinomatous glands. This observation was supported later by Harding and Samuels[45] in rat ventral prostates performed *in vivo* with

Table 19.2
Total, Bound, and Free Androgens in Untreated Prostatic Carcinoma Patients and Age-Matched Control Individuals[a]

Group	Steroid[b]	Total (ng/100 ml)	Albumin-bound (ng/100 ml)	%	SHBG-bound (ng/100 ml)	%	Free Hormone (ng/100 ml)	%
Prostatic carcinoma (n = 41)	TESTO	437.6 ± 174	264 ± 111	60.3	163 ± 82.7	37.3	10.6 ± 4.3	2.4
	DHT	41.8 ± 14.1	14.3 ± 7.2	34.2	26.6 ± 10.1	63.6	0.9 ± 0.5	2.2
	ADIOL	15.1 ± 5.3	12.7 ± 4.2	84.2	0.8 ± 0.4	5.3	1.6 ± 0.5	10.5
Age-matched controls (n = 19)	TESTO	360.9 ± 145	247 ± 107	68.5	104 ± 55	28.8	9.9 ± 4.2	2.7
	DHT	36.4 ± 7.3	15.1 ± 4.7	41.5	19.9 ± 6.9	54.7	1.4 ± 0.6	3.8
	ADIOL	29.5 ± 9.3	24.3 ± 7.3	82.4	1.1 ± 0.7	3.7	4.1 ± 2.3	13.9
Young controls (n = 21)	TESTO	507 ± 177	329 ± 130	64.9	153 ± 76.7	30.2	25 ± 5.7	4.9
	DHT	56.2 ± 8.8	22.7 ± 8.0	40.4	32.8 ± 8.2	58.4	0.7 ± 0.08	1.2
	ADIOL	15.2 ± 5.3	12.3 ± 4.3	80.9	0.5 ± 0.2	3.3	2.4 ± 0.9	15.7

[a] From G. H. Jacobi et al.[37]
[b] TESTO, testosterone; DHT, 5 α-dihydrotestosterone; ADIOL, 5α-androstane-3α,17β-diol.

Table 19.3
Mean Serum Levels of Free Androgens Related to Separate and Combined Histological Grading and Clinical Staging in 41 Patients with Untreated Prostatic Adenocarcinoma[a]

Androgens (ng/100 ml)	Differentiated[b]		Stage[c]		Highly Diff. Stage B + C (n = 29)	Poorly Diff. Stage D (n = 12)
	Highly (n = 24)	Poorly (n = 17)	B + C (n = 24)	D (n = 17)		
Testosterone	11.3	9.7	11.4	8.6	12.6	9.5
Dihydrotestosterone	1.3	1.2	1.3	0.9	1.1	1.0
Androstanediol	2.2	2.5	2.4	2.3	2.3	2.4
Total free androgens	14.8	13.4	15.1	11.8	16.0	12.9

[a] Modified from G. H. Jacobi et al.[37]
[b] Predominant grade in biopsy.
[c] According to Whitmore (1956).

labelled testosterone. On the other hand, Pearlman and Pearlman[46], on infusing rats with labelled androstenedione, found higher concentrations of testosterone, 5α- and 5β-androstane-3α-ol-17-one, and 5α-androstane-dione in the prostate than in the blood.

According to Prout et al.[47] there is a profound difference in DHT formation between benign prostatic hyperplasia and prostatic cancer, the latter producing much less, while both groups have relatively similar uptake of [³H]-testosterone. These findings indicate that there has been loss or repression of 5α-reductase activity in the tissues of prostatic carcinoma when compared to BPH. The observation that the DHT formation in metastatic nodes of untreated men is diminished made these investigators conclude that at the time of diagnosis there are autonomous cells that cannot convert testosterone to DHT to a normal extent and presumably have a reduced requirement for DHT. Kliman et al.[48] also observed altered androgen metabolism in metastatic prostate cancer, where DHT formation was reduced by 76% in the metastases compared to primary tissues.

Altwein et al.,[49] on the other hand, detected 60% of the recovered radioactivity to be associated with 5α-reduced metabolites of testosterone in BPH. Besides these androstenedione was found to be the only important steroid. Gloyna and Wilson[50] demonstrated an active transformation of testosterone into DHT by BPH tissue, and Collins et al.[51] reported that in simple adenoma of the prostate androstenedione can be converted into testosterone and DHT. Di Silverio et al.[52] using labelled dehydroepian-drosterone-sulphate observed that 3β-ol-dehydrogenase and 5α-reductase activity in neoplastic tissue was very low or completely absent.

The 3α-reduction of DHT is also an important step in the bioconversion of androgens by prostatic tissue, and the enzyme responsible for this is located in both the particulate and the soluble fractions of human prostatic tissues. Although Baulieu and Robel[53] found that growth and activity of the prostatic cells can only be stimulated by 3β-androstanediol, 3α-epimer was found to stimulate the activity of the DNA polymerase enzyme isolated from the dog prostate.[54] Jacobi and Wilson[55] demonstrated the formation of 3α-androstanediol and its 3β-epimer in cytosol and in microsomes obtained from human prostate. These investigators observed the formation of a significantly higher amount of androstanediol from hypertrophic than from normal glands, which contradicts the earlier observations of Shida et al.[56] These findings indicate that the enzymes that form both androstanediols are higher in the glandular rather than in the stromal elements of the gland. These investigators[55] postulated that as hypertrophic nodule contains an increase in the ratio of stromal to glandular elements, the acute increase in enzyme per glandular cell might be greater than appears to be the case when the findings are reported on a *per milligram protein* or *per gram wet weight* basis.

Our own findings[57] using simultaneously labelled testosterone and androstenedione demonstrated greatest amount of radioactivity associated with DHT and androstanediol in human BPH tissue. In contrast, carcinomatous tissue showed a negligible amount of radioactivity associated with androstanediol and converted less testosterone to DHT than do BPH and normal tissues. These results are consistent with those of other investigators.[47, 48, 55]

More extensive study[57a] of the relationship between bioconversion of testosterone and tissue condition confirmed the occurrence of an elevated 5α-reductase enzyme in the BPH patients, whether in the glandular or in the adenomatous prostatic TUR slices (Fig. 19.2), which was significantly higher than those found in the glandular sections obtained from either young healthy men ($p = 0.01$) or cancer patients ($p = 0.001$). Although the glandular and adenomatous prostatic slices from the cancer patients

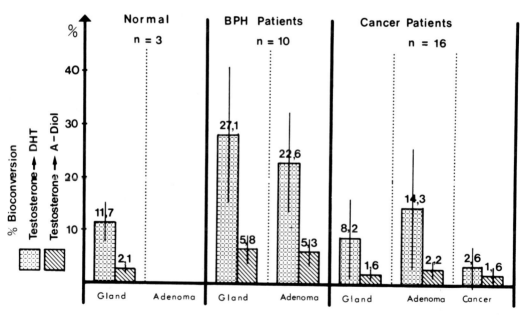

Figure 19.2 Testosterone bioconversion in glandular adenomatous (benign hyperplastic) and carcinomatous prostatic TUR slices obtained from healthy young men and patients with previously untreated benign prostatic hyperplasia (BPH) or prostatic carcinoma; data given as percent of total radioactivity recovered. *DHT*, 5α-dihydrotestosterone; *A-Diol*, 5α-androstane-3α, 17β-diol. (Reproduced from St. H. Flüchter et al.[57a])

did not differ significantly from the glandular slices of young adults, the carcinoma tissues were virtually lacking in this enzyme. Thus, a change in the enzyme constellation following the onset of carcinoma may be postulated.

Furthermore, the patients with *incidental* carcinoma in their glandular and adenomatous prostatic slices registered adequate and similar 5α-reductase activity (Fig. 19.3). The analysis of individual postbioconversion steroid patterns of the cancer patients graded as stages B through D registered two distinctly different groups, on the basis of the high and low 5α-reductase activity. Ten subjects demonstrated ample bioconversion of the precursor testosterone to DHT by their glandular and adenomatous tissues, while their carcinomatous slices recorded lack of this enzyme. Three patients, however, showed complete lack of 5α-reductase activity in each type of their prostatic slices. This condition may be cited in support of the postulation for differentiating subjects as hormone-sensitive and those who are refractory to such treatment.

Cyproterone Acetate

Clinical experience concerning the use of antiandrogens such as cyproterone acetate in the treatment of BPH or prostate adenocarcinoma is rather limited (see Chapter 15). Belham and Neal[58] did not observe any

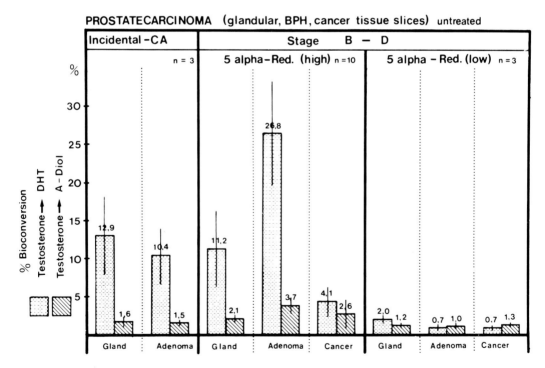

Figure 19.3 Testosterone bioconversion in glandular adenomatous (benign hyperplastic), and carcinomatous prostatic TUR slices from 16 patients with previously untreated prostatic carcinoma. Data given as percent of total radioactivity recovered. *DHT*, 5α-dihydrotestosterone; *A-Diol*, 5α-androstane-3α, 17β-diol. (Reproduced from St. H. Flüchter *et al.*[57a])

effect, whereas Walsh and Korenman[59] postulated that this antiandrogen is a potent inhibitor of the binding of DHT to the prostatic cell nucleus, but having no inhibitory effect on androgen metabolism (for details see Chapter 14).

Our own findings[57] confirmed that cyproterone acetate whether *in vivo* or *in vitro* can greatly reduce the formation of the 5α-reduced compounds from both precursors, testosterone and andostanedione, which are in agreement with the reported data.[60, 61]

The inhibition in the formation of DHT from androstenedione was somewhat less than having testosterone as precursor, but this difference was not significant. When the drastic fall in the formation of DHT and androstanediol with the addition of cyproterone acetate in the *in vitro* studies was compared to the therapeutic action of the drug, different patterns of metabolism emerged. The metabolic pattern in the carcinomatous tissue from subjects treated with cyproterone acetate *in vivo* was similar but not consistently in agreement with the findings seen after the addition of the substance *in vitro*. Treatment with cyproterone acetate *in vivo* always resulted in lesser decrease of 5α-reductase activity than seen in the *in vitro* studies.

According to Scott[62] and Scott and Wade,[63] who conducted a study of 13 patients, there had been definite clinical improvement with cyproterone acetate in relation to the concentration of acid phosphatase and a decrease in size of the primary lesion. Jones[64] observed cyproterone acetate suppressed fructose secretion in the prostate whereas Grants and Stitch[65] postulated that this antiandrogen might impair the transformation of progesterone to 17-hydroxyprogesterone and possibly side chain cleavage of 17-hydroxyprogesterone to androstenedione. According to Hansson and Tveter[66] the average reduction in the uptake of [^{3}H]-testosterone caused by cyproterone acetate was 27%. It is probable that the improved clinical findings are related to the reduced uptake of androgen and the depressed formation of androgen-receptor complexes in prostate caused by cyproterone acetate (see Chapter 14).

ANDROGEN RECEPTORS

In view of the foregoing discussions which amply demonstrated that the prostate gland is heavily dependent upon the androgens for normal growth and function, in recent years intensive studies have been carried out to sort out the mechanism by which androgens exert their effects on prostatic tissue. Evidence for the existence of a specific androgen-binding receptor protein in the human prostate has been presented by a number of investigators[67-70] as further outlined in Chapter 20. Androgen receptors found in the human prostate have physicochemical properties very similar to those described in rats.[71] These proteins are precipitated with 40% ammonium sulphate, have a sedimentation coefficient of about 8 s, and are eluted in the void volume from sephadex G-200 columns. Androgen receptors in all human tissues are easily destroyed by heat and by sulfhydryl reagents. Binding to human androgen receptors is prevented by antiandrogens, such as cyptroterone or *SKF 7690*. These investigators[71] also examined the androgen receptors obtained from human prostatic hyperplasia and cancer, but could not demonstrate any physicochemical differences between the two groups of tissues. All the receptors were found to have the same size, stability, and steroid binding properties.

In contrast to the above observations Karr et al.[72] were able to identify and differentiate specific receptors for DHT in BPH specimens having lowest binding sites (4.1 and 14.3 fmoles) when compared to normal specimens the values of which were within the limits of those reported by other groups.[73]

Most of the earlier studies[68–70] on the androgen receptors in human prostate have been carried out with labelled DHT that unfortunately has a high affinity for sex hormone binding globulin (SHBG) in plasma. This creates a potential source of error during receptor quantitation. Investigating upon this problem Mobbs et al.[74] concluded that the steroid specificity of the binding occurring in human prostate tissue appeared closer to that of SHBG than to that of the androgen receptor in rat prostate. To overcome these difficulties a synthetic androgen, methyltrienolone (R 1881), which binds specifically to the androgen receptor but not to plasma SHBG[75, 76] has been utilized as a ligand on characteristics of the androgen receptor in human prostate with BPH and carcinoma by Snochowski et al.[77] These authors found five of eight BPH tissue specimens had high affinity and low capacity binding of [³H] R 1881 varying from 9.1 to 19.6 fmoles of binding sites per milligram of protein, whereas the remaining three did not show any specific binding. One carcinomatous tissue with a low degree of differentiation showed the highest number of specific binding sites (26.3 fmoles/mg protein), while another carcinomatous tissue with a higher degree of differentiation contained only 13.6 fmoles of specific binding sites per milligram of protein.[77] Ekman et al.[78] also used this synthetic androgen methyltrienolone (R 1881) in the study of androgen receptors in the prostatic tissue. They found that this substance binds to both androgen and progestin receptors and concluded that an androgen receptor assay of BPH specimens utilizing R 1881 as ligand is not specific. Although specific binding sites for R 1881 were present in all normal and hyperplastic prostates, in a number of BPH tissues there was a lack of measurable progestin receptors.[78] The cancerous tissues, on the other hand, in several metastatic carcinomatous specimens were found to be R 1881 receptor-negative. These authors[78] therefore postulated that perhaps benign androgen-dependent tissues such as normal and hyperplastic prostates always contain androgen receptors, whereas malignant prostatic tissues with a more variable hormone sensitivity show a more heterogenous steroid receptor profile.

Recently Mobbs et al.[79] assayed DHT in 84 prostatic specimens from patients with BPH and prostatic carcinoma. They have attempted clinical response to hormonal manipulation in 11 patients whose tumors were reported to have over 60% malignant involvement. Their investigations indicate that patients with low levels of androgen receptor in tumor cytosol were insensitive to hormonal therapy.

In a very important recent report Sidh et al.[80] measured androgen as well as estrogen receptors in 40 patients with carcinoma of the prostate before and during hormonal manipulation. Of 15 patients who showed both subjective and objective regression of disease, 13 had estradiol receptors (2.6 to 126.0 *fmoles*/mg cytosol protein), nine had DHT receptors (9.2 to 170.4 *fmoles*/mg), and one had unusually high DHT receptor (2543.0 *fmoles*/mg). Analysis of the receptor protein concentration for 18 patients whose disease progressed subjectively as well as objectively showed significantly higher DHT binding compared to estradiol binding in all but one patient. In seven of these patients no measurable estradiol receptor protein was detected.

From these findings the authors[80] postulated that there are perhaps significant differences in the type of receptor protein among patients who are endocrine-sensitive and those who are refractory to such treatment. The former, it appears, are rich in estradiol receptor and the latter in DHT receptor proteins.

CONCLUSION

In view of the above discussions it may be suggested that a better knowledge of the hormonal profile, whether blood or tissue concentrations, bioconversion of the androgens, or binding components in human prostate is of pathophysiological importance. The indications are that with the help of these studies it may be possible to differentiate the endocrine-refractory patients from hormone-sensitive ones. In fact in recent studies Sinha *et al.*[81, 82] have demonstrated two types of cells in prostatic epithelium; one binds with estrogen and the other does not bind with estrogen. Ultrastructurally also they have detected two distinct types of basal cells, light type and dark type, in the acini of cancerous prostate. Patients who subsequently become refractory to endocrine manipulation show more dark cells than do hormone-sensitive patients. Therefore, a thorough investigative procedure regarding hormonal status of a patient during hormonal therapy may be a valuable diagnostic tool in choosing the most appropriate form of therapy for his disease.

REFERENCES

1. Moore, R. A. The evolution and involution of the prostate gland. *Am. J. Pathol. 12:* 599, 1935.
2. Zuckerman, S., and Groome, J. R. The aetiology of benign enlargement of the prostate in the dog. *J. Pathol. Bacteriol. 44:* 113, 1937.
3. Denung, C. L., and Wolf, J. S. The anatomical origin of benign prostatic enlargement. *J. Urol. 42:* 566, 1939.
4. Huggins, C. The etiology of benign prostatic hyperplasia. *Bull. N.Y. Acad. Med. 23:* 696, 1947.
5. Bruchovsky, N., and Wilson, J. D. The intranuclear binding of testosterone and 5α-androstane-17β-ol-3-one by rat prostate. *J. Biol. Chem. 243:* 5953, 1968.
6. Baulieu, E.-E., Lasnitzki, I., and Robel, P. Metabolism of testosterone and action of metabolites on prostate glands grown in organ culture. *Nature 219:* 1155, 1968.
7. Wilson, J. D., and Gloyna, R. E. Intranuclear metabolism of testosterone in the accessory organs of reproduction. *Recent Prog. Horm. Res. 26:* 309, 1970.

8. King, R. J. B., and Mainwaring., W. I. P. *Steroid-Cell Interactions.* University Park Press, Baltimore, 1975.

9. Dorfman, R. I., and Shipley, R. A. *Androgens: Biochemistry, Physiology and Clinical Significance.* Wiley, New York, 1956.

10. Baulieu, E.-E., and Jung, I. A prostatic cytosol receptor. *Biochem. Biophys. Res. Commun. 38:* 599, 1970.

11. Fang, S., and Liao, S. A. Androgen receptors. Steroid- and tissue-specific retention of a 17β-hydroxy-5α-androstan-3-one-protein complex by the cell nuclei of ventral prostate. *J. Biol. Chem. 246:* 16, 1971.

12. Mainwaring, W. I. P., and Peterken, B. M. A reconstituted cell-free system for the specific transfer of steroid receptor complexes into nuclear chromatin isolated from rat ventral prostate gland. *Biochem. J. 125:* 285, 1971.

13. Lieberburg, I., and McEwen, B. S. Brain cell nuclear-retention of testosterone metabolites, 5α-dihydrotestosterone and estradiol-17β, in adult rats. *Endocrinology 100:* 588, 1977.

14. Vermeulen, A., Rubens, R., and Verdonck, L. Testosterone secretion and metabolism in male senescence. *J. Clin. Endocrinol. 34:* 730, 1972.

15. Stearns, E. L., MacDonnell, J. A., Kaufman, B. J., Padua, R., Lucman, T. S., Winter, J. S. D., and Faiman, C. Declining testicular function with age: hormonal and clinical correlates. *Am. J. Med. 57:* 671, 1974.

16. Gupta, D., Jacobi, G. H., Blank, B., and Altwein, J. E. Hormonal investigation in prostate cancer, in press 1982.

17. Swyer, G. M. Post-natal growth changes in the human prostate. *J. Anat. 78:* 130, 1944.

18. Siiteri, P. K., and Wilson, J. D. Dihydrotestosterone in prostatic hypertrophy. 1. The formation and content of dihydrotestosterone in the hypertrophic prostate of man. *J. Clin. Invest. 49:* 1737, 1970.

19. Hammond, G. L. Endogenous steroid levels in the human prostate from birth to old age: a comparison of normal and diseased tissues. *J. Endocrinol. 78:* 7, 1978.

20. Albert, J., Geller, J., Geller, S., and Lopez, D. Prostate concentrations of endogenous androgens by radioimmunoassay. *J. Steroid Biochem. 7:* 301, 1976.

21. Millington, D. S., Bnoy, M. E., Brooks, G., Harper, M. E., and Griffiths, K. Thin-layer chromatography and high resolution selected ion monitoring for the analysis of C_{19}-steroids in human hyperplastic prostate tissue. *Biomed. Mass Spectrometry 2:* 219, 1975.

22. Malathi, K., and Gurpide, E. Metabolism of 5α-dihydrotestosterone in human benign hyperplastic prostate. *J. Steroid Biochem. 8:* 141, 1977.

23. Geller, J., Albert, J., Lopez, D., Geller, S., and Niwayama, G. Comparison of androgen metabolites in benign prostatic hypertrophy (BPH) and normal prostate. *J. Clin. Endocrinol. 43:* 686, 1976.

24. Habib, F. K., Lee, I. R., Stitch, S. R., and Smith, P. H. Androgen levels in the plasma and prostatic tissues of patients with benign hypertrophy and carcinoma of the prostate. *J. Endocrinol. 71:* 99, 1976.

25. Mahoudeau, J. A., Delasalle, A., and Bricaire, H. Secretion of dihydrotestosterone by human prostate in benign prostatic hypertrophy. *Acta Endocrinol. 77:* 401, 1974.

26. Pazzagli, M., Forti, G., Cappellini, A., and Serio, M. Radioimmunoassay of plasma dihydrotestosterone in normal and hypogonadal men. *Clin. Endocrinol. 4:* 513, 1975.

27. Horton, R., Hsieh, P., Barberia, J., Pages, L., and Cosgrove, M. Altered blood androgens in elderly men with prostatic hyperplasia. *J. Clin. Endocrinol. 41:* 793, 1975.

28. Sciarra, F., Sorcini, G., Di Silverio, F., and Gagliardi, V. Testosterone and 4-androstenedione concentration in peripheral and spermatic venous blood of patients with prostatic adenocarcinoma. Effects of diethylstilbesterol and cyproterone acetate therapy. *J. Steroid Biochem. 2:* 313, 1971.

29. Yamaguchi, K., Kasai, H., Minesita, T., Kotoh, K., and Matsumoto, K. 5α-reduction and binding of testosterone in androgen-dependent and independent mouse mammary tumours. *Endocrinology 95:* 1424, 1974.

30. Ishimaru, T., Pages, L., and Horton, R. Altered metabolism of androgens in elderly men with benign prostatic hyperplasia. *J. Clin. Endocrinol. 45:* 695, 1977.

31. Chisholm, G. D., and Ghanadian, R. Comparison between the changes in serum 5α-dihydrotestosterone and testosterone in normal men and patients with benign prostatic hypertrophy. Proceedings of the V. International Congress of Endocrinology, p. 186, 1976.

32. Vermeulen, A., and De Sy, W. Androgens in patients with benign prostatic hyperplasia before and after prostatectomy. *J. Clin. Endocrinol. 43:* 1250, 1976.

33. Bird, C. E., and Clark, A. F. Kinetics of ³H-5α-dihydrotestosterone metabolism in normal men and men with prostatic carcinoma: effects of estrogen administration in men. *J. Clin. Endocrinol. 34:* 467, 1972.

34. Pazzagli, M., Borrelli, D., Forti, G., and Serio, M. Dihydrotestosterone in human spermatic venous plasma. *Acta Endocrinol. (Kbh). 76:* 388, 1974.

35. Kinouchi, T., and Horton, R. 3α-Androstanediol kinetics in man. *J. Clin. Endocrinol. 54:* 646, 1974.

36. Jacobi, G. H., Kurth, K. H., Gupta, D., and Altwein, J. E. Endocrine profile in patients with untreated staged and graded prostatic carcinoma based on nine hormone parameters. Presented at the 73rd Annual Meeting of the American Urological Association, Washington, D.C., May 21–25, 1978.

37. Jacobi, G. H., Gupta, D., Rathgen, G. H., and Altwein, J. E. Hormone dependence of prostatic carcinoma: serum androgens, plasma SHBG, and prostatic androstanediol formation in untreated patients. In *Steroid Receptors and Hormone-Dependent Neoplasia*, edited by J. L. Wittliff and O. Dapunt. Masson Publ., New York, 1980, pp. 155–160.

38. Vermeulen, A. Testicular hormonal secretion and aging in males. In *Benign Prostatic Hyperplasia*, edited by J. T. Grayhack, J. D. Wilson, and M. J. Scherbenske. DHEW Publication (NIH 76-1113), Bethesda, 1975, pp. 177–182.

39. Rosenfield, R. L. Plasma testosterone binding globuline and indexes of the concentration of unbound plasma androgens in normal and hirsute subjects. *J. Clin. Endocrinol. 32:* 717, 1971.

40. Blank, B., Attanasio, A., Rager, K., and Gupta, D. Determination of serum sex hormone binding globulin (SHBG) in preadolescent and adolescent boys. *J. Steroids Biochem 9:* 121, 1978.

41. Houghton, A. L., Turner, R., and Cooper, E. H. Sex hormone binding globulin in carcinoma of the prostate. *Br. J. Urol. 49:* 227, 1977.

42. Dennis, M., Horst, H.-J., Krieg, M., and Voigt, K. D. Plasma sex hormone binding capacity in benign prostatic hypertrophy and prostatic carcinoma: comparison with an age dependent rise in normal human males. *Acta Endocrinol. (Kbh) 84:* 207, 1972.

43. Bartsch, W., Horst, H.-J., Becker, H., and Nehse, G. Sex hormone binding globulin binding capacity, testosterone, 5α-dihydrotestosterone, oestradiol and prolactin in plasma of patients with prostatic carcinoma under various types of hormonal treatment. *Acta Endocrinol. (Kbh) 85:* 650, 1977.

44. Wotiz, H. H., and Lemon, H. M. Studies in steroid metabolism: I. Metabolism of testosterone by human prostatic tissue slices. *J. Biol. Chem. 206:* 525, 1954.

45 Harding, B. W., and Samuels, L. T. Uptake and subcellular distribution of C¹⁴-labelled steroid in rat ventral prostate following in vivo administration of testosterone-4-C¹⁴. *Endocrinology 70:* 109, 1962.

46. Pearlman, W. H., and Pearlman, M. R. J. Metabolism in vivo of delta-4-androstene-3,17-dione-7-H³: its localization in ventral prostate and other tissues of rat. *J. Biol. Chem. 236:* 1321, 1961.

47. Prout, G. R., Jr., Kliman, B., Daly, J. J., MacLaughlin, R. A., and Griffin, P. P. In vitro uptake of ³H testosterone and its conversion to dihydrotestosterone by prostatic carcinoma and other tissues. *J. Urol. 116:* 603, 1976.

48. Kliman, B., Prout, G. R., Jr., MacLaughlin, R. A., Daly, J. J., and Griffin, P. P. Altered androgen metabolism in metastatic prostate cancer. *J. Urol. 117:* 623, 1978.

49. Altwein, J. E., Rubin, A., Klose, K., Knapstein, P., and Orestano, F. Kinetik der 5-alpha-Reduktase im Prostataadenom in Gegenwart von Östradiol, Diäthylstilböstrol, Progesteron und Gestonoron-Capronat (Depostat). *Urologe A 13:* 41, 1974.

50. Gloyna, R. E., and Wilson, S. D. A comparative study of the conversion of testosterone to 17α-hydroxy-5-androstan-3-one (dihydrotestosterone) by prostate and epididymis. *J. Clin. Endocrinol. 29:* 970, 1969.

51. Collins, W. P., Koullapis, E. N., Bridges, C. E., and Sommerville, I. F. Studies on steroid metabolism in human prostatic tissue. *J. Steroid Biochem. 1:* 195, 1970.

52. Di Silverio, F., Gagliardi, V., Sorcini, G., and Sciarra, F. Biosynthesis and metabolism of androgenic hormones in cancer of the prostate. *Invest. Urol. 15:* 286, 1976.

53. Baulieu, E.-E., and Robel, P. Testosterone metabolites: their receptors, metabolism and action in the rat ventral prostate. In *Some Aspects of the Aetiology & Biochemistry of Prostatic Cancer*, edited by K. Griffiths and C. G. Pierrepoint. Alpha-Omega-Alpha. Publishing Co., Cardiff, Wales, 1970, pp. 74–81.

54. Harper, M. E., Pierrepoint, C. G., Fahmy, A. R., and Griffiths, K. The metabolism of steroids in the canine prostate and testis. *J. Endocrinol. 49:* 213, 1971.

55. Jacobi, G. H., and Wilson, J. D. Formation of 5α-androstane-3α,17β-diol by normal and hypertrophic human prostate. *J. Clin. Endocrinol. Metab. 44:* 107, 1977.

56. Shida, K., Shimazaki, J., Ito, Y., Yamanaka, H., and Nagai-Yuasa, H. 3α-reduction of dihydrotestosterone in human normal and hypertrophic prostate tissues. *Invest. Urol. 13:* 241, 1975.

57. Gupta, D., Rager, K., Ziegler, H., and Voelter, D. *In vivo* and *in vitro* effects of cyproterone acetate on androgen metabolism by human carcinomatous prostatic tissue, in press 1982.

57a. Flüchter, St. H., Grun, W., Harzmann, R., Bichler, K.-H. and Gupta, D. Comparative studies of *in vitro* testosterone metabolism in various types of tissue sections in healthy and diseased prostates, in press 1982.

58. Belham, J. E., and Neal, G. E. Testosterone action in the rat ventral prostate. The effects of diethylstilbestrol and cyproterone acetate on the metabolism of ³H-testosterone and the retention of labelled metabolites by rat ventral prostate in vivo and in vitro. *Biochem. J. 125:* 81, 1971.

59. Walsh, P. C., and Korenman, S. G. Action of the antiandrogens: preservation of 5α-reductase activity and inhibition of chromatin-dihydrotestosterone complex formation. *Clin. Res. 18:* 126, 1970.

60. Wein, A. J., and Murphy, J. J. Experience in the treatment of prostatic carcinoma with cyproterone acetate. *J. Urol. 109:* 68, 1973.

61. Smith, R. B., Walsh, P. C., and Goodwin, W. E. Cyproterone acetate in the treatment of advanced carcinoma of the prostate. *J. Urol. 110:* 106, 1973.

62. Scott, W. W. Cyproterone acetate treatment of disseminated prostatic cancer and benign nodular hyperplasia. In *International Symposium on the Treatment of Carcinoma of the Prostate*, edited by G. Raspé and W. Brosig. Pergamon Press, Oxford, 1971, pp. 161–163.

63. Scott, W. W., and Wade, J. C. Medical treatment of benign nodular prostatic hyperplasia with cyproterone acetate. *J. Urol. 101:* 81, 1969.

64. Jones, R. Effects of testosterone, testosterone metabolites and antiandrogens on the function of the male accessory glands in the rabbit and rat. *J. Endocrinol. 74:* 75, 1977.

65. Grants, A., and Stitch, S. R. The effect of cyproterone acetate on androgen biosynthesis by the rabbit testis. *J. Endocrinol. 57:* 597, 1973.

66. Hansson, V., and Tveter, K. J. Effect of anti-androgens on the uptake and binding of androgen by human benign nodular prostatic hyperplasia in vitro. *Acta Endocrinol. (Kbh) 68:* 69, 1971.

67. Mainwaring, W. I. P., and Milroy, E. J. G. Characterization of the specific androgen receptors in the human prostate gland. *J. Endocrinol. 57:* 371, 1973.

68. Rosen, V., Jung, I., Baulieu, E.-E., and Robel, P. Androgen-binding proteins in human benign prostatic hypertrophy. *J. Clin. Endocrinol. 41:* 761, 1975.

69. Geller, J., Cantor, T., and Albert, J. Evidence for a specific dihydrotestosterone-binding cytosol receptor in the human prostate. *J. Clin. Endocrinol. 41:* 854, 1975.

70. Attramadal, A., Tveter, K. J., Weddington, S. C., Djøseland, O., Naess, O., Hansson, V., and Torgersen, O. Androgen binding and metabolism in the human prostate. *Vitam. Horm. 33:* 247, 1975.

71. Attramadal, A., Weddington, S. C., Naess, O. Djøseland, O., and Hansson, V. Androgen receptors in male sex tissues of rats and humans. In *Prostatic Disease*, edited by H. Marberger, H. Haschek, H. K. A. Schirmer, J. A. C. Colston, and E. Witkin. Alan R. Liss, New York, 1976, pp. 189–203.

72. Karr, J. P., Wajsman, Z., Madajewicz, S., Kirdani, R. Y., Murphy, G. P., and Sandberg, A. A. Steroid hormone receptors in the prostate. *J. Urol. 122:* 170, 1979.

73. Menon, M., Tananis, C. E., McLoughlin, M. G., and Walsh, P. C. Androgen receptors in human prostatic tissue: a review. *Cancer Treat. Rep. 61:* 265, 1977.

74. Mobbs, B. G., Johnson, I. E., and Connolly, J. G. In vitro assay of androgen binding by human prostate. *J. Steroid Biochem. 6:* 453, 1975.

75. Bonne, C., and Raynaud, J.-P. Methyltrienolone, a specific ligand for cellular androgen receptors. *Steroids 26:* 227, 1975.

76. Bonne, C., and Raynaud, J.-P. Assay of androgen binding sites by exchange with methyltrienolone (R1881). *Steroids 27:* 497, 1976.

77. Snochowski, M., Pousette, Å., Ekman, P., Bression, D., Andersson, L., Högberg, B., and Gustafsson, J.-Å. Characterization and measurement of the androgen receptor in human benign prostatic hyperplasia and prostatic carcinoma. *J. Clin. Endocrinol. 45:* 920, 1977.

78. Ekman, P., Snochowski, M., Dahlberg, E., Bression, D., Högberg, B., and Gustafsson, J.-Å. Steroid receptor content in cytosol from normal and hyperplastic human prostates. *J. Clin. Endocrinol. 49:* 205, 1979.

79. Mobbs, B. G., Johnson, I. E., Connolly, J. G., and Clark, A. F. Androgen receptor assay in human benign and malignant prostatic tumor cytosol using protamine sulphate precipitation. *J. Steroid Biochem. 9:* 289, 1978.

80. Sidh, S. M., Young, J. D., Jr., Karmi, S. A., Powder, J. R., and Bashirelahi, N. Adenocarcinoma of prostate: role of 17β-estradiol and 5α-dihydrotestosterone binding proteins. *Urology 13:* 597, 1979.

81. Sinha, A. A., Blackard, C. E., Doe, R. P., and Seal, U. S. The in vitro localization of ^{3}H-estradiol in human prostatic carcinoma. *Cancer 31:* 682, 1973.

82. Sinha, A. A., Blackard, C. E., and Seal, U. S. A critical analysis of tumour morphology and hormone treatments in the untreated and estrogen-treated responsive and refractory human prostatic carcinoma. *Cancer 40:* 2836, 1977.

20

Steroid Receptor Measurements in Prostate Cancer Tissue

H. J. deVoogt, M.D.

INTRODUCTION

Since we know that the prostate can be considered as a target organ for androgenic and probably also for estrogenic hormones, the study of intracellular steroid action has gained enormous interest. The theoretical concept and the actual demonstration of cytoplasmic and nuclear steroid receptors during the last two decades have contributed remarkably to our understanding of the intracellular metabolic processes of steroids in target organs. At least for breast cancer the determination of the presence of estrogen receptors has proved to be of clinical importance in the treatment of this tumor.[1] The clinical relevance of steroid receptors for prostatic cancer, however, has yet to be determined.

In the early 1960s Jensen and Jacobson[2, 3] were the first to demonstrate that estrogen target tissues accumulate and retain estradiol (E_2) which indicates that these tissues must contain specific binding components. Talwar et al.[4] and Toft and Gorski[5] were able to extract these binding proteins, called "receptors," from the cytoplasmic fraction of homogenized tissue (cytosol), while Jungblut et al.[6] found such a macromolecular binding protein in the nuclear fraction. The cytosol receptor sedimented at 8 S* in sucrose density gradient centrifugation and the nuclear receptor at 5 S. Jensen et al.[7, 8] discovered that the cytosol receptor in high ionic salt solution sedimented at 4 S.

The E_2-receptor became also a well studied binding protein, and most of the data of the properties of this receptor can generally be applied to androgenic and other steroid receptors as well. Receptors are extremely

---

* S, *Svedberg units* of sedimentation coefficient.

labile proteins, and so far all attempts to isolate pure receptor have been unsuccessful. The molecular weight is about 7 to 8×10^4. In the presence of estradiol the cytosolic receptor is transformed by a heat-dependent process from 4 S to 5 S, and Little et al.[9, 10] demonstrated that this transformation is the result of dimerization of two identical receptor subunits. This dimer seems to be an activated form which is translocated to the nucleus where it binds tightly to chromatin structures. The 5 S nuclear receptor could be transformed back to the 4 S form by proton addition or hyaluronidase.[11, 12] Receptors are destroyed by proteolytic enzymes, but not by RNAse or DNAse.[13] They are also destroyed by heat. This means that the indirect measurements of receptors and their association constants have to be done at low temperatures of 0 to 4°C preferably.

MODELS FOR THE ROLE OF STEROID RECEPTORS

Three models have been suggested for the physiological role of receptors:

1. Receptors are transport and storage proteins, which protect steroids against enzymatic attacks or loss by nonspecific binding and which in the nucleus release trace amounts of steroids for specific acceptor regions of the genome. The steroids are then the initiators of biological effects.

2. Receptors have a latent functional activity. The steroid modifies the protein during binding by a conformational change. This then leads to dimerization and translocation to the nucleus. The steroid-receptor complex as a whole is the most important component that induces biosynthetic effects.[9, 14, 15]

3. The receptor protein itself induces biological effects and is in fact a transcription-regulating protein. Steroid hormones only amplify the receptor action and thereby control the rate of biological processes.[11]

Receptor proteins are not the only specific steroid-binding molecules. An important role is played by SHBG (Sex Hormone Binding Globulin) in the plasma, which serves as a transport protein for steroids (see Chapter 19). The affinity and specificity of SHBG is much lower than that of the receptor, but it is much more stable. The small physical differences between SHBG and receptors demand very sensitive and specific assessment procedures that can discriminate between the two; this is one of the problems that has greatly interfered with the determination of androgen receptors in human prostatic tissue.

Although the role of androgen receptors in target tissues can be assumed to be generally the same as that of estrogen receptors, there is a major difference. The naturally circulating androgen, testosterone, is not the most active or potent androgen in most of the target tissues. Bruchovsky and Wilson[16, 17] demonstrated in rats that testosterone as well as the other naturally occurring androgens (from testicular as well as adrenal origin) were converted intracellularly into 5α-dihydrotestosteron (DHT) which can be considered the principal potent androgen. The enzyme 5α-reductase plays a very important role in this process.[18, 19]

It is the DHT that binds to the receptor of the target cell cytoplasm and is then translocated to the nucleus and in this way initiates or activates the biological effect. Recently Bruchovsky et al.[20, 21] noted that the nucleus retains relatively large amounts of DHT, more than accounts for cytosolic receptor binding. The significance of this has yet to be established.

ANIMAL STUDIES

Liao and co-workers,[22-25] in the search for the specific androgen receptor proteins in rats, found two fractions, which they called α- and β-proteins. The β-protein seemed to fulfill all requirements for specific receptor action, translocation to the nucleus and binding to the chromatin structures, after which protein synthesis is initiated and receptor proteins are also formed. Liao's original concept of androgen-receptor cycling is illustrated by Figure 20.1. The present concept of steroid metabolism in a prostatic cell is illustrated by the still simplified model of Ekman et al.[26] in Figure 20.2.

Later Gustafsson et al.[27] and Heyns and de Moor[28] described another binding protein in the prostate cytosol, which is largely connected with the secreting activity of prostatic glandular cells. There is increasing evidence that Liao's α-protein and the prostatic secretion protein are one and the same.[29]

The transfer from animal experiments (mostly in rats) to the human prostate proved to be a difficult step as far as receptor determination was concerned. The difficulties encountered are given in Table 20.1.

Normal prostate is hard to define and even more difficult to obtain fresh for this purpose. Hyperplastic tissue of the prostate (BPH) is

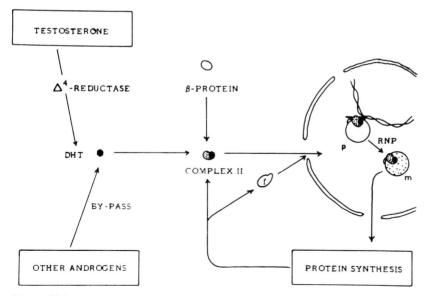

Figure 20.1 A model for androgen-receptor cycling. (Reproduced with permission from S. Liao et al.[29])

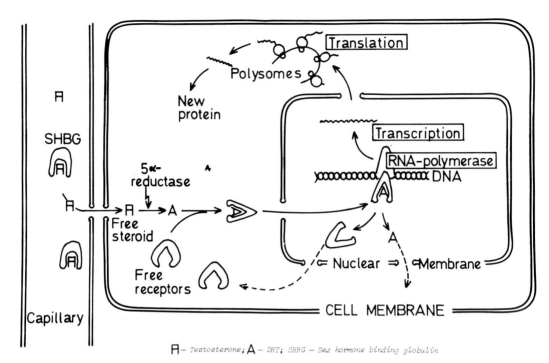

R− *Testosterone*; A − *DHT*; *SHBG − Sex hormone binding globulin*

Figure 20.2 Simplified model of the interaction of androgens within a prostatic cell. (Reproduced with permission from P. Ekman et al.[26])

Table 20.1
Difficulties Encountered Regarding Receptor Determination in Experiments with the Human Prostate

1. Normal prostatic tissue usually not readily available.
2. Therefore only BPH tissue available for comparison.
3. How to get enough and "proper" cancer tissue?
4. The endogenous androgens and plasma contaminants (SHBG).
5. The relation of stromal to epithelial elements in any given piece of prostatic tissue.

available in large quantities, but this is neoplastic in itself and may be the result of endocrine disorder. Prostatic carcinoma can usually be obtained only by needle biopsies or *tr*ansu*r*ethral *r*esection (TUR). The amount of a needle biopsy is usually considered too small for the biochemical assay, and TUR material is rejected by most scientists because the receptor proteins could be destroyed by heat. However, Dingjan[30] demonstrated that even in the small amount of a needle biopsy (50 to 100 mg) receptor proteins can be detected (Fig. 20.3), and he also demonstrated that TUR material can be used for receptor assay.

It is known that normally the amount of circulating endogenous androgens in men is high. This means that most of the androgen receptors (free binding sites) in target cells will be occupied by these endogenous androgens, and only a few can be determined by our indirect biochemical assays. It explains why in patients with prostatic carcinoma who are

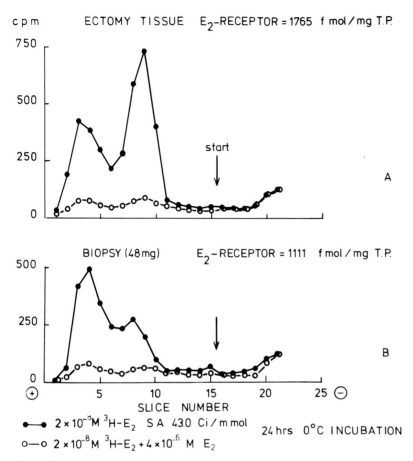

Figure 20.3 Agar electrophoresis in benign prostate hypertrophy. Comparison of receptor determination in tissue of BPH, obtained by biopsy as well as by prostatectomy. (Reproduced with permission from P. G. Dingjan.[30])

treated by estrogens, many more free binding sites can be found. To overcome this problem exchange incubation techniques have been developed, in which total receptor content and nuclear receptors are determined and the cytoplasmic receptor content is found by subtraction.[31–33] More important, however, is the fact that the tissue in a biopsy is nearly always very heterogeneous in composition: a mixture of stromal and glandular cells of which the latter can be normal, hyperplastic, as well as carcinomatous. This means that most of the results of receptor determinations have to be regarded critically in this respect.

STUDIES IN THE HUMAN

Tveter et al.[34] was the first to determine androgen receptors in human prostate. Others were Hsu et al.,[35] Mainwaring and Milroy,[36, 37] and Hansson et al.[38] But these studies did not pay much attention to the aforementioned problems. Wagner[39, 40] was the first to describe a method, the cold agar-gel-electrophoresis, which, using natural tritiated steroids as ligands, can discriminate clearly between SHBG-bound and receptor-bound steroids (Figs. 20.4 and 20.5). As SHBG is a contaminant of all human tissue samples, this method is preferable above all other methods, like the sucrose density gradient centrifugation, protamine sulfate precipitation assay, polyacrilamide gel electrophoresis, and others that lack this ability. Surprisingly enough this method never was adopted (as far as can be gathered from published data) in the USA, where such a large amount of fundamental research in the field of receptors was done. In my opinion this partly explains the controversial results of U.S. and European research on this matter.[41, 42]

Another method, which has gained more attention recently, is the use of artificial ligands which were created in the Uclaff-Roussel-Laboratories

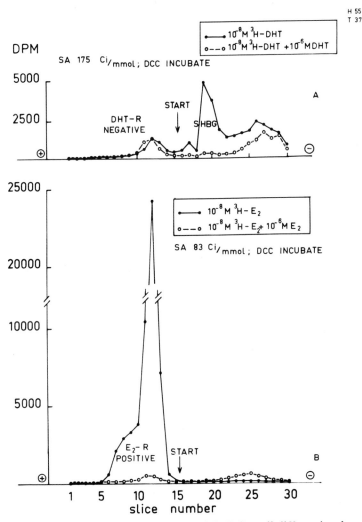

Figure 20.4 Determination of DHT-R and E_2-R in well differentiated prostatic adenocarcinoma by agar-gel electrophoresis. (Reproduced with permission from H. J. de Voogt and P. G. Dingjan.[60])

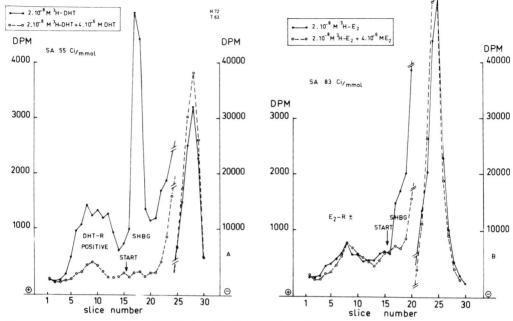

Figure 20.5 Determination of DHT-R and E_2-R in poorly differentiated prostatic adenocarcinoma by agar-gel electrophoresis. (Reproduced with permission from H. J. de Voogt and P. G. Dingjan.[60])

and first reported by Velluz et al.[43] Raynaud and co-workers[44, 45] published several reports on the use of these ligands for steroid-receptor assays. The principal advantages of these probes are that they do not bind to SHBG and are not metabolized during incubation. They allow for direct measurement of total receptors as well as for indirect exchange incubation techniques to measure cytoplasmic and nuclear receptors separately. It seems that quantitative measurement of cytoplasmic and nuclear receptors is necessary for maximal diagnostic or prognostic accuracy.[46] However, when we see how strongly determination of receptor (binding) sites diverges in many published data and how many different ways of reproduction of results are used, the conclusion forces itself on us that standardization is requested urgently.[47–49]

Ekman,[50] using these ligands, could identify DHT-receptor in prostatic cancer and eventually found a correlation between receptor content and response to endocrine therapy. Thus far he is the only one, for most other studies and particularly the ones using agar-gel electrophoresis, who failed to find such a correlation.[30, 48, 51, 52] Bashirelahi and co-workers[53] recently found exactly the opposite of Ekman. One explanation is that Ekman used mainly metastatic cancer tissue, which contains homogeneous cancer cells. Another possiblity is the method used by Bashirelahi's group (Sidh et al.[53]), namely the dextran-coated charcoal extraction, which is known to remove large amounts of specific (receptor-bound) steroids.[30]

The problem of the heterogeneity of the prostatic tissue was tackled by doing morphometric analysis of the tissue involved[30, 55] or by separating stroma from epithelial cells and doing receptor-assays in both.[56, 57]

In regard to the common use of estrogens for the treatment of advanced prostatic cancer, many of the investigators looked for estrogen receptors in prostatic tissue. Here again the results were far from uniform. Estrophilic proteins were definitely found by some[30, 54, 58, 59] and regarded as nonexistent by others.[50] De Voogt and Dingjan[60, 61] demonstrated by statistical analysis that their E_2-receptor was mainly located in stromal cells. This is in accordance with the findings of Schweikert et al.[57] who noted that stromal cells of the prostate have their own steroid metabolism, in which even androgens can be converted into estrogens. Also, the experiments of Lasnitzki and co-workers[62] have to be memorized, as they pointed to the specific role of genital stroma for the development of secondary sex organs.

Lastly, progesterone and corticosteroid receptors have been found in prostatic tissue, but so far they have not contributed much to the understanding of the relationship between endocrine therapy and steroid metabolism in prostatic tissues.

PRESENT SITUATION AND CONCLUSION

When we finally survey the subject of steroid receptors in prostatic cancer, the following conclusions are derived:

1. Androgen receptors (*i.e. DHT-r*) exist in prostatic tissue and play a major role in metabolism of glandular cells. The differences in *DHT-r* content between BPH and prostatic cancer indicate a certain diagnostic significance. However, as to a prognosis for endocrine manipulation the results of receptor-assays are still controversial.

2. Estrogen receptors are found in BPH as well as in prostatic cancer. Their significance is mainly connected with stromal (fibrous and smooth muscle) cells. Prediction of response to estrogen therapy, however, is not yet related with E_2-receptor assays.

3. The knowledge about other steroid receptors is at the moment still scanty, which does not preclude a possible significance in the future.

4. There is much need for standardization of methodology of receptor determination in prostatic tissue, as well as for the development of micromethods, which can make use of the small amount of a needle biopsy or preferably of the material obtained by aspiration biopsy. If a cytochemical method becomes available, this would signify a considerable progress. At present there are already attempts to purify receptor protein and develop antibodies against it.[63-65] Of these the method using monoclonal hybridoma cells[66] is very promising for the future, but also the immunofluorescence methods[67, 68] have to be watched carefully.

5. Steroid receptors have contributed greatly to our understanding of steroid metabolism in target cells and also have provided a physiological basis for endocrine manipulation of prostatic cancer. However, the unexpressed desire that they would unveil some of the etiology or prostatic cancer has not been fulfilled.[36]

REFERENCES

1. Jensen, E. V. Estrogen receptors in hormone-dependent breast cancers. *Cancer Res. 35:* 3362, 1975.
2. Jensen, E. V., and Jacobson, H. I. *Biological Activities of Steroids in Relation to Cancer*, edited by G. Pincus, and E. P. Vollmer. Academic Press, New York, 1960, p. 161.
3. Jensen, E. V., and Jacobson, H. I. Basic guides to the mechanism of estrogen action. *Recent Prog. Horm. Res. 18:* 387, 1962.
4. Talwar, G. P., Segal, S. J., Evans, A., and Davidson, O. W. The binding of oestradiol in the uterus. A mechanism for depression of RNA-synthesis. *Proc. Natl. Acad. Sci. USA 52:* 1059, 1964.
5. Toft, D., Gorski, J. A receptor molecule for oestrogens: isolation from the rat uterus and preliminary characterization. *Proc. Natl. Acad. Sci. USA 55:* 1574, 1966.
6. Jungblut, P. W., Hätzel, I., de Sombre, E. R., and Jensen, E. V. Die oestrogen-bindenden Prinzipien der Erfolgsorgane. *Colloq. Ges. Physiol. Chem. 18:* 58, 1967.
7. Jensen, E. V., Suzuki, T., Nutama, M., Smith, S., and de Sombre, E. R. Estrogen-binding substances of target tissue. *Steroids 13:* 417, 1969.
8. Jensen, E. V., Numata, M., Smith, S., Suzuki, T., Brechner, P. I., and de Sombre, E. R. Estrogen-receptor interaction in target tissues. *Dev. Biol. Suppl. 3:* 151 1969.
9. Little, M., Szendro, P. I., and Jungblut, P. W. Hormone-mediated dimerisation of microsomal oestradiol receptor. *Hoppe Seyler's Z. Physiol. Chem. 354:* 1599, 1973.
10. Little, M., Szendro, P., Teran, C., Hughes, A., and Jungblut, P. W. Biosynthesis and transformation of microsomal and cytosol estradiol receptors. *J. Steroid Biochem. 6:* 493, 1975.
11. Jungblut, P. W., Gaues, J., Hughes, A., Kallweit, E., Sierralta, W., Szendro, P., and Wagner, R. K. Activation of transcription-regulating proteins by steroids. *J. Steroid Biochem. 7:* 1109, 1976.
12. Jungblut, P. W., Meyer, H. H. P., and Wagner, R. K. The interrelationship of estrogen receptors extracted from various subcellular compartments. Abstr. Internat. Symp. Perspectives in Steroid Receptor Research. Sorrento, 1979.
13. Gorski, J., Toft, D., Shyamala, G., Smith, D., and Notides, A. Hormone receptors: studies on the interaction of estrogen with the uterus. *Recent Prog. Horm. Res. 24:* 45, 1968.
14. Mainwaring, W. I. P. The mechanism of action of androgens: a survey. In *Monographs on Endocrinology*, Vol. 10. Springer, New York, 1977.
15. Buller, R. E., and O'Malley, B. W. The biology and mechanism of steroid hormone receptor interaction with the eukariotic nucleus. *Biochem. Pharmacol. 25:* 1, 1976.
16. Bruchovsky, N., and Wilson, J. D. The intranuclear binding of testosterone and 5α-androstan-17β-ol-3-one by rat prostate. *J. Biol. Chem. 243:* 5953, 1968.
17. Bruchovsky, N., and Wilson, J. D. The conversion of testosterone to 5α-androstan-17β-ol-3-one by rat prostate in vivo and in vitro. *J. Biol. Chem. 243:* 2012, 1968.
18. Moore, R. J., and Wilson, J. D. Localization of the reduced nicotinamide adenine dinucleotide phosphate: Δ^4-3-ketosteroid 5α-oxido-reductase in the nuclear membrane of the rat ventral prostate. *J. Biol. Chem. 247:* 958, 1972.
19. Moore, R. J., and Wilson, J. D. The effect of androgenic hormones on the reduced nicotinamide adenine dinucleotide phosphate Δ^4-3-ketosteroid 5α-oxido-reductase in the nuclear membrane of the rat ventral prostate. *Endocrinology 93:* 581, 1973.
20. Bruchovsky, N., Rennie, P. S., and Wilkin, R. P. New aspects of androgen action in prostatic cells: stromal localization of 5α-reductase, nuclear abundance of androstanolone and binding of receptor to linker deoxyribonucleic acid. In *Steroid Receptors, Metabolism and Prostatic Cancer*, edited by F. H. Schröder and H. J. de Voogt. Excerpta Medica, Amsterdam, 1980, pp. 57–76.
21. Bruchovsky, N., Rennie, P. S., and Vanson, A. Studies on the regulation of the concentration of androgens and androgen receptors in nuclei of prostatic cells. Elsevier Scientific Publishing Co., Amsterdam, 1980.
22. Anderson, K. M., and Liao, S. Selective retention of dihydrotestosterone by prostatic nuclei. *Nature 219:* 277, 1968.

23. Liao, S., and Fang, S. Receptor-proteins for androgens and the mode of action of androgens on gene transcription in ventral prostate. *Vitam. Horm. 27:* 17, 1969.

24. Fang, S., Anderson, K. M., and Liao, S. Receptor proteins for androgens. *J. Biol. Chem 244:* 6584, 1969.

25. Fang, S., and Liao, S. Androgen receptors steroid- and tissue-specific retention of a 17β-hydroxy-5α-androstan-3-one protein complex by the cell nuclei of ventral prostate. *J. Biol. Chem. 246:* 16, 1971.

26. Ekman, P., Snochowski, M., Dahlberg, E., and Gustafsson, J. A. Steroid receptors in metastatic carcinoma of the human prostate. *Eur. J. Cancer 15:* 257, 1979.

27. Gustafsson, J. Å., Björk, P., Carlsröm, K., Forsgren, B., Hökfelt, T., Poussette, Å., and Högberg, B. On the presence of a major protein, prostatic secretion protein or estramustine-binding protein, in the rat ventral prostate and in the human prostate. In *Steroid Receptors, Metabolism and Prostatic Cancer*, edited by F. H. Schröder and H. J. de Voogt. Excerpta Medica, Amsterdam, 1980, pp. 86–101.

28. Heyns, W., and de Moor, P. Prostatic binding protein. A steroid-binding protein secreted by rat prostate. *Eur. J. Biochem. 78:* 221, 1977.

29. Liao, S., Chen, C., Loor, R., and Hiipakka, R. A. Androgen-sensitive protein in rat ventral prostate: a specific intracellular protein and a secretory protein. In *Steroid Receptors, Metabolism and Prostatic Cancer*, edited by F. H. Schröder and H. J. de Voogt. Excerpta Medica, Amsterdam, 1980, pp. 13–21.

30. Dingjan, P. G. Steroid Hormoon Receptoren in Humaan Prostaatweefsel. Dissertation, University of Leiden, The Netherlands, 1978.

31. Rosen, V., Jung, I., Beaulieu, E.-E., and Robel, P. Androgen-binding proteins in human BPH. *J. Clin. Endocrinol. Metab. 41:* 761, 1975.

32. Shain, S. A., and Boesel, R. W. Androgen receptor content of the normal and hyperplastic canine prostate. *J. Clin. Invest. 61:* 654, 1978.

33. Sirret, D. A. N., and Grant, J. K. Androgen binding in cytosols and nuclei of human benign hyperplastic prostatic tissue. *J. Endocrinol. 77:* 101, 1978

34. Tveter, K. J., Unjhem, O., Attramadal, A., Åakvaag, A., and Hansson, V. Androgenic receptors in rat and human prostate. *Adv. Biosci. 7:* 193, 1971.

35. Hsu, R. S., Middleton, R. G., and Fang, S. Androgen receptors in human prostate. In *Normal and Abnormal Growth of the Prostate*, edited by M. Goland. Charles C Thomas, Springfield, Ill., 1975, pp. 663–675.

36. Mainwaring, W. I. P. *Some Aspects of the Aetiology and Biochemistry of Prostatic Cancer*, edited by K. Griffiths and C. G. Pierrepoint. Alpha Omega Alpha Press, Cardiff, 1970, p. 109.

37. Mainwaring, W. I. P., and Milroy, E. J. G. Characterization of the specific androgen receptors in the human prostate gland. *J. Endocrinol. 57:* 371, 1973.

38. Hansson, V., Larsen, J., and Rensch, E. Physiochemical properties of the 5α-dihydrotestosterone binding protein in human male serum. *Steroids 20:* 555, 1973.

39. Wagner, R. K. *The Assay of Steroid Hormone Receptors by Agar Electrophoresis, Principle and Application*, Schoeller-Junkmann-Preis, Schering AG, West Berlin, 1972.

40. Wagner, R. K. Characterization and assay of steroid hormone receptors and steroid-binding serum proteins by agar gel electrophoresis at low temperature. *Hoppe Seyler's Z. Physiol. Chem. 353:* 1235, 1972b.

41. Menon, M., Tananis, C. E., McLoughlin, M. G., and Walsh, P. C. Androgen receptors in human prostatic tissue: a review. *Cancer Treat. Rep. 61:* 265, 1977.

42. Menon, M., Tananis, C. E., McLoughlin, M. G., Lippman, M. E., and Walsh, P. C. The measurement of androgen receptors in human prostatic tissue utilizing sucrose density centrifugation and a protamine precipitation assay. *J. Urol. 117:* 309, 1977.

43. Velluz, L., Nominé, G., Bucourt, R., and Mathieu, J. Un analogue triénique de la méthyltestostérone. *C. R. Hebd. Seances Acad. Sci. 257:* 569, 1963.

44. Bonne, C., and Raynaud, J. B. Methyltrienolone, a specific ligand for cellular androgen receptors. *Steroids 26:* 227, 1975.

45. Bonne, C., and Raynaud, J. P. Assay of androgen binding sites by exchange with R 1881. *Steroids 27:* 497, 1976.

46. Shain, S. A., and Boesel, R. W. Human prostate steroid hormone receptor quantitation.

Invest. Urol. 16: 169, 1978.

47. Menon, M., Tananis, C. E., Hicks, L. L., Hawkins, E. F., McLoughlin, M. G., and Walsh, P. C. Characterization of the binding of a potent synthetic androgen, methyltrienolone, to human tissues. *J. Clin. Invest. 61:* 150, 1978.

48. Krieg, M., Bartsch, W., Janssen, W., and Voigt, K. D. A comparative study of binding, metabolism and endogenous levels of androgens in normal, hyperplastic and carcinomatous human prostate. *J. Steroid Biochem. 11:* 615, 1979.

49. Karr, J. P., Wajsman, Z., Madajewicz, S., Kirdani, R. Y., Murphy, G. P., and Sandberg, A. A. Steroid hormone receptors in the prostate. *J. Urol. 122:* 1970, 1979.

50. Ekman, P. Steroid receptors in the human prostate. Thesis, University of Stockholm, 1978.

51. Wagner, R. K. Extracellular and intracellular steroid binding proteins. Properties, discrimination, assay and clinical applications. *Acta Endocrinol. 88[Suppl.] 218:* 1, 1978.

52. Pfitzenmayer, N., Schmid, W., and Röhl, L. Is there a correlation between receptor content and response to endocrine therapy in prostatic cancer? In *Steroid Receptors, Metabolism and Prostatic Cancer*, edited by F. H. Schröder and H. J. de Voogt. Excerpta Medica, Amsterdam, 1980, pp 199–201.

53. Sidh, S. M., Young, J. D., Karmi, S. A. Powder, J. R., and Bashirelahi, N. Adenocarcinoma of prostate: role of 17β-estradiol and 5α-dihydrotestosterone binding proteins. *Urology, 13:* 597, 1979.

54. Bashirelahi, N., and Young, J. D. Specific binding protein for 17β-estradiol in prostate with adenocarcinoma. *Urology 8:* 553, 1976.

55. Bartsch, G., and Rohr, H. P. Ultrastructural stereology: a new approach to the study of prostatic function. *Invest. Urol. 14:* 301, 1977.

56. Romijn, J. C., Oishi, K., Schweikert, H. U., Mulder, E., Schröder, F. H., and Bolt-de Vries, J. Androgen metabolism and androgen receptors in separated epithelium and stroma of the human prostate. In *Steroid Receptors, Metabolism and Prostatic Cancer*, edited by F. H. Schröder and H. J. de Voogt. Excerpta Medica, Amsterdam, 1980, pp. 134–143.

57. Schweikert, H. U., Hein, H. J., and Schröder, F. H. Androgen metabolism in fibroblasts from human benign prostatic hyperplasia, prostatic carcinoma, and nongenital skin. In *Steroid Receptors, Metabolism and Prostatic Cancer*, edited by F. H. Schröder and H. J. de Voogt. Excerpta Medica, Amsterdam, 1980, pp. 126–133.

58. Hawkins, E. F., Nijs, M., Brassine, C., and Tagnon, H. J. Steroid receptors in the human prostate. I. Estradiol-17β binding in benign prostatic hypertrophy. *Steroids 26:* 458, 1975.

59. Jungblut, P. W., Hughes, S. F., Görlich, L., Gowers, U., and Wagner, R. K. Simultaneous occurrence of individual oestrogen- and androgen receptors in female and male target organs. *Hoppe Seyler's Z. Physiol. Chem. 352:* 1603, 1971.

60. de Voogt, H. J., and Dingjan, P. G. Steroid receptors in human prostatic cancer. *Urol. Res. 6:* 151, 1978.

61. de Voogt, H. J., and Dingjan, P. G. Is there a place for the assay of cytoplasmic steroid receptors in the endocrine treatment of prostatic cancer? In *Steroid Receptors, Metabolism and Prostatic Cancer*, edited by F. H. Schröder and H. J. de Voogt. Excerpta Medica, Amsterdam, 1980, pp. 265–271.

62. Bard, D. R., Lasnitzki, I., and Mizuno, T. The role of testosterone metabolism in the mesenchymal induction of the rat prostate gland in vitro. In *Steroid Receptors, Metabolism and Prostatic Cancer*, edited by F. H. Schröder and H. J. de Voogt. Excerpta Medica, Amsterdam, 1980, pp. 44–52.

63. Hicks, L. L., and Walsh, P. C. A micro-assay for the measurement of androgen receptors in human prostatic tissue. *Steroids 33:* 389, 1979.

64. Greene, G. L., Closs, L. E., Fleming, H., de Sombre, E. R., and Jensen, E. V. Antibodies to estrogen receptor: immunochemical similarity of estrophilin from various mammalian species. *Proc. Natl. Acad. Sci. USA 74:* 3681, 1977.

65. Fishman, J., and Fishman, J. H. Competitive binding assay for estradiol receptor using immobilized antibody. *J. Clin. Endocrin. Metab. 39:* 603, 1974.

66. Jensen, E. V., Greene, G. L., and de Sombre, E. R. Immunochemical probes for receptor

structure and function. Abstract of the International Symposium on Perspectives in Steroid Receptor Research, Sorrento, 1979.

67. Nenci, I. Receptor and centriole pathways of steroid action in normal and neoplastic cells. *Cancer Res. 38:* 4204, 1978.

68. Pertschuk, L. P., Zava, D. T., Tobin, E. H., Brigati, T. J., Gaetjens, E., Macchia, R. J., Wise, G. J., Wax, H. S., and Kim, D. S. Histochemical detection of steroid hormone receptors in the human prostate. In *Prostate Cancer and Hormone Receptors*, edited by G. P. Murphy and A. A. Sandberg, Progr. Clin. Biol. Res., Vol. 33. Liss, New York, 1979, pp. 113–132.

Editorial Comment to Chapter 20

For clinicians, the major question arising from the variety of receptor studies is whether numerical data expressed in *femtomoles per milligram nuclear protein* or simply keyed as *receptor-positive versus negative* may be of any value in predicting hormone responsiveness from the beginning, or in indicating the need to change therapy.

Since under hormonal therapy the receptor content of the prostate greatly changes (Martelli *et al.* (1980), Mobbs *et al.* (1980)), Mobbs *et al.* (1980) stated that, "a high concentration of cytosolic androgen receptor does not necessarily indicate responsiveness to contrasexual hormonal treatment." Consequently, the use of such tests in laboratory medicine must be based on clinical usefulness and not primarily on academic medicine (Schwartz, 1979). Broad overviews on the subject are given by Murphy and Sandberg (1979) and Leavitt and Clark (1979).

G. H. J.

REFERENCES

Leavitt, W. W., and Clark, J. H. Steroid hormone receptor systems. *Adv. Exp. Med. Biol.* Vol. *117*. Plenum Press, New York, 1979.

Martelli, A., Soli, M., Bercovich, E., Prodi, G., Grilli, S., de Giovanni, C., and Galli, M. C. Correlation between clinical response to antiandrogenic therapy and occurrence of receptors in human prostatic cancer. *Urology 16:* 245, 1980.

Mobbs, B. G., Johnson, I. E., and Connolly, J. G. The effect of therapy o the concentration and occupancy of androgen receptors in human prostatic cytosol. *Prostate 1*: 37, 1980.

Murphy, G. P., and Sandberg, A. A. Prostate cancer and hormone receptors. *Prog. Clin. Biol. Res., 33*, 1979.

Schwartz, M. K. Relevance of steroid receptor measurements in the diagnosis and therapeutic management of cancer patients. In Prostate cancer and hormone receptors. *Prog. Clin. Biol. Res.*, Vol. 33. Liss, New York, 1979, pp. 201–208.

21

Protein Hormones and Prostate Cancer

M. E. Harper, B.Sc., Ph.D.
K. Griffiths, B.Sc., Ph.D.

Early studies in animals indicated that pituitary hormones could influence prostatic growth and function, a more marked atrophy of the rat prostate gland being observed after both hypophysectomy and castration, than after castration alone.[1] Furthermore, an impaired uptake of testosterone into the ventral prostate was also reported in hypophysectomized rats.[2] There was, however, some confusion as to which of the pituitary hormones were involved, partly due to the impurity of the hormone preparations available at that time.[3-5] Although prolactin emerged as a protein hormone, with evidence sufficiently convincing to suggest it had a direct effect on prostatic tissue, it appears however to have a role that is synergistic with that of testosterone.[6] Increased steroid uptake into prostatic tissue *in vitro* in the presence of prolactin has been shown by several investigators,[7-9] and zinc uptake and distribution are also influenced by this hormone.[10] Opinions are divided on the hormone's capacity to stimulate the activity of prostatic adenylcyclase.[11] Although studies with rats given the prolactin inhibitor bromocriptine, and also implanted with prolactin-secreting tumors, have failed to show significant changes in prostatic growth,[12, 13] nevertheless, specific binding sites for prolactin have been demonstrated in prostatic tissue.[14, 15] Growth hormone, ACTH and the gonadotropins LH and FSH, do not appear to have a direct effect on prostatic tissue, although their influence on available plasma androgen levels will profoundly affect prostate growth. Testicular androgen synthesis is dependent on adequate LH stimulation and adrenal C_{19}-steroid synthesis on ACTH. Prolactin may influence the availability of androgens by virtue of its synergistic action with LH on the testis[16] and by influencing adrenal C_{19}-steroid synthesis *per se*.[17] (Chapter 22).

PLASMA PITUITARY HORMONE CONCENTRATIONS

Asano,[18] using a bioassay, first reported elevated urinary prolactin concentrations in patients with prostatic cancer, and this early suggestion of this hormone's relationship to prostatic disease was further investigated by the analysis of plasma protein hormone concentrations. In an original study from this laboratory, the concentration of plasma prolactin in prostatic cancer patients was not significantly different from normal, although it was raised when compared to those levels found in patients with benign prostatic hyperplasia (BPH).[19] Other investigations similarly failed to find a consistently elevated level, Bartsch et al.[20] reporting that only 50% of their patients had raised plasma prolactin levels. Hammond et al.[21] and recently Jacobi and co-workers[22] also failed to find significantly different values in BPH or prostatic cancer patients and normal individuals. In the latter study, no correlation was found between plasma testosterone and prolactin concentrations, thereby agreeing with the data obtained by the *British Prostate Study Group*.[23] In this study, it was found that prolactin did not correlate with age, nor with the plasma concentration of testosterone, estradiol-17β, LH or FSH, but did appear to correlate with plasma growth hormone in the metastasis-free M_0-category of prostatic cancer patients.[23] A feature of the results obtained for patients and normals in these studies was the very wide variation encountered in hormone levels. Age-related changes in this elderly population, particularly in the plasma gonadotropin levels, was not surprising, since testicular atrophy can occur at any time throughout this age range. The dramatic hormonal differences associated with aging occur to the same extent in BPH, prostatic cancer patients, and clinically asymptomatic individuals.

Although these hormones may not be actively concerned in the initiation of prostatic carcinogenesis, a permissive role should not be overlooked, and one particular endocrine milieu might well promote tumor growth and dissemination. Clinical experience of prostatic cancer clearly indicates that prostate cancer is androgen-dependent. Alternatively, tumor size and spread could affect the secretion of the stress-related hormones such as ACTH, growth hormone, prolactin, or cortisol. Moreover, abnormal levels of steroid metabolites such as the 5α-androstanediols, synthesized by the prostatic tumor, could effect the release of pituitary hormones, and consequently the plasma hormone profile may be related to tumor size and development. The *British Prostate Study Group* investigated the relationship between primary tumor stage and metastatic status, and the plasma hormone levels. Using both Mann-Whitney statistics and canonical variate analysis, the only significant difference found was in the growth hormone concentrations of patients with and without metastases, the latter having lower levels. Further studies on the influence of growth hormone in prostatic tumor dissemination could be of interest.

PROTEIN HORMONES AND TREATMENT

As a consequence of the androgen-dependent nature of the majority of prostatic cancers, either estrogen treatment, often in the form of diethylstilbestrol or orchiectomy, provide the principal form of therapy, although permanent clinical control of the disease is rarely accomplished. One possible factor that might appear to be related to the relapse of the patient on high-dose estrogen therapy is the concomitant rise observed in plasma

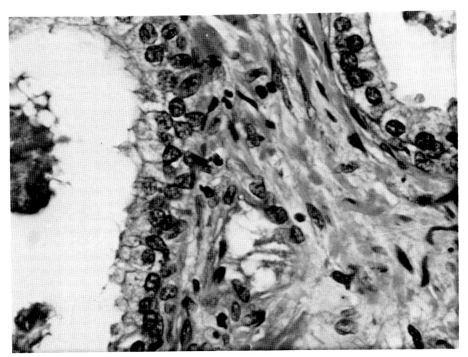

Figure 21.1 Consecutive sections from a patient (R. M.) with histologically diagnosed benign prostatic hyperplasia (Figs. 21.1 to 21.5). Hematoxylin and eosin. Part of two glandular acini can be seen separated by stroma containing a capillary.

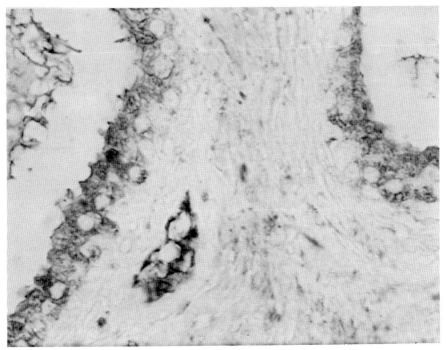

Figure 21.2 Human *prolactin* antiserum (1/500). Intense stain intracellularly located in the cytoplasm of epithelial cells with the nuclei clearly unstained. Acini secretions and elements in the stroma, particularly a capillary, contain reaction product.

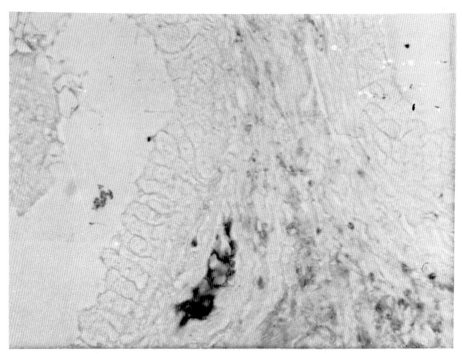

Figure 21.3 Human *growth hormone* antiserum (1/100). Staining is confined to stromal areas, notably a capillary.

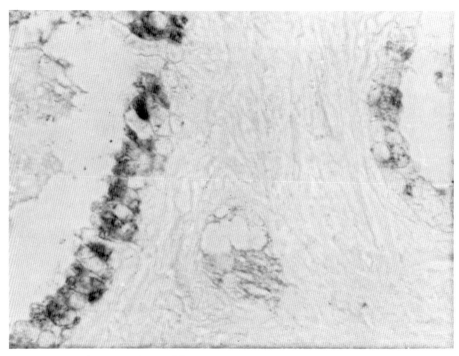

Figure 21.4 Human *FSH* antiserum (1/100). Strong stain is visible in the cytoplasm of some epithelial cells with the nuclei unstained. Little reaction product is present in the stroma.

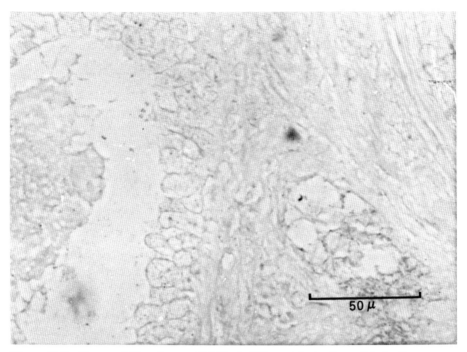

Figure 21.5 Human *LH* antiserum (1/50). A diffuse stain is discernible in the epithelium and stroma.

prolactin levels,[19] which could therefore influence androgen uptake into the prostate, and also adrenal steroid synthesis. This would to some extent counteract the beneficial and required reduction in the secretion of testosterone by the testes, achieved with estrogen treatment (see also Chapter 22). Alternative forms of therapy, such as orchiectomy and antiandrogen treatment in which prolactin levels are unchanged, would be expected to be more successful; however, this does not appear to be the case. The use of estrogens in combination with drugs that inhibit prolactin secretion, such as bromocriptine (CB 154) have also been investigated,[24] and the results in patients who have developed endocrine resistance look promising. Changes in androgen dynamics and prostatic steroid metabolism have also been reported in patients receiving CB 154.[25] Treatment of prostatic cancer patients with CB 154 alone has not, however, met with much success,[26] but relief of bone pain has been reported in patients receiving L-dopa,[27] a drug which also reduces prolactin concentrations.

Gonadotropin levels are raised in patients after orchiectomy, whereas they are considerably lower during estrogen therapy. Since both forms of treatment produce a similar clinical response, it is apparent that the consequent decrease in plasma androgen concentration produced is the important factor, and the resulting gonadotropin levels are of little consequence.

PROTEIN HORMONES AT THE CELLULAR LEVEL

Qualitative and quantitative analysis of steroids and steroid hormone receptors in hormone-responsive tumors have been shown to be useful in clinical practice. Protein hormone receptor analysis has not yet attracted as much attention, partly due to the techniques available and also to be limited evidence that they are involved in human breast and prostatic cancer. It may well be, however, that a convenient method for the analysis of protein hormones, or their receptors, may be afforded by immunocytochemistry. The advantage of this technique lies in the small amount of tissue required and its ability to identify those cells which contain either hormone or hormone receptor, in what is usually a heterologous population of normal and cancer cells. In this laboratory histologically, fixed, human BPH tissue has been examined using the technique essentially as described by Sternberger[28] and antisera raised against human growth hormone, prolactin, LH, and FSH. Figures 21.1 to 21.5 show typical results obtained with these various antisera, the staining indicating the probable localization of protein hormones or their subunits in prostatic tissue sections. Staining of the epithelial cell cytoplasm was observed using the prolactin antiserum (Fig. 21.2), whereas with growth hormone antiserum (Fig. 21.3) this area was unstained. Both antisera gave intense staining in various components of the stroma, particularly in capillaries and with blood cells. Strong epithelial cytoplasmic staining was obtained in a large number of the acini with the FSH antiserum (Fig. 21.4), whereas the stromal components were unstained. Very diffuse staining was observed with the LH antiserum over the whole of the tissue section (Fig. 21.5). This pattern of localization for the four antisera was evident in the specimens obtained from 11 BPH patients, but the preliminary data obtained with prostatic cancer specimens differed in certain aspects and is currently being collated. These findings were consistent with the apparent internalization of protein hormones and their receptors in target tissues.[29] Such data should provide valuable information on the relationship of protein hormones to prostatic dysfunction and may possibly find clinical application in therapy decisions. The approach could also be of value in identifying the role of protein hormones in the etiology of prostate cancer.

REFERENCES

1. Lostroh, A. J., and Li, C. H. Stimulation of the sex accessories of hypophysectomised male rats by non-gonadotrophic hormones of the pituitary gland. *Acta Endocrinol. (Kbh)* 25: 1, 1957.
2. Lawrence, A. M., and Landau, R. L. Impaired ventral prostate affinity for testosterone in hypophysectomized rats. *Endocrinology* 73: 1119, 1965.
3. Chase, M. D., Geschwind, I. I., and Bern, H. A. Synergistic role of prolactin in response of male rat sex accessories to androgen. *Proc. Soc. Exp. Biol. Med.* 94: 680, 1957.
4. Tullner, W. W. Hormonal factors in the adrenal-dependent growth of the rat ventral prostate. *Natl. Cancer Inst. Monogr.* 12: 211, 1963.
5. Asano, M. Basic experimental studies of the pituitary prolactin-prostate interrelationships. *J. Urol.* 93: 87, 1965.
6. Grayhack, J. T., and Lebowitz, J. M. Effect of prolactin on citric acid of lateral lobe of the prostate of Sprague-Dawley rat. *Invest. Urol.* 5: 87, 1967.
7. Farnsworth, W. E. Role of lactogen in prostatic physiology. *Urol. Res.* 3: 129, 1975.
8. Lasnitzki, I. The effect of prolactin on rat prostate glands in organ culture. In *Prolactin and Carcinogenesis*, edited by A. R. Boyns and K. Griffiths. Alpha Omega Alpha, Cardiff, Wales, 1972, p. 200–206.

9. Lloyd, J. W., Thomas, J. A., and Mawhinney, M. G. A difference in the in vitro accumulation and metabolism of testosterone-1,2 [3]-H by the rat prostate gland incubation with ovine or bovine prolactin. *Steroids 22:* 473, 1973.

10. Gunn, S. A., Gould, T. C., and Anderson, W. A. D. The effect of growth hormone and prolactin preparations on the control by interstitial cell stimulating hormone of uptake of [65]Zn by the rat dorsal lateral prostate. *J. Endocrinol. 32:* 205, 1965.

11. Golder, M. P., Boyns, A. R., Harper, M. E., and Griffiths, K. An effect of prolactin on prostatic adenylate cyclase activity. *Biochem. J. 128:* 725, 1972.

12. Harper, M. E., Danutra, V., Chandler, J. A., and Griffiths, K. The effect of 2-bromo-α-ergocryptine (CB154) administration on the hormone levels, organ weights, prostatic morphology and zinc concentrations in the male rat. *Acta Endocrinol. (Kbh) 83:* 211, 1976.

13. Bartke, A., and Lloyd, C. W. The influence of pituitary homografts on the weight of the accessory reproductive organs in castrated male mice and rats and on the mating behaviour in male mice. *J. Endocrinol. 46:* 313, 1970.

14. Aragona, C., and Friesen, H. G. Specific prolactin binding sites in the prostate and testis of rats. *Endocrinology 97:* 677, 1975.

15. Kledzik, G. S., Marshall, S., Campbell, G. A., and Gelato, M. Effects of castration, testosterone, estradiol and prolactin on specific prolactin-binding activity in ventral prostate of male rats. *Endocrinology 33:* 873, 1971.

16. Hafiez, A. A., Bartke, A., and Lloyd, C. W. The role of prolactin in the regulation of testis function. *Endocrinology 53:* 223, 1972.

17. Jones, T., Brownsey, B. G., Cowley, T. H., and Griffiths, K. *Tissue Culture in Medical Research*, edited by F. Jacoby and K. T. Rajan. Heinemann, London, 1974, pp. 263–272.

18. Asano, M. Studies on urinary prolactin with special reference to carcinoma of the prostate. *Jpn. J. Urol. 53:* 901, 1962.

19. Harper, M. E., Peeling, W. B., Cowley, T., Brownsey, B. G., Phillips, M. E. A., Groom, G., Fahmy, D. R., and Griffiths, K. Plasma steroid and protein hormone concentrations in patients with prostatic carcinoma before and during oestrogen therapy. *Acta Endocrinol. (Kbh) 81:* 409, 1976.

20. Bartsch, W., Horst, H. J., Becker, H., and Nehse, G. Sex hormone binding globulin capacity, testosterone, 5α-dihydrotestosterone, oestradiol and prolactin in plasma of patients with prostatic carcinoma under various types of hormonal treatment. *Acta Endocrinol. (Kbh) 85:* 650, 1977.

21. Hammond, G. L., Kontturi, M., Maattala, P., Puuka, M., and Vihko, R. Serum FSH, LH and prolactin in normal males and patients with prostatic diseases. *Clin. Endocrinol. 7:* 129, 1977.

22. Jacobi, G. H., Altwein, J. E., and Rathgen, G. H. Serum prolactin and tumors of the prostate: unchanged basal levels and lack of correlation to serum testosterone. *J. Endocr. Invest. 3:* 15, 1980.

23. British Prostate Study Group: Elevation of plasma hormone concentrations in relation to clinical staging in patients with prostatic cancer. *Br. J. Urol. 51:* 382, 1979.

24. Jacobi, G. H., Altwein, J. E., and Hohenfellner, R. Adjunct bromocriptine treatment as palliation for prostatic cancer: experimental and clinical evaluation *Scand. J. Urol. Nephrol. Suppl. 55:* 107, 1980.

25. Jacobi, G. H., Altwein, J. E., and Hohenfeller, R. Alterations of peripheral testosterone metabolism after induced hypoprolactinemia in patients with prostatic carcinoma. *Klin. Wochenschr. 57:* 49, 1979.

26. Coune, A., and Smith, P. Clinical trial of 2-bromo-α-ergocryptine (NSC-169774) in human prostatic cancer. *Cancer Chemother. Rep. 59:* 209, 1975.

27. Sadoughi, N., Razvi, M., Busch, I., Albin, R., and Guinan, P. Cancer of prostate, relief of bone pain with levodopa. *Urology 4:* 107, 1974.

28. Sternberger, L. A. *Foundations of Immunology.* Prentice-Hall, Englewood Cliffs, New Jersey, 1974, pp. 129–171.

29. Conn, P. M., Conti, M., Harwood, J. P., Dufau, M. L., and Catt, K. J. Internalization of gonadotrophin-receptor complex in ovarian luteal cells. *Nature 274:* 598, 1978.

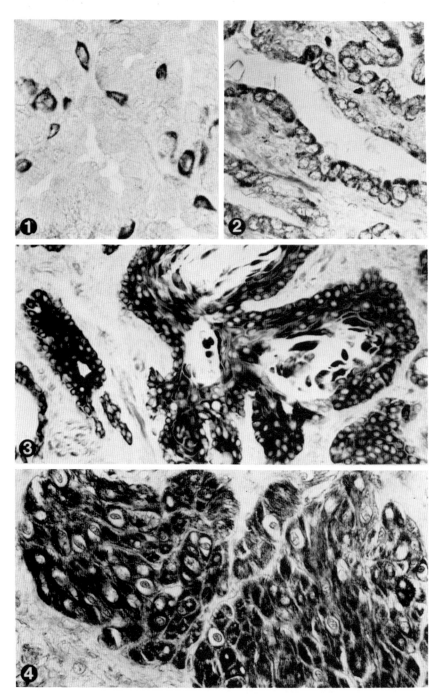

Figure 21.6 Histological sections of prostate glands of castrated dogs. The sections were treated with the immunoperoxidase technique to localize prolactin (PRL)-dependent staining. **1**, A dog treated for 6 months with 5α-androstane-3α, 17β-diol (75 mg/week IM). PRL-dependent staining was localized only in basal cells, but not in glandular epithelium. ×560. **2**, A dog treated for 6 months with 5α-androstane-3α, 17β-diol (75 mg/week IM). Focal glandular cystic hyperplasia showing intracellular PRL-dependent staining distributed throughout the cyto-

Editorial Comment to Chapter 21

As will further be outlined in Chapter 22, with the demonstration of prolactin binding in various prostatic tissues of animals and man, we have a tool to qualitatively and perhaps quantitatively characterize the physiological and possibly pathophysiological role of prolactin on the prostate. The *Tenovus Group* has herein demonstrated binding of prolactin and apparently also of LH and FSH to human BPH tissue, data that are still difficult to interpret today. In the dog, however, a species in which benign prostatic hyperplasia can be induced by androgens plus estrogens, prolactin binding patterns change during this kind of hormone manipulation. We are indebted to Professor El Etreby (Berlin) for letting us reproduce some of his results, illustrated in Figure 21.6. The addition of estrogens to androgens in the induction of canine BPH clearly increases prolactin binding.

M. E. Harper and K. Griffiths have outlined and recently accentuated (Sibley *et al.*, 1981) prostatic prolactin binding studies by applying the immunoperoxidase methodology, which is being increasingly applied to the human malignant (Witorsch, 1979) and benign (Becht *et al.* 1981) condition.

G. H. J.

REFERENCES

Becht, E., Baba, S., and Jacobi, G. H. Prolaktinbindung in der benignen Prostatahyperplasie des Menschen. In *Die Prostatahyperplasie, Klin. Exp. Urol.*, Vol. 4, edited by K. Bandhauer, H. Toggenburg, and H.W. Bauer. Zuckschwerdt Verlag, München, 1981, pp. 53–59.

Sibley, P. E. C., Harper, M. E., Joyce, B.G., Peeling, W. B., and Griffiths, K. The immunocytochemical detection of protein hormones in human prostatic tissues. *Prostate* 2: 175, 1981.

Witorsch, R. J. The application of immunoperoxidase methodology for the visualization of prolactin binding sites in human prostate tissue. *Hum. Pathol. 10:* 521, 1979.

plasm of most cells. Selected cells are either lightly stained or unstained, indicating a deficiency in intracellular PRL. ×560. (**1** and **2**, Reproduced with permission from M. F. El Etreby and A. T. Mahrous. *Histochemistry* 64: 279–286, 1979. **3**, A dog treated for 6 months with 5α-androstane-3α, 17β-diol (75 mg/week IM) and 17β-estradiol (0.75 mg/week IM). Intracellular PRL-dependent staining in hyperplastic and squamous metaplastic epithelium. Cytoplasm of most cells is darkly stained, indicating high intracellular PRL. ×220. **4**, A dog treated for 6 months with 5α-androstane-3α, 17β-diol (75 mg/week IM), 17β-estradiol (0.75 mg/week IM), and cyproterone acetate (600 mg/week subcutaneously). Highly active muscular tissue shows marked PRL staining. ×560. (**3** and **4**, Reproduced with permission from M. F. El Etreby *et al. Cell Tissue Res.* 204: 367–378, 1979.)

22

Experimental Rationale for the Investigation of Antiprolactins as Palliative Treatment for Prostate Cancer

G. H. Jacobi, M.D.

INTRODUCTION

Besides the variety of contrasexual measures, such as surgical *ablation* of the main androgen source by orchiectomy or *additive* androgen suppression by natural and synthetic estrogen preparations, the use of more specific antihormonal substances with a more selective action on the periphery and/or on the target site itself, has been introduced for palliation of advanced stages of prostate cancer. In the case of cyproterone acetate, for example, a considerable body of evidence is available to date indicating that this *antiandrogen* is effective in estrogen-relapsed cases (Chapter 15). It was the clinically as well as experimentally still obscure estrogen escape phenomenon which justified in the past the search for new antihormones.

In the somewhat vague play of speculations about the mechanisms and pathogenetic factors possibly involved in the phenomenon of acquired hormone resistance after an uncertain period of response to estrogens (for definition see Chapter 3), the discussion of *prolactin*, another hormone with obviously *prostatotrophic* functions, arose rather early. The development of the concept that prolactin, a pituitary hormone with well-established functions in the female, may also have some sort of "nutritive" function in the prostate gland was based on extensive animal studies. This effect of prolactin was considered to either be associated with its own receptor-mediated mode of action at a membrane level of the target cell, or associated with some supportive influence of prolactin on the supply and utilization of androgens. Using a variety of animal models and different experimental approaches, a number of investigators have accumulated straightforward evidence that prolactin has various stimulatory effects on prostatic growth, on a direct prostatic as well as on an indirect testicular and adrenal level.

CO-ANDROGENIC EFFECTS OF PROLACTIN

Two different routes of androgenic influence of prolactin have been studied extensively.

1. *Via the testis:* The currently reported effects of prolactin augmentation or suppression on testicular steroidogenesis are summarized in Table 22.1. In reviewing these data[25] it becomes clear that prolactin promotes androgen synthesis in several enzymatic steps, in the rat and mouse[4, 19] and that prolactin may have some co-function on the LH-receptor of Leydig cells.[2, 6] The results of Rubin and co-workers[40] and Magrini and associates[33] may at first also give the impression that this mediatory role of prolactin to androgens could be applied to the human condition.

2. *Via the adrenals:* In contrast to the situation on the testicular level, for which experimental data derive almost exclusively from animal studies, the mode of action of prolactin in altering *adrenal* steroid

Table 22.1
Prolactin Actions on the Testis: Stimulatory (↑) and Suppressive (↓) Effects on Leydig Cell Metabolism

Author[a]	Effects		Condition
Bartke (1971)[a] Bartke (1973)[a]	Cholesterol ester stores	↑	Mouse, *in vivo*
Bartke (1974)[a]	Cholesterol stores	↓	By PRL-inhibition
Hafiez *et al.* (1972)[a]	Acetate → testosterone	↑	LH + PRL synergism, *in vivo*
Mathur *et al.* (1975)[a]	Δ4,5-Isomerase -3β-hydroxy-steroid dehydrogenase (DHEA → 4Δ)	↑	Mouse, *in vitro*
Musto *et al.* (1972)[a]	17β-Hydroxysteroid dehydrogenase (4Δ → testosterone)	↑	Mouse, *in vitro*
Hafiez *et al.* (1971)[a]	3β-Hydroxysteroid-dehydrogenase	↑	Mouse, rat, *in vivo*
Aragona *et al.*[2]	LH-receptors	↑	Rat
Bex and Bartke[6]	LH-receptors	↑	Hamster
Bartke (1973)[a]	Testosterone in serum	↓	PRL-suppression, rat, mouse
Hafiez *et al.*[19]	Testosterone in serum androstenedione in serum	↑ ↑	By PRL + LH, rat
Bartke (1971)[a]	Spermiogenesis	↑	PRL↑, mouse
Rubin *et al.*[40]	Testosterone/PRL parallelism		Circadian rhythm, man
Magrini *et al.*[33]	Dihydrotestosterone	↓	PRL ↑ by sulpiride

[a] These references taken from G. H. Jacobi.[25]

formation derive from clinical studies in men. Not only androgens[44] but also corticosteroids and mineralocorticoids show some significant changes during clinical states of hyperprolactinemia or after pharmacological alterations of prolactin release (Table 22.2).

THE PROSTATE AS PROLACTIN TARGET

Huggins and Russell[23] first discovered in 1946 that hypophysectomy combined with castration results in a more pronounced involution of dog

Table 22.2
Stimulatory (↑) and Suppressive (↓) Effects of Long-Term Hyperprolactinemia on Adrenocortical Steroid Hormone Metabolism

Author[a]	Effects[b]		Condition
Vermeulen et al.[44]	DHEA i.s.; DHEA-S i.s.	↑ ↑	Prolactinoma, sulpiride, phenothiazine
Vermeulen and Ando (1978)[a]	DHEA-S i.s.	↑	After long time PRL ↑
Bassi et al. (1977)[a]	DHEA i.u.	↑	PRL ↑ -amenorrhea
Carter et al. (1977)[a]	DHEA + DHEA-S i.s.; DHEA + DHEA-S i.s.	↑ ↓	Galactorrhea-amenorrhea- syndrome by bromocriptine
Büber (1978)[a]	Cortisol i.s.; testosterone i.s.	↓ →	After bromocriptine in PRL ↑ hirsutism
Ingvarsson (1969)[a]	Corticosteroids i.s.	↑	By PRL in ACTH refractory patients with rheumatism
Donabedian et al. (1976)[a]	17-Ketosteroids i.u.	↑	PRL ↑ -amenorrhea
Uberti et al. (1979)[a]	Aldosterone i.s.; renin i.s.; cortisol i.s.	↓ ↓ →	After bromocriptine in healthy men
Edwards et al. (1975)[a]	Aldosterone i.s.		Furosemide-induced in- crease, by bromocriptine reversible
Edwards and Jeffcoate (1976)[a]	Aldosterone i.s.	↓	By bromocriptine in prim. hyperaldosteronism
Manku et al. (1972)[a]	ADH i.s.	↑	By PRL under H_2O-loading
Boyns et al.[8]	Androstenedione; testosterone	↑ ↑	By PRL in explanted human adrenals
Lichtenstein et al. (1976)[a]	Aldosterone	↑	By PRL in rat adrenal in vi- tro
Lis et al. (1973)[a]	Corticosterone	↑	By PRL in isolated rat adre- nal
Winters et al. (1975)[a]	Fetal adrenal growth		Correlates with PRL-levels
Kandeel et al. (1978)[a]	DHEA-S. i.s.; 3β-ol-dehydrogenase- isomerase (5Δ → 4Δ)	↑ ↓	PRL ↑ in females, by bromo- criptine reversible

[a] These references taken from G. H. Jacobi.[25]
[b] Abbreviations used are: i.s., in serum; i.u., in urine.

prostate than castration alone, and these authors speculated that some unknown pituitary-promoting factor might be involved. Consequently, Grayhack and his co-workers[16–18] investigated the influence of prolactin and other pituitary factors on prostatic response to androgens, on prostatic growth and differentiation, and on prostatic citric acid content. The essential information obtained from the more than 40 publications that have appeared in the meantime can be summarized as follows: prolactin modulates prostatic androgen uptake, affects intracellular metabolism and utilization, thus promoting differentiation, growth, and function of the prostate.[3, 8, 13, 34, 35, 37, 42, 46] Also, in terms of pathological prostatic growth, data from our laboratory clearly show that in the dog model for benign prostatic hyperplasia[45] prolactin also affects the stimulatory properties of exogenically administered androgens and estrogens.[28] The animal prostate has the highest number of prolactin-binding sites among androgen target organs.[1] Since prolactin binding to specific receptor sites at the target cell is under some regulation of sex hormones,[30] it is conceivable that the mechanism involved in the intraprostatic actions of androgens is mediated by a complex connection of both the prolactin and the steroid hormone receptor machineries (Fig. 22.1). Prolactin binding has been demonstrated by immunohistochemical as well as biochemical means in normal and malignant prostate tissue of animals and man[29, 48, 49]; the binding of prolactin to human benign prostatic hyperplasia has already been illustrated in Chapter 21. However, the data presented by Ron et al.,[39] suggesting that increasing peripheral prolactin levels during prostatectomy are indicative of an accumulation of prolactin in hyperplastic prostatic tissue which could then be released by operative squeezing of the organ, are at the least questionable: peripheral prolactin levels are dependent on numerous exogenic and endogenous stimuli.[12, 38, 43]

PROLACTIN-ANDROGEN RELATIONSHIP IN MAN

The two main questions arising from the aforementioned data are whether in the normal state the androgen environment is dependent on peripheral prolactin levels and whether in pathologic prostate conditions of man the prolactin environment is altered.

Birkhoff and co-workers[7] have studied prolactin levels in patients with different prostate conditions and did not find significant differences in the subjects with benign prostatic hyperplasia. Prolactin levels do not differ in patients with prostatic carcinoma as compared to age-matched control individuals.[10, 26] Furthermore, in a large group of untreated prostatic carcinoma patients, prolactin levels are not discriminated by tumor stage or grade (Table 22.3). There is no statistically significant linear correlation between the individual prolactin values and the levels of androgens and estradiol.[25] Since suppression of prolactin by bromocriptine or stimulation by chlorpromazine does not alter the 24-hour pattern of plasma testosterone (Fig. 22.2a), nor the response of plasma testosterone to HCG stimulation (Fig. 22.2b), it can be stated that the peripheral

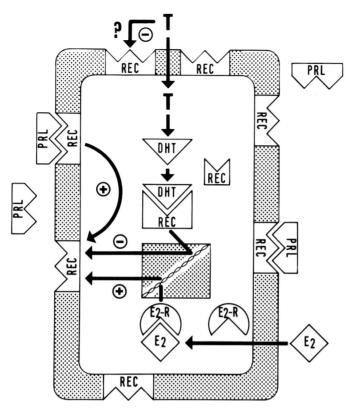

Figure 22.1 Intracellular receptor-mediated prolactin binding at the target cell; testosterone (T) is taken up through the membrane, reduced to dihydrotestosterone (DHT) and bound to a specific receptor (REC). Estradiol (E_2) also binds to a specific cytoplasmic receptor (E_2-R); prolactin (*PRL*) binds to membrane receptor sites, receptor-bound PRL stimulates its receptor formation (+). While androgens negatively influence prolactin receptor binding, estradiol has a positive influence on the prolactin-binding mechanism.

Table 22.3
Prolactin Levels of 73 Patients with Untreated Prostatic Carcinoma analyzed according to Clinical Stage and Histological Grade[a]

Classification (UICC, 1978)	No. ($n = 73$)	Plasma-Prolactin (ng/ml)	±SD	Significance[b] (if $p < 0.01$)
Stage[c]				
M_0	41	8.2	2.7 ⎤	
M_1	32	10.4	2.9 ⎦	N.S.
Grade[d]				
G_1	19	10.5	3.1 ⎤	N.S. ⎤
G_2	30	7.9	2.5 ⎦ N.S.	⎦ N.S. ⎤ N.S.
G_3	24	8.1	2.2	⎦

[a] From G. H. Jacobi.[25]
[b] None of the differences was statistically significant (N.S.)
[c] M_0, without distant metastasis; M_1, with distant metastasis, UICC, 1978.
[d] G_1, highly differentiated; G_2, moderately to poorly differentiated; G_3, undifferentiated, anaplastic or cribriform pattern.

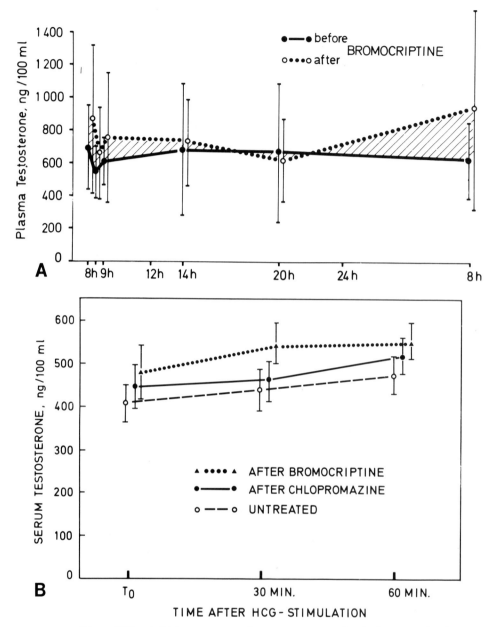

Figure 22.2 *A*, 24-hour pattern of testosterone secretion before and after bromo-criptine-induced prolactin suppression in four patients with untreated prostate cancer. A 6-day oral treatment with 15 mg bromocriptine per day resulted in a drop of prolactin from 10.4 ± 5.9 to 1.6 ± 0.3 ng/ml ($p < 0.01$); plasma testosterone was not altered significantly. *B*, Plasma testosterone before (T_0) and during a 60-minute stimulation with 5000 IU HCG in nine patients with untreated prostatic cancer; studies were performed before (untreated), as well as after prolactin suppression by bromocriptine (prolactin 5.3 ± 0.6 to 2.0 ± 0.4 ng/ml), or after prolactin stimulation by chlorpromazine (prolactin to 8.2 ± 1.6 ng/ml); testicular response to HCG was not altered significantly by prolactin manipulations.

prolactin levels do not alter the peripheral androgen environment in man. Support is given by the fact that testosterone is not altered under stimulatory conditions with LH-RH and TRH, when the study is performed before or after prolactin suppression with bromocriptine.[47]

These data are contradictory to preliminary results reported by Giuliani et al.[15] on an increased pituitary reserve of prolactin release in patients with prostatic carcinoma. Thus, we are left with the conclusion that in man, in contrast to the animal condition, peripheral androgens are not related to the peripheral prolactin environment, and prostatic cancer patients behave as age-matched controls as far as peripheral prolactin supply is concerned.

ESTROGEN TREATMENT AND PROLACTIN ENVIRONMENT

After the numerous experimental data derived from studies using hypophysectomy, immunological prolactin inactivation by prolactin antisera, pharmacological prolactin suppression by ergot alkaloids, and using hereditary prolactin-deficient animals, a *clinical observation* gave support to further consideration of prolactin as a significant factor in prostate cancer maintenance. This was the increase of prolactin release by estrogens first discovered by Ratner et al.[36] Hanafy and co-workers[20] then speculated that the prolonged hyperprolactinemia induced by long-term estrogen treatment may be responsible for the so-called estrogen escape phenomenon.

In terms of prolactin alteration, estradiol acts threefold on the hypothalamus-pituitary axis[32]; via a "short-loop," estradiol stimulates dopamine receptors at the hypothalamus, and this dopaminergic effect results in a prolactin suppression. Via a pituitary "long-loop," dopamine receptors are inhibited and TRH receptors stimulated, both resulting in a strong prolactin release (Fig. 22.3). The net effect of these hypothalamic-pituitary estrogen actions is a hyperprolactinemia as encountered during the menstrual cycle and pregnancy.

After an increase of peripheral prolactin during long-term estrogen treatment was demonstrated by the Tenovus Group,[9, 21] a systematic evaluation of this issue was initiated by our laboratory. It was shown that not only estrogens, but also antiandrogens with a gestagenic component of action increased prolactin.[27] Figure 22.4 demonstrates the wave-like augmentation of prolactin after treatment of prostatic carcinoma with an estrogen depot preparation, while Figure 22.5A shows the continuous hyperprolactinemia during daily treatment with diethylstilbestrol. This event can be circumvented by drugs specifically suppressing prolactin release. Two different agents have been investigated: bromocriptine, a lysergic acid derivative[12] and lisuride, an aminoergoline derivative.[22] In Figure 22.5B the prompt prolactin suppression by bromocriptine treatment is demonstrated in patients with high prolactin levels after oral DES therapy, as well as the prevention of hyperprolactinemia if bromocriptine

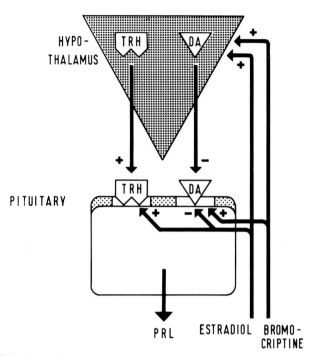

Figure 22.3 Hypothalamic-pituitary mode of action of estrogens on prolactin release. The influence on the dopaminergic receptors (DA) of the hypothalamus (+) and the pituitary (−) has as net effect an increased prolactin release; stimulation of TRH-receptors at the pituitary further increases prolactin secretion. Bromocriptine, on the other hand, positively stimulates dopamine receptors at both levels, thus suppressing prolactin secretion.

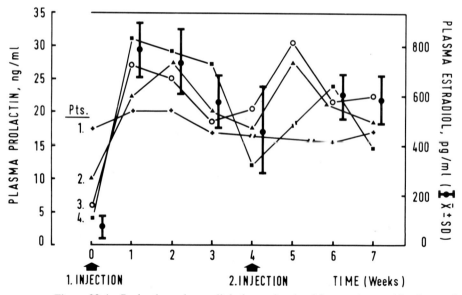

Figure 22.4 Prolactin and estradiol plasma levels of four patients with advanced prostatic carcinoma before and during long-term depot estrogen treatment with 80 mg polyestradiol phosphate/month IM; individual prolactin values increased after the first and second estrogen injection; estradiol values given as mean ± standard deviation.

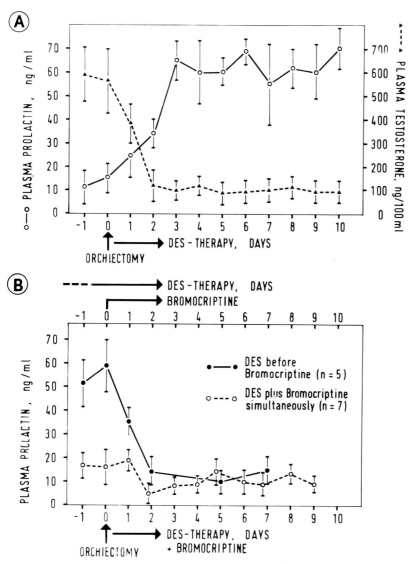

Figure 22.5 *A*, Influence of orchiectomy plus immediate beginning of diethyl-stilbestrol-diphosphate (HONVAN) treatment (1.2 gm/day IV) on plasma testos-terone and plasma prolactin; testosterone drop and prolactin rise are statistically significant ($p < 0.001$). *B, Upper curve:* oral long-term DES-diphosphate (HON-VAN) treatment has induced a hyperprolactinemia ($d_1 + T_0$) which is suppressed within 2 days by a daily dose of 15 mg bromocriptine (mean ± standard deviation in five patients). *Lower curve,* In previously untreated patients, bromocriptine is given initially together with DES-diphosphate after orchiectomy; bromocriptine prevents prolactin stimulation (*A*) when given in a daily dose of 15 mg/day (mean ± standard deviation of seven patients).

is given at the time of initiation of DES treatment. In Figure 22.6 the potent prolactin-suppressing effect of lisuride on high prolactin levels induced by long-term depot estrogen treatment is illustrated. In further studies it has been shown that prolactin elevation is an almost universal feature during long-term treatment with a variety of synthetic estrogen

ANTIPROLACTINS AS PALLIATIVE TREATMENT   427

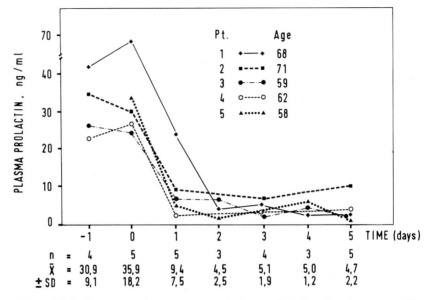

Figure 22.6 Long-term depot estrogens (polyestradiol phosphate) in a monthly IM dose of 80 mg has induced a hyperprolactinemia (first prolactin determination 2 weeks after the last estrogen injection (d_1); initiation of antiprolactin treatment with lisuride (300 μg/day) at time T_0 results in a prompt suppression of prolactin within 1 day.

preparations and estradiol. Castration does not alter prolactin levels, nor do peripheral prolactin changes influence the castration-induced androgen decrease.

CLINICAL APPLICATION

In light of the aforementioned data, it was the idea of Harper et al.[21] and Farnsworth and Gonder[14] to combine estrogens with antiprolactins when applying palliative treatment to prostatic carcinoma patients. While Sadoughi et al.[41] have subjectively influenced such patients with prolactin suppression by L-dopa, Jacobi et al.[27] subjectively and objectively improved the situation with bromocriptine, Klosterhalfen and co-workers[31] with lisuride. Coune and Smith[11] did not yield a beneficial effect when bromocriptine was given as a single agent.

The facts that bromocriptine treatment suppresses androgen uptake in prostatic carcinoma tissue *in vivo*[14a, 24] and that there is significant prolactin binding in prostatic carcinoma tissue[29, 48] would at least justify further evaluation of antiprolactins in randomized controlled clinical trials. It is only this approach which could confirm whether the observation by Berry and co-workers[5], that a high prolactin level is a certain risk factor associated with a worse prognosis of prostatic cancer, is true. The present experimental and clinical basis for palliative treatment of prostate cancer by antiprolactins is summarized in Table 22.4. At present, the statement made by Witorsch[48] that, "an estimation of prolactin binding activity may

Table 22.4
Experimental and Clinical Basis for the Application of Antiprolactins in Palliative Treatment of Advanced Prostate Cancer

Author	Evidence[a] Gained	
	Experimentally	Clinically
Hanafy et al.[20]	+	
Boyns et al.[9]	+	+
Sadoughi et al.[41]		+[b]
Plumpton and Morales[35a]		+[b]
Coune and Smith[11]		−[c]
Harper et al.[21]	+[c]	+[c]
Farnsworth and Gonder[14]		+[b]
Jacobi et al.[24]	+[c]	
Jacobi et al.[24a]	+[c]	
Jacobi et al.[24b]	+[c]	
Klosterhalfen et al.[31]		+[d]
Jacobi et al.[27]	+[c]	+[c]
Witorsch[48]	+	
Farnsworth et al.[14a]	+	

[a] +, pro; −, contra.
[b] L-Dopa treatment.
[c] Bromocriptine treatment.
[d] Lisuride treatment.

be of potential value in the diagnosis and treatment planning of prostatic cancer" seems attractive, but is still a speculation.

REFERENCES

1. Aragona, C., and Friesen, H. G. Specific prolactin binding sites in the prostate and testis of rats. *Endocrinology 97:* 677, 1975.
2. Aragona, C., Bohnet, H. G., and Friesen, H. G. Localization of prolactin binding on prostate and testis. The role of serum prolactin concentration on the testicular LH receptor. *Acta Endocrinol. 84:* 402, 1977.
3. Asano, M. Basic experimental studies on the pituitary prolactin-prostate interrelationships. *J. Urol. 93:* 87, 1965.
4. Bartke, A. Effects of inhibitors of pituitary prolactin release on testicular cholesterol stores, seminal vesicle weight, fertility and lactation in mice. *Biol. Reprod. 11:* 319, 1974.
5. Berry, W. R., Laszlo, J., Cox, E., Walker, A., and Paulson, D. Prognostic factors in metastatic and hormonally unresponsive carcinoma of the prostate. *Cancer 44:* 763, 1979.
6. Bex, F. J., and Bartke, A. Testicular LH binding in the hamster: modification by photoperiod and prolactin. *Endocrinology 100:* 1223, 1977.
7. Birkhoff, J. D., Lattimer, J. K., and Frantz, A. G. Role of prolactin in benign prostatic hypertrophy. *Urology 4:* 557, 1974.
8. Boyns, A. R., Cole, E. N., Golder, M. P., Danutra, V., Harper, M. E., Brownsey, B., Cowley, T., Jones, G. E., and Griffiths, K. Prolactin studies with the prostate. In *Prolactin and Carcinogenesis,* edited by A. R. Boyns and K. Griffiths. Alpha-Omega-Alpha, Cardiff, Wales, 1972, pp. 207–216.
9. Boyns, A. R., Cole, E. N., Phillips, M. E. A., Hillier, S. G., Cameron, E. H. D., Griffiths, K., Shahmanesh, M., Feneley, R. C. L., and Hartog, M. Plasma prolactin, GH, LH, FSH, TSH and testosterone during treatment of prostatic carcinoma with oestrogens. *Eur. J. Cancer 10:* 445, 1974.
10. British Prostate Study Group. Evaluation of plasma hormone concentrations in relation to clinical staging in patients with prostatic cancer. *Br. J. Urol. 51:* 382, 1979.
11. Coune, A., and Smith, P. Clinical trial of 2-bromo-α-ergocryptine (NSC-169774) in

human prostatic cancer. *Cancer Chemother. Rep. 59:* 209, 1975.

12. Del Pozo, E., and Brownell, J. Prolactin, I. Mechanism of control, peripheral actions and modification by drugs. *Horm. Res. 10:* 143, 1979.

13. Farnsworth, W. E. Prolactin and androgen mobilization. In *Normal and Abnormal Growth of the Prostate*, edited by M. Goland. Charles C Thomas, Springfield, ILL., 1975, pp. 502–508.

14. Farnsworth, W. E., and Gonder, M. J. Prolactin and prostate cancer. *Urology 10:* 33, 1977.

14a. Farnsworth, W. E., Slaunwhite, W. R., Jr., Sharma, M., Oseko, F., Brown, J. R., Gonder, M. J., and Cartagena, R. Interaction of prolactin and testosterone in human prostate. *Urol. Res. 9:* 79, 1981.

15. Giuliani, L., Pescatore, D., Martorana, G., Giberti, C., Barreca, T., and Rolandi, E. Increased serum prolactin pituitary reserve in patients with prostatic neoplasms. *Br. J. Urol. 51:* 390, 1979.

16. Grayhack, J. T., Bunce, P. L., Kearns, J. W., and Scott, W. W. Influence of the pituitary on prostatic response to androgen in the rat. *Bull. Johns Hopkins Hosp. 96:* 154, 1955.

17. Grayhack, J. T. Pituitary factors influencing growth of the prostate. *Natl. Cancer Inst. Monogr. 12:* 189, 1963.

18. Grayhack, J. T., and Lebowitz, J. M. Effect of prolactin on citric acid of lateral lobe of prostate of Sprague-Dawley rat. *Invest. Urol. 5:* 87, 1967.

19. Hafiez, A. A., Lloyd, C. W., and Bartke, A. The role of prolactin in the regulation of testis function: the effects of prolactin and luteinizing hormone on the plasma levels of testosterone and androstenedione in hypophysectomized rats. *J. Endocrinol. 52:* 327, 1972.

20. Hanafy, H. M., Gursel, E., and Veenema, R. J. A possible role of Sertoli cells in prostatic cancer refractory to estrogen: a preliminary report. *J. Urol. 108:* 914, 1972.

21. Harper, M. E., Peeling, W. B., Cowley, T., Brownsey, B. G., Phillips, M. E. A., Groom, G., Fahmy, D. R., and Griffiths, K. Plasma steroid and protein hormone concentrations in patients with prostatic carcinoma before and during oestrogen therapy. *Acta Endocrinol. 81:* 409, 1976.

22. Horowski, R., Wendt, H., and Gräf, K.-J. Prolactin lowering effect of low doses of lisuride in man. *Acta Endocrinol. 87:* 234, 1978.

23. Huggins, C., and Russell, P. S. Quantitative effects of hypophysectomy on testis and prostate of dogs. *Endocrinology 39:* 1, 1946.

24. Jacobi, G. H., Sinterhauf, K., Kurth, K. H., and Altwein, J. E. Bromocriptine and prostatic carcinoma: Plasma kinetics, production and tissue uptake of ^{3}H-testosterone in vivo. *J. Urol. 119:* 240, 1978.

24a. Jacobi, G. H., Kurth, K. H., and Altwein, J. E., Bromocriptine and prostatic carcinoma: testosterone metabolism in relation to tumor grading. *Urologe A 18:* 91, 1979.

24b. Jacobi, G. H., Altwein, J. E., and Hohenfellner, R. Alterations of peripheral testosterone metabolism after induced hypoprolactinemia in patients with prostatic carcinoma. *Klin. Wochenschr. 57:* 49, 1979.

25. Jacobi, G. H. *Palliativtherapie des Prostatakarzinoms. Endokrinologische Grundlagen, klinische Situation, Prolaktin—ein neues Prinzip.* W. Zuckschwerdt-Verlag, München, 1980.

26. Jacobi, G. H., Altwein, J. E., and Rathgen, G. H. Serum prolactin and tumors of the prostate: unchanged basal levels and lack of correlation to serum testosterone. *J. Endocrinol. Invest. 3:* 15, 1980.

27. Jacobi, G. H., Altwein, J. E., and Hohenfellner, R. Adjunct bromocriptine treatment as palliation for prostate cancer: experimental and clinical evaluation. *Scand. J. Urol. Nephrol. Suppl. 55:* 107, 1980.

28. Janetschek, G., Becht, E., and Jacobi, G. H. The role of prolactin on steroid-induced benign prostatic hyperplasia in the dog. In *Hormone Cell Interactions in Reproductive Tissue*, edited by J. L. Wittliff and O. Dapunt. Masson Publ., New York, 1982.

29. Keenan, E. J., Kemp, E. D., Ramsey, E. E., Garrison, L. B., Pearse, H. D., and Hodges, C. V. Specific binding of prolactin by the prostate gland of the rat and man. *J. Urol. 122:* 43, 1979.

30. Kledzik, G. S., Marshall, S., Campbell, G. A., Gelato, M., and Meites, J. Effects of

castration, testosterone, estradiol and prolactin on specific prolactin binding activity in ventral prostate of male rats. *Endocrinology 98:* 373, 1976.

31. Klosterhalfen, H., Becker, H., and Krieg, M. Antiprolactin treatment in metastasizing prostatic cancer. First International Congress on Hormones and Cancer, Rome, October 3–6, 1979.

32. Labrie, F., Beaulieu, M., Caron, M. G., and Raymond, V. The adenohypophyseal dopamine receptor: specificity and modulation of its activity by estradiol. In *Progress in Prolactin Physiology and Pathology*, edited by C. Robyn and M. Harter. Elsevier/North-Holland Biomedical Press, Amsterdam-New York, 1978, pp. 121–136.

33. Magrini, G., Ebiner, J. R., Burckhardt, P., and Felber, J. P. Study on the relationship between plasma prolactin levels and androgen metabolism in man. *J. Clin. Endocrinol. Metab. 43:* 944, 1976.

34. Manandhar, M. S., and Thomas, J. A. Effect of prolactin on the metabolism of androgens by the rat ventral prostate in vitro. *Invest. Urol. 14:* 20, 1976.

35. Moger, W. H., and Geschwind, I. I. The action of prolactin on the sex accessory glands of the male rat. *Proc. Soc. Exp. Biol. Med. 141:* 1017, 1972.

35a. Plumpton, K., and Morales, A. Levodopa in cancer of the prostate (Letter to the Editor) *J. Urol. 114:* 482, 1975.

36. Ratner, A., Talwalker, P. K., and Meites, J. Effect of estrogen administration in vivo on prolactin release by rat pituitary in vitro. *Proc. Soc. Exp. Biol. Med. 112:* 12, 1963.

37. Resnick, M. I., Walvoord, D. J., and Grayhack, J. T. Effect of prolactin on testosterone uptake by the perfused canine prostate. *Surg. Forum 25:* 70, 1974.

38. Robyn, C., and Harter, M. *Progress in Prolactin Physiology and Pathology*. Elsevier/North-Holland Biomedical Press, Amsterdam–New York, 1978.

39. Ron, M., Shapiro, A., Caine, M., Ben-David, M., and Palti, Z. Serum prolactin levels in men during retropubic prostatectomy *Urology 15:* 150, 1980.

40. Rubin, R. T., Gouin, P. R., Lubin, A., Poland, R. E., and Pirke, K. M. Nocturnal increase of plasma testosterone in men: relation to gonadotropins and prolactin. *J. Clin. Endocrinol. Metab. 40:* 1027, 1975.

41. Sadoughi, N., Razvi, M., Busch, I., Ablin, R., and Guinan, P. Cancer of the prostate, relief of bone pain with levodopa. *Urology 4:* 107, 1974.

42. Thomas, J. A., and Keenan, E. J. Prolactin influences upon androgen action in male accessory sex organs. *Adv. Sex Horm. Res. 2:* 425, 1976.

43. Turkington, R. W. Prolactin secretion in patients treated with various drugs. *Arch. Intern. Med. 130:* 349, 1972.

44. Vermeulen, A., Suy, E., and Rubens, R. Effect of prolactin on plasma DHEA(S) levels. *J. Clin. Endocrinol. Metab. 44:* 1222, 1977.

45. Walsh, P. C., and Wilson, J. D. The induction of prostatic hypertrophy in the dog with androstanediol. *J. Clin. Invest. 57:* 1093, 1976.

46. Walvoord, D. J., Resnick, M. I., and Grayhack, J. T. Effect of testosterone, dihydrotestosterone, estradiol, and prolactin on the weight and citric acid content of the lateral lobe of the rat prostate. *Invest. Urol. 14:* 60, 1976.

47. Wenderoth, U., and Jacobi, G. H. The possible prolactin-testosterone interrelationship in patients with prostate cancer. *Neuro-Endocrinol. Lett. 1:* 19, 1979.

48. Witorsch, R. J. The application of immunoperoxidase methodology for the visualization of prolactin binding sites in human prostate tissue. *Hum. Pathol. 10:* 521, 1979.

49. Witorsch, R. J. Immunohistochemical localization of prolactin-binding sites in R 3327 rat prostatic cancer cells. *Horm. Res.*, in press 1982.

23

Stereology—A New Method to Assess Normal and Pathological Growth of the Prostate

G. Bartsch, M.D.
H. P. Rohr, M.D.

In general, morphologic evaluation of prostatic tissue especially of human biopsy specimens is based on qualitative description obtained on the light and/or electron microscopic level. This descriptive morphology is of primary and undisputed importance. Although a considerable amount of biochemical data is now available, the morphological investigations of the prostate have been restricted to descriptive findings. However, in order to establish structure-function relationships these morphological methods should be complemented by quantitative techniques which would yield objective and reproducible values for any morphological structure allowing statistically defined comparisons. This can be achieved by stereological methods.

Stereology, a term coined by the *International Society of Stereology* in 1961, is based on geometric probability and allows to quantitate three-dimensional structures by extrapolation from measurements of two-dimensional cross-sections thereof. Morphometry is the application of stereologic axioms[30,37,39] which allows to quantitate the volume (V), the surface (S), and number (N) of tissue and cell components by light and/or electron microscopy (Fig. 23.1).

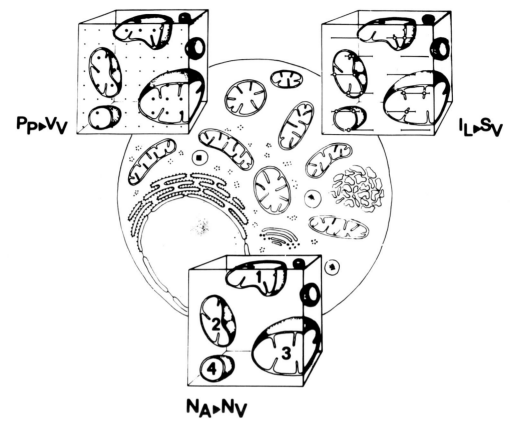

Figure 23.1 Measurements of the three main parameters. Volume density (V_v) (*top left*), Fraction of test points laying over profiles of a given particle equals volume density. Surface density (S_v) (*top right*), Surface density is calculated from the intersection of membrane traces with test lines. Numerical density (N_v) (*bottom*), Number or profiles (1 to 4) in the test area is converted to N_v by a formular including correction factors for shape and inhomogeneous distribution.

STEREOLOGICAL METHODS

Definition*

Quantitative morphological information can be obtained from electron micrographs by applying stereological techniques. These stereological procedures provide values for volumes, surfaces, and number of tissue or cellular components, as the nucleus, the rough endoplasmic reticulum, the Golgi apparatus, the mitochondria, lysosomes, and secretory granules. The stereological data (amount of volume, surface area, and number) of these cell structures are expressed always as the density found within a reference (containing) system. For instance, the membranes of the rough endoplasmic reticulum can be described as the amount of the membrane

---

* Abbreviations not defined in text are VPL (P), ventral prostatic lobe; GC, C, glandular cell; ORG, organelles; GS, ground substance; G, Golgi apparatus; Ly, lysosomes; SD, secretory droplets; F, fat droplets; MF, myofilament; Comp, compartment; A_T, test area.

surface area found within a cubic centimeter of tissue; the tissue in this case is the reference system.

In general, the following parameters for a tissue or cellular compartment (i) can be determined:

Volume density (V_{Vi}) = volume of the component i within the unit volume of a given reference space.

Surface density (S_{Vi}) = surface of the component i within the volume of a given reference space.

Numerical density (N_{Vi}) = number of the component i within the unit volume of a given reference space.

By appropriate calculations[30] this "density" can be related to different reference spaces: volume of prostatic tissue; volume of acinar parenchyma; volume of glandular cell cytoplasm, and absolute volume of an average glandular cell.

Preconditions for Stereological Analysis

1. The structure to be analyzed must be distributed homogeneously in the reference space.
2. The study must be done on a representative number of strictly randomized sections or micrographs to perform statistical analysis. As a rule the standard error for a compartment should be less than 10% of the mean, otherwise the sampling volume has to be increased.
3. For the determination of volume or surface densities the cellular compartments can be simple or complicated structures, discrete or continuous, large or small or variable in size.[37] However, for the determination of the numerical density the shape of the cellular component must be geometrically defined.
4. Standardization of fixation, buffering and embedding procedures should be observed, especially in comparative studies.

Theoretical Basis of Stereology

In which way can these different densities be determined? For the determination of volume densities, the French geologist Delesse in 1847 demonstrated the equivalence of area and volume fractions, by showing that the area occupied by a mineral component was proportional to its volume in the entire rock. Glagoleff[15] and Chalkley[12] extended the Delesse principle by establishing the basis for the currently applied so-called point counting procedures: the fraction of test points lying on profiles of a cellular component is proportional to its volume density ($P_P = V_V$ in Fig. 23.1).

With respect to surface density, Tomkeieff[34] demonstrated that surface density (S_{Vi}) can be calculated from the number of intersections (I_L) formed by the membrane traces of the structure i with a test line system ($I_L \rightarrow S_V$ in Fig. 23.1).

The numerical particle density (N_{Vi}) is evaluated by counting the number of particle profiles in the test area ($N_A \rightarrow N_V$ in Fig. 23.1). The value is dependent on the shape and the size distribution of the particle in question. Therefore, correction factors, *e.g.* for the shape, have to be introduced. For spherical particles, such as normal nuclei, the shape factor is usually well definable, whereas for complicated structures, *e.g.* for distorted mitochondria, the reliability of related calculations is reduced. The values for the numerical densities must be regarded as estimates in most cases.

In practice, stereological analysis is based on counting of points (for V_{Vi}), intersection points (for S_{Vi}), and particle profiles (for N_{Vi}) as illustrated in Figure 23.1. Detailed information on stereological theory and practice (choice of test lines, point sets, and sample size) is given by Weibel *et al.*,[37-41] Bolender,[11] and Rohr *et al.*[30]

STEREOLOGICAL MODEL

Ventral Lobe of Rat Prostate

To evaluate the prostatic gland and its components in stereological terms a morphometric model of the rat ventral prostatic lobe was developed.[2] Figure 23.2 shows how the ventral lobe of the rat prostate was divided into morphologically defined compartments. Essentially the model has two major divisions—the *interacinar* (= stromal) *tissue (IT)*, including connective tissue, blood vessels, nerves and smooth muscle fibers and the *acinar parenchyma (AP)*, including the lumina of the acini and the glandular epithelial cells. The latter were divided into the nuclei and the various cytoplasmic compartments.

The stereological analysis, then, must be performed at several magnification levels, since the cellular components have a broad range of their size and frequency. Three magnification levels are used in the determination of the different parameters listed as follows:

Level I, primary magnification 1:90 *(light microscopy)*.
Level II, primary magnification 1:1,300 *(electron microscopy)*.
Level III, primary magnification 1:4,100 *(electron microscopy)*.

STEREOLOGICAL CALCULATIONS

Level I

Counted: test points on

$$P_C^I \quad \text{(fine lattice, } P_T = 1,089)$$
$$P_{AL}^I \quad \text{(course lattice, } P_T = 121)$$
$$P_{IT}^I \quad \text{(course lattice, } P_T = 121)$$

Calculated:

$$P_P = \tfrac{1}{9}\, P_C + P_{AL} + P_{IT}$$
$$P_{AP} = \tfrac{1}{9}\, P_C + P_{AL}$$

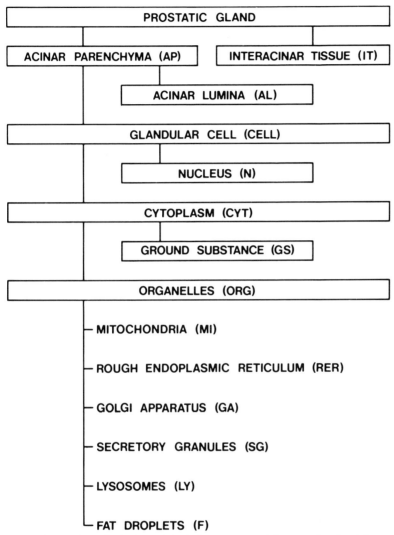

Figure 23.2 Stereological model of the prostate and prostatic glandular cells. Level I, For stereological measurements four paraffin-embedded HE-stained sections were selected from each human prostatic gland biopsy specimen. For each section at least 30 randomized test areas were analyzed (120 test areas per prostatic gland biopsy specimen). Level II, At least three tissue blocks for each human prostatic gland biopsy specimen were sectioned. The areas to be evaluated were selected according to a systematic sampling procedure by photographing at level II and III in regular steps in predetermined corners of the meshes of the supporting copper grid. The test systems applied to the three sampling levels were as follows: Level I (X90), multipurpose test lattice ($P_T = 100$)[37]; level II (X1,200), multipurpose test lattice ($P_T = 100$)[37]; level III (X4,100), double square lattice system (1:9, 121:1,089), where 1:9 signifies the ratio of coarse to fine points and 121:1,089 the number of coarse to fine points.[37]

Volume densities of C, AL, or IT in prostate (P) and *acinar parenchyma* (AP), respectively, *e.g.*:

$$AL : P_{VAL,P} = \frac{P_{AL}}{P_P} \quad \text{and}$$

$$C : V_{VC,P} = \frac{P_C}{9 \cdot P_P} \quad \text{and finally}$$

$$V_{VAL,AP} = \frac{P_{AL}}{P_{AP}} \, ;$$

$$V_{VC,AP} = \frac{P_C}{9 \cdot P_{AP}} \, .$$

Level II

Counted:

$$P_N^{\text{II}}$$

$$P_{IT}^{\text{II}} \qquad P_T = 100$$

$$P_{AL}^{\text{II}}$$

and the number of nuclear profiles (N_N^{II}) within the test area (A_T).
Calculated: $P_C = P_T - (P_{IT}^{\text{II}} + P_{AL}^{\text{II}})$.
Volume density of nuclei (N) in acinar cell (C):

$$V_{VN,C} = \frac{P_N^{\text{II}}}{P_C} = \frac{P_N^{\text{II}}}{P_T - (P_{IT}^{\text{II}} + P_{AL}^{\text{II}})}$$

The *numerical density of the nuclei ($N_{VN,C}$)* was calculated according to Weibel and Gomez.[41]

$$N_{VN,C} = \frac{1}{\beta} \cdot \frac{(N_{AN,C})^{3/2}}{(V_{VN,C})^{1/2}} , \quad \text{whereby}$$

$$N_{AN,C} = \frac{N_N^{\text{II}}}{A_T} \cdot \frac{P_T}{P_C^{\text{II}}}$$

Level III

Counted:
Coarse test points ($P_T = 121$)

$$P_N^{\text{III}} + P_{IT}^{\text{III}} + P_{AL}^{\text{III}}$$

$$P_{RER}^{\text{III}}$$

Fine test points ($P_T = 1,089$)

$$P_G^{\text{III}} + P_M^{\text{III}} + P_{LY}^{\text{III}} + P_F^{\text{III}} + P_{GS}^{\text{III}}.$$

Intersections of both horizontal and vertical 22 coarse lines with rough endoplasmic reticulum: I_{RER}.
Number of mitochondrial profiles N_M per test area A_T.
Calculated:

$$P_{CYT} = P_T - (P_N^{\text{III}} + P_{IT}^{\text{III}} + P_{AL}^{\text{III}})$$

$$P_{CYT} = P_{RER}^{\text{III}} + \tfrac{1}{9} (P_G^{\text{III}} + P_M^{\text{III}} + P_{LY}^{\text{III}} + P_F^{\text{III}} + P_{GS}^{\text{III}}).$$

Volume of rough endoplasmic reticulum (RER) in cytoplasm (CYT):

$$V_{VRER,CYT} = \frac{P_{RER}^{III}}{P_{CYT}}, \quad \text{or}$$

$$V_{VM,CYT} = \frac{P_M^{III}}{9 \cdot P_{CYT}}.$$

Surface density of RER in cytoplasm (CYT).

$$S_{VER,CYT} = \frac{2 \cdot I_{RER}}{L_{T,CYT}} = \frac{I_{RER}}{d \cdot P_{CYT}}$$

The *numerical density of mitochondria* ($N_{VM,CYT}$) was calculated according to Weibel and Gomez.[41]

$$N_{VM,CYT} = \frac{1}{\beta} \cdot \frac{(N_{AM,CYT})^{3/2}}{(V_{VM,CYT})^{1/2}}, \quad \text{whereby}$$

$$N_{AM,CYT} = \frac{N_M^{II}}{A_T} \cdot \frac{P_T}{P_{CYT}^{II}}$$

Absolute Values

The mean *single volume of an "average prostatic acinar cell,"* V_C was calculated as follows:

$$V_C = \frac{1}{N_{VN,C}}.$$

The *volume of mitochondria (M)* per average cell was then obtained as

$$V_{M,C} = V_{VM,C} \cdot V_C$$

and the *average volume of a single mitochondria (M)* as

$$V_M = \frac{V_{VM,CYT}}{N_{VM,CYT}}$$

and finally the *mean number of mitochondria* per acinar cell as

$$N_{M,C} = \frac{N_{VM,C}}{N_{VN,C}}.$$

HUMAN PROSTATIC GLAND: STEREOLOGICAL MODEL

For the general stereological procedure we refer to Weibel[37] and Rohr et al.[30] The model of the human prostatic gland outlined in Figure 23.2 is similar to that of the ventral lobe of the rat prostate. Essentially the model has three major divisions: *acinar parenchyma* (AP), *acinar lumina* (AL), and *interstitial tissue* (IT), including connective tissue, blood vessels, and smooth muscle cells. The acinar parenchyma was not further subdivided into different cell types I to III.

The acinar parenchymal cells were divided into the nucleus and the different cellular compartments (Fig. 23.2) which were defined as the aggregate of all cellular elements of a given component.[11]

Basically three reference systems were introduced in the stereological model of the human prostatic gland: (1) 1 cm^3 of benign prostatic hyperplastic tissue (BPH-T); (2) 1 cm³ of acinar parenchyma (AP), and (3) 1 cm³ of the acinar parenchymal cell (C).

A stereological model of prostatic smooth muscle cells is shown in Figure 23.3.

Multistage Sampling (Weibel[37])

The different cellular components could not be evaluated at a single stage of magnification due to the broad differences in shape, size, and frequencies of these components. Therefore, sampling was done at three magnifications to establish an adequate relationship between the size of the components and the point or test line sets. The different cellular components counted at these three stages are shown and further described in Figure 23.2.

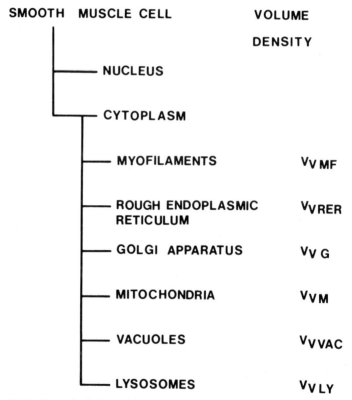

Figure 23.3 Stereological model of prostatic smooth muscle cell. Human smooth muscle cells (SMC), stage I (X4,100):

$$P_{SM} = P_T - P_{EX} = P_{COMP} + P_N$$

$$P_{COMP} = P_{MF} + P_G + P_M + P_{RER} + P_{VES}$$

$$P_{SMCYT} = P_T - (P_{EX} + P_N)$$

$$P_{COMP,SMCYT} = \frac{P_G}{P_{SMCYT}} = \frac{P_G}{P_T - (P_{EX} + P_N)}$$

APPLICATIONS

Five examples are presented to illustrate how quantitative morphology can be applied to assess normal and pathological growth of the prostate.

1. Stereology, an Objective Method to Assess the Effect of Steroids and Antihormones on Prostatic Tissue (for Example on the Rat Ventral Prostatic Lobe)

LIGHT AND ELECTRON MICROSCOPIC ANALYSIS OF THE NORMAL VENTRAL PROSTATIC LOBE OF THE RAT

As previously shown the glandular part contributes 75% of the whole ventral prostatic lobe; the acinar lumina represent 52% of the rat ventral prostatic lobe, the glandular cells 23%.[2] The stromal part (= interacinar tissue) amounts to 25% of the whole glandular volume. The rough endoplasmic reticulum makes up 31% of the unit volume of cytoplasm; the Golgi apparatus amounts to 8%. The compartment of lysosomes is defined to contain primarily lysosomes and secretory granules.

Using this approach of the first quantitative data of the prostatic gland the influence of various steroids on the fine structure of the rat glandular prostatic cell was studied. Two examples are demonstrated. The administration of *17-ethyl-19-nortestosterone* in a daily dosage of 180 µg/day for 3 months leads to a reduction of the acinar parenchyma, the glandular cell, and its various subcellular compartments. The volume density of the stromal tissue (= interacinar tissue) is not changed. Related to the unit volume of prostatic tissue there is a significant decrease of the acinar parenchyma, the nucleus, and the cytoplasm, as well as of the various subcellular organelles of the glandular cell (Fig. 23.4). Related to the unit volume of cytoplasm there is a significant decrease of the rough endoplasmic reticulum, while the volume densities of the Golgi apparatus, the mitochondria, and the lysosomes remain constant (Fig. 23.5).

The fine structure of the ventral prostatic gland of the rat after administration of a low dosage of progestin for a long time is not similar to that after castration or administration of a high dosage of estrogen.[7, 18] Whereas castration or estrogen administration is followed by a marked and sustained collapse and depletion of the rough endoplasmic reticulum and by a diminution of the Golgi apparatus,[18] these morphometric findings after 3 months of progestin administration support the assumption of persistence of the cell compartments involved in enzyme and protein synthesis. Secretion still occurs in the glandular cell.

The administration of the *antiestrogen tamoxifen* for 28 days in a daily dosage of 0.6 mg/kg body weight leads to an activation of the acinar parenchyma, the glandular cell, and the cellular compartments. As shown in Fig. 23.6 the volume density of the glandular cells related to the unit volume of prostatic tissue (= 100%) is increased by 45% compared to that of the controls, whereas the volume density of the acinar lumina becomes significantly smaller in amount. The relative volume of the interacinar

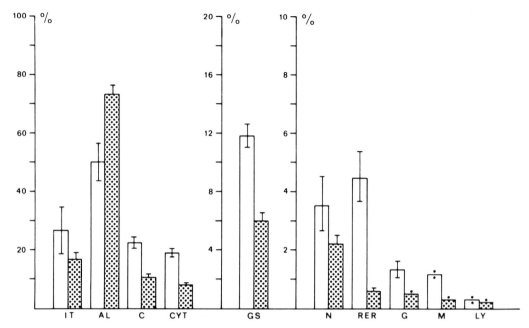

Figure 23.4 Tissue components and glandular cell compartments of the ventral prostatic lobe of the rat are expressed as percentage of the total prostatic gland volume. The values of the progestin-treated animals are seen in *dotted bars*, control animals as *open bars*. Standard errors of the mean are indicated; abbreviations are given on page 434 and in text.

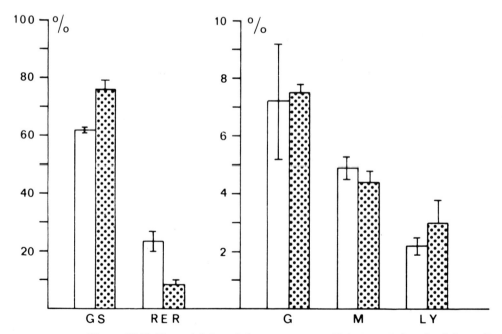

Figure 23.5 Ventral lobe of the rat prostate. Volumes of the glandular cell compartments are expressed as a percentage of total glandular cell cytoplasm volume. The values of the progestin-treated animals are seen in *dotted bars*, control animals as *open bars*. Standard errors of the mean are indicated.

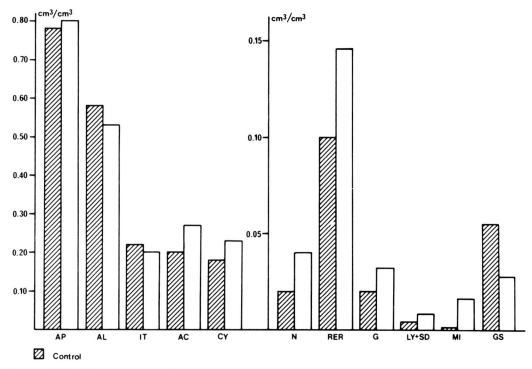

Figure 23.6 Effect of tamoxifen on volume densities of tissue and cellular components per unit volume of prostatic tissue; abbreviations are given on page 434 and in text.

tissue has not changed. Related to the unit volume of cytoplasm, the volume density of the rough endoplasmic reticulum is decreased (0.47, controls: 0.58), while that of the Golgi apparatus (0.17), the mitochondria (0.06) and of the lysosomes and the secretory droplets (0.03) are elevated (Fig. 23.7) (controls: Golgi apparatus, 0.10; mitochondria, 0.05; lysosomes and secretory droplets, 0.02).

After stimulation of the *hypothalamic-pituitary-gonadal* axis by administration of the antiestrogen tamoxifen the fine structure of the ventral prostatic gland of the rat is similar to that of adult male rats after treating them with a high dosage of testosterone.[16] The stereological data suggest a proliferation of the glandular epithelim. This fact is demonstrated by a significant increase in the volume density of the glandular cells and their nuclei as well as by a significant increase in the number of nuclear profiles of the glandular cells. Unfortunately, the effect of testosterone metabolism on prostatic subcellular organelles is still unknown. The significant increase in the volume of the Golgi apparatus is possibly an indication that this cell compartment plays a key role in testosterone metabolism.

2. Synergistic Effect of Estrogens and Androgens on Prostatic Growth (Light Microscopic Stereological Analysis of Steroid-Induced Canine Prostatic Hyperplasia)

Walsh and Wilson[36] showed that 17β-estradiol in combination with 5α-androstane-3α,17β-diol (= 3α-A) has a synergistic effect on prostatic

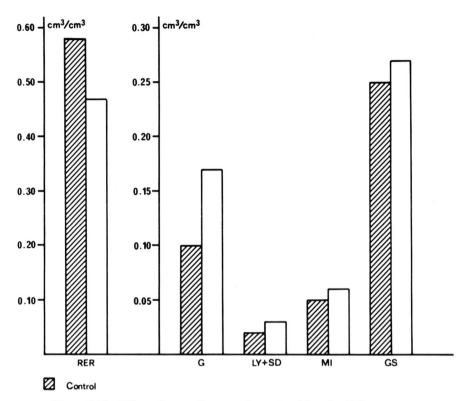

Figure 23.7 Effect of tamoxifen on volume densities of cellular components per unit volume of glandular cell cytoplasm; abbreviations are given on page 434 and in text.

growth. The administration of 17β-estradiol stimulates the stromal growth of the prostate in castrated dogs.[28] Recently it has been shown that 5α-dihydrotestosterone (= *5α-DHT*) and 3α-A in combination with 17β-estradiol induce prostatic hyperplasia in intact and castrated dogs.[22] In order to evaluate the canine prostatic gland and its tissue components in stereological terms a stereological model of the dog was developed; thus the relative and absolute volumes of the following tissue compartments were determined: glandular part, glandular cells, stromal part, and smooth muscle cells.

The dog experiment has been performed at the Brady Urological Institute of the Johns Hopkins University.[22] Young beagles (109, average age: 2.3 ± 0.3 years) with a body weight of 11.3 ± 2.2 kg were used. The steroids were administered by IM injections (androgens: 25 mg/ml triolein, 17β-estradiol: 0.25 mg/ml triolein) over a period of 4 months; following castration all animals were allowed 1 month for recovery and involution of the prostate before starting the treatment.

The stereological model has two divisions: AP = glandular part, including the glandular cells (AC) and the lumina of the acini (AL), and ST = stromal part, including the remaining stromal tissue and the smooth muscle cells (SMC). The light microscopic analysis was performed at two magnification levels: level 1, 1 × 125; level 2, 1 × 400. For each prostate a total of at least 20 sections was analyzed; a total of at least 20 visual fields per section was evaluated with a multipurpose test screen.

As regards the relative amounts of glandular and stromal tissue in castrated dogs treated with androgens, and in castrated and intact dogs treated with testosterone and 17β-estradiol the stereological analysis of steroid-induced dog prostatic hyperplasia shows a glandular *versus* stromal ratio which corresponds to that of intact animals (Fig. 23.8); however, 5α-DHT or 3α-A in combination with 17β-estradiol leads to an increase in the glandular part which resembles that of spontaneous canine prostatic hyperplasia (Fig. 23.8).

Regarding the absolute amount of the glandular part no difference can be found between the testosterone, 3α-A, and 5α-DHT treated castrated dogs; in the castrated animals treatment with 3α-A or 5α-DHT in combination with 17β-estradiol induces a 4-fold increase in the glandular part compared to the animals treated with androgens only (Fig. 23.8). If the testes are left intact, either 5α-DHT or 3α-A induces an increase in the glandular part and the glandular cells; however, if combined with 17β-estradiol a high absolute increase in the glandular part and glandular cells is observed. Combined treatment of testosterone and 17β-estradiol fails to increase the glandular part in both intact and castrated dogs; however, the same amount of glandular and stromal tissue can be observed as in intact or androgen-substituted castrated dogs (Fig. 23.8).

These stereological analyses of steroid-induced prostatic hyperplasia show a synergistic effect of 17β-estradiol on 5α-DHT or 3α-A induced

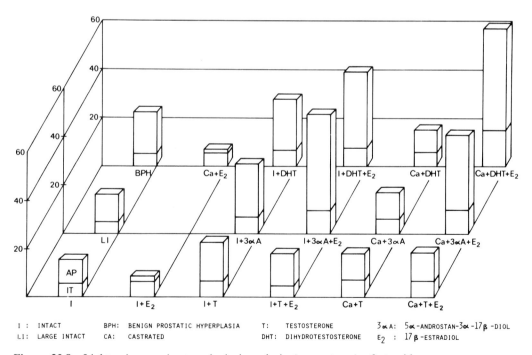

I : INTACT   BPH: BENIGN PROSTATIC HYPERPLASIA   T: TESTOSTERONE   3αA: 5α-ANDROSTAN-3α-17β-DIOL
LI: LARGE INTACT   CA: CASTRATED   DHT: DIHYDROTESTOSTERONE   E$_2$: 17β-ESTRADIOL

Figure 23.8 Light microscopic stereological analysis (percentages) of steroid-induced dog prostatic hyperplasia.

growth of the glandular part of the prostate in intact and castrated dogs; compared to the dogs treated with androgens only, a 4-fold increase in the glandular part and glandular cells can be observed. Conversely, 17β-estradiol does not enhance testosterone-induced glandular growth in castrated and intact dogs; as regards tissue distribution there is no difference between intact dogs and those treated with testosterone and 17β-estradiol, whereas the group treated with 5α-DHT or 3α-A plus 17β-estradiol shows a tissue pattern similar to that of spontaneous hyperplasia. As has previously been shown in castrated dogs 17β-estradiol leads to an induction of the stromal part with an activation of the smooth muscle cells.[28] Glandular hyperplasia in the 5α-DHT or 3α-A plus 17β-estradiol treated group is possibly the cause of a primary estradiol-induced stromal change, which in the presence of normal androgen stimulation by stromal glandular interactions may lead to glandular hyperplasia. The mechanism, the molecular basis of these stromal glandular interactions is unknown; however, enhancement of ^{3}H-DHT binding in the prostate cytosol after administering 17β-estradiol to the castrated dog has previously been described.[24]

3. Human BPH—a Stromal Disease (Light and Electron Microscopic Stereological Analysis of Normal Human Prostate and of Benign Prostatic Hyperplasia)

There is some evidence that interactions between stromal and epithelial cells play a crucial role in the regulation of coordinated growth of the prostatic gland. Since the separation of prostatic acinar parenchyma and stroma is difficult—whenever possible—and the common biochemical practice consists in homogenizing the prostatic tissue prior to biochemical assays, most biochemists overlooked the cellular elements of the stromal tissue.

Therefore, an understanding of stromal function regarding hormonal response is virtually absent. Despite the fact that receptor proteins have been found for estradiol, progesterone, testosterone, and dihydrotestoster-one[1, 17, 21, 23] the action site of these steroids in the different glandular and stromal cell components has not been demonstrated. Thus the role of glandular and stromal elements of the prostate gland in steroid metabolism is still almost unclear. A better understanding of these unknown stromal-epithelial interactions will be of prime importance for future medical control in human BPH. One possible approach for the demonstration of tissue distribution patterns of receptor-proteins is the dry-mount high-resolution autoradiography.[33] Another very promising approach by which the response of glandular and stromal elements can be assessed will be quantitative morphology, stereology.

METHODOLOGICAL CONSIDERATIONS

One of the most serious restrictions when performing stereological studies on human biopsy specimens is the small amount of tissue available. Therefore, a light microscopic stereological analysis of needle biopsy material cannot be performed. Contrary to needle biopsies, light and electron microscopic stereological analysis can be performed on prostatectomy specimens.

In view of the difficulties (inhomogeneity of material) encountered in stereological analysis of human biopsy specimens in contrast to experimental studies on animals, the following strategies may be considered (Fig. 23.9).[29]

1. Evaluation of a healthy volunteer group as performed in the present study, in which the mean and the physiologic variations are calculated. In addition, each individual of this group may be compared with the mean of the whole group and/or with any single individual of this group (evaluation 1).
2. Evaluation of a number of individual patients before and after treatment (evaluated B1 and B2).
3. Comparison of an entire group of patients before and after treatment with strict consideration of variability (evaluation C1).
4. Comparison of a normal volunteer group with a group of patients before (evaluation C2) and after treatment (evaluation C3).
5. Comparison of every single patient before and after treatment with the mean of the volunteer group (evaluation D1 and D2).
6. In focal cell alterations, the specific lesion may be compared with the rest of the parenchyma in a given biopsy (evaluation E1) and the control group (evaluation E2).

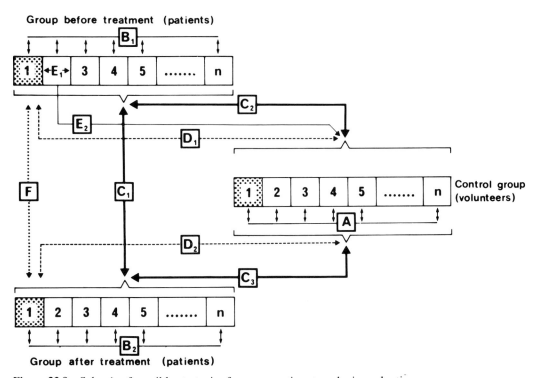

Figure 23.9 Scheme of possible strategies for comparative stereologic evaluation of human biopsy specimens (for details see text).

7. Evaluation of a single patient compared morphometrically before and after treatment (evaluation F).

According to our experience, stereological analysis on human material is of restricted, if of any, diagnostic value. However, stereological analysis can be of primary importance in time-sequence studies in order to get some further information about the pathogenesis of a disease. In considering special sample strategies, it has been shown previously by Hess *et al.*[19] and Rohr *et al.*[30] that a stereological analysis is also successful with needle biopsies; so far *the stereological methods are also practicable to study the normal human prostatic gland.*

OWN STUDIES: NORMAL HUMAN PROSTATE

Using a Vim-Silverman needle, perineal prostate biopsies were performed in five young voluntary men, aged 21 to 29 years, who underwent vasectomy. All five patients have had no history of a foregoing disease of the genitourinary tract, especially no history of inflammation of the prostate. The testosterone, 17β-estradiol, LH, FSH, and prolactin levels in all five patients were within the normal range, indicating no pathological lesions of the pituitary gonadal system in these patients.

BENIGN PROSTATIC HYPERPLASIA

Portions of specimens, obtained by suprapubic prostatectomy from five patients, were used. All five patients have had a history of long lasting bladder neck obstruction symptoms and have had no endocrine therapy for BPH; the weight of the enucleated hyperplasia ranged from 70 to 95 gm.

LIGHT MICROSCOPIC STEREOLOGICAL ANALYSIS

As shown in Fig. 23.10 and Table 23.1 the stromal part of the normal human prostate contributes 45% of the tissue, whereas the glandular cells represent 21%. Compared to the normal human prostate in benign prostatic hyperplasia a statistically significant increase of the stromal tissue and a statistically significant decrease of the glandular part compared to the normal human prostate is indicated (Fig. 23.10, Tables 23.1 and 23.2).

ULTRASTRUCTURAL FINDINGS

In the normal human prostate the glandular cells are mostly tall columnar in shape. In the apical region numerous electron-dense secretory droplets and lysosomes can be observed. A moderate number of mitochondria are interspersed between rough endoplasmatic reticulum and Golgi apparatus (Fig. 23.11*A*). In benign prostatic hyperplasia the glandular cells are reduced in height; the amount of secretory droplets is diminished, wheras the rough endoplasmic reticulum, Golgi apparatus, and mitochondria do not differ significantly from the normal human prostate (Fig. 23.11*B*). The smooth muscle cells in the normal human prostate are spindle shaped. Most of the organelles are located near the

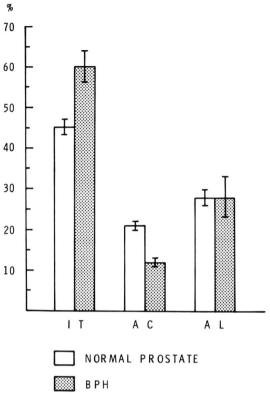

Figure 23.10 Light microscopic stereological analysis of normal human prostate and human benign prostatic hyperplasia. *IT*, interacinar (stromal) tissue; *AC*, acinar cells; *AL*, acinar lumina.

Table 23.1
Volume Densities of the Stromal Tissue (V_{VST}), the Glandular Cells (V_{VCG}), and the Acinar Lumina (V_{VAL}) in the Normal Human Prostate and in Benign Prostatic Hyperplasia (BPH)

		V_{VST}	V_{VCG}	V_{VAL}
Normal human prostate	Mean	0.45	0.21	0.34
(N = 9)	S.E.	0.02	0.01	0.02
Benign prostatic hyperplasia	Mean	0.60	0.12	0.28
(N = 7)	S.E.	0.04	0.01	0.05
Analysis of significance[a]		S.	S.	N.S.

[a] Differences are only significant (S.) if the error of probability $2p$ was < 0.05.

Table 23.2
Absolute Weights (gm) of the Stromal and Glandular Part of the Normal Human Prostate and of Benign Prostatic Hyperplasia

	Stromal Part	Glandular Part	Luminal Part
Normal human prostate	11.25	5.25	8.5
Benign prostatic hyperplasia	45.0	9	21

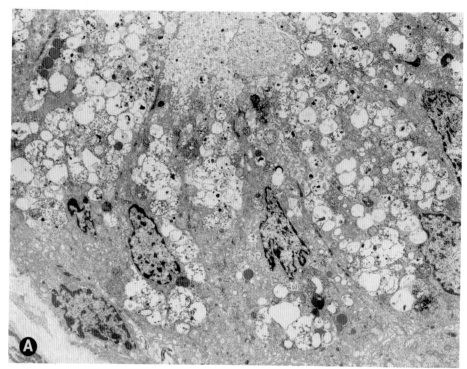

Figure 23.11 *A,* Glandular cells of normal human prostate. Note the large amount of secretory droplets and lysosomes. ×3,280.

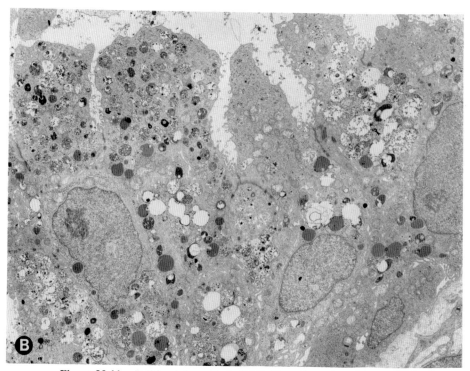

Figure 23.11 *B,* Glandular cells in BPH. Note the reduced amount of secretory droplets and lysosomes. ×3,280.

nucleus or in small clusters in the cell periphery. The largest portion of the cytoplasm is occupied by myofilaments. The rough endoplasmic reticulum consists of a few profiles of membranes and a great part is often seen devoid of ribosomes; sometimes a small Golgi apparatus and mitochondria can be observed (Fig. 23.12A). Contrary to these findings in benign prostatic hyperplasia, the perinuclear zone is markedly increased. The abundant rough endoplasmatic reticula show enlarged cisternae, studded with ribosomes. The Golgi apparatus is enlarged too and contains more vesical than cisternal elements (Fig. 23.12B).

STEREOLOGICAL DATA

Data for the various glandular and smooth muscle cell compartments are given in Figure 23.13 and Table 23.3. Related to the unit volume of glandular cell cytoplasm in the normal human prostate, the volume fraction of secretory droplets and lysosomes was estimated to comprise 35% of the whole cytoplasm (rough endoplasmic reticulum, 13%; Golgi apparatus, 4%; mitochondria, 5% (Fig. 23.13). In human prostatic hyperplasia the following relative amounts of cell compartments were found: rough endoplasmic reticulum, 17.8%; Golgi apparatus, 2.6%; secretory droplets, 25.3%; mitochondria, 8.4% (Fig. 23.13). Regarding the smooth muscle cell in benign prostatic hyperplasia compared to the normal human prostate, there is a statistically significant increase in the volume fraction of the rough endoplasmic reticulum, mitochondria, and Golgi apparatus (normal, 5%; BPH, 14%, Table 23.3).

These light and electron microscopic measurements show that tissue overgrowth in human BPH is mostly due to an increase of stromal tissue, as shown by the electron microscopic measurements in the BPH-changed prostatic tissue; an activated smooth muscle cell is observed, which possibly plays a key role in the pathogenesis of human BPH. Contrary to these stromal changes the glandular part in the human BPH, compared to the normal human prostate, is diminished, seen from its relative volumetric amount of prostatic tissue.

4. The Effect of Antihormones on BPH Stromal Tissue (Electron Microscopic Stereological Analysis)

Human BPH was shown to be predominantly a stromal disease with secondary interactions of the glandular part of the hyperplastic prostatic tissue.[3,4] It was shown that in the stromal part of the prostate (guinea pig) the endogenous concentration of estrogens exceeds that of plasma; this findings supports the theory that endogenous estrogens may be of importance in the regulation of stromal function[10], however, 5α-reductase activity was demonstrated predominantly in the stroma of BPH.[13] To study the action of endogenous androgens and estrogens on stromal tissue, selective androgen and estrogen antagonists as well as bromocriptine, an antiprolactin, were used.

Fifteen patients (aged 64 to 80 years) were included in the study on medical treatment of BPH; the weight of the suprapubically enucleated prostate ranged from 55 to 92 gm. Prior to treatment perineal prostate

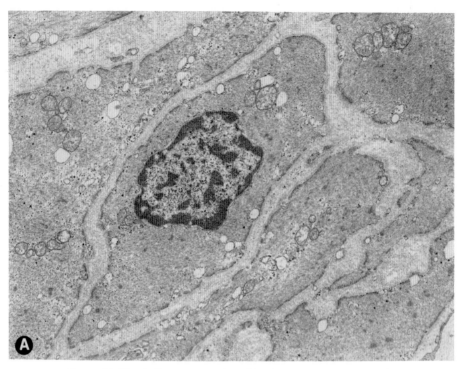

Figure 23.12 *A*, Smooth muscle cell in the normal human prostate. ×3,280.

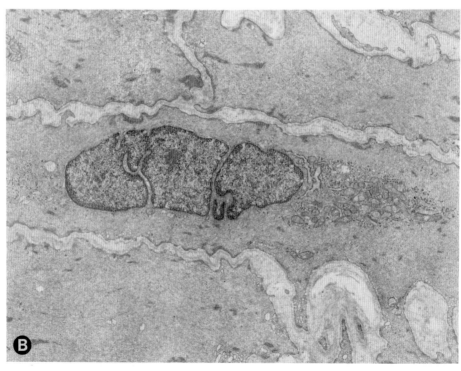

Figure 23.12 *B*, Smooth muscle cell in BPH. An enlargement of the RER, Golgi apparatus, and mitochondria can be seen. ×3,280.

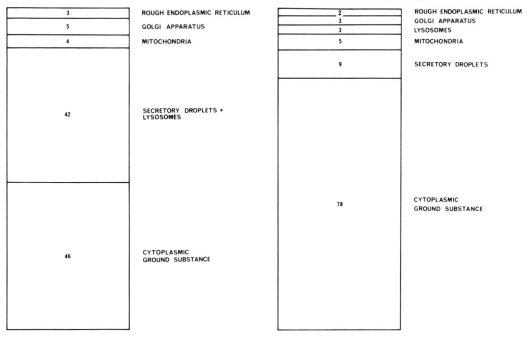

Figure 23.13 Volumes of the glandular cell compartments for normal human prostate and of human benign prostatic hyperplasia are expressed as percent of total glandular cell cytoplasm (= 100 %).

Table 23.3
Volume Densities of Smooth Muscle Cells in the Normal Human Prostate and Benign Prostatic Hyperplasia

	Golgi Apparatus[a]	Organelles[a]	Myofilaments[a]
Normal human prostate (5 pts.)			
Mean	0.002	0.048	0.950
Standard error	0.001	0.005	0.026
Benign prostatic hyperplasia (5 pts.)			
Mean	0.013	0.134	0.853
Standard error	0.001	0.006	0.032

[a] Analysis of variance—signficant.

biopsies were performed. The patients were medicated for 8 weeks with the following antagonists: *antiestrogen*: tamoxifen (40 mg daily p.o.); *antiandrogen:* cyproterone acetate (100 mg daily p.o.); *antiprolactin,* bromocriptine (starting with 2.5 mg for days 1 to 7, continuing with 5 mg for days 8 to 14, from the 15th day 15 mg daily p.o.). From the suprapubically enucleated tissue of BPH light and electron microscopic stereological analyses were performed (Fig. 23.14).

The administration of the antiestrogen *tamoxifen* did not show an alteration compared to the values before treatment (Fig. 23.14*A*), whereas the application of *cyproterone acetate* led to a reduced volumetric amount of the smooth muscle cell organelles (54% related to the pretreatment

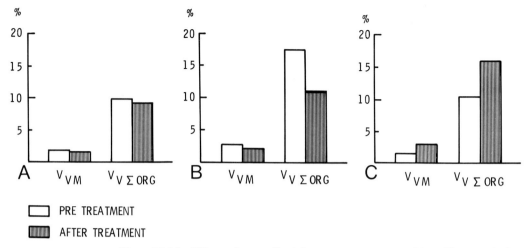

% 20 15 10 5

Figure 23.14 Effects of *tamoxifen* (*A*), cyproterone acetate (*B*) and bromocriptine (*C*) on volume densities of cellular components per unit volume of smooth muscle cell cytoplasm.

volume, Fig. 23.14*B*). Following *bromocriptine* medication a further activation of the smooth muscle cells was observed (a 60% increase in the cell organelles compared to the pretreatment values, Fig. 23.14*C*). These investigations show that the stromal tissue is possibly sensitive to estrogens and androgens; however, it is still not known whether estrogens and/or androgens lead to smooth muscle cell activation in human BPH. The physiological or pathophysiological role of the antiprolactin is unknown in this regard.

5. The Contribution of Stereology in Biochemical Studies on Human Prostatic Specimens (Correlative Biochemical and Light Microscopic Stereological Study on Human Prostatic Specimens of Normal Prostate, Benign Prostatic Hyperplasia, Prostatic Cancer*)

5α-Reductase and *3α-hydroxysteroid oxidoreductase* activities were shown to be metabolic parameters the change of which indicates success or failure of hormonal treatment of prostatic cancer.[20,26] Testosterone uptake, 5α-dihydrotestosterone and 5α-androstane-3α,17β-diol formation were investigated in treated and untreated local tumors and metastases by Prout *et al.*[26] These authors found a significantly decreased or absent 5α-reductase enzyme activity in primary hormone-insensitive and hormone-resistant prostatic carcinoma. They stated that 5α-reductase should serve as a parameter for the individual hormone responsiveness of prostatic cancer. Morfin[25] as well as Jacobi[20] and their co-workers showed a diminished *3α-hydroxysteroid oxidoreductase* activity in poorly differentiated prostatic carcinomas. In undifferentiated prostatic carcinoma testosterone is metabolized to androstenedion by the oxidative pathway instead of being metabolized to 5α-dihydrotestosterone and 5α-andros-

---

* This study was performed together with Dr. H. U. Schweikert, Department of Internal Medicine, Bonn, Federal Republic of Germany.

tane-$3\alpha,17\beta$-diol by the reductive pathway. The interpretation of these biochemical results is difficult, since the quantitative distribution of the different tissue components (prostatic carcinoma, stromal tissue, unchanged BPH, or normal glandular cells) is unknown in these studies. It is well known that the range of the relative amount of prostatic cancer, glandular and stromal cells varies from biopsy to biopsy from only a few percent to 90%.

From kidney donor patients normal prostates were used; from patients who underwent transurethral resection or open prostatectomy BPH samples were used to correlate biochemical results and stereological data. The separation and identification of 5α-dihydrotestosterone and 5α-androstane-$3\alpha,17\beta$-diol was done by thin-layer chromatography. The metabolism of testosterone was calculated in *pmol* per 100 mg prostatic tissue per 1 hour of incubation time.[31] After steroid extraction the biopsy material was fixed in formalin and embedded in paraffin. A morphometric analysis of the same biopsy material which was analyzed biochemically for testosterone metabolism was performed, thus calculating the stromal and glandular parts of the prostatic biopsy material (= 100 %).

These correlating biochemical and morphometric data show that the *5α-reductase* and *3α-hydroxysteroid oxidoreductase* of the stromal part in the normal human prostate as well as in prostatic hyperplasia was found to occur to a similar extent as in the glandular part (Fig. 23.15). Enzyme assays of biopsy specimens have to be interpreted very cautiously since *5α-reductase* or *3α-hydroxysteroid oxidoreductase* activities may result from the stromal or the glandular part of the biopsy specimen. Therefore, accurate correlations between these biochemical assays and quantitative morphological data on tissue distribution should be performed in future.

COLLABORATION BETWEEN THE CLINICIAN, THE BIOCHEMIST, AND THE MORPHOLOGIST

Five applications have been presented to show how stereology can be used to obtain information from light microscopic slides and electron micrographs of normal and pathological growth of prostatic tissue. Stereological methods can be very helpful in interdisciplinary work. However, some serious hurdles have to be overcome and warnings observed in the stereological day-to-day work in order not to discredit this quantitative morphological approach.[27,30]

In attempting a relation between morphological and biochemical data, these quantitative morphological data permit us to determine from intact tissue the relative, partial, and the absolute amounts of tissue and cell compartments of prostatic tissue. For example, a microsomal fraction of the rat prostatic tissue, containing rough endoplasmic reticulum and Golgi apparatus, would be expected of about 80% rough endoplasmic reticulum and 20% Golgi apparatus.

Under some restrictions quantitative morphological data can also be obtained from homogenates, thus making possible a comparison of the stereological data of the homogenates with the cell fractions.[11] By means

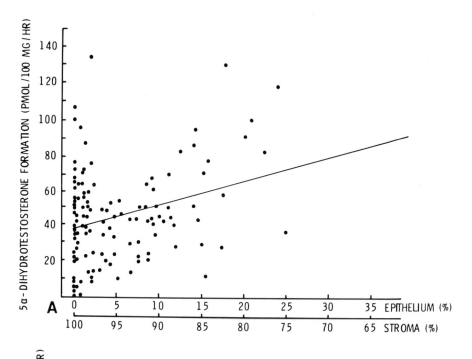

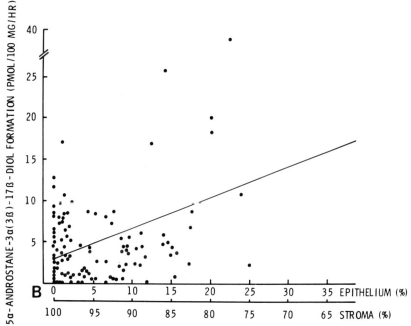

Figure 23.15 *A*, Correlative biochemical and morphometric study on human biopsy specimens. 5α-Reductase activity is correlated to the amount of stromal and glandular tissue of the biopsy specimen (=100%). *B*, Correlative biochemical and morphometric study on human biopsy specimens. 3α-Hydroxysteroid-oxidoreductase activity is correlated to the amount of stromal and glandular tissue of the biopsy specimen (=100%)

of stereological methods a differentiation of the two parts of the prostate (glandular and stromal) as well as a differentiation of the various cells (glandular cells, smooth muscle cell) is possible where biochemistry fails. Therefore, especially in the example of the human prostate with a high volumetric amount of stromal tissue it must be expected that subcellular fractions derived from homogenized tissue will contain a large amount of organelles and membranes from cells other than the glandular cells. Such considerations may be very important for the biochemist and are possibly responsible for the contradictory biochemical results obtained from human prostatic tissue homogenates, especially in benign prostatic hyperplasia. As has been shown in the correlative biochemical and light microscopic stereological study on human prostatic specimens, enzyme activity assays of biopsy material have to be interpreted very cautiously; accurate correlation between these *biochemical* assays and *quantitative morphological* data on tissue distribution of biopsy specimens are now under way.

Acknowledgment. This work was supported by the Swiss National Science Foundation (grant 3.286.78), *Switzerland* and by the "Fonds zur Förderung der wissenschaftlichen Forschung (Nr. 3278 and 4030), *Austria*.

REFERENCES

1. Atger, M., and Baulieu, E. An investigation of progesterone receptors in guinea pig, vagina, uterine cervix, mammary glands, pituitary and hypothalamus. *Endocrinology 94:* 161, 1974.
2. Bartsch, G., Fischer, E., and Rohr, H. P. Ultrastructural morphometric analysis of the rat prostate (ventral lobe). *Urol. Res. 3:* 1, 1975.
3. Bartsch, G., Frick, J., Rüegg, I., Bucher, M., Holliger, O., Oberholzer, M., and Rohr, H. P. Electron microscopic stereological analysis of the normal human prostate and of benign prostate hyperplasia. *J. Urol. 122:* 481, 1979.
4. Bartsch, G., Müller, H. R., Oberholzer, M., and Rohr, H. P. Light microscopic stereological analysis of the normal human prostate and of benign prostate hyperplasia. *J. Urol. 122:* 487, 1979.
5. Bartsch, G., and Rohr, H. P. Ultrastructural stereology: a new approach to the study of prostatic function. *Invest. Urol. 14:* 301, 1977.
6. Bartsch, G., Hindermann, Ch., and Rohr, H. P. The effect of a synthetic progestine on the fine structure of rat prostate (ultrastructural-morphometric analysis). *Exp. Mol. Pathol. 23:* 188, 1975.
7. Brandes, D. The fine structure and histochemistry of prostatic glands in relation to sex hormones. *Int. Rev. Cytol. 20:* 207, 1966.
8. Brandes, D., Kirchheim, D., and Scott, W. W. Ultrastructure of the human prostate: normal and neoplastic. *Lab. Invest. 13:* 1541, 1964.
9. Brandes, D. Histochemical and ultrastructural observations on prostatic epithelium of old rats. *Lab. Invest. 12:* 290, 1963.
10. Blume, D. Ch., and Mawhinney, M. G. Endogenous concentrations of 17β-estradiol in the male guinea pig. *J. Steroid Biochem. 9:* 515, 1978.
11. Bolender, R. P. Stereological analysis of the guinea pig pancreas. *J. Cell Biol. 61:* 269, 1974.
12. Chalkley, H. W. Method for the quantitative morphological analysis of tissues. *J. Natl. Cancer Inst. 4:* 47, 1943.
13. Cowan, R. A., Cowan, S. K., Grant, J. K., and Elder, H. Y. Biochemical investigations of separated epithelium and stroma from benign prostatic hyperplastic tissue. *J. Endocrinol. 74:* 111, 1977.

14. Delesse, M. A. Procédé mécanique pour déterminer la composition des roches. *C. R. Acad. Sci.* [D] (Paris) *25:* 544, 1947.

15. Glagoleff, A. A. On the geometrical methods of quantitative mineralogic analysis of rocks. *Trans. Inst. Econ. Mineral (Moscow)* 1933, p. 59.

16. Gysin-Kellerhals, P. The effect of a high dosage of testosterone in the fine structure of rat prostate (Unpublished data, 1979).

17. Harrison, R. W., and Taft, D. O. Estrogen receptors in the chick oviduct. *Endocrinology 96:* 199, 1975.

18. Helminen, H. J., and Ericsson, J. L. E. Ultrastructural studies on prostatic involution in the rat. Changes in secretory pathways. *J. Ultrastruct. Res. 40:* 152, 1972.

19. Hess, F. A., Weibel, E. R., and Preisig, R. Morphometry of dog liver. Normal base line data. *Virchows Arch.[B Cell Pathol.] 12:* 303, 1973.

20. Jacobi, G. H., and Altwein, J. E. Androgenstoffwechsel im Prostatakarzinom: 3-Hydroxysteroid-Dehydrogenase-Aktivitat in Abhängigkeit vom Tumor-Differenzierungsgrad. *Urol. Intern. 35:* 194, 1980.

21. Jensen, E. V. Suzuku, T., and Numata, M. Estrogen binding substances of target tissues. *Steroids 13:* 317, 1969.

22. De Klerk, D. P., Coffey, D. S., Ewing, L. L., McDermott, I. R., Reiner, W. G., Robinson, C. H. Scott, W. W., Standberg, J. D., Talakay, P., Walsh P. C., Wheaton, L. G., and Zirkin, B. R. A comparison of spontaneous and experimentally induced canine prostatic hyperplasia. *J. Clin. Invest 63:* 842, 1979.

23. Liao, s., Fang, S., Tymoczko, J. L., and Liang, T. In *Male Accessory Sex Organs: Structure and Function in Mammals,* edited by D. Brandes. Academic Press, New York, 1974, pp. 237-265.

24. Moore, R. J., Gazak, J. M., and Wilson, J. D. Regulation of cytoplasmic dihydrotestosterone binding in dog prostate by 17β-estradiol. *J. Clin. Invest. 63:* 351, 1979.

25. Morfin, R. F., Leav, I., Chavles, J. F., Cavazos, L. F., Ofner, P., and Floch, H. H. Correlative study of the morphology and C_{19}-steroid metabolism of benign and cancerous human prostatic tissue. *Cancer 39:* 1517, 1977.

26. Prout, G. R., Jr., Kliman, B., Daly, J. J., MacLaughlin, R. A., and Griffin, P.D. In vitro uptake of ^{3}H testosterone and its conversion to dihydrotestosterone by prostatic carcinoma and other tissues. *J. Urol. 116:* 603, 1976.

27. Reith, A., Barnard, T., and Rohr, H. P. Stereology of cellular reaction patterns. CRC *Crit. Rev. Toxicol. 4:* 219, 1976.

28. Rohr, H. P., Naev, H. F., Holliger, O., Oberholzer, M., Ibach, B., Weissbach, L., and Bartsch, G. The effect of estrogen on stromal growth of the dog prostate. *Urol. Res. 9:* 201, 1981.

29. Rohr, H. P., Lüthy, L., Gudat, F., Oberholzer, M., Gysin, G., Stadler, G., and Bianchi, L. Stereology: a new supplement to the study of human liver biopsy specimens. In *Progress in Liver Diseases,* edited by H. Popper and F. Schaffner. Grune & Stratton, New York, 1975, pp. 41-56.

30. Rohr, H. P., Oberholzer, M., Bartsch, G., and Keller, M. Morphometry in experimental pathology (Methods, Baseline data and Applications). *Int. Rev. Exp. Pathol. 15:* 233, 1976.

31. Schweikert, H. U., and Wilson, J. D. Regulation of human hair growth by steroid hormones. I. Testosterone metabolism in isolated hairs. J. Clin. Endocrinol. Metab. *38:* 811, 1974.

32. Schweikert, H. U., and Wilson, J. D. Regulation of human hair growth by steroid hormones. II. Androstenedion metabolism in isolated hairs. *J. Clin. Endocrinol. Metab. 39:* 1012, 1974.

33. Stumpf, W. E. Nuclear concentration of ^{3}H-estradiol in target tissues. Dry-mount autoradiography of vagina, oviduct, testis, mammary tumor, liver and adrenal. *Endocrinology 85:* 31, 1969.

34. Tomkeieff, S. I. Linear intercepts, areas and volumes. *Nature (Lond.), 155:* 107, 1945.

35. Voigt, W., Fernandez, E. P., and Hsia, S. L. Transformation of testosterone into 17β-hydroxy-5-α-androstan-3-one by microsomal preparations of human skin. *Chemistry 245:* 5594, 1970.

36. Walsh, P. C., and Wilson, J. D. The induction of prostatic hypertrophy in the dog with

androstanediol. *J. Clin. Invest. 57:* 1093, 1976.

37. Weibel, E. R. Stereological principles for morphometry in electron microscopy cytology. *Int. Rev. Cytol. 26:* 35, 1969.
38. Weibel, E. R. Stereological techniques for electron microscopic morphometry. In *Principles and Techniques of Electron Microscopy,* edited by M. A. Hayat, Vol. 3. Van Nostrand Reinhold Publishing Co., New York, 1973, pp. 237–296.
39. Weibel, E. R., Kistler, G. S., and Scherle, W. F. Practical stereological methods for morphometric cytology. *J. Cell. Biol. 30:* 23, 1966.
40. Weibel, E. R. Selection of the best method in stereology. *J. Microsc. 100:* 261, 1974.
41. Weibel, E. R., and Gomez, D. M. A principle for counting tissue structures on random sections. *J. Appl. Physiol. 17:* 343, 1962.

Editorial Comment to Chapter 23

The paramount contribution of these authors to the improved under-standing of prostatic disease by applying highly sophisticated morpho-metric techniques was acknowledged by receipt of the C. E. Alken Award of the *Carl-Erich-Alken-Foundation* in 1978.

R. H.

24

Prostate Cancer: Value of Histophotometric Tissue Diagnosis

K. H. Kurth, M.D.
A. Binder, Ph.D.
F. J. W. ten Kate, M.D.

INTRODUCTION

The goal of this communication is to report results obtained by application of *histophotometry* to human prostatic tissue and lymph nodes. These results are correlated with proposals for routine clinical diagnosis.

There is a large and steadily growing number of attempts to develop methods for automated rapid diagnosis of tumors. Coherent optical probing,[1] light scattering methods,[2-5] fluorescence methods,[5, 6] light absorption methods,[3, 7] coulter volume methods,[8] and computerized microdissection of cellular images[9] are used to determine cellular morphological parameters and cellular contents. However, up to now these are only screening methods using cell-by-cell discriminating devices. The application to solid tissue samples is quite artificial. It is necessary to separate single cells from solid material. Thus, manipulation and possible secondary effects cannot be avoided.

The method described herein is applicable to solid tissue. The examination is performed without manipulation and preparation. About 1-mm thick tissue slices are used. Cells are only damaged on the slice surfaces. The number of these cells is very small when compared with the undamaged cells of the interior which are included in the examination in a similar way as the cells on the surfaces. Thus, the results are decided by undamaged cells. In cytological methods, on the contrary, cell debris and slightly damaged cells give inaccurate results.

METHODOLOGICAL CONSIDERATIONS

The results reported in this communication were obtained partly by a simple experimental set-up and partly by a more sophisticated fully automated device called *Histomat*. The main advantages of the *Histomat* are its simple application and its rapidity. *Histomat* is commercially manufactured now (Hytec, Seeheim-Jugenheim, West Germany).

An illustration of the method can be given in a simple way by description of the experimental set-up. For the measurements the tissue slice is squeezed between two plane-parallel glass slides. Spacers fix the distance of the two slides at about 0.3 mm. The original thickness of the tissue is not critical but can range from 0.9 to 2.0 mm. The sample, mounted in the center of a goniometer, is irradiated perpendicularly with a focused monochromatic ultraviolet (UV) beam (Fig. 24.1).

The UV light has a wave-length of 366 nm. A stabilized superpressure mercury lamp (Osram HBO 200) produces the UV light. A semiconductor UV detector measures the angular distribution of the light emerging from the sample. The detector is fixed on the mobile part of the goniometer. Transmission of fluorescent light from the sample to the detector is inhibited by a filter. From the detector the signals are transmitted via an integrating digital voltmeter to a computer. The computer calculates a parameter which is a regular function of the ratio of cell nuclear volume to the amount of nucleic acids per cell. This parameter is called the *diagnostic parameter D*.

The cross-section of the light beam impinging on the tissue sample has an area of 2×0.4 mm^2. This provides information averaged over several hundred thousand cells. In the computer evaluation the dark response of

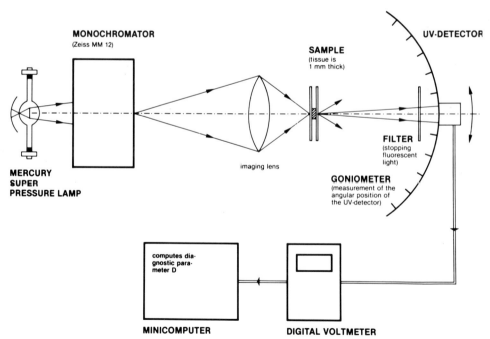

Figure 24.1   The scheme of the experimental set-up (principle) is shown. This experimental set-up was a cheap possibility to test histophotometry. Disadvantages of the set-up were its complicated handling and the long time necessary to obtain results.

the system and the effects on the measurements of the reflecting and refracting slide surfaces are considered and corrected. Lastly, the measurements are corrected for the finite size of the detector.

Based on the experience with the experimental set-up a fully automated device for rapid tissue diagnosis was developed (Figs. 24.2 and 24.3). This *Histomat* gives normally the *diagnostic parameters D* within 25 seconds after the tissue sample is fixed in the apparatus. If it is necessary, the diagnosis time of the *Histomat* can be drastically shortened.

In solid tissue the cells are normally packed closely together, and light scattering at the cell boundaries is small when compared with the light scattering at the cell nuclei. In this case the determination of the averaged cell nuclear volume is possible with the help of light scattering. It is well established by other investigators that the volume of a particle is proportional to forward scattering.[10–12] Therefore, the averaged cell nuclear volume is proportional to the forward scattering coefficient of the examined tissue. The amount of nucleic acids per cell is proportional to the extinction coefficient. This is valid for a wave length of 366 nm. In physics, forward scattering and extinction coefficient are defined for a thin layer. These coefficients are now introduced into the radiative transfer theory of thick tissue layers.

It follows from the preceding that the averaged ratio of cell nuclear volume to the amount of nucleic acids per cell is proportional to the ratio of forward scattering *versus* the extinction coefficient.

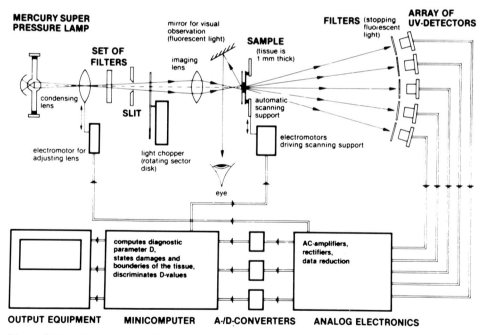

Figure 24.2 The prototype *Histomat* (principle) is drawn schematically. Most of the described histophotometrical results are obtained by this device. Main advantages of the *Histomat* are its simple handling and the short diagnosis time of 25 seconds. This time could drastically be reduced, if it would be necessary.

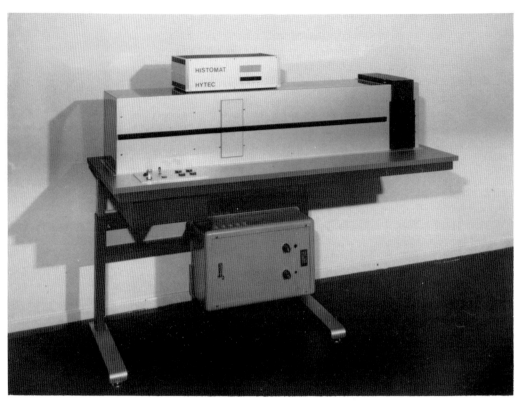

Figure 24.3 The outer appearance of the *Histomat* is shown. The longish box on the table is the optical part. The sample chamber in this optical part is closed by the flap in the middle. Above can be seen the minicomputer with LED-displays.

The radiation distribution in a thick layer with uniformly distributed scattering and absorption centers is described by the classical radiative transfer equation.[13] This equation was combined with the extended light conduction theory and with considerations about radiative transfer through solid inhomogeneous layers. Thus, a theory of radiative transfer through a thick tissue slice was developed. It takes into account the interaction of radiation with cells, with blood and lymphatic vessels, and also with glandular ducts which are not too densely incorporated into the tissue. Light conduction is caused by ducts and vessels.

Formulas for the determination of the so-called *diagnostic parameter D* were obtained. The *D*-value is normally a regular function of the averaged ratio of forward scattering to extinction coefficient. So, *D*-value is normally also a regular function of the averaged ratio of cell nuclear volume to the amount of nucleic acids per cell. This ratio is characteristic for benign or malignant tissues.[14-16]

Special tissues characterized by a high density of glandular ducts or inclosures give a *diagnostic parameter D* which is altered in a characteristic way when compared with the same tissue without inclosures or with a low density of glandular ducts. In the case of this special tissue the *D-value* is not exactly a regular function of the averaged ratio of forward scattering to the extinction coefficient. The characteristic alteration of D is very advantageous for the diagnosis of these special tissue properties (for example tissue with edema).

The theory shows that it is necessary to squeeze the tissue sample. After squeezing, the *D-value* can be determined from measurements of the emerging radiation in the angular interval between $12°$ and $-12°$. This theory is confirmed by experimental findings. A more detailed discussion has been previously published.[17]

OWN STUDIES WITH HUMAN PROSTATE

Prostatic specimens were harvested by transurethral resection or ectomy of prostatic hyperplasia and prostatic carcinoma.

Two categories of tissue samples were examined by histophotometry: (1) fresh unprepared tissue; (2) formalin-fixed tissue (4% formalin, unbuffered). The fixed tissue samples were examined partly by the experimental set-up and partly by the *Histomat*. Fresh tissue was tested only by the *Histomat*.

Measurements were made on 72 samples (34 patients) of fixed tissue and on 67 samples (26 patients) of fresh tissue. Parameter D was calculated and then compared with the clinical and histological diagnosis for the

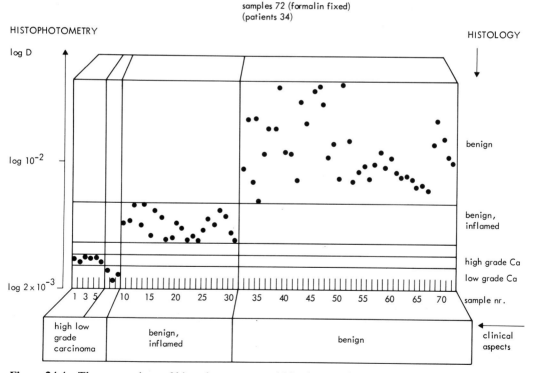

Figure 24.4 The comparison of histophotometry and histology of the prostate is shown by a graph. It is valid for fixed tissue. On the *left* is drawn the histophotometrical result (logarithmic scale), on the *right* the correlated histology. Below, the sample numbers are given.

same sample. The results of this simple blind study are seen in Figures 24.4 and 24.5, and in Tables 24.1 and 24.2. As is demonstrated in Figures 24.4 and 24.5 the histological diagnoses for benign prostatic hyperplasia, benign prostatic hyperplasia together with prostatitis, and prostatic carcinoma of different histological grades could be clearly related to the histophotometrical measurements. Each tissue sample was first measured and then examined histologically.

The different histological diagnoses are, without ambiguities, associated with different nonoverlapping numerical intervals of the *diagnostic parameter D*. A very important result is that carcinomas of different histological grades give vastly different values of the *parameter D*. This can be demonstrated for fixed as well as for fresh tissue. In the case of fresh tissue the minimal relative distance between the *D-intervals* of cribriform and small gland (solid) carcinomas is about 463% (Fig. 24.5, Table 24.2). In the case of fixed tissue, the minimal relative distance between the *D-values* of high and low grade carcinomas is about 26% (Fig. 24.4, Table 24.1). The D-values of cribriform carcinomas (Fig. 24.4, Table 24.1) are found between those of high and low grade carcinomas. Some of the examined samples were harvested from mixed (pluriform) tumors. It could be shown that different parts of such mixed tumors could be distinguished by histophotometry.

It was further possible to distinguish histophotometrically between tissues altered by inflammation (prostatitis) and tissues without inflammatory reaction (Figs. 24.4 and 24.5, Tables 24.1 and 24.2). The tissue

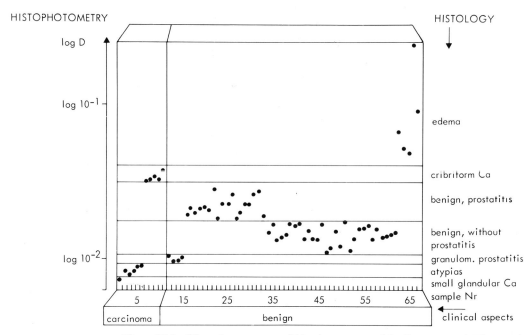

Figure 24.5 Histophotometry and histology are graphically compared. The graph is valid for fresh unprepared prostatic tissue. On the *left* is drawn the histophotometrical result (logarithmic scale), on the *right* the correlated histology. Below, the sample numbers are given.

Table 24.1
Prostate, *Fixed Tissue*: Comparison of Histophotometry and Histology.[a]

Histophotometry		Histology of Prostate
Parameter *D*		
0.00603 .... 0.0259		Benign prostatic hyperplasia (BPH)
0.00373 .... 0.00548		BPH + prostatitis
0.00226 .... 0.00302		Carcinoma
0.00285 .... 0.00302		High grade carcinoma
0.00240		Cribriform carcinoma
0.00226		Low grade part of a carcinoma
0.00257		Cribriform part of a carcinoma
0.00396		BPH + prostatitis in a tumor-bearing prostate
0.00502		"
0.00411		"

[a] Numerical intervals of the *diagnostic parameter D* are correlated with histological diagnosis.

Table 24.2
Prostate, *Fresh Tissue*: Comparison of Histophotometry and Histology.[a]

Histophotometry		Histology of Prostate
.... 0.00710		Small gland carcinoma
0.00710 ... 0.00900		Small gland carcinoma + connective tissue, atypias
0.00900 .... 0.0100		Granulomatous prostatitis
0.0100 .... 0.0205		Benign prostatic hyperplasia (BPH)
0.0205 .... 0.0370		BPH + prostatitis
0.0400 .... 0.0600		Cribriform carcinoma
0.0400 .... 0.0600		Lymph node metastases of cribriform carcinomas

[a] Numerical intervals of the *diagnostic parameter D* are correlated with histological diagnosis.

components of the prostate (muscle, connective tissue, tissue with glandular ducts) can be differentiated by histophotometry. However, the accuracy of this differentiation is not known, because normal histology as a reference method is not very exact.

Fresh tissue samples harvested from lymph nodes of patients lymphadenectomized for prostatic carcinoma were additionally examined by histophotometry. It could be shown in this way that the *D-values* of lymph node metastases are exactly the same as those of the prostatic primary tumor. These *D-values* are completely different from *D-values* of lymph nodes without metastases.

DISCUSSION AND CONCLUSION

The results demonstrate that solid tissue samples can be examined rapidly (diagnosis time 25 seconds by the *Histomat*) and in a simple way by histophotometry. The method is called *histophotometry* because the results are obtained from thick solid tissue samples and because the topography of a tumor can be determined. Development has been started of a device to interpret fully automatically the *D-values* obtained by rapid scanning. Histological experience can be stored in this device to suppress inadequate values. For example, only two glandular ducts with a cribriform pattern in a sample with proliferative hyperplasia cannot justify the diagnosis "carcinoma." The Histomat resolves such glandular ducts. If there are only two such glandular ducts in a sample, the automated interpretation device would suppress the *D-value* for these ducts and would not give the diagnosis "carcinoma." Another advantage of such an interpretation device is that critical regions of a sample can be shown graphically on a TV monitor. Cytophotometry cannot give these advantages.

The numerical results obtained by histophotometry could without ambiguities be associated with histological diagnoses. The correlation of a certain histological diagnosis to a certain *D-interval* provides the possibility of a definite histophotometrical diagnosis for tissue of known origin. If such a correlation is determined for all tissues, it should be possible to give a histological diagnosis in a histophotometrical way.

Indeed, we have found the same clear correlation between histophotometry and histology for bladder,[17] kidney,[18] and testis[19] tissues also, but the borders between benign and malignant tissues are different for materials from different organs. This means that numerical histophotometrical results are not equal for benign tissues form different sites; the same is true for malignant samples. These differences are obviously caused by the different tissue functions of the various organs. Thus, the histophotometrical results for every organ have first—to set up a standard—to be compared with the histological diagnoses.

Up to now, we have encountered no differences between histophotometrical diagnsis and histology. Therefore, it is to be expected that histophotometry and histology have similar reliability. However, experience with histophotometry is limited. More data have to be collected.

Experience shows that histophotometry can differentiate better than a pathologist during routine examination. In some cases tissue properties which were not noted by the examining pathologist were detected by the *Histomat*. After this detection by the *Histomat* these properties were stated as corrected diagnoses by the examining pathologist. It has also been found that the *Histomat* is able to detect prostatic carcinomas of very low grade. These carcinomas are only slightly different from normal prostatic tissue. Another point seems to be important. Histophotometry gives a quantitative histological grading which is independent of subjective criteria. In cases where different histological grades were stated by different pathologists for the same tissue sample, histophotometry could be helpful: The device delivers *D-values* which are without ambiguities characteristic for one predominant grade of prostatic carcinoma.

Histophotometrical devices can also be used for basic research. For example, whole organs like prostate can be examined in a rapid and simple way by the *Histomat*. This is an inexpensive method to determine accurately the local tumor extension in a prostate harvested by radical surgery, and to state for a multiform tumor the local distribution of tumor parts with different histological grades (pluriformity). Furthermore the local distribution of the benign tissue components of the prostate can be determined. For more accuracy, this research can be done on fresh unprepared tissue. In our experience, fresh tissue shows no significant change during a time interval of 6 hours after harvesting. This time interval is in many cases sufficient for an extensive examination by the *Histomat*. On the other hand, formaline fixed tissue is altered when compared with fresh tissue. Therefore, fixed tissue does not give very accurate results in some cases of a quantitative study.

Another application of the *Histomat* could be to examine the whole mass of the prostatic resection material of a patient. This could be done on fresh unprepared tissue. It would be a simple and cheap method to diagnose incidental carcinomas in whole BPH specimens.

For the future, a clinical application of histophotometry should be expected. Two categories of such an application seem to be possible. *First*, the *Histomat* could be used for rapid and simple intraoperative tissue diagnosis. It would be advantageous that a circa 1-mm thick tissue slice could be examined. In conventional frozen section techniques used commonly for normal intraoperative diagnosis, about 50 sections of such a thick tissue slice should be cut. Instead of 50 sections, only about 10 sections are routinely cut to shorten the diagnosis time. In some cases, tumors were not detected by this routine application of the frozen section technique. Examples can be given that such tumors are detected by the *Histomat*. In these cases, the *Histomat* is more exact than routine histology. *Second*, the *Histomat* could be used for clinical routine histology on fixed tissue. It would reduce the routine work of the pathologist.

In summarizing the following can be stated: It has been shown in a blind study that the diagnosis of prostatic carcinoma can be made with the use of histophotometry with great accuracy. The malignant lesion can be discriminated from BPH and prostatitis. Very small amounts of tumor can be detected with great speed and reliability. Grading of prostatic cancer also seems to be possible and the figures obtained are reproducible.

The main goal for the future is to standardize the diagnostic device *Histomat* on the basis of a great number of histophotometrically investigated and histologically reconfirmed tissue samples of one given organ and of a variety of tumor entities.

References

1. Kopp, R. E., Lisa, J., Mendelsohn, J., Pernick, B., Stone, H., and Wohlers, R. Coherent optical processing of cervical cytologic samples. *J. Histochem. Cytochem. 24:* 122, 1976.
2. Fercher, A. F. Modellrechnungen zum Beugungsbild biologischer Zellen mit Hilfe der Mieschen-Theorie. *Optik 43:* 129, 1975.
3. Meyer, R. A., and Brunsting, A. Light scattering from nucleated biological cells. *Biophys. J. 15:* 191, 1975.
4. Salzman, G. C., Crowell, J. M., Goad, C. A., Hansen, K. M., Hierbert, R. D., La Bauve, P. M., Martin, J. C., Ingram, M. L., and Mullaney, P. F. A flow-system multiangle light scattering instrument for cell characterization. *Clin. Chem. 21:* 1297, 1975.
5. Salzman, G. C., Crowell, J. M., Hansen, K. M., Ingram, M. L., and Mullaney, P. F. Gynecological specimen analysis by multiangle light scattering in a flow-system. *J. Histochem. Cytochem. 24:* 308, 1976.

6. Wheeless, L. L., and Patten, S. F. Slit-scan cytofluorometry. *Acta Cytol. 17:* 333, 1973.
7. Kamentsky, L. A., Melamed, M. R., and Derman, H. Spectrophotometer: new instrument for rapid cell analysis. *Science 166:* 747, 1965.
8. Grover, N. B., Naaman, J., Ben-Sassons, S., Doljanski, F., and Nadav, E. Electrical sizing of particles in suspensions. *Biophys. J. 9:* 1398, 1969.
9. Wied, G. L., Bahr, G. F., Bibbo, M., Puls, J. H., Taylor, J. Jr., and Bartels, P. H. The TICAS-RTCIP real time cell identification processor. *Acta Cytol. 19:* 286, 1975.
10. Arndt-Jovin, D. J., and Jovin, T. M. Computer-controlled multiparameter analysis and sorting of cells and particles. *J. Histochem. Cytochem. 22:* 622, 1974.
11. Kattawar, G. W., and Plass, G. N. Electromagnetic scattering from absorbing spheres. *Appl. Opt. 6:* 1371, 1967.
12. Loken, R. M., Sweet, R. G., and Herzenberg, L. A. Cell discrimination by multiangle light scattering. *J. Histochem. Cytochem. 24:* 284, 1976.
13. Chandrasekhar, S. Radiative transfer. Dover Publications, New York, 1960.
14. Goerttler, K. L., Haag, D., and Tasca, C. Cytophotometrische Untersuchungen an Zellkernen von experimentell erzeugten Neoplasmen. *Z. Krebsforsch. 76:* 155, 1971.
15. Haag, D., Schlieter, F., Ehemann, V., and Goerttler, Kl. Cytological and cytophotometric studies on DMBA-induced changes for the conjunctival epithelium in Syrian golden hamsters. *Z. Krebsforsch. 89:* 201, 1977.
16. Tasca, C., Haag, D., and Goerttler, K. L. Cytophotometrische Befunde in der Trachealschleimhaut und in DÄNA-behandelten Trachealpapillomen beim syrischen Goldhamster. *Z. Krebsforsch. 74:* 355, 1970.
17. Kurth, K. H., Binder, A., Jacobi, G. H., and Schneider, H. M. Histophotometry: a new method for automated histological examination of solid tissue samples demonstrated on bladder cancer. *Urol. Res. 7:* 113, 1979.
18. Kurth, K. H., Binder, A., Jacobi, G. H., and Schneider, H. M. Histophotometry: a new method for automated histological examination. Its application to solid GU-tract tissue. Abstract, Third Congress of the European Association of Urology, Monte Carlo, 1978.
19. Kurth, K. H., Binder, A., Jacobi, G. H., and Schneider, H. M. Histophotometrische Untersuchungen an Lymphadenektomiepräparaten germinaler Hodentumoren. *Verh. Dtsch. Ges. Urol.* Springer, Heidelberg, 1979, pp. 301–304.

Editorial Comment to Chapter 24

For this most promising contribution to the field of automated tumor characterization, the author of this chapter and his first co-author were awarded the C. E. Alken prize of the *Carl-Erich-Alken Foundation in 1978.*

R. H.

25

Nucleic Acid Determinations as Therapy Monitoring of Prostate Cancer

W. Leistenschneider, M.D.

INTRODUCTION

Through systematic biopsies, the inoperable, conservatively treated prostatic carcinoma offers, in the optimal form, the opportunity for monitoring therapy-induced changes of the local tumor. In this way, along with morphological examinations, histo- or cytochemical studies can be performed of the removed tumor cell material to determine the therapy-induced regression and the biological behavior of the tumor. The cytophotometric analysis of the nuclear DNA content appears to be especially suited for this approach. DNA is namely of main importance for cell kinetic studies. The cytophotometric DNA analysis quantifies the amount of DNA. According to their DNA content, the particular cells, *i.e.* cell nuclei, are categorized into the different cell cycle phases in a given cell population. Changes in the cell kinetics lead to respective changes in the DNA cytophotograms.

Since the studies done by Sandritter[14] as well as those done by Leuchtenberger *et al.*[12], it is known that tumor cell populations compared with normal tissue show a higher DNA content in relation to the changes in the number of chromosomes, in the sense of an aneuploidy. This observation was later confirmed by studies of different organs, especially of breast,[6] lung,[3] and urinary bladder[8, 12] and can also be applied to prostatic carcinoma. According to single cell photometric studies, there is a significant statistical difference between the DNA content in the tumor nuclei of carcinoma and of benign prostatic hyperplasia.[10, 15, 18]

As of now, there is little known about the DNA content of prostatic carcinomas as a result of therapy and its prognostic as well as biological significance for the carcinoma. Our first studies[9] showed that with DNA cytophotometry it is apparently possible to predict the capability of a prostatic carcinoma to change the degree of proliferation during therapy.

This chapter will, on the basis of further studies in this field, elaborate on the meaning of the nuclear DNA analysis for the evaluation of the treatment's effectiveness.

AUTHOR'S EXPERIENCE

Between 1 week and at the most 36 weeks after beginning therapy (in one instance up to five times), prospective repeated nuclear DNA analysis was performed in 20 cases of patients under different treatments for dedifferentiated prostatic carcinomas.

1. Primary hormone therapy, five patients.
2. Primary Estracyt therapy, three patients.
3. Secondary Estracyt therapy, seven patients.
4. Secondary chemotherapy, one patient.
5. Tertiary chemotherapy (cyclophosphamide as monotherapy), four patients.

Skeletal metastases were diagnosed in one patient from the *hormone group*, two patients from the *primary Estracyt group*, three patients from the *secondary Estracyt group*, and all of the patients from the *chemotherapy group*.

The samples were obtained by aspiration biopsy according to Franzén (see Chapter 5). A cytological smear was prepared from half of the aspiration, fixed, and stained according to Papanicolaou. The degree of regression was cytomorphologically diagnosed (see Chapter 6). The other half of the aspiration was mounted on fat-free slides, smeared, and, in order to prevent the cell material from floating away, fixed horizontally in Carnoy's solution. After fixation, the nuclear reaction according to Feulgen and Rossenbeck[2] with a 30-minute hydrolysis at room temperature was performed. Only preparations with the typical scarlet-red coloring of the DNA were used for measurement.

The identification of approximately 100 tumor cell nuclei was made according to strict morphological criteria. The DNA content of these nuclei was determined with the use of single cell absorption photometry. The measurements were made using the fine scanning technique with the MPV-2-cytophotometer (Leitz, Wetzlar). The steering of the scanning-table, the measuring process, and the registration of the absorption were controlled by a *pdp-8a* digital computer. The data (total extinction, nuclear surface) along with the mean, standard deviation, variance, and variation coefficient were printed out by a teletype.

The determination of the *2c-value, i.e.* DNA content, which is equivalent to a normal diploid chromosome number, was done by using human leukocytes or normal prostatic cell nuclei as diploid calibration populations. The nuclear DNA content is defined as euploid or polyploid when it is within ±25% of the average of the diploid calibration population or when its multiplicator lies within the range of ±25%. All other nuclei which are outside the euploid or polyploid range are defined as aneuploid. The DNA content of approximately 100 nuclei are shown together in a DNA cytophotogram. The DNA-content is given in *AU* (*arbitrary units*), the number of the cytophotometrically measured nuclei in "*n*."

RESULTS

1. Primary Hormone Therapy

At the beginning of treatment, all five of the carcinomas displayed DNA frequency peaks in the tetraploid or hypertetraploid region with

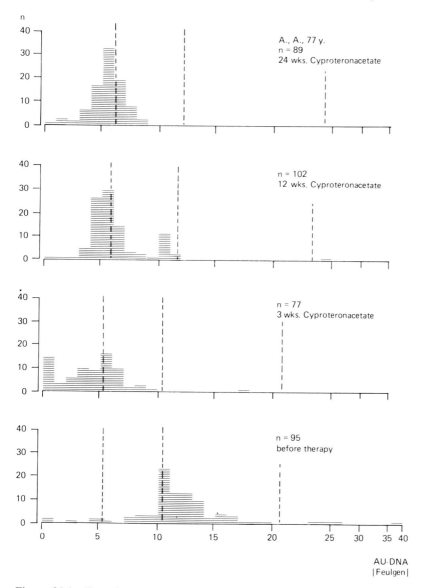

Figure 25.1 Cytophotogram of a prostatic carcinoma under primary hormone treatment (for details, see text).

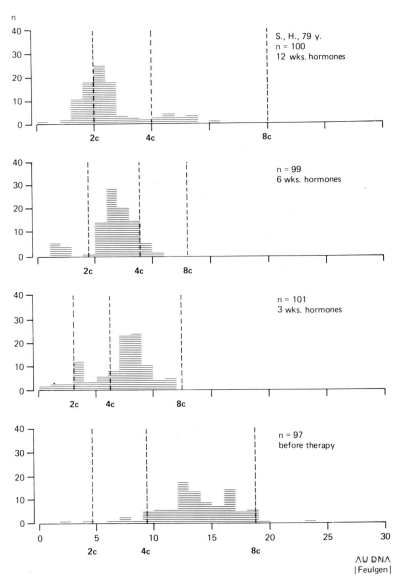

Figure 25.2 Cytophotogram of a prostatic carcinoma under primary hormone treatment (for details, see text).

scattered values partially reaching octaploid. In one case (Fig. 25.1) the values were beyond the octaploid region (*8c*). In three cases under treatment there was a definite reduction of the DNA frequency peaks to *2c*, which is within the diploid region; statistically this was highly significant ($p < 0.001$). Figure 25.1 shows that in the case of these patients as early as 3 and 12 weeks after beginning therapy a peak at *2c* could be detected. The difference between these measurements and the cytophotogram made at the beginning of therapy was statistically significant. Scattered values still strayed into the *4c* region though. Then, after being

476   PROSTATE CANCER

under treatment for 24 weeks, there was a pronounced DNA frequency peak in the diploid region.

Figure 25.2 shows another example. Three weeks after starting with hormone therapy, there was still a distinct peaking in the *4c* to *5c* border region; however, along with this, there was a second peak at *2c*. This difference, compared to the findings before treatment, was statistically highly significant. Six weeks after beginning treatment, a definite DNA frequency peak at *3c* with part of the values at *2c* and lower was achieved. Twelve weeks after beginning treatment there was finally a DNA fre-

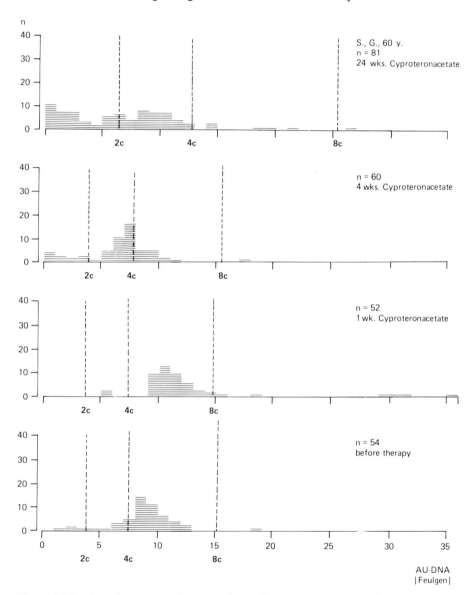

Figure 25.3 Cytophotogram of a prostatic carcinoma under primary hormone treatment (for details, see text).

quency peak reached at *2c*. Only very few of the values still rose above *4c*. In spite of skeletal metastases, this patient is objectively stable 1 year after starting therapy. In the meantime, the other patient with dedifferentiated carcinoma and without skeletal metastases before treatment has been clinically completely inconspicuous for 2 years.

In comparison Figure 25.3 shows a different behavior. One week after beginning treatment with cyproterone acetate, there was a definite DNA frequency peak at *5c* with scattered values up to *8c*, so that a shifting to the right can be seen ($p < 0.05$). Four weeks after beginning treatment, the peaking was back at *4c* with scattered values down to *2c*; this however was not statistically significant. After 24 weeks of treatment, another nuclear DNA analysis showed a very wide range of DNA values from *1c* to *4c* and singular values reaching the octaploid region. The numerous values at *3c*, *i.e.* in the region of the synthesis phase, were conspicuous. Five months later objective progression with the formation of metastases could already be observed in this case.

The other two patients from the primary hormone group showed no reduction of nuclear DNA content after being under treatment for 6 and

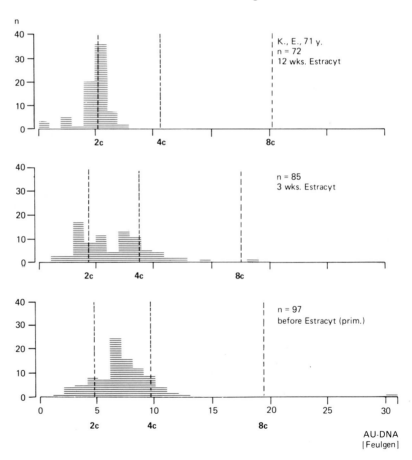

Figure 25.4 Cytophotogram of a prostatic carcinoma under primary treatment with Estracyt (estramustine phosphate) (for details, see text).

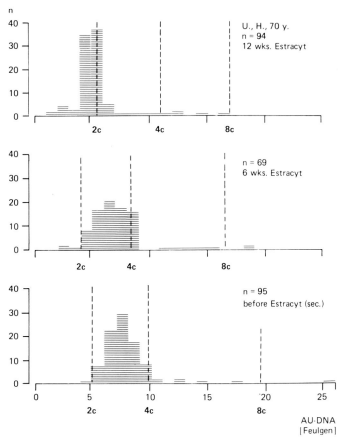

Figure 25.5 Cytophotogram of a prostatic carcinoma under secondary treatment with Estracyt (estramustine phosphate) after estrogen failure (for details, see text).

12 weeks, respectively. In these two patients the DNA values scattered up to *8c* with peak in *4c* before therapy. Four months after beginning therapy, both patients were still stable.

2. Primary Estracyt Therapy

In all three cases a pronounced DNA frequency peak in the *2c* region could be seen 12 weeks after starting the primary Estracyt therapy ($p <$ 0.0001). Figure 25.4 shows one example. As early as 3 weeks after treatment a distinct peak at *2c* could be recognized. However, the values were still straying into the tetraploid region. After being under treatment for 12 weeks, the peak at *2c* was definite, and numerous values were even under *2c*.

During the course of therapy and in spite of generalized bone metastases, one patient with such a drastic reduction of the nuclear DNA content under Estracyt treatment showed improvement of a metastatic paraplegia. It was 2¼ years later that an objective progression first reappeared. The other two patients are objectively clinically stable after 5 months and 2 years, respectively.

3. Secondary Estracyt Therapy

In these seven patients, a sequential nuclear DNA analysis was made at least once and up to four times, at the latest 36 weeks after beginning therapy. Before therapy there was a definite DNA frequency peak at *4c* in six cases, in one case at *3c*. The values continually spread into the octaploid region (*8c*) so that before beginning the secondary Estracyt therapy a distinct aneuploidy of the tumor could be seen. After being under treatment for 12 weeks, in three cases a considerable reduction in the nuclear DNA content with a high peak in the *2c* region could be ascertained ($p < 0.001$) (Fig. 25.5). When a shifting to the right in the cytophotogram could be seen which meant a distribution of the measured values in the *4c* region and above, a renewed progression was also clinically confirmed. Figure 25.6 shows one example: 24 weeks after beginning the secondary Estracyt therapy, the DNA frequency peak was in the *4c* region and the values spread above *8c*.

Two further patients from the group treated with Estracyt displayed a reduction in the nuclear DNA content without, however, a peak in the *2c* region, but rather between *2c* and *3c*. Both patients showed no progression

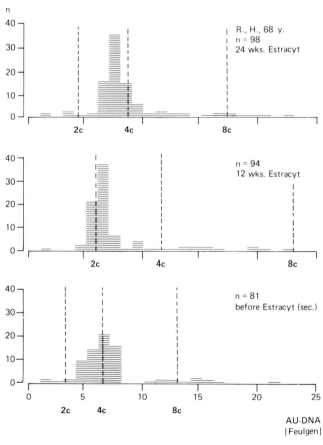

Figure 25.6 Cytophotogram of a prostatic carcinoma under secondary treatment with Estracyt (estramustine phosphate) after estrogen failure (for details, see text).

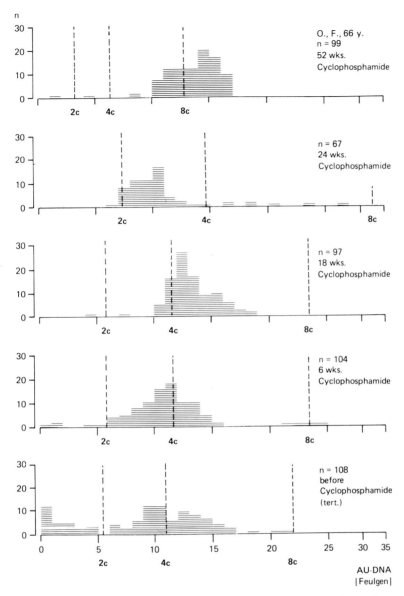

Figure 25.7 Cytophotogram of a prostatic carcinoma under chemotherapy (cyclophosphamide) after hormone failure (for more details, see text).

within the observation period after beginning therapy (maximal 36 weeks). Two other patients in this group had no significant reduction in the DNA content, and within half a year after beginning therapy were definitely in objective progression.

4. Secondary and Tertiary Chemotherapy

One patient was treated with cyclophosphamide as a secondary form of therapy after tumor progression with metastatic spread. After 6 weeks of treatment there was a statistically highly significant reduction of the nuclear DNA content with peak at *2c* ($p < 0.001$). Twelve weeks after beginning treatment further nuclear DNA analysis showed an increase in the DNA content with peaking and conglomeration of the values at *4c* and spreading to *8c*. Six weeks later the patient was in objective clinical progression.

Three patients previously treated with cyclophosphamide were given 5-fluorouracil as a tertiary form of therapy, and the nuclear DNA content of the tumor was sequentially examined. Before beginning this therapy, all of the patients demonstrated high aneuploid DNA values. There was no significant reduction of the nuclear DNA of the tumors in any of these cases. Within the first 12 weeks of treatment, all patients were clinically progressive.

Figure 25.7 shows a typical example. Before therapy values peaked at *4c* with wide scattering of the values above *4c*. After 6 weeks of treatment with cyclophosphamide a practically unchanged picture was seen; the same was true after 18 weeks of treatment. Twenty-four weeks after beginning therapy, a slight shift to the left with peaking at *3c* occurred, but there were scattered values at *4c* and above, as compared to findings before treatment.

One year after treatment with cyclophosphamide there was a massive conglomeration of values in the *8c* region, here with extreme polyploidy of the tumor. As the year passed, this patient was increasingly progressive with continuous deterioration of the skeletal metastases, which were generalized 52 weeks after beginning therapy.

DISCUSSION AND CONCLUSION

The results presented here show that a significant reduction in the nuclear DNA content of prostatic carcinoma and a respectively marked DNA frequency peaking in the euploid region (*2c*) could be achieved with treatment. Sprenger *et al.*[16] were the first to report on such single photometric findings in a patient with prostatic carcinoma treated with estrogens. On the other hand, Haag *et al.*[4] could show a significant increase in the average nuclear DNA content in the conjunctive sack of Syrian gold hamsters under the influence of dimethylbencanthracene (DMBA), using DNA single cell cytophotometry according to Feulgen.

In relation to the cell cycle, the achievement of DNA distribution peaking at *2c* by the treatment means that the majority of the carcinoma nuclei are in the G_1-*phase*. Moreover, this DNA distribution pattern corresponds to that of prostatic hyperplasia.[11, 14] The nuclei in the G_1-*phase* are probably in arrest so that progression from G_1 to S is hindered. It is therefore not surprising that the clinical course of all patients with such a significant decrease in DNA frequency peaks is more favorable than vice versa by an increase. In all cases, independent of the chosen form of therapy, by conglomeration of measurement values at *3c*, *4c*, or even higher, there was a poor clinical course of the disease.

Measurement values in the *3c* region mean that the nuclei are in the synthesis (*s*)-*phase*. Such DNA cytophotograms were found by rapidly proliferating cell populations as in material from cell cultures in the growth phase.[17] Measurement values at *4c* and above can be compared to the *G₂*- and *M-phase* and indicate a strong aneuploidy of the tumors.[1] In addition, by using an autoradiography, the accumulation of values in this region could also be examined to determine whether a prolongation of the *G₂-phase* was evident.

At the end, however, the presence of such an aneuploidy under treatment apparently indicates that the biological behavior of the tumor before treatment has an almost identical DNA cytophotogram and remains dedifferentiated morphologically. According to several authors, this tumor population will, without any treatment, constantly display a definite aneuploidy.[10, 15, 18] If this does not change under therapy, unfavorable clinical progress can soon be expected.

By retrospective DNA analysis under treatment, Zetterberg[19] confirmed these findings and pointed out the good correlation between the DNA content and clinical progress.

The results of the nuclear DNA analysis show that the cytochemical behavior in the nuclei has an enormous significance for predicting the biological behavior of prostatic carcinoma. Since caryometric research has shown that a correlation exists between the size of the nucleus and the DNA content, it can also be assumed that in the morphological examinations of prostatic carcinomas, the cell nucleus, especially its size as well as the consistency of the chromatin and nucleoli, have more significance than has until now been given them. In this context, the account of Harada *et al.*[5] deserves special attention. According to these investigators the prognosis of prostatic carcinoma correlates closely to the size of the tumor nuclei.

Until now our own results could not definitely answer the question of how far the nuclear DNA content documented before therapy could prognostically reflect the possible therapeutic influence. At present it can only be said that, especially in carcinomas with peaking of the DNA distribution in the tetraploid region and heavy scattering of the values into the octaploid region, a therapy resistance can be expected immediately or shortly after treatment begins, as was the case in all of the patients treated with cyclophosphamide. These tumors are clearly aneuploid and therefore apparently have a rapid proliferation tendency.

Further measurements must show whether the prognosis of prostatic carcinomas, which quickly achieve a diploid value of the DNA distribution under treatment, is favorable in the long run. In the future, prospective studies could help clarify which form of therapy is best for reducing the proliferation of the prostatic carcinoma, especially those of poor differentiation. This viewpoint is currently of special interest since the renewed increase in the application of cytotoxic therapy in treating prostatic carcinomas.

Exact statements about the DNA content of prostatic carcinoma nuclei, before or during treatment, can only be made by scanning single cell cytophotometry as applied here. This is the only method which makes it possible to bring the individual nucleus, identified as a carcinoma cell nucleus, exactly into the field of measurement. However, it takes between 90 and 120 minutes to measure approximately 100 nuclei. The fast flow cytophotometry used by other authors[7, 20] for determining the nuclear DNA content of prostatic carcinomas is, with a time of 15 minutes for the same measurement, in contrast with the single cell cytophotometry certainly quicker, but as of now it is not as reliable. This is especially important for control studies of the DNA content of patients under treatment, because with this method the relation of the measured DNA content to the morphology of the cell, *i.e.* the nucleus, cannot be determined.

In contrast to single cell cytophotometry it is never really clear in fast flow cytophotometry from which cell nucleus in the prepared cell suspension the measured DNA content originates. Since an accurate cell sorting system does not exist at the present, damaged cell nuclei or white blood cells such as lymphocytes or leukocytes can continually be taken into the inexact cytophotogram during measurement.

In the near future exact nuclear DNA analysis will only be attainable with single cell cytophotometry; the complete automation of this process remains a goal to be achieved. The possibility of being able to tell more about the natural history by using this method certainly compensates for the large amount of time it consumes. In general, the results presented here show that the examination of the *local tumor* itself may be of importance for the diagnosis of the progress and the prognosis of prostatic carcinoma as *a whole*.

SUMMARY

Sequential nuclear DNA analysis was performed on 20 patients with dedifferentiated prostatic carcinomas during treatment with different forms of therapy. Before therapy a nuclear DNA analysis was performed on all patients using single cell cytophotometry. It could be shown that under all forms of treatment (hormone therapy, Estracyt as a primary or secondary form of therapy, and cyclophosphamide as a secondary form of therapy), except tertiary chemotherapy with cyclophosphamide, a highly significant shifting to the left, from aneuploid to diploid, of the DNA distribution could be achieved.

The clinical prognosis correlated closely to the DNA content measured under therapy. Prostatic carcinoma with high peaking of the DNA distribution at *4c* and scattering of the measurement values to *8c* must be considered as potentially therapy-resistant.

The scanning single cell cytophotometry which was used here to ascertain the nuclear DNA content under therapy is certainly time-consuming; however, at the moment, it is the only exact method available for these study purposes. In comparison, the fast flow cytophotometry is considerably faster, but not as accurate.

REFERENCES

1. Andreef, M. *Zellkinetik des Tumorwachstums. Grundlagen—Methoden—Experimente.* Georg Thieme, Stuttgart, 1977.
2. Feulgen, R., and Rossenbeck, H. Mikroskopisch-chemischer Nachweis einer Thymus-nukleinsaüre und die darauf beruhende elektive Förderung von Zellkernen in mikroskopischen Präparaten. *Z. Physiol. Chem. 135:* 203, 1924.
3. Greisen, O. Deoxyribonucleic acid content in bronchogenetic carcinoma with special reference to polyploid cell nuclei. *Acta Pathol. Microbiol. Scand. 77:* 177, 1969.
4. Haag, D., Schlieter, F., Ehemann, V., and Goerttler, K. Cytological and cytophotometric studies on DMBA-induced changes of the conjunctival epithelium in Syrian golden hamsters. *Z. Krebsforsch. 89:* 201, 1977.
5. Harada, M., Mostofi, F. K., Corle, D. K., Byar, D. P., and Trump, B. F. Preliminary studies of histologic prognosis in cancer of the prostate. *Cancer Treat. Rep. 61:* 223, 1977.
6. Kallenberger, A., Hagmann, A., Meier-Ruge, W., and Descoeudres, Cl. Beziehungen zwischen See-Chromatinvorkommen, Kerngrösse und DNS Werten in Mammatumoren und ihre Bedeutung für die Überlebenszeit. *Schweiz. Med. Wochenschr. 97:* 678, 1967.
7. Jaer, T. B., Thommesen, P., Fredrikson, P., and Bichel, P. DNA content in cells aspirated from carcinoma of the prostate treated with oestrogenic compounds. *Urol. Res. 7:* 249, 1979.
8. Lederer, B., Mikuz, G., Gütterer, W., and Zur Nedden, S. Zytophotometrische Untersuchungen von Tumoren des Übergangsepithels der Harnblase. Vergleich zytophotometrischer Untersuchungsergebnisse mit dem histologischen Grading. *Beitr. Pathol. 147:* 379, 1972.
9. Leistenschneider, W., and Nagel, R. Bestimmung des DNS-Gehaltes des behandelten Prostatakarzinoms mit Scanning-Zytophotometrie. *Verh. Dtsch. Ges. Urol.* Springer, Berlin, 1979, pp. 399–401.
10. Leistenschneider, W., and Nagel, R. Zellkern-DNS-Analyse am unbehandelten und behandelten Prostatakarzinom mit Scanning—Einzelzellzytophotometrie. *Akt. Urol. 10:* 353, 1979.
11. Leistenschneider, W., and Nagel, R. Untersuchungen zum DNS-Gehalt von Prostata-adenomen und -karzinomen. Vortr. 31. Kongress Dtsch. Ges. Urol., München, October 17–20, 1979.
12. Leuchtenberger, C., Leuchtenberger, R., and Davis, A. M. A microspectrophotometric study of the deoxyribose nucleic acid (DNA) content in cells of normal and malignant human tissues. *Am. J. Pathol. 30:* 65, 1954.
13. Levi, P. E., Cooper, E. H., Anderson, C. K., Path, M. C., and Williams, R. E. Analysis of DNA content, nuclear size and cell proliferation of transitional cell carcinoma in man. *Cancer 23:* 1074, 1969.
14. Sandritter, W. Über den Nucleinsäuregehalt in verschiedenen Tumoren. *Frankf. Z. Pathol. 63:* 423, 1952.
15. Sprenger, E., Volk, L., and Michaelis, W. E. Die Aussagekraft der Zellkern-DNS-Bestimmung bei der Diagnostik des Prostatakarzinoms. *Beitr. Pathol. 153:* 370, 1974.
16. Sprenger, E., Michaelis, W. E., Vogt-Schaden, M., and Otto, C. The significance of DNA flow through fluorescence cytophotometry for the diagnosis of prostate carcinoma. *Beitr. Pathol. 159:* 292, 1976.
17. Sprenger, E. Anwendungsmöglichkeiten der Durchflussphotometrie in der zytologischen Diagnostik. In *Moderne Untersuchungsmethoden in der Zytologie, 2. Auflage,* edited by S. Witte and F. Ruch. Gerhard Witzstrock, Baden-Baden, 1979.
18. Zetterberg, A., and Esposti, P. L. Cytophotometric DNA-analysis of aspirated cells from prostatic carcinoma. *Acta Cytol. (Baltimore) 20:* 46, 1976.
19. Zetterberg, A. Cytochemical method of malignancy grading. WHO-Collaborating Centre Meeting on Prostatic Cancer. Stockholm, March 12–15, 1979.
20. Zimmermann, A., and Truss, F. Vergleichende zytologische und impulszytophotometrische Untersuchungen an Prostatazellen. *Urologe [A] 17:* 391, 1978.

Index